Immunology of Aging

Immunology of Aging

Edited by Isla Pierce

hayle
medical

New York

Hayle Medical,
750 Third Avenue, 9th Floor,
New York, NY 10017, USA

Visit us on the World Wide Web at:
www.haylemedical.com

ISBN: 978-1-63241-642-1

Cataloging-in-Publication Data

Immunology of aging / edited by Isla Pierce.
    p. cm.
Includes bibliographical references and index.
ISBN 978-1-63241-642-1
1. Aging--Immunological aspects. 2. Older people--Diseases--Immunological aspects.
3. Geriatrics. 4. Gerontology. I. Pierce, Isla.
RC952.5 .I46 2019
618.97--dc23

Table of Contents

Preface...IX

Chapter 1 **Cellular immune activity biomarker neopterin is associated**
hyperlipidemia: results from a large population-based study........................ 1
Shu-Chun Chuang, Heiner Boeing, Stein Emil Vollset, Øivind Midttun,
Per Magne Ueland, Bas Bueno-de-Mesquita, Martin Lajous, Guy Fagherazzi,
Marie-Christine Boutron-Ruault, Rudolf Kaaks, Tilman Küehn, Tobias Pischon,
Dagmar Drogan, Anne Tjønneland, Kim Overvad, J Ramón Quirós,
Antonio Agudo, Esther Molina-Montes, Miren Dorronsoro, José María Huerta,
Aurelio Barricarte, Kay-Tee Khaw, Nicholas J. Wareham, Ruth C. Travis,
Antonia Trichopoulou, Pagona Lagiou, Dimitrios Trichopoulos, Giovanna Masala,
Claudia Agnoli, Rosario Tumino, Amalia Mattiello, Petra H Peeters,
Elisabete Weiderpass, Richard Palmqvist, Ingrid Ljuslinder, Marc Gunter,
Yunxia Lu, Amanda J. Cross, Elio Riboli, Paolo Vineis and Krasimira Aleksandrova

Chapter 2 **Transcriptomic profiles of aging in naïve and memory CD4+ cells from mice** 12
Jackson Taylor, Lindsay Reynolds, Li Hou, Kurt Lohman, Wei Cui,
Stephen Kritchevsky, Charles McCall and Yongmei Liu

Chapter 3 **The insulin receptor substrate Chico regulates antibacterial immune**
function in *Drosophila* 26
Sarah McCormack, Shruti Yadav, Upasana Shokal, Eric Kenney,
Dustin Cooper and Ioannis Eleftherianos

Chapter 4 **Frailty has a stronger association with inflammation than age in older veterans** 37
P. Van Epps, D. Oswald, P. A. Higgins, T. R. Hornick, H. Aung, R. E. Banks,
B. M. Wilson, C. Burant, S. Gravenstein and D. H. Canaday

Chapter 5 **The anti-ageing molecule sirt1 mediates beneficial effects of cardiac**
rehabilitation.. 46
Giusy Russomanno, Graziamaria Corbi, Valentina Manzo, Nicola Ferrara,
Giuseppe Rengo, Annibale A. Puca, Salvatore Latte, Albino Carrizzo,
Maria Consiglia Calabrese, Ramaroson Andriantsitohaina, Walter Filippelli,
Carmine Vecchione, Amelia Filippelli and Valeria Conti

Chapter 6 **HCV monoinfection and HIV/HCV coinfection enhance T-cell immune**
senescence in injecting drug users early during infection.............................. 54
Bart P. X. Grady, Nening M. Nanlohy and Debbie van Baarle

Chapter 7 **Herpes virus seroepidemiology in the adult Swedish population**.......................... 65
Jan Olsson, Eloise Kok, Rolf Adolfsson, Hugo Lövheim and Fredrik Elgh

Chapter 8 **Changes in peripheral immune cell numbers and functions in octogenarian**
walkers – an acute exercise study... 71
Kornelis S. M. van der Geest, Qi Wang, Thijs M. H. Eijsvogels,
Hans J. P. Koenen, Irma Joosten, Elisabeth Brouwer, Maria T. E. Hopman,
Joannes F. M. Jacobs and Annemieke M. H. Boots

Chapter 9   **Age dependent accumulation patterns of advanced glycation end product receptor (RAGE) ligands and binding intensities between RAGE and its ligands differ in the liver, kidney and skeletal muscle**................................. 84
Myeongjoo Son, Wook-Jin Chung, Seyeon Oh, Hyosang Ahn,
Chang Hu Choi, Suntaek Hong, Kook Yang Park, Kuk Hui Son and
Kyunghee Byun

Chapter 10   **Interleukin-6 and C-reactive protein, successful aging, and mortality: the PolSenior study** 92
Monika Puzianowska-Kuźnicka, Magdalena Owczarz,
Katarzyna Wieczorowska-Tobis, Pawel Nadrowski, Jerzy Chudek,
Przemyslaw Slusarczyk, Anna Skalska, Marta Jonas,
Edward Franek and Malgorzata Mossakowska

Chapter 11   **Effect of a synbiotic on the response to seasonal influenza vaccination is strongly influenced by degree of immunosenescence** 104
Agnieszka Przemska-Kosicka, Caroline E. Childs, Sumia Enani,
Catherine Maidens, Honglin Dong, Iman Bin Dayel, Kieran Tuohy,
Susan Todd, Margot A. Gosney and Parveen Yaqoob

Chapter 12   **pERK-dependent defective TCR-mediated activation of CD4+ T cells in end-stage renal disease patients** 116
Ling Huang, Nicolle H. R. Litjens, Nynke M. Kannegieter, Mariska Klepper,
Carla C. Baan and Michiel G. H. Betjes

Chapter 13   **Changes in blood lymphocyte numbers with age in vivo and their association with the levels of cytokines/cytokine receptors** 130
Yun Lin, Jiewan Kim, E. Jeffrey Metter, Huy Nguyen, Thai Truong,
Ana Lustig, Luigi Ferrucci and Nan-ping Weng

Chapter 14   **Human longevity: Genetics or Lifestyle? It takes two to tango** 139
Giuseppe Passarino, Francesco De Rango and Alberto Montesanto

Chapter 15   **Transcriptomic evidence of a para-inflammatory state in the middle aged lumbar spinal cord** 145
William Galbavy, Yong Lu, Martin Kaczocha, Michelino Puopolo,
Lixin Liu and Mario J. Rebecchi

Chapter 16   **β-glucans: ex vivo inflammatory and oxidative stress results after pasta intake** 155
Annalisa Barera, Silvio Buscemi, Roberto Monastero, Calogero Caruso,
Rosalia Caldarella, Marcello Ciaccio and Sonya Vasto

Chapter 17   **Prescription database analyses indicates that the asthma medicine montelukast might protect against dementia: a hypothesis to be verified** 161
Bjørn Grinde and Bo Engdahl

Chapter 18   **ESRD-associated immune phenotype depends on dialysis modality and iron status: clinical implications** 168
Didier Ducloux, Mathieu Legendre, Jamal Bamoulid, Jean-Michel Rebibou,
Philippe Saas, Cécile Courivaud and Thomas Crepin

Chapter 19   **Molecular changes associated with increased TNF-α-induced apoptotis in naïve (T_N) and central memory (T_{CM}) CD8+ T cells in aged humans** 178
Sudhir Gupta, Houfen Su, Sudhanshu Agrawal and Sastry Gollapudi

Chapter 20   Gene and protein expression of *CXCR4* in adult and elderly patients with
chronic rhinitis, pharyngitis or sinusitis undergoing thermal
water nasal inhalations 188
Monica Neri, Luigi Sansone, Luisa Pietrasanta, Aliaksei Kisialiou,
Eloisa Cabano, Marina Martini, Matteo A. Russo, Donatella Ugolini,
Marco Tafani and Stefano Bonassi

Chapter 21   Thymus and activation-regulated chemokine (TARC)/CCL17 and IgE are
associated with elderly asthmatics 202
Kyung Mi Jo, Hyo Kyung Lim, Jae Woong Sull, Eugene Choi, Ji-Sook Lee,
Mee Ae Cheong, Min Hwa Hong, Yoori Kim and In Sik Kim

Chapter 22   Vaccines for the elderly: current use and future challenges 209
Birgit Weinberger

Chapter 23   Immune response to influenza vaccination in the elderly is altered by
chronic medication use 217
Divyansh Agarwal, Kenneth E. Schmader, Andrew V. Kossenkov, Susan Doyle,
Raj Kurupati and Hildegund C. J. Ertl

Chapter 24   Antibodies against 1940s era a/H1N1 influenza strains a/Weiss/43 and
a/FM/1/47 and heterotypic responses after seasonal vaccination of an elderly
Spanish population 230
Ivan Sanz, Silvia Rojo, Sonia Tamames, Jose María Eiros and
Raúl Ortiz de Lejarazu

Chapter 25   The baseline levels and risk factors for high-sensitive C-reactive protein in
Chinese healthy population 240
Ying Tang, Peifen Liang, Junzhe Chen, Sha Fu, Bo Liu, Min Feng,
Baojuan Lin, Ben Lee, Anping Xu and Hui Y. Lan

Chapter 26   Interventions to restore appropriate immune function in the elderly 248
Richard Aspinall and Pierre Olivier Lang

Chapter 27   Chlorinative stress in age-related diseases 256
Marco Casciaro, Eleonora Di Salvo, Elisabetta Pace, Elvira Ventura-Spagnolo,
Michele Navarra and Sebastiano Gangemi

Chapter 28   A comprehensive characterization of aggravated aging-related changes in
T lymphocytes and monocytes in end-stage renal disease: the iESRD study 263
Yen-Ling Chiu, Kai-Hsiang Shu, Feng-Jung Yang, Tzu-Ying Chou,
Ping-Min Chen, Fang-Yun Lay, Szu-Yu Pan, Cheng-Jui Lin, Nicolle H R Litjens,
Michiel G H Betjes, Selma Bermudez, Kung-Chi Kao, Jean-San Chia,
George Wang, Yu-Sen Peng and Yi-Fang Chuang

Permissions

List of Contributors

Index

Preface

The gradual decline in the functioning ability of the immune system to respond to the pathogens, brought on by natural age advancement is called immunosenescence. It includes a decline in the host's capacity to respond to infections and the deterioration of the development of long-term immune memory. It is a major cause of increased frequency of morbidity and mortality among older adults. It may result due to unavoidable exposure to a wide variety of antigens, including virus and bacteria. It is believed that a decline in the hormone levels with advancement in age is also responsible for weakened immune responses in aging individuals. This book includes some of the vital pieces of work being conducted across the world, on various topics related to the immunology of aging. It aims to shed light on some of the unexplored aspects of the immunology of aging and the recent researches in the subject. The extensive content of this book provides the readers with a thorough understanding of the subject.

This book unites the global concepts and researches in an organized manner for a comprehensive understanding of the subject. It is a ripe text for all researchers, students, scientists or anyone else who is interested in acquiring a better knowledge of this dynamic field.

I extend my sincere thanks to the contributors for such eloquent research chapters. Finally, I thank my family for being a source of support and help.

Editor

Cellular immune activity biomarker neopterin is associated hyperlipidemia: results from a large population-based study

Shu-Chun Chuang[1,2]* (iD), Heiner Boeing[3], Stein Emil Vollset[4,5], Øivind Midttun[6], Per Magne Ueland[7,8],
Bas Bueno-de-Mesquita[2,9,10,11], Martin Lajous[12,13,14], Guy Fagherazzi[12,13,14], Marie-Christine Boutron-Ruault[12,13,14],
Rudolf Kaaks[15], Tilman Küehn[15], Tobias Pischon[16], Dagmar Drogan[17], Anne Tjønneland[18], Kim Overvad[19],
J Ramón Quirós[20], Antonio Agudo[21], Esther Molina-Montes[22,23], Miren Dorronsoro[24], José María Huerta[23,25],
Aurelio Barricarte[26], Kay-Tee Khaw[27], Nicholas J. Wareham[28], Ruth C. Travis[29], Antonia Trichopoulou[29,30],
Pagona Lagiou[31,32,33], Dimitrios Trichopoulos[30,32^], Giovanna Masala[34], Claudia Agnoli[35], Rosario Tumino[36],
Amalia Mattiello[37], Petra H Peeters[2,38], Elisabete Weiderpass[39,40,41,42], Richard Palmqvist[43], Ingrid Ljuslinder[44],
Marc Gunter[2], Yunxia Lu[2], Amanda J. Cross[2], Elio Riboli[2], Paolo Vineis[2] and Krasimira Aleksandrova[45]

Abstract

Background: Increased serum neopterin had been described in older age two decades ago. Neopterin is a biomarker of systemic adaptive immune activation that could be potentially implicated in metabolic syndrome (MetS). Measurements of waist circumference, triglycerides, high-density lipoprotein cholesterol (HDLC), systolic and diastolic blood pressure, glycated hemoglobin as components of MetS definition, and plasma total neopterin concentrations were performed in 594 participants recruited in the European Prospective Investigation into Cancer and Nutrition (EPIC).

Results: Higher total neopterin concentrations were associated with reduced HDLC (9.7 %, $p < 0.01$ for men and 9.2 %, $p < 0.01$ for women), whereas no association was observed with the rest of the MetS components as well as with MetS overall (per 10 nmol/L: OR = 1.42, 95 % CI = 0.85-2.39 for men and OR = 1.38, 95 % CI = 0.79-2.43).

Conclusions: These data suggest that high total neopterin concentrations are cross-sectionally associated with reduced HDLC, but not with overall MetS.

Keywords: Neopterin, Cell-mediated immunity, Metabolic syndrome

Background

Neopterin, a biomarker of systemic adaptive immune activation, is synthesized by monocyte-derived macrophages and dendritic cells upon stimulation of interferon-gamma (IFN-γ) and is considered a reliable proxy to assess the rate of IFN-γ production [1–4]. The concentrations of neopterin increase with the dose of interferon, thereby help to monitor the activity of INF-γ inducible inflammation. Thus, the measurement of neopterin concentrations in body fluids provides information about activation of T-helper cell derived systemic adaptive immune activation [5]. As high neopterin is associated with increased production of reactive oxygen species, neopterin can also be regarded as an indicator for oxidative stress due to immune activation [6].

Neopterin has been used clinically in the assessment of bacterial and viral infections, autoimmune diseases, and malignant conditions [7]. Increased blood neopterin concentrations had been described in older age

* Correspondence: scchuang@nhri.org.tw
Dimitrios Trichopoulos Deceased.
^Deceased
[1]Institute of Population Health Sciences, National Health Research Institutes, 35 Keyan Road, Zhunan, Miaoli County 35053, Taiwan
[2]Department of Epidemiology and Biostatistics, School of Public Health, Imperial College London, London, UK
Full list of author information is available at the end of the article

[8, 9] and have been positively related to aging-related chronic disorders, including metabolic syndrome (MetS) [3], cancer, cardio-vascular disease, as well as overall mortality [2–4, 10–13].

An emerging field of research - immunometabolism - recognizes the existence of an interplay between immunity, inflammation, and impaired metabolism [14]. Central to this theory, inflammation and immune activation are involved in the development of obesity, insulin resistance and potentially also in MetS [14–16]. Despite biological plausibility, only a few epidemiological studies have explored the relation between neopterin and selected metabolic factors. In a study of 3946 patients with acute coronary syndrome, higher plasma concentrations of neopterin were associated with older age, a prior history of hypertension or diabetes, lower low-density lipoprotein cholesterol levels, and higher high-sensitivity C-reactive protein (hsCRP) levels [17]. In another study among 592 patients with high prevalence of MetS, plasma neopterin concentrations were correlated, though weakly, with abdominal obesity, high-density lipoprotein cholesterol (HDLC), and insulin resistance [2]. Similarly, a weak correlation between neopterin and abdominal obesity was reported in another patient cohort of 477 middle-aged and older white individuals at high risk for type 2 diabetes and cardiovascular disease [18].

It remains unclear whether the potential association of neopterin with MetS and its components, may be independent of age and markers of chronic inflammation such as hsCRP. Such knowledge may provide important insights into the potential link between immune activation and impaired metabolism. Therefore, the aim of the study was to investigate the association of plasma total neopterin concentrations with MetS and its components in the European Prospective Investigation into Cancer and Nutrition (EPIC) cohort.

Results

Overall, the geometric mean of total neopterin concentrations in the study population were 18.74 (standard deviations, SD: 1.50) for men and 18.63 (SD: 1.40) for women. Table 1 shows the characteristics of the study population.

Table 2 presents the Spearman's partial correlation coefficients of clinical markers of MetS and total neopterin concentrations. Total neopterin was inversely correlated with pyridoxal 5′-phosphate (PLP) and HDLC but positively correlated with hsCRP.

High total neopterin concentrations were associated with lower HDLC, but not with other components of MetS (Table 3). After mutual adjustment, the mean total neopterin concentrations remained different according to HDLC categories (p < 0.01 for both men and women). Figure 1 shows the adjusted means and 95 % CI of total neopterin

by increasing number of MetS components. The average differences per component was 4.0 % ($P_{difference} = 0.07$) for men and 0.8 % ($P_{difference} = 0.64$) for women.

In our study, increased total neopterin was associated with reduced HDLC (OR $_{per\ 10\ nmol/L}$ = 2.22, 95 % CI = 1.24-3.97 for men and OR $_{per\ 10\ nmol/L}$ = 2.82, 95 % CI = 1.68-4.73 for women), and these associations were independent of PLP (Table 4). Further adjustment for hsCRP did not change the results (OR $_{per\ 10\ nmol/L}$ = 2.14, 95 % CI = 1.17-3.91 for men and OR $_{per\ 10\ nmol/L}$ = 2.70, 95 % CI = 1.58-4.61, data not shown). Increased plasma total neopterin was not associated with overall MetS, defined as presence of any three of the MetS components (OR $_{per\ 10\ nmol/L}$ = 1.42, 95 % CI = 0.85-2.39 for men and OR $_{per\ 10\ nmol/L}$ = 1.38, 95 % CI = 0.79-2.43 for women).

Discussion

In this study, high total neopterin concentrations were associated with reduced HDLC, but not with overall MetS. These data indicate that immune activation may be related to lipid changes; however, the cross-sectional nature of the study does not provide sufficient information for interpreting the direction of these relations.

Previously only three studies investigated the association of neopterin concentrations with clinical markers of MetS; however, these studies were conducted in participants with underlying diseases, including cardiovascular disease, type 2 diabetes and MetS [2, 18, 19]. In agreement with the study of Oxengrug et al. 2011 [2], we observed an inverse association of total neopterin with HDLC.

Our data suggest an inverse association of total neopterin with HDLC, as well as low-density lipoprotein cholesterol and total cholesterol. This association was independent of age, sex, EPIC study center and smoking status as well as PLP and hsCRP levels. Similar findings have been reported, in patients with HIV infection [20], cardiovascular diseases [4] and MetS [2]. HDLC helps to remove excess cholesterol from peripheral tissue and transport it to the liver for excretion. The functions of HDL include anti-inflammatory and anti-oxidant activities [21]. If the function is impaired, cholesterol accumulates in peripheral tissue and causes inflammation and atherosclerosis. Despite the concept of HDL dysfunction evolved over the last decades, little is known on factors that underline possible alterations between functional and dysfunctional HDL. Recently, immunity was suggested as one of the main pathophysiological pathways of HDLC functionality via modulating cholesterol content in immune cells [22]. It has been shown that inhibition of cholesterol efflux mechanisms in macrophages promotes an inflammatory phenotype in these cells [23]. The raised neopterin levels may indicate activated immune response in individuals

Table 1 Characteristics of the study population

	Total		Men		Women	
	N	%	N	%	N	%
Age, mean (SD)	57.59	(8.24)	58.24	(7.81)	57.04	(8.55)
Education						
None or primary school completed	247	42	118	44	129	40
Technical/professional school	123	21	58	21	65	20
Secondary school	83	14	16	6	67	21
Longer education	119	20	66	24	53	16
Not specified	22	4	12	4	10	3
Smoking status						
Never	273	46	80	30	193	60
Former	196	33	125	46	71	22
Current	118	20	61	23	57	18
Unknown	7	1	4	1	3	1
Physical activity						
Low	102	17	60	22	42	13
Medium	121	20	62	23	59	18
High	139	23	53	20	86	27
Very high	205	35	77	29	128	40
Missing	27	5	18	7	9	3
Waist circumference, cm, mean (SD)	87.22	(11.83)	94.37	(9.33)	81.41	(10.38)
Tryglicerides, mmol/L, mean (SD)	1.19	(0.94)	1.29	(1.07)	1.10	(0.80)
High-density lipoprotein cholesterol, mmol/L, mean (SD)	1.43	(0.39)	1.29	(0.36)	1.54	(0.38)
Systolic blood pressure, mmHg, mean (SD)	128.93	(16.77)	131.41	(15.70)	127.14	(17.31)
Diastolic blood pressure, mmHg, mean (SD)	79.72	(9.84)	81.94	(9.76)	78.12	(9.60)
HbA1c (%), mean (SD)	5.74	(0.61)	5.77	(0.63)	5.71	(0.60)
Nopterin (nmol/L) , mean (SD)	20.07	(7.90)	20.39	(8.37)	19.81	(7.49)

with low HDL cholesterol levels. Neopterin had been associated with cardiovascular events [4, 24, 25], suggesting a potential involvement of adaptive immunity and inflammation in modulating the association between cholesterol metabolism and cardio-metabolic risk. From a practical perspective, measurement of neopterin in addition to HDLC may aid in identifying HDL anti-inflammatory/proinflammatory function and could likely yield important additional information beyond that available from simple measurement of HDLC in an individual. However, future studies are needed in order to evaluate potential practical implication of these findings. Of note, despite the association with HDLC, we observed no association with previous diagnosis of hyperlipidemia (data not shown). This can be partly explained by the observation that total neopterin concentrations were lower in those who used lipid-lowering drugs [4].

Previous studies have reported positive associations between neopterin and waist circumference [2, 10, 18, 26, 27]. In one of these; however, such association disappeared after adjustment for other metabolic biomarkers [18]. Thewissen et al. (2011) reported that the association between abdominal fat and neopterin - considered a marker of adaptive immune activation - was mediated, by elevations in hsCRP and other immune activation markers [18]. They hypothesized that it is not merely an increased mass of adipose tissue that directly leads to attenuation of insulin action, but rather adipose tissue inflammation mediated by activated immune system in obese individuals that leads to insulin resistance. In our study, we only observed a non-statistically significant marginal association between abdominal obesity and total neopterin concentrations. Further prospective studies are needed to test this hypothesis.

Similarly to a previous report [4], we found no association between total neopterin concentrations and triglycerides (TG). There was no association between total neopterin concentrations and measured systolic or diastolic blood pressure (BP), including pre-defined cutoffs for hypertension. There have been reports suggesting

Table 2 Spearman partial correlation coefficients (r)[1] between total neopterin, pyridoxal 5'-phosphate (PLP) and markers of metabolic factors

	PLP, μmol/L		Waist circumference, cm		Tryglicerides, mmol/L		High-density lipoprotein cholesterol, mmol/L		Systolic blood pressure (mmHg)		Diastolic blood pressure, mmHg		HbA1c (%)		hsCRP, mg/L	
	ρ	p	ρ	p	ρ	p	ρ	p	ρ	p	ρ	p	ρ	p	ρ	p
Men																
Neopterin, nmol/L	-0.13	0.04	0.24	<0.01	-0.07	0.29	-0.18	0.01	0.09	0.22	0.16	0.04	0.01	0.91	0.18	0.01
PLP, μmol/L			0.08	0.24	-0.04	0.55	0.21	<0.01	-0.18	0.07	-0.05	0.57	-0.09	0.35	-0.11	0.11
Waist circumference, cm					0.26	<0.01	-0.23	<0.01	0.26	<0.01	0.28	<0.01	0.12	0.15	0.21	0.02
Tryglicerides, mmol/L							-0.35	<0.01	0.15	0.04	0.24	0.00	0.06	0.50	0.02	0.79
High-density lipoprotein cholesterol, mmol/L									-0.18	0.01	-0.17	0.02	0.04	0.58	-0.17	0.01
Systolic blood pressure, mmHg											0.66	<0.01	0.11	0.27	0.08	0.29
Diastolic blood pressure, mmHg													-0.01	0.89	0.07	0.36
HbA1c (%)															0.07	0.45
Women																
Neopterin, nmol/L	-0.15	0.01	0.10	0.09	0.02	0.68	-0.24	<0.01	-0.05	0.43	-0.07	0.28	-0.11	0.23	0.15	0.01
PLP, μmol/L			-0.06	0.29	-0.08	0.17	0.14	0.02	-0.08	0.44	-0.03	0.78	0.25	0.01	-0.20	<0.01
Waist circumference, cm					0.31	<0.01	-0.28	<0.01	0.25	<0.01	0.21	<0.01	0.14	0.15	0.27	<0.01
Tryglicerides, mmol/L							-0.35	<0.01	0.16	0.01	0.13	0.03	0.07	0.50	0.15	0.12
High-density lipoprotein cholesterol, mmol/L									-0.04	0.48	0.01	0.89	0.14	0.12	-0.09	0.12
Systolic blood pressure, mmHg											0.64	<0.01	0.01	0.95	0.19	<0.01
Diastolic blood pressure, mmHg													0.03	0.76	0.04	0.56
HbA1c (%)															0.00	0.99

[1]The partial correlation coefficients were adjusted for age at blood collection (years), sex, EPIC study centers, and smoking status (never, former, current, and unknown)
Abbreviations: PLP pyridoxal 5'-phosphate, *WC* waist circumference, *TG* triglycerides, *HDLC* high-density lipoprotein cholesterol, *SBP* systolic blood pressure, *DBP* diastolic blood pressure, *hsCRP* high-sensitivity C-reactive protein, *HbA1c* glycatred hemoglobin

Table 3 Adjusted geometric means and 95 % confidence intervals (95 % CI) of the means of total neopterin by levels of pyridoxal 5'-phosphate (PLP) and markers of metabolic factors

	Men				Women				
	Mean[1]	95 % CI		Difference[2]	p	Mean[1]	95 % CI		Difference[2]	p
PLP, μmol/L										
T1 (M: <=28.1 (Median:21.4); F: <=24.5 (Median:19.6))	18.09	15.67	20.89			15.53	13.42	17.98		
T2 (M: 28.1-44.9 (Median:34.7); F: 24.5-38.9 (Median:30.4))	17.26	14.81	20.11	−4.7 %	0.43	14.68	12.81	16.83	−7.3 %	0.11
T3 (M: >44.9 (Median:63.5); F: >38.9 (Median:53.9))	16.72	14.52	19.24	−7.9 %	0.18	16.71	14.60	19.13	−13.0 %	0.01
Per tertile				−3.9 %	0.18				−6.5 %	0.01
Waist circumference (cm)										
T1 (M: <=91.01 (Median:86.45); F: <=76.77 (Median:71.50))	17.26	14.90	19.98			16.03	13.77	18.67		
T2 (M: 91.01-98.71 (Median:95); F: 76.77-85.51 (Median:80.50))	18.93	16.37	21.89	9.2 %	0.12	16.25	13.91	18.98	1.3 %	0.77
T3 (M: >98.71 (Median:104); F: >85.51 (Median:93))	19.17	16.44	22.37	10.5 %	0.11	16.93	14.62	19.61	5.4 %	0.26
Per tertile				5.3 %	0.11				2.7 %	0.27
Triglyceride (mmol/L)										
<1.7	17.07	14.95	19.49			16.24	13.94	18.92		
1.7-3.4	17.09	14.62	19.99	0.2 %	0.98	16.21	14.01	18.75	−3.7 %	0.53
> = 3.4	21.66	16.99	27.61	23.8 %	0.03	16.29	13.94	19.03	9.3 %	0.48
Per mmol/L				5.9 %	0.03				2.3 %	0.56
High-density lipoprotein cholesterol (mmol/L)										
T1 (M: <=1.10 (median:0.98); F: <=1.33 (median:1.18))	19.72	17.09	22.75			18.52	15.97	21.47		
T2 (M: 1.10-1.34 (median:1.21); F: 1.33-1.62 (median:1.49))	16.52	14.33	19.04	−17.7 %	0.00	15.73	13.62	18.15	−16.4 %	0.00
T3 (M: >1.34 (median:1.60); F: >1.62 (median:1.87))	16.29	14.15	18.75	−19.1 %	0.00	15.44	13.36	17.85	−18.2 %	<0.01
Per tertile				−9.7 %	0.00				−9.2 %	<0.01
Low-density lipoprotein cholesterol (mmol/L)										
Q1 (M: <3.88 (median:3.37); F: <3.88 (median:3.34))	18.96	16.39	21.94			16.65	14.49	19.14		
Q2 (M: 3.88-4.70 (median:4.25); F: 3.88-4.90 (median:4.34))	16.79	14.64	19.27	−12.2 %	0.03	15.60	13.59	17.92	−6.5 %	0.17
Q3 (M: ≥4.70 (median:5.29); F: ≥4.90 (median:5.55))	16.63	14.37	19.26	−13.1 %	0.03	14.76	12.83	16.98	−12.1 %	0.02
Per tertile				−6.6 %	0.03				−6.0 %	0.02
Total cholesterol (mmol/L)										
Q1 (M: <5.74 (median:5.16); F: <5.94 (median:5.29))	19.19	16.58	22.21			16.61	14.43	19.12		
Q2 (M: 5.74-6.59 (median:6.17); F: 5.94-6.99 (median:6.49))	16.61	14.48	19.06	−14.4 %	0.01	15.47	13.46	17.79	−7.1 %	0.15
Q3 (M: ≥6.59 (median:7.32); F: ≥6.99 (median:7.69))	16.85	14.53	19.54	−13.0 %	0.03	15.03	13.07	17.29	−10.0 %	0.05
Per tertile				−6.8 %	0.03				−4.9 %	0.05
Blood pressure										
Systolic BP										
<=123	16.87	14.59	19.51			16.20	13.68	19.18		
123-139	17.01	14.66	19.74	0.8 %	0.89	16.15	13.66	19.09	−0.3 %	0.95
>139	18.14	15.50	21.24	7.3 %	0.28	15.75	13.31	18.64	−2.8 %	0.61
Per tertile				3.6 %	0.27				−1.4 %	0.60
Diastolic BP										
<=76	16.76	14.53	19.34			16.43	13.88	19.46		
76-85	16.93	14.59	19.65	1.0 %	0.87	16.11	13.68	18.98	−0.02	0.70
>85	18.50	15.85	21.60	9.9 %	0.12	15.32	12.90	18.19	−0.07	0.19
Per tertile				4.9 %	0.11				−3.5 %	0.19

Table 3 Adjusted geometric means and 95 % confidence intervals (95 % CI) of the means of total neopterin by levels of pyridoxal 5'-phosphate (PLP) and markers of metabolic factors *(Continued)*

	Mean	Low	High	Diff	P	Mean	Low	High	Diff	P
Systolic BP ≥130 or diastolic BP ≥85 mmHg or diagnosis for hypertension										
No	16.89	14.60	19.54			16.01	14.06	18.25		
Yes	17.29	14.83	20.15	2.3 %	0.66	14.90	12.94	17.16	−7.2 %	0.08
HbA1C										
T1 (M < 5.5; F < 5.5)	17.96	15.72	20.50			18.24	14.72	22.60		
T2 (M: 5.5-5.9; F: 5.5-5.8)	17.00	14.81	19.51	−5.5 %	0.43	17.75	14.18	22.22	−2.7 %	0.67
T3 (M ≥ 5.9; F ≥ 5.8)	17.51	15.07	20.34	−2.5 %	0.74	16.73	13.29	21.06	−8.7 %	0.22
Per tertile				−1.4 %	0.71				−4.2 %	0.23
<5.7 %	17.77	15.61	20.24		0.67	17.85	14.44	22.08		0.84
≥5.7 %	17.32	15.30	19.62	−2.6 %		17.66	14.19	21.98	−1.1 %	
HbA1C ≥5.7 % or diagnosis for diabetes										
No	16.99	14.74	19.59		0.80	15.78	13.81	18.05		0.37
Yes	17.21	14.67	20.18	1.3 %		15.16	13.09	17.57	−4.0 %	

[1] The means were calculated by exponentiating the natural-log transformed means, which were estimated from multiple linear regression and adjusted for age at blood collection (years), sex, country, education (none or primary school completed, technical or professional school, secondary school, above secondary school, and not specified), smoking status (never, former, current, and unknown), and physical activity (low, medium, high, very high, missing)

[2] The differences compared to the first category of each variable

Abbreviations: T tertile, PLP pyridoxal 5'-phosphate, BP blood pressure, HbA1C glycated hemoglobin

that neopterin could be a predictive marker for cardiovascular events [4, 19, 24, 25, 28–31], including an elevated diastolic BP [29, 32]. However, its associations with hypertension (or BP) have been inconsistent across studies. In this context, our results might suggest that although hypertension is an important component of cardiovascular diseases, it might not be directly associated with inflammation or IFN-γ mediated inflammation.

Previous studies have also reported that neopterin concentrations were positively associated with glucose

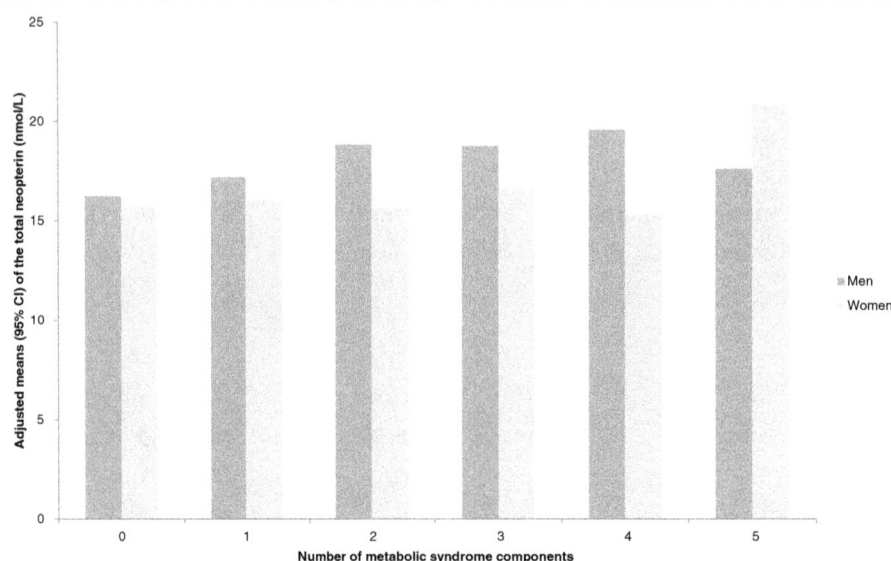

Fig. 1 Adjusted means[1] and 95 % confidence intervals of total neopterin by increasing number of metabolic syndrome components[2]. 1. The means were calculated by exponentiating the natural-log transformed means, which were estimated from multiple linear regression and adjusted for age at blood collection (years), sex, education (none or primary school completed, technical or professional school, secondary school, above secondary school, and not specified), smoking status (never, former, current, and unknown), and physical activity (low, medium, high, very high, missing). 2. The markers were considered abnormal when waist circumference ≥94 cm in men and ≥88 in women; triglycerides ≥1.7 mmol/L; high-density lipoprotein cholesterol <1.03 in men, <1.29 mmol/L in women; systolic blood pressure ≥130 or diastolic ≥85 mmHg; and HbA1c ≥5.7 % or self-reported ever physician diagnosed diabetes

Table 4 Association between total neopterin and metabolic syndrome (MetS)[1] and its components

MetS components	T1[2]			T2[2]				T3[2]				Per 10 nmol/L		
	Normal	Abnormal	OR[4]	Normal	Abnormal	OR[4]	95% CI	Normal	Abnormal	OR[4]	95% CI	OR[4]	95% CI	P_{trend}
Total Neopterin, nmol/L, Men														
Waist circumference ≥94 cm in men	52	37	1.00	39	51	2.00	(1.00, 3.99)	31	49	2.12	(1.01, 4.42)	1.64	(0.99, 2.73)	0.05
Triglycerides ≥1.7 mmol/L	77	22	1.00	67	22	1.21	(0.57, 2.56)	58	22	1.14	(0.52, 2.50)	1.08	(0.64, 1.84)	0.77
High-density lipoprotein cholesterol ,<1.03 in men	90	9	1.00	69	21	2.75	(1.13, 6.70)	56	24	3.71	(1.48, 9.32)	2.22	(1.24, 3.97)	0.01
Systolic blood pressure ≥130 or diastolic ≥85 mmHg or diagnosis for hypertension	49	50	1.00	50	40	0.93	(0.43, 2.04)	37	43	0.82	(0.34, 1.95)	0.87	(0.48, 1.59)	0.65
HbA1c ≥5.7 % or self-reported ever physician diagnosed diabetes	69	30	1.00	53	37	1.62	(0.83, 3.15)	50	30	1.47	(0.72, 3.01)	1.28	(0.79, 2.08)	0.32
Any three of the above	86	13	1.00	73	18	2.02	(0.95, 4.30)	61	19	1.82	(0.83, 3.99)	1.42	(0.85, 2.39)	0.18
Total Neopterin, nmol/L, Women														
Waist circumference ≥80 cm in women[3]	68	51	1.00	49	57	1.48	(0.83, 2.61)	44	50	1.27	(0.70, 2.31)	1.21	(0.76, 1.94)	0.43
Triglycerides ≥1.7 mmol/L	104	17	1.00	90	15	0.97	(0.43, 2.16)	80	15	0.87	(0.38, 2.00)	0.89	(0.46, 1.73)	0.74
High-density lipoprotein cholesterol, <1.29 mmol/L in women	102	19	1.00	72	34	2.90	(1.48, 5.70)	58	37	4.05	(2.04, 8.03)	2.82	(1.68, 4.73)	<0.01
Systolic blood pressure ≥130 or diastolic ≥85 mmHg or diagnosis for hypertension	73	50	1.00	64	42	0.80	(0.43, 1.51)	60	35	0.66	(0.33, 1.30)	0.72	(0.42, 1.23)	0.22
HbA1c ≥5.7 % or self-reported ever physician diagnosed diabetes	90	30	1.00	80	24	0.90	(0.46, 1.74)	70	25	1.08	(0.55, 2.10)	1.06	(0.62, 1.81)	0.83
Any three of the above	109	14	1.00	90	16	1.43	(0.71, 2.91)	77	18	1.53	(0.74, 3.16)	1.38	(0.79, 2.43)	0.26

[1] Metabolic syndrome is defined based on the joint interim statement of the International Diabetes Federation Task Force on Epidemiology and Prevention; National Heart, Lung, and Blood Institute; American Heart Association; World Heart Federation; International Atherosclerosis Society; and International Association for the Study of Obesity. Analysis is based on an alternate MetS definition modified to include HbA1C instead of glucose as a marker for impaired glucose metabolism (22)

[2] Tertile 1 (T1, nmol/L): ≤17.20 for men and ≤16.30 for women; tertile 2 (T2): 17.20-22.60 for men and 16.30-21.90 for women; tertile 3 (T3): >22.60 for men and >21.90 for women. Medians (nmol/L): 13.70 for men and 14.18 for women in T1, 19.60 for men and 19.65 for women in T2, and 28.20 for men and 26.80 for women in T3

[3] Recent American Heart Association/National Heart, Lung, and Blood Institute guidelines for metabolic syndrome recognize an increased risk for CVD and diabetes at waist-circumference thresholds of ≥94 cm in men and ≥80 cm in women and identify these as optional cut points for individuals or populations with increased insulin resistance (22)

[4] ORs were adjusted for age at blood collection (years), sex, country, education (none or primary school completed, technical or professional school, secondary school, above secondary school, and not specified), smoking status (never, former, current, and unknown), and physical activity (low, medium, high, very high, missing)

Abbreviations: MetS metabolic syndrome, T tertile, OR odds ratio

concentrations [10]. However, we did not observe an association between total neopterin concentrations and diabetes, either using the glycated haemoglobin (HbA1C), a marker of long-term blood glucose levels, or with self-reported diabetes. Similar findings have been obtained in a small saline-controlled crossover study on six healthy men (mean age 22 years) for IFN-γ [33].

Limitations of the present study have to be taken into account. First, the mean and median concentrations of total neopterin in this study population was somewhat higher than previously reported [2, 27]. An explanation is that our assay measures total neopterin, which is the sum of 7,8-dihydroneopterin and neopterin, in contrast to ELISA method which measures only neopterin. Nevertheless, both neopterin and total neopterin reflect inflammation and the associations between total neopterin and hsCRP, as well as the other metabolic biomarkers were comparable with previous reports (9). In addition, in our data no unexpected correlations between neopterin and basic characteristics were observed, as well as main findings were also in line with the previous reports. Secondly, the study population included controls of a nested case–control study; therefore, it may not be representative of the general population. However, when compared to the overall EPIC population, we have not seen major differences according to baseline characteristics, except for that our study population was slightly older, included a higher proportion of men, and a higher proportion of smokers. The range of the concentration of total neopterin reported here may not be fully representative of the general population. Thirdly, the relation between total neopterin and MetS components was assessed within the context of a cross-sectional study design, which does not allow inference about the direction of the associations. Finally, about 70 % of the study participants provided non-fasting blood samples, which may have affected the TG levels; however, we have been accounting for fasting status and found essentially the same results after excluding non-fasting participants.

Conclusions

In conclusion, high total neopterin concentrations are associated with reduced HDLC, but not with overall MetS. These data support the emerging knowledge on the interplay of immune response and cholesterol metabolism. Future studies are warranted to better understand the potential role of these interrelations in chronic disease development.

Methods
Study population
The design of the EPIC cohort has been described previously [34]. In brief, EPIC recruited 518,408 volunteers from 23 centers in 10 countries (Sweden, Denmark, Norway, the Netherlands, United Kingdom, France, Germany, Spain, Italy, and Greece) between 1992 and 2000. The eligibility criteria for participation was primarily decided within each cohort. In general, apparently healthy, middle-aged subjects who agreed to participate in the study and to have their health status followed up for the rest of their lives, were recruited. The questionnaires were completed and the blood samples were taken at recruitment.

Assessment of anthropometry and lifestyle data
The lifestyle questionnaires, which were completed by participants, included questions on diet, education, occupation, previous illnesses, alcohol, tobacco consumption, and physical activity. Informed consent forms were filled at each local center and the study was approved by the Institutional Review Board at the International Agency for Research on Cancer (IARC) and the local ethics committees. Waist circumference was measured either at the narrowest torso circumference or at the midpoint between the lower ribs and iliac crest. Systolic BP and diastolic BP were measured by trained personnel. Two readings were performed on the right arm in a sitting position (spaced by 1–5 minutes) by use of a standard mercury manometer or oscillometric device. To avoid any possible white coat effect, we used the second reading, and when unavailable, the first reading.

Definition of MetS
The definition of MetS and its components have been described previously [35]. In general, we followed the harmonized definition published by Alberti et al. in 2009 [36] with slight modification in determining abnormal glucose metabolism. Briefly, MetS was defined as having any three of the following five components: 1) abdominal obesity, i.e. waist circumference is greater than or equal to 94 cm in men or 80 cm in women; 2) elevated TG, i.e. greater than or equal to 1.7 mmol/L, after correction for the fasting status of the study subjects; that is, subtracting the sex-specific geometric mean difference between non-fasting and fasting subjects from the individual levels of non-fasting subjects; 3) reduced HDLC, i.e. less than 1.03 mmol/L in men and 1.29 mmol/L in women; 4) elevated BP, i.e. systolic BP 130 mmHg or more or diastolic BP 85 mmHg or more or self-reported physician diagnosed hypertension; and 5) abnormal glucose metabolism, i.e. self-reported physician diagnosed diabetes status or HbA1c of 5.7 %, which corresponds to fasting plasma glucose levels of 100 mg/dL .

Laboratory assays
Plasma concentration of total neopterin (7,8-dihydroneopterin + neopterin) and PLP was determined by liquid chromatography-tandem mass spectrometry (LC-MS/MS) [37] at Bevital A/S (http://www.bevital.no), Bergen, Norway.

Serum hsCRP was measured by a high-sensitivity assay (Beckman-Coulter, Woerden, the Netherlands), and the HDLC and TG concentrations by a colorimetric method, on a Synchron LX-20 Pro autoanalyzer (Beckman-Coulter, [38]). Measurements of HbA1c in erythrocyte hemolysate were carried out using high-performance liquid chromatography with a Bio-Rad Variant II instrument (Bio-Rad Laboratories, Hercules, California) [39]. The within and between day coefficients of variance (CV) were 3-10 % for total neopterin and PLP [37]. The inter-assay CV were 6.0 % and 6.5 % at CRP concentrations of 1.16 and 1.89 mg/L, respectively, 4.1 %, 3.4 %, and 3.6 % at HDLC concentrations of 0.62, 1.20, and 1.65 mmol/L, respectively, and 3.3 %, 2.1 %, and 2.0 % at TG concentrations at 86.6, 165.9, and 227.0 mg/dL, respectively. The intra-batch CV was 2.5 % for HbA1c [39].

Statistical analysis

The current analysis is based on 845 subjects (375 men and 470 women) who served as controls in matched case–control studies of colorectal cancer nested within the EPIC. The original aims of the nested case–control studies were to explore the risk of colon and rectal cancer in relation to MetS [35] and one-carbon metabolism biomarkers [40, 41]. MetS component measurements were not available subjects from Norway and Malmo center of Sweden. We further excluded 207 subjects who received treatment or the treatment information were missing for hyperlipidemia (n = 94), hypertension (n = 175), or diabetes (n = 15). Additional 44 subjects were excluded because their total neopterin measurements were not available. The final sample size for the analysis was 594.

The correlation between total neopterin and components were examined by Spearman's partial correlation coefficients (r), adjusted for age, sex, country, and smoking status. Adjusted means for total neopterin according to tertiles of each MetS component were calculated using multiple linear regression models. Because the range of the middle category of TG is narrow, we categorized TG at 1.7 and 3.4 mmol/L. The dependent variable, total neopterin concentrations, was natural log-transformed and the normality assumption was tested by graphic examination of the residual distribution. The models were adjusted for age at blood collection (years), sex, country, education (none or primary school completed, technical or professional school, secondary school, above secondary school, and not specified), smoking status (never, former, current, and unknown), and physical activity (low, medium, high, very high, and missing). The adjusted means were also assessed by mutual adjustment for the other MetS components as well as PLP, due to its role in INF-γ stimulated inflammatory responses [2, 27] and hsCRP, due to its association with low-grade inflammation. The adjusted means were then back-transformed by exponentiating the natural-log transformed means from the model. The associations between total neopterin and pre-defined cutoffs of each component of MetS and the composite MetS were also examined by calculating odds ratios (OR) and 95 % confidence intervals (CI) in logistic regression analysis, adjusted for age at blood collection (years), sex, country, education (none or primary school completed, technical or professional school, secondary school, above secondary school, and not specified), smoking status (never, former, current, and unknown), and physical activity (low, medium, high, very high, missing). Total neopterin was modeled in three categories according to sex-specific tertiles. Tests for trend were performed by modelling the median values of each category as a continuous variable. Subgroup analyses were performed by age (<55, 50–65, and ≥65 years old), sex, and body mass index (BMI, <30 and ≥30 kg/m^2).

Analyses were performed using SAS 9.3. All tests were two sided and statistical significance was assessed at the level of 0.05.

Abbreviation

AGM: BP: blood pressure; CI: confidence interval; CV: coefficients of variance; EPIC: European Prospective Investigation into Cancer and Nutrition; HbA1c: glycated haemoglobin; HDLC: high-density lipoprotein cholesterol; hsCRP: high-sensitivity C-reactive protein; IFN-γ: Interferon-gamma; MetS: metabolic syndrome; OR: odds ratio; PLP: pyridoxal 5′-phosphate; TG: Triglycerides.

Competing interests

The authors declare that they have no competing interest.

Authors' contributions

SCC, SEV, ØM, PMU, BB, PV, and KA participated in the data analysis, manuscript writing, and interpretation of the results. BB, ML, GF, MB, RK, TK, TP, DD, ATjønneland, KO, JQ, AA, EM, MD, JMH, AB, KTK, NJW, RT, ATrichopoulou, PL, DT, GM, CA, RT, AM, PHP, EW, RP, IL, MG, YL, AJC, ER, and PV were involved in data collection and interpretation of the results. All authors read and approved the final manuscript.

Acknowledgements

We thank the participants, study and administrative staff, and researchers in the European Prospective Investigation into Cancer and Nutrition (EPIC) Cohort for their outstanding cooperation.

Contributors

We would like to specifically acknowledge the contribution of Joyce Kong and Heinz Freisling (International Agency for Research on Cancer IARC-WHO, Lyon, France) for critical revision of the manuscript, and to Ellen Kohlsdorf (German Institute of Human Nutrition) and Bertrand Hemon (International Agency for Research on Cancer IARC-WHO, Lyon, France) for data management.

Funding

The EPIC cohort is supported by the Europe Against Cancer Program of the European Commission (SANCO). The individual centers also received funding from: Denmark: Danish Cancer Society; France: Ligue centre le Cancer, Institut Gustave Roussy, Mutuelle Générale de l'Education Nationale, Institut National de la Santé et de la Recherche Médicale (INSERM); Greece: the Hellenic Health Foundation, the Stavros Niarchos Foundation, and the Hellenic Ministry of Health and Social Solidarity; Germany : German Cancer Aid, and Federal Ministry of Education and Research; Italy: Italian Association for Research on Cancer and the National Research Council; The Netherlands: Dutch Ministry of Public Health, Welfare and Sports (VWS), Netherlands Cancer Registry (NKR), LK Research Funds, Dutch Prevention Funds, Dutch ZON (Zorg Onderzoek Nederland), World Cancer Research Fund (WCRF), Statistics Netherlands; Norway: Helga – Nordforsk centre of excellence in food, nutrition and health and The Norwegian Extra Foundation for Health and Rehabilitation, The Norwegian Cancer Society; Spain: Health Research Fund (FIS) of the Spanish Ministry of Health (Exp 96/0032, RETICC DR06/0020), the Spanish Regional Governments of Andalusia, Asturias, Basque Country, Murcia (N^0 6236), and the Navarra and the Catalan Institute of Oncology; Sweden: Swedish Cancer Society, Swedish Scientific Council, and Regional Governments of Skane and Västerbotten; UK: Cancer Research UK and Medical Research Council.

Grant supports for the biochemical measurements: HDL-C and TG were analysed with additional support from the Ministry of Public Health, Welfare and Sports, the Netherlands,German Cancer Aid, Federal Ministry for Education and Research, European Union, European Union and AIRC-ITALY , German Cancer Aid, Federal Ministry for Education and Research, European Union, Stavros Niarchos Foundation , Hellenic Ministry of Health, Hellenic Health Foundation, MRC and Cancer Research UK;Hba1c was analysed with additional support from National Cancer Institute grant 1RO1CA102460 and data analyses on CRP were performed with support from World Cancer Research Fund International and Wereld Kanker Onderzoek Fonds (WCRF NL).

The funders played no role in designing or conducting the study or in the collection, management, analysis, and interpretation of the data, nor did they have any input into the preparation, review, or approval of this manuscript.

Author details

[1]Institute of Population Health Sciences, National Health Research Institutes, 35 Keyan Road, Zhunan, Miaoli County 35053, Taiwan. [2]Department of Epidemiology and Biostatistics, School of Public Health, Imperial College London, London, UK. [3]Department of Epidemiology, German Institute of Human Nutrition Potsdam-Rehbruecke, Nuthetal, Germany. [4]Department of Public Health and Primary Health Care, University of Bergen, Bergen, Norway. [5]Division of Epidemiology, Norwegian Institute of Public Health, Bergen, Norway. [6]Bevital AS, Bergen, Norway. [7]Department of Clinical Science, University of Bergen, Bergen, Norway. [8]Laboratory of Clinical Biochemistry, Haukeland University Hospital, Bergen, Norway. [9]The National Institute for Public Health and the Environment (RIVM), Bilthoven, The Netherlands. [10]Department of Gastroenterology and Hepatology, University Medical Centre, Utrecht, The Netherlands. [11]Department of Social and Preventive Medicine, Faculty of Medicine, University of Malaya, Kuala Lumpur, Malaysia. [12]Inserm, Centre for research in Epidemiology and Population Health (CESP), U1018, Nutrition, Hormones and Women's Health team, F-94805 Villejuif, France. [13]University of Paris Sud, UMRS 1018, F-94805 Villejuif, France. [14]IGR, F-94805, Villejuif, France. [15]Division of Cancer Epidemiology, German Cancer Research Center, Heidelberg, Germany. [16]Molecular Epidemiology Group, Max Delbrueck Center for Molecular Medicine (MDC), Berlin-Buch, Germany. [17]Department of Epidemiology, German Institute of Human Nutrition Potsdam-Rehbrücke, Nuthetal, Germany. [18]Diet, Genes and Environment, Danish Cancer Society Research Center, Copenhagen, Denmark. [19]Department of Public Health, Section for Epidemiology, Aarhus University, Aarhus, Denmark. [20]Public Health Directorate, Asturias, Oviedo, Spain. [21]Unit of Nutrition, Environment and Cancer, Catalan Institute of Oncology-ICO, IDIBELL, L'Hospitalet de Llobregat, Barcelona, Spain. [22]Escuela Andaluza de Salud Pública. Instituto de Investigación Biosanitaria de Granada (Granada.ibs), Granada, Spain. [23]Consortium for Biomedical Research in Epidemiology and Public Health (CIBER Epidemiología y Salud Pública-CIBERESP), Madrid, Spain. [24]Epidemiology and Health Information, Public Health Division of Gipuzkoa, Basque Regional Health Department, San Sebastian, Spain. [25]Department of Epidemiology, Murcia Regional Health Council, Murcia, Spain. [26]Navarre Public Health Institute, Pamplona, Spain. [27]Clinical Gerontology Unit, Addenbrooke's Hospital, University of Cambridge School of Clinical Medicine, Cambridge, UK. [28]MRC Epidemiology Unit, Institute of Metabolic Science, University of Cambridge School of Clinical Medicine, Cambridge, UK. [29]Cancer Epidemiology Unit, Nuffield Department of Population Health, University of Oxford, Oxford, UK. [30]Hellenic Health Foundation, Athens, Greece. [31]Bureau of Epidemiologic Research, Academy of Athens, Athens, Greece. [32]Department of Hygiene, Epidemiology and Medical Statistics, University of Athens Medical School, Athens, Greece. [33]Department of Epidemiology, Harvard School of Public Health, Boston, USA. [34]Molecular and Nutritional Epidemiology Unit, Cancer Research and Prevention Institute – ISPO, Florence, Italy. [35]Epidemiology and Prevention Unit, Fondazione IRCCS Istituto Nazionale dei Tumori, Milan, Italy. [36]Cancer Registry and Histopathology Unit, "Civic - M.P. Arezzo" Hospital, ASP Ragusa, Italy. [37]Dipartamento di Medicina Clinica e Chirurgia, Federico II University, Naples, Italy. [38]Julius Center for Health Sciences and Primary Care, University Medical Center Utrecht, Utrecht, The Netherlands. [39]Department of Community Medicine, Faculty of Health Sciences, University of Tromso, Tromsø, Norway. [40]Department of Research, Cancer Registry of Norway, Oslo, Norway. [41]Department of Medical Epidemiology and Biostatistics, Karolinska Institutet, Stockholm, Sweden. [42]Samfundet Folkhälsan, Helsinki, Finland. [43]Department of Medical Biosciences, Pathology, Umeå University, Umeå, Sweden. [44]Department of Radiation Sciences, Oncology, Umeå University, Umeå, Sweden. [45]Nutrition, Immunity and Metabolism Start-up Lab, Department of Epidemiology, German Institute of Human Nutrition Potsdam-Rehbruecke, Nuthetal, Germany.

Reference

1. Sucher R, Schroecksnadel K, Weiss G, Margreiter R, Fuchs D, Brandacher G. Neopterin, a prognostic marker in human malignancies. Cancer Lett. 2010; 287:13–22.

2. Oxenkrug G, Tucker KL, Requintina P, Summergrad P. Neopterin, a marker of interferon-gamma-inducible inflammation, correlates with pyridoxal-5'-phosphate, waist circumference, hdl-cholesterol, insulin resistance and mortality risk in adult boston community dwellers of Puerto Rican origin. Am J Neuroprot Neuroregen. 2011;3:48–52.

3. Oxenkrug GF. Interferon-gamma-inducible kynurenines/pteridines inflammation cascade: implications for aging and aging-associated psychiatric and medical disorders. J Neural Transm. 2011;118:75–85.

4. Grammer TB, Fuchs D, Boehm BO, Winkelmann BR, Maerz W. Neopterin as a predictor of total and cardiovascular mortality in individuals undergoing angiography in the Ludwigshafen risk and cardiovascular health study. Clin Chem. 2009;55:1135–46.

5. Murr C, Widner B, Wirleitner B, Fuchs D. Neopterin as a marker for immune system activation. Curr Drug Metab. 2002;3:175–87.

6. Weiss G, Widner B, Zoller H, Schobersberger W, Fuchs D. Immune response and iron metabolism. Br J Anaesth. 1998;81 Suppl 1:6–9.

7. Hoffmann G, Wirleitner B, Fuchs D. Potential role of immune system activation-associated production of neopterin derivatives in humans. Inflamm Res. 2003;52:313–21.

8. Oxenkrug G. Interferon-gamma - inducible inflammation: contribution to aging and aging-associated psychiatric disorders. Aging Dis. 2011;2:474–86.

9. Capuron L, Geisler S, Kurz K, Leblhuber F, Sperner-Unterweger B, Fuchs D. Activated immune system and inflammation in healthy ageing: relevance for tryptophan and neopterin metabolism. Curr Pharm Des. 2014;20:6048–57.

10. Ledochowski M, Murr C, Widner B, Fuchs D. Association between insulin resistance, body mass and neopterin concentrations. Clin Chim Acta. 1999;282:115–23.

11. Spencer ME, Jain A, Matteini A, Beamer BA, Wang NY, Leng SX, et al. Serum levels of the immune activation marker neopterin change with age and gender and are modified by race, BMI, and percentage of body fat. J Gerontol A Biol Sci Med Sci. 2010;65:858–65.

12. Oxenkrug GF. Metabolic syndrome, age-associated neuroendocrine disorders, and dysregulation of tryptophan-kynurenine metabolism. Ann N Y Acad Sci. 2010;1199:1–14.

13. Avanzas P, Arroyo-Espliguero R, Kaski JC. Neopterin and cardiovascular disease: growing evidence for a role in patient risk stratification. Clin Chem. 2009;55:1056–7.

14. Mathis D, Shoelson SE. Immunometabolism: an emerging frontier. Nat Rev Immunol. 2011;11:81.

15. Odegaard JI, Chawla A. The immune system as a sensor of the metabolic state. Immunity. 2013;38:644–54.

16. Osborn O, Olefsky JM. The cellular and signaling networks linking the immune system and metabolism in disease. Nat Med. 2012;18:363–74.

17. Ray KK, Morrow DA, Sabatine MS, Shui A, Rifai N, Cannon CP, et al. Long-term prognostic value of neopterin: a novel marker of monocyte activation in patients with acute coronary syndrome. Circulation. 2007;115:3071–8.

18. Thewissen MM, Damoiseaux JG, Duijvestijn AM, van Greevenbroek MM, van der Kallen CJ, Feskens EJ, et al. Abdominal fat mass is associated with adaptive immune activation: the CODAM Study. Obesity (Silver Spring). 2011;19:1690–8.

19. Kaski JC, Consuegra-Sanchez L, Fernandez-Berges DJ, Cruz-Fernandez JM, Garcia-Moll X, Marrugat J, et al. Elevated serum neopterin levels and adverse cardiac events at 6 months follow-up in Mediterranean patients with non-ST-segment elevation acute coronary syndrome. Atherosclerosis. 2008;201:176–83.

20. Zangerle R, Sarcletti M, Gallati H, Reibnegger G, Wachter H, Fuchs D. Decreased plasma concentrations of HDL cholesterol in HIV-infected individuals are associated with immune activation. J Acquir Immune Defic Syndr. 1994;7:1149–56.

21. Eren E, Yilmaz N, Aydin O. High density lipoprotein and it's dysfunction. Open Biochem J. 2012;6:78–93.

22. Norata GD, Pirillo A, Ammirati E, Catapano AL. Emerging role of high density lipoproteins as a player in the immune system. Atherosclerosis. 2012;220:11–21.

23. Holven KB, Retterstol K, Ueland T, Ulven SM, Nenseter MS, Sandvik M, et al. Subjects with low plasma HDL cholesterol levels are characterized by an inflammatory and oxidative phenotype. PLoS One. 2013;8, e78241.

24. Garcia-Moll X, Cole D, Zouridakis E, Kaski JC. Increased serum neopterin: a marker of coronary artery disease activity in women. Heart. 2000;83:346–50.

25. Sulo G, Vollset SE, Nygard O, Midttun O, Ueland PM, Eussen SJ, et al. Neopterin and kynurenine-tryptophan ratio as predictors of coronary events in older adults, the Hordaland Health Study. Int J Cardiol. 2013;168(2):1435–40.

26. Ursavas A, Karadag M, Oral AY, Demirdogen E, Oral HB, Ege E. Association between serum neopterin, obesity and daytime sleepiness in patients with obstructive sleep apnea. Respir Med. 2008;102:1193–7.

27. Theofylaktopoulou D, Midttun O, Ulvik A, Ueland PM, Tell GS, Vollset SE, et al. A community-based study on determinants of circulating markers of cellular immune activation and kynurenines: the Hordaland Health Study. Clin Exp Immunol. 2013;173:121–30.

28. van Haelst PL, Liem A, van Boven AJ, Veeger NJ, van Veldhuisen DJ, Tervaert JW, et al. Usefulness of elevated neopterin and C-reactive protein levels in predicting cardiovascular events in patients with non-Q-wave myocardial infarction. Am J Cardiol. 2003;92:1201–3.

29. Avanzas P, Arroyo-Espliguero R, Cosin-Sales J, Quiles J, Zouridakis E, Kaski JC. Prognostic value of neopterin levels in treated patients with hypertension and chest pain but without obstructive coronary artery disease. Am J Cardiol. 2004;93:627–9.

30. Avanzas P, Arroyo-Espliguero R, Quiles J, Roy D, Kaski JC. Elevated serum neopterin predicts future adverse cardiac events in patients with chronic stable angina pectoris. Eur Heart J. 2005;26:457–63.

31. Pacileo M, Cirillo P, De RS, Ucci G, Petrillo G, Musto DS, et al. The role of neopterin in cardiovascular disease. Monaldi Arch Chest Dis. 2007;68:68–73.

32. Schennach H, Murr C, Gachter E, Mayersbach P, Schonitzer D, Fuchs D. Factors influencing serum neopterin concentrations in a population of blood donors. Clin Chem. 2002;48:643–5.

33. de Metz J, Sprangers F, Endert E, Ackermans MT, ten Berge IJ, Sauerwein HP, et al. Interferon-gamma has immunomodulatory effects with minor endocrine and metabolic effects in humans. J Appl Physiol. 1999;86:517–22.

34. Riboli E, Hunt KJ, Slimani N, Ferrari P, Norat T, Fahey M, et al. European Prospective Investigation into Cancer and Nutrition (EPIC): study populations and data collection. Public Health Nutr. 2002;5:1113–24.

35. Aleksandrova K, Boeing H, Jenab M, Bas Bueno-de-Mesquita H, Jansen E, van Duijnhoven FJ, et al. Metabolic syndrome and risks of colon and rectal cancer: the European prospective investigation into cancer and nutrition study. Cancer Prev Res (Phila). 2011;4:1873–83.

36. Alberti KG, Eckel RH, Grundy SM, Zimmet PZ, Cleeman JI, Donato KA, et al. Harmonizing the metabolic syndrome: a joint interim statement of the International Diabetes Federation Task Force on Epidemiology and Prevention; National Heart, Lung, and Blood Institute; American Heart Association; World Heart Federation; International Atherosclerosis Society; and International Association for the Study of Obesity. Circulation. 2009;120:1640–5.

37. Midttun O, Hustad S, Ueland PM. Quantitative profiling of biomarkers related to B-vitamin status, tryptophan metabolism and inflammation in human plasma by liquid chromatography/tandem mass spectrometry. Rapid Commun Mass Spectrom. 2009;23:1371–9.

38. van Duijnhoven FJ, Bueno-de-Mesquita HB, Calligaro M, Jenab M, Pischon T, Jansen EH, et al. Blood lipid and lipoprotein concentrations and colorectal cancer risk in the European prospective investigation into cancer and nutrition. Gut. 2011;60:1094–102.

39. Rinaldi S, Rohrmann S, Jenab M, Biessy C, Sieri S, Palli D, et al. Glycosylated hemoglobin and risk of colorectal cancer in men and women, the European prospective investigation into cancer and nutrition. Cancer Epidemiol Biomarkers Prev. 2008;17:3108–15.

40. Eussen SJ, Vollset SE, Igland J, Meyer K, Fredriksen A, Ueland PM, et al. Plasma folate, related genetic variants, and colorectal cancer risk in EPIC. Cancer Epidemiol Biomarkers Prev. 2010;19:1328–40.

41. Eussen SJ, Vollset SE, Hustad S, Midttun O, Meyer K, Fredriksen A, et al. Plasma vitamins B2, B6, and B12, and related genetic variants as predictors of colorectal cancer risk. Cancer Epidemiol Biomarkers Prev. 2010;19:2549–61.

Transcriptomic profiles of aging in naïve and memory CD4$^+$ cells from mice

Jackson Taylor[1,2,3*], Lindsay Reynolds[1], Li Hou[1], Kurt Lohman[1], Wei Cui[1], Stephen Kritchevsky[2], Charles McCall[2] and Yongmei Liu[1]

Abstract

Background: CD4+ T cells can be broadly divided into naïve and memory subsets, each of which are differentially impaired by the aging process. It is unclear if and how these differences are reflected at the transcriptomic level. We performed microarray profiling on RNA derived from naïve (CD44^{low}) and memory (CD44^{high}) CD4+ T cells derived from young (2–3 month) and old (28 month) mice, in order to better understand the mechanisms of age-related functional alterations in both subsets. We also performed follow-up bioinformatic analyses in order to determine the functional consequences of gene expression changes in both of these subsets, and identify regulatory factors potentially responsible for these changes.

Results: We found 185 and 328 genes differentially expressed (FDR ≤ 0.05) in young vs. old naïve and memory cells, respectively, with 50 genes differentially expressed in both subsets. Functional annotation analyses highlighted an increase in genes involved in apoptosis specific to aged naïve cells. Both subsets shared age-related increases in inflammatory signaling genes, along with a decrease in oxidative phosphorylation genes. Cis-regulatory analyses revealed enrichment of multiple transcription factor binding sites near genes with age-associated expression, in particular NF-κB and several forkhead box transcription factors. Enhancer associated histone modifications were enriched near genes down-regulated in naïve cells. Comparison of our results with previous mouse and human datasets indicates few overlapping genes overall, but suggest consistent up-regulation of *Casp1* and *Il1r2*, and down-regulation of *Foxp1* in both mouse and human CD4+ T cells.

Conclusions: The transcriptomes of naïve and memory CD4+ T cells are distinctly affected by the aging process. However, both subsets exhibit a common increase inflammatory genes and decrease in oxidative phosphorylation genes. NF-κB, forkhead box, and Myc transcription factors are implicated as upstream regulators of these gene expression changes in both subsets, with enhancer histone modifications potentially driving unique changes unique to naïve cells. Finally we conclude that there is little overlap in age-related gene expression changes between humans and mice; however, age-related alterations in a small subset of genes may be conserved.

Keywords: Aging, T cells, CD4+, Transcriptomic, NFKB, Enhancer, Inflammation

Background

T cells are critical mediators of the body's immune response to infection and tumor formation. Advanced age is linked to a number of functional impairments in human T cells [1], many of which are also observed in laboratory animals [2]. The primary consequence of age-related decline in T cell function is an increased risk of mortality from infection in elderly individuals, which stems from both an impaired adaptive immune response [1, 2] and a decreased effectiveness of vaccination [3]. Impaired function of aged T cells may also contribute to increased incidence of cancer in the elderly [1]. Further, T cells are thought to exhibit increased autoimmune activity with age [4], which contributes to chronic inflammatory disorders such as rheumatoid arthritis. The ability to prevent or reverse age-related changes in T cells is therefore of great importance for the treatment of human disease. However the molecular underpinnings of

---

* Correspondence: Jackson_taylor@brown.edu
[1]Department of Epidemiology & Prevention, Public Health Sciences, Wake Forest School of Medicine, Winston-Salem, NC 27157, USA
[2]Department of Internal Medicine, Wake Forest School of Medicine, Winston-Salem, NC 27157, USA
Full list of author information is available at the end of the article

age-related functional impairment in T cells are not fully understood.

T cells exist in a variety of subsets, which are classified according to function and surface protein expression. The two major classes are CD4$^+$ (helper) and CD8$^+$ (cytotoxic) T cells-both of which are further divided into naïve (never exposed to cognate antigen) and memory (previously exposed to cognate antigen) subsets. A number of well-characterized aging phenotypes have been observed in general T cell populations including: decreased proportion of naïve T cells [2], decreased proliferation in response to antigen stimulation [5], altered apoptotic signaling [6, 7], decreased T cell receptor (TCR) diversity [8], and altered cytokine production [9]. Naïve and memory subsets are also differentially affected by the aging process. For example, memory CD4$^+$ T cells do not exhibit age-related impairment in cytokine-mediated proliferation, while naïve CD4$^+$ T cells do [10]. In addition, memory cells generated from young naïve cells function well even into old age, while memory cells generated from aged naïve cells function poorly [9]. The turnover rate and replicative capacity of both subsets is also different. Naïve T cells have a 10-fold lower turnover rate than memory [10] and also possess longer telomeres [11] - which allows naïve T cell to divide a far greater number of times than memory cells before entering replicative senescence. In addition, the lifespan of naïve CD4$^+$ cells increases with age in mice and this enhanced longevity has been proposed to cause functional deficits during the aging process [7].

What underlies these general and subset-specific aging phenotypes in CD4+ T cells? A probable driving force is changes in gene expression. A number of individual genes have been demonstrated to change expression levels between young and aged T cells. Perhaps the most consistent finding in T cells (both CD4+ and CD8+) is age-related loss of the co-stimulatory surface protein CD28, which is attributed to diminished transcription of the CD28 gene [12], leading to reduced TCR diversity and antigen-induced proliferation. Additionally, transcript expression of the tumor suppressor $p16^{INK4a}$ show a positive correlation with donor age in human CD4+ T cells [13], which is associated with increased IL-6 expression. The functional consequence of increased $p16^{INK4a}$ expression with age is unclear but it appears to be a useful predictor of chronological age and may be connected to clinical markers of frailty and cellular senescence. Decline in expression of the microRNA miR-181a in human CD4+ T cells leads to increased expression of DUSP6, which impairs ERK signaling and subsequently impairs T cell activation, proliferation, and differentiation [14].

Whole-transcriptome profiling with microarray and RNA-seq technologies has allowed a more in depth look at the molecular basis of T cell aging. Widespread alteration of mRNA expression levels is a hallmark of T cell aging in mice and humans [15], with changes in specific genes providing a logical source for some of the observed age-related phenotypes. An initial microarray study of age-related changes in mouse CD4$^+$ T cells found that aging was associated with increased expression of multiple chemokine receptor gene transcripts [16]-a finding that was confirmed in a later study [17]. An age-related decrease in expression of several cell cycle genes with pro-proliferative function has also been reported from microarray analysis of young and aged T cells from mice [17, 18]. Further, increased mRNA expression of both pro- and anti-apoptotic genes has also been reported [17], which may underlie the complex changes in apoptotic signaling observed in aged T cells [6, 7, 19]. In humans, a previous transcriptomic profiling of young and old CD4$^+$ T cells revealed an enrichment of genes induced by NF-κB that were up-regulated in aged individuals [20]. Our group recently performed global gene expression profiling on purified CD4$^+$ T cells and CD14$^+$ monocytes from a large human cohort, aged 55–91 [21]. In CD4$^+$ T cells, we found suggestive evidence for enrichment for immune function amongst gene transcripts up-regulated with age and enrichment for ribonucleoprotein complex involvement in genes down-regulated with age.

Although our results and those from others offer a molecular basis for some of the more general phenotypes observed during aging in CD4+ T cells, they did not compare individual subsets and are unable to offer insight into gene expression changes which may underlie subset-specific age-related phenotypes. We sought to determine to what degree age-related transcriptomic changes in CD4+ T cells were unique to naïve and memory subsets, respectively, and whether these changes could be linked to their respective phenotypes. To this end, we utilized whole-genome microarray analyses to identify transcriptomic changes that occur during aging in naïve and memory CD4$^+$ populations. Using these data, we also performed comprehensive bioinformatic analyses in order to elucidate biological consequences of altered gene expression and identify up-stream cis-regulators of age-affected genes. Finally, we compared our results in mouse with previous published mouse and human data sets to identify key genes which show conserved and reproducible alterations during aging. Our results identify molecular targets which may drive age-related functional decline in naïve and memory CD4 + cells and suggest some of these targets are conserved in humans.

Results

Naïve T cells up-regulate the surface protein CD44 indefinitely upon exposure to a cognate antigen, and thus high expression of CD44 is a well-established marker of memory cells [22–24]. We isolated splenocytes from young and aged mice, and used fluorescent activated cell sorting (FACS) to collect naïve (CD4$^+$/CD44$^{low/intermediate}$) and memory (CD4$^+$/CD44^{high}) cells from each animal (Additional file 1; Figure S1). We then purified total RNA from each sample and conducted microarray analysis using Illumina MouseWG-6 v2.0 Expression BeadChips (Fig. 1a). Using an initial false discovery rate (FDR) threshold of ≤ 0.05, we identified 185 unique genes that were differentially expressed between young and old naïve CD4$^+$ cells, and 328 unique genes that were differentially expressed between young and memory CD4$^+$ cells (Fig. 1b, Additional file 2: Tables S1 and S2). Of these, 121 and 256 genes were up-regulated during aging in naïve and memory cells, respectively, 41 of which were up-regulated in both populations (Additional file 2: Tables S1 and S2). In turn, 64 and 98 genes were down-regulated during aging in naïve and memory cells, respectively, 9 of which were down-regulated in both populations (Fig. 1b, Additional file 2: Tables S1 and S2). In agreement with our previous results using this microarray technology on human CD4+ T cells [21], fold change in expression was generally modest, ranging from ≈ 1.2–2.8 fold in naïve cells and ≈ 1.1–8 fold in memory cells.

Because the number of genes passing significance cutoff at FDR ≤ 0.05 was relatively small compared to previous mouse results [17], and smaller gene lists sometimes limit the effectiveness of bioinformatic tools, we also created an expanded set of differentially expressed genes using a FDR threshold of ≤ 0.1 for supplemental use. Using this expanded FDR, we identified 548 unique genes that were differentially expressed between young and old naïve CD4$^+$ cells, and 693 unique genes that were differentially expressed between young and old memory CD4$^+$ cells (Fig. 1c, Additional file 2: Tables S1 and S2). Of these, 320 and 413 genes were up-regulated during aging in naïve and memory cells, respectively, 104 of which were up-regulated in both populations (Fig. 1c, Additional file 2: Tables S1 and S2). In turn, 228 and 280 genes were down-regulated during aging in naïve and memory cells, respectively, 38 of which were down-regulated in both populations (Fig. 1c, Additional file 2: Tables S1 and S2).

Functional annotation of Age-genes

We first wanted to see if differentially expressed genes identified in naïve and memory cells would show enrichment for specific functional annotations and if so, whether these annotations would be shared or unique between the two subsets. To address these questions, we first performed singular enrichment analysis (using DAVID Bioinformatic Resources v6.7) for enriched Gene Ontology (GO) and functional terms (e.g., KEGG

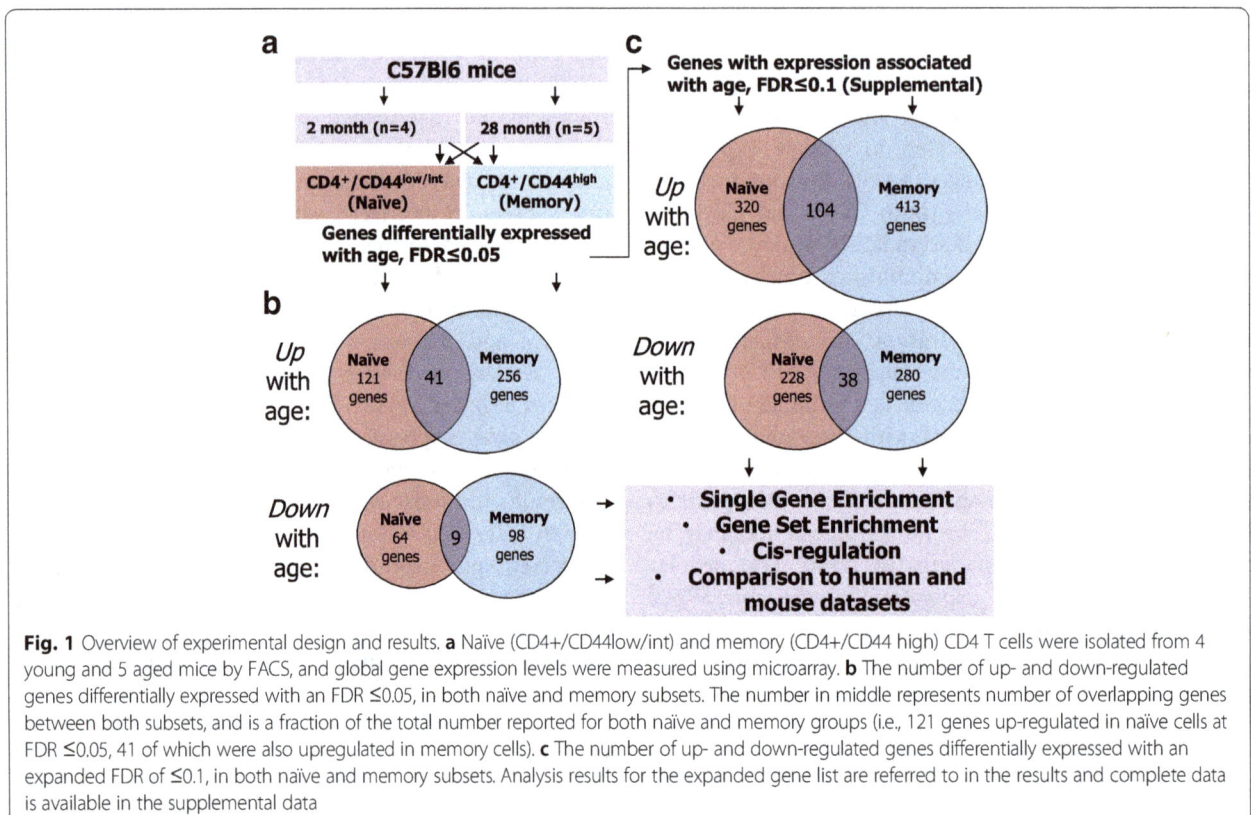

Fig. 1 Overview of experimental design and results. a Naïve (CD4+/CD44low/int) and memory (CD4+/CD44 high) CD4 T cells were isolated from 4 young and 5 aged mice by FACS, and global gene expression levels were measured using microarray. b The number of up- and down-regulated genes differentially expressed with an FDR ≤0.05, in both naïve and memory subsets. The number in middle represents number of overlapping genes between both subsets, and is a fraction of the total number reported for both naïve and memory groups (i.e., 121 genes up-regulated in naïve cells at FDR ≤0.05, 41 of which were also upregulated in memory cells). c The number of up- and down-regulated genes differentially expressed with an expanded FDR of ≤0.1, in both naïve and memory subsets. Analysis results for the expanded gene list are referred to in the results and complete data is available in the supplemental data

pathway) on our lists of genes that were up and down-regulated (FDR ≤ 0.05) in naïve and memory cells (Table 1). Among genes up-regulated with age in naïve cells, significant (FDR ≤ 0.05) enrichment was found for genes involved in immune response, cytokine-cytokine receptor interaction, and regulation of apoptosis (6 classified as positive and 4 as negative regulators of apoptosis per GO annotation). Genes up-regulated in memory T cells were also enriched for cytokine-cytokine receptor interaction (four of these, *Ccl5*, *Cxcr5*, *Tnfrs4*, and *Bmp7*, were also part of this term for naïve cells), as well as endopeptidase inhibitor activity, regulation of interleukin-10 production, positive regulation of immune system processes, and lymphocyte and B cell activation. Enrichment from our expanded gene list (FDR ≤ 0.1) provided similar results (Additional file 3). No significant enrichment was found among genes down-regulated during aging in naïve or memory subsets, although in the expanded gene list (FDR ≤ 0.1) down-regulated genes in naïve cells were enriched for RNA polymerase II transcription factor activity and transcriptional activator activity (Additional file 4). These findings indicate that gene expression changes that occur during aging of naïve and memory CD4$^+$ T cells reflect specific functional programs that are both shared and distinct between the two subsets.

To enhance our understanding of the functional consequences of age-related gene expression in naïve and memory CD4$^+$ T cells, we next performed Gene Set Enrichment Analysis (GSEA) on our samples from both subsets (Table 2). Rather than classifying genes based on pre-defined statistical cutoffs, GSEA is performed on all of the detectable probes measured within each sample, and ranks how well genes correlate with each phenotype (e.g., young and old), and then looks for over-representation of genes from predefined categories (e.g., oxidative phosphorylation) near the top or bottom of these lists. The major advantage of this method is that it can identify functional groups comprised of many genes with small fold-changes in the same direction that would otherwise be excluded by traditional statistical cutoffs. Gene transcripts down-regulated with age in naïve cells were enriched for Myc target genes, oxidative phosphorylation, DNA repair, epigenetic regulation of gene expression, and ribonucleoprotein complex. Genes up-regulated with age in naïve cells were enriched for a variety of different functions. Many gene sets up-regulated in naïve cells were involved in specific cytokine signaling pathways, including genes involved in TNFα signaling via NF-κB and genes activated by STAT5 in response to IL-2 signaling. GSEA also reiterated the increase in apoptosis genes in aged naïve T cells, although this was also accompanied by an increase in pro-proliferative genes. Memory cells showed similar enrichment of many of the same gene sets as naïve cells, with oxidative phosphorylation and Myc target genes being down-regulated with age, and genes involved in TNFα signaling via NF-κB, IL-2/STAT5 signaling, and IFNγ response (*Ifng* gene expression itself was up-regulated in aged memory cells, but not in naïve) being up-regulated with age. Together these results suggest that down-regulation of oxidative phosphorylation and MYC target genes and up-regulation of particular cytokine signaling pathways during aging is shared by

Table 1 Singular Enrichment Analysis results from DAVID v6.7

Gene list	Category	Term	Count	P Value	FDR
Naïve Up	GOTERM_BP_FAT	GO:0006955 ~ immune response	13	1.72E-05	0.000266
	GOTERM_CC_FAT	GO:0005576 ~ extracellular region	15	4.64E-05	0.000517
	KEGG_PATHWAY	mmu04060:Cytokine-cytokine receptor interaction	8	1.41E-04	0.001418
	GOTERM_BP_FAT	GO:0042981 ~ regulation of apoptosis	13	3.17E-04	0.004887
Naïve Down	N/A	N/A	N/A	N/A	
Memory Up	KEGG_PATHWAY	mmu04060:Cytokine-cytokine receptor interaction	12	1.34E-05	0.000151
	GOTERM_MF_FAT	GO:0004866 ~ endopeptidase inhibitor activity	7	9.61E-05	0.001289
	INTERPRO	IPR007110:Immunoglobulin-like	13	2.07E-04	0.002886
	GOTERM_CC_FAT	GO:0016021 ~ integral to membrane	58	3.68E-04	0.004519
	GOTERM_BP_FAT	GO:0032653 ~ regulation of interleukin-10 production	4	6.05E-04	0.00977
	GOTERM_BP_FAT	GO:0002684 ~ positive regulation of immune system process	11	8.28E-04	0.01335
	GOTERM_BP_FAT	GO:0051249 ~ regulation of lymphocyte activation	9	0.001606	0.025729
	GOTERM_BP_FAT	GO:0050871 ~ positive regulation of B cell activation	5	0.00307	0.048641
Memory Down	N/A	N/A	N/A	N/A	N/A

Lists of genes differentially expressed between young and old mice at FDR ≤0.05 in naïve and memory CD4+ T cells were used as input, with all expressed genes in naïve and memory cells used as background. Broad terms such as "signal" and "disulfide bond" were excluded. A FDR of 0.05 was used as a threshold for enriched terms. No terms were significantly enriched in down-regulated gene lists

Table 2 Gene Set Enrichment Analysis results

Enriched in Naïve Young (vs. Naïve Old) Hallmarks	SIZE	FDR	Enriched in Memory Young (vs. Memory Old) Hallmarks	SIZE	FDR
MYC_TARGETS_V1	155	0.001215	OXIDATIVE_PHOSPHORYLATION	163	0.001571
MYC_TARGETS_V2	40	0.002431	G2M_CHECKPOINT	128	0.011848
OXIDATIVE_PHOSPHORYLATION	162	0.002438	E2F_TARGETS	144	0.017543
DNA_REPAIR[a]	119	0.056895	MYC_TARGETS_V1	157	0.022091
			ANDROGEN_RESPONSE	64	0.02355
Enriched in Naïve Young (vs. Naïve Old)	SIZE	FDR	Enriched in Memory Young (vs. Memory Young) GO terms	SIZE	FDR
REGULATION_OF_GENE_EXPRESSION_EPIGENETIC	19	0.040616	N/A	N/A	N/A
RIBONUCLEOPROTEIN_COMPLEX[a]	95	0.057685			
Enriched in Naïve Old (vs. Naïve Young)	SIZE	FDR	Enriched in Memory Old (vs. Memory Young) Hallmarks	SIZE	FDR
IL2_STAT5_SIGNALING	128	0	TNFA_SIGNALING_VIA_NFKB	118	0.00186
TNFA_SIGNALING_VIA_NFKB	112	0	IL2_STAT5_SIGNALING	142	0.002496
INTERFERON_GAMMA_RESPONSE	130	0	INTERFERON_GAMMA_RESPONSE	135	0.010827
COMPLEMENT	92	2.19E-04	KRAS_SIGNALING_UP	80	0.029101
IL6_JAK_STAT3_SIGNALING	44	2.74E-04	IL6_JAK_STAT3_SIGNALING	52	0.035991
INFLAMMATORY_RESPONSE	92	7.16E-04	ALLOGRAFT_REJECTION	129	0.039874
KRAS_SIGNALING_UP	79	7.53E-04	INFLAMMATORY_RESPONSE	98	0.046285
ALLOGRAFT_REJECTION	126	0.001159			
APOPTOSIS	100	0.012965			
ESTROGEN_RESPONSE_EARLY	80	0.015578			
EPITHELIAL_MESENCHYMAL_TRANSITION	53	0.030826			
CHOLESTEROL_HOMEOSTASIS	40	0.045692			
Enriched in Naïve Old (vs. Naïve Young)	SIZE	FDR	Enriched in Memory Old (vs. Memory Young) GO Terms	SIZE	FDR
IMMUNE_RESPONSE	122	0.002943	N/A	N/A	N/A
CYTOKINE_ACTIVITY	26	0.014125			
CYTOKINE_BINDING	25	0.014879			
VIRAL_REPRODUCTIVE_PROCESS	22	0.045368			
PROTEIN_TYROSINE_KINASE_ACTIVITY	21	0.045902			
TRANSMEMBRANE_RECEPTOR_ACTIVITY	70	0.046233			
CYSTEINE_TYPE_ENDOPEPTIDASE_ACTIVITY	24	0.051925			
POSITIVE_REGULATION_OF_CELL_PROLIFERATION[a]	59	0.055409			

Association of a term with phenotype (i.e., Young or Old) indicates genes which comprise that term are more highly expressed within the phenotype (i.e., MYC_TARGETS_V1 are more highly expressed in young naïve cells than in old naïve cells). Size indicates number of genes from each term that were enriched within phenotype. "Hallmarks" and "GO terms" indicate gene sets database used for analysis
[a]indicates terms that were slightly above significance cutoff (FDR 0.05) but were included in results because of previously established relevance to T cell aging

epigenetic regulator and ribonucleoprotein complex genes, and age-related increase in apoptotic and cell proliferation genes.

Cis-regulators of naïve and memory age-genes
To determine potential upstream regulators of genes whose expression was altered by age, we next utilized i-cisTarget [25], a web tool which allows analysis of the regulatory regions of gene lists for enrichment of transcription factor binding sites (TFBSs; consensus DNA sequence to which a transcription factor binds;

cataloged as position weight matrices [PWM]), previously mapped ChIP-seq results, and previously mapped histone modifications (Table 3). In naïve cells, genes up-regulated with age were most enriched for ChIP-seq peaks from the CHD1 transcription factor, although this dataset was from experiments performed in the CH12 (mouse B-cell lymphoma) cell line. The next top hits were all derived from archived consensus TFBSs, and indicate enrichment for NFκB/Rel, Runx family, and Gapb1 (Pu.1) TFBSs near genes up-regulated with age in naïve cells. Interestingly, the top 3 enriched features of

Table 3 Cis-regulatory analysis of genes differentially expressed (FDR ≤0.05) during aging by i-cisTarget

Naïve Up-regulated			
Possible Transcription Factors/Histone Mods	**NES**	**P-value**	**Logo**
CHD1 (ChIP-seq on CH12 cells)	9.93	3.27E-14	N/A
Nfkb1, Rela (PWM)	5.39	4.61E-08	tfdimers-MD00267
Runx2, Runx3, Runx1, Cbfb, Runx1t1 (PWM)	4.89	5.48E-11	homer-M00159
Gabpb1, Sfpi1, Irf4 (PWM)	4.68	7.31E-11	transfac_pro-M00769
Naïve Down-regulated			
Possible Transcription Factors/Histone Mods	**NES**	**P-value**	**Logo**
H3K27ac (ChIP-seq on 8-week mouse thymus)	11.3	1.14E-26	N/A
EP300 (ChIP-seq on 8-week mouse heart)	6.56	8.56E-08	N/A
H3K4me1 (ChIP-seq on 8-week mouse thymus)	5.48	2.24E-21	N/A
Foxo3, Foxo1, Foxo6, Foxo4 (PWM)	4.55	2.48E-11	actorgurvey-foxo_SANGER_10_FBgn0038
Memory Up-regulated			
Possible Transcription Factors/Histone Mods	**NES**	**P-value**	**Logo**
Foxd3 (PWM)	4.70	9.85E-10	taipale-NRNWAAYRTTKNYN-FOXD3-DBD
Memory Down-Regulated			
Possible Transcription Factors/Histone Mods	**NES**	**P-value**	**Logo**
N/A	N/A	N/A	N/A

Table shows transcription factor binding sites and histone modifications found to be enriched in +/− 10 kb regions flanking transcription start site of target genes (excluding coding regions). Parenthesis indicate database from which enriched feature was derived. NES = Normalized Enrichment Score. PWM = Positional Weight Matrix. P-value calculated using hypergeometric test

genes down-regulated with age in naïve T cells all dealt with histone acetylation, particular in regards to epigenetic enhancer function. The top feature was H3K27ac (a mark of active enhancers [26]) ChIP-seq peaks from mouse thymus and the third ranked feature was H3K4me1 (a general mark of poised or active enhancers) ChIP-seq peaks from mouse thymus. The second ranked feature was ChIP-seq peaks for the histone acetyltransferase EP300, which also indicates enhancer regions [27], although these ChIP-seq peaks were collected from mouse heart tissue and thus the relevance to T cells is more uncertain. The sole nucleotide motif which passed our enrichment threshold (see methods) for genes down-regulated with age in naïve cells was a TFBS for

several class O forkhead box (Foxo) transcription factors. In memory T cells, genes that changed with age were associated with fewer features. Up-regulated genes were only enriched for a Foxd3 TFBS, and down-regulated genes did not show any enriched features. Similar results were achieved with our expanded FDR (FDR ≤ 0.1) gene list (Additional file 5), although NF-κB became the top feature for genes up-regulated in memory cells and Foxo and Foxd3 TFBSs were no longer enriched near genes up-regulated in naïve and down-regulated in memory cells, respectively.

We also used the webtool oPOSSUM3 [28], which conducts similar analyses of gene lists based on PWM scoring (see methods for description), to analyze the cis-regulator regions of genes differentially expressed with age (Table 4). For genes up-regulated in naïve cells, no specific TFBS passed our enrichment threshold (Z-score ≥ 7, Fisher p-value ≤ 0.01; see methods); however, NF-κB was the top ranked TFBS by Fisher score and had a Z-score (Z-score = 6.6) just below our cutoff. Thus two independent methods identified enrichment of NF-κB binding sites in the regulatory regions of genes up-regulated during aging in naïve T cells. Genes down-regulated in naïve cells showed enrichment for a number of TFBSs, including interleukin responsive transcription factors Nfil3 and Gfi, and forkhead box transcription factors Foxo3 (also identified by i-cisTarget), FoxI1, and Foxq1. In memory cells, the binding site for IRF-1 (Interferon regulatory factor 1) was highly enriched amongst up-regulated genes as a function of both z-score and Fisher score (Z-score = 15.9;

Fisher p-value = 4.7E-08). IRF-1 functions both as a tumor suppressor and regulator of immune response, and is required for IFNγ-mediated T_H1 differentiation in CD4$^+$ T cells [29]. Although they fell slightly below our Z or F-score cutoffs, we also found marginal enrichment for NF-κB, Foxq1, and Foxd3 (the top TFBS for up-regulated memory genes identified by i-cisTarget) binding sites near genes up-regulated in memory cells. Like naïve cells, genes down-regulated in memory cells were enriched for a larger variety of TFBSs than up-regulated genes, including several that were also enriched near genes down-regulated in naïve cells (Gfi, Nfil3, ELF5, and Prrx2). Similar results were achieved with our expanded FDR (FDR ≤ 0.1) gene list (Additional file 6) although, as with i-cisTarget results, NF-κB TFBSs became more enriched near up-regulated memory genes and Foxo and Foxd3 TFBSs were no longer

Table 4 Cis-regulatory analysis of genes differentially expressed (FDR ≤0.05) during aging by oPOSSUM-3

Cell Type	Direction	TFBS	# of Targets	Z-score	F p-value	Cell Type	Direction	TFBS	# of Targets	Z-score	F p-value
Naïve	Up	NF-kappaB*	56	6.6	0.00197	Memory	Up	IRF1	82	15.916	4.7098E-08
Naïve	Up	Ar*	6	10.673	0.01202	Memory	Up	HOXA5	170	15.025	0.00065615
						Memory	Up	Ar	12	13.167	0.00010069
						Memory	Up	HNF1B	42	11.353	0.00990832
						Memory	Up	PPARG::RXRA	72	7.257	0.00070307
						Memory	Up	Gata1	152	6.963	0.00028379
						Memory	Up	NFKB1*	45	6.94	0.00058749
						Memory	Up	Foxq1*	92	6.759	6.2087E-05
						Memory	Up	Foxd3*	113	9.875	0.08090959
Cell Type	Direction	TFBS	# of Targets	Z-score	F p-value	Cell Type	Direction	TFBS	# of Targets	Z-score	F p-value
Naïve	Down	Prrx2	46	19.911	0.00112	Memory	Down	TP53	1	12.016	0.0043451
Naïve	Down	FOXI1	39	16.131	0.004315	Memory	Down	Gfi	64	11.621	0.00210378
Naïve	Down	Nobox	43	15.018	0.002301	Memory	Down	Ar	7	9.839	6.9823E-05
Naïve	Down	NFIL3	23	14.324	0.009441	Memory	Down	TEAD1	38	9.762	3.2211E-09
Naïve	Down	Gfi	45	13.979	0.000217	Memory	Down	TBP	59	9.326	4.8641E-08
Naïve	Down	Sox17	45	13.953	0.002388	Memory	Down	FEV	73	9.251	7.0307E-06
Naïve	Down	FOXO3	44	13.693	0.006281	Memory	Down	NFIL3	37	9.063	0.00019231
Naïve	Down	Foxq1	27	13.092	0.007568	Memory	Down	Lhx3	28	8.971	0.00107152
Naïve	Down	HLF	23	12.977	0.000107	Memory	Down	Pdx1	69	8.883	0.00365595
Naïve	Down	Gata1	47	12.834	0.000198	Memory	Down	FOXF2	25	8.74	8.3946E-05
Naïve	Down	Tal1::Gata1	24	12.074	0.001469	Memory	Down	NR3C1	19	8.273	7.9799E-06
Naïve	Down	CEBPA	41	10.428	0.004955	Memory	Down	Stat3	53	7.515	9.2897E-05
Naïve	Down	TBP	35	9.593	0.004688	Memory	Down	SPI1	74	7.368	1.3183E-05
Naïve	Down	SOX9	40	9.21	0.001014	Memory	Down	ELF5	77	7.248	4.14E-08
Naïve	Down	Myb	44	9.044	0.002547	Memory	Down	Egr1	37	7.203	7.4131E-06
Naïve	Down	RREB1	7	7.524	0.004571	Memory	Down	Prrx2	69	7.103	9.1411E-05
Naïve	Down	ELF5	51	7.382	3.47E-05						

Table shows transcription factor binding sites found to be enriched in +/− 10 kb regions flanking transcription start site of target genes (excluding coding regions). See Methods for explanation of Z-score and Fisher p-value

enriched near naïve up and memory down-regulated genes, respectively.

In summary, our cis-regulatory analyses suggest that altered activity and/or expression of several transcription factors and histone modifications may underlie the altered expression of these genes. In particular, our results point to increased NF-κB activity as a cause of increased gene expression in naïve and memory cells, a finding supported by our GSEA enrichment results (Table 2). Both analysis programs also identified Foxd3 binding sites near genes up-regulated in memory cells and Foxo binding sites near genes down-regulated in naïve cells. Finally, we identified enrichment of enhancer marks H3K27ac and H3K4me1 from thymus in the regulatory regions of genes down-regulated with age in naïve cells. Although enhancer marks are highly tissue specific [27], the fact that these marks were mapped in thymic tissue suggests a genuine involvement in T cell gene-regulation.

Comparison to previous mouse and human results

A previous microarray study identified over 2,000 genes that were differentially expressed in naïve CD4+ T cells from young and aged mice [17] and we recently reported 186 genes with age-associated expression in human CD4+ T cells (FDR ≤0.01) [21]. We wanted to see which of the genes identified in the current study overlapped with previous results in mice and humans, in order to identify high confidence genes for future study-particularly those with relevance to human aging which can be studied in mouse models. Genes that were up- or down-regulated in more than one study are listed in in Table 5 (FDR ≤ 0.05) and Additional file 6 (FDR ≤ 0.1). Because CD4+ cells used in our human study contained a mixture of naïve and memory cells, we separately compared human results (converted to mouse orthologues, see Methods) to genes differentially expressed in naïve and memory CD4+ cells from the current study. We also calculated the probability of the observed vs. expected level of overlap in each comparison. In general, up-regulated genes showed more significant (hypergeometric test) overlap between datasets, especially between genes up-regulated in naïve cells from both mouse studies (p < 1.866e-15). The pro-inflammatory enzyme *Casp1* (Caspase-1) gene was up-regulated with age in all four datasets, and *Il1r2* (type 2 IL-1 receptor) was up-regulated in human CD4+ cells as well as both naïve and memory cells from our current experiments. Interestingly, *Casp1* and *Il1r2* have biologically antagonistic roles, with Casp1 protein functioning to cleave pro-IL-1β into the mature pro-inflammatory cytokine IL-1β, and IL-1r2 acting as a soluble decoy receptor that sequesters pro-IL-1β [30]. Also noteworthy is the up-regulation of *Dusp6* (dual specific phosphatase 6) transcripts in both of our naïve and memory groups along with our previous human results. Dusp6 is a phosphatase that was previously reported to increase with age in naïve human CD4+ T cells and cause defects in TCR signaling [14]. While there was little consistency amongst datasets for down-

Table 5 Comparison with previous mouse and human results

Dataset 1	Dataset 2	Direction	Genes	P-value
Human CD4+ (118)	Mouse Naïve (119)	Up	**Casp1**, Dusp6, Rgs1,	p < 0.021
Human CD4+ (118)	Mouse Naïve (Mirza et al., 2011) (734)	Up	Acvr2a, Aqp9, Arrdc4, Bcl2l2, **Casp1**, Cd86, Fcgr2b, Fgl2, Fndc3b, **Il1r2**, Ltb4r1, Rgs12, Lyn	p < 6.225e-05
Human CD4+ (118)	Mouse Memory (237)	Up	Bcl6, **Casp1**, Cyp4v3, Dusp6, **Il1r2**, Plcb2,	p < 0.001
Mouse Naïve (119)	Mouse Naïve (Mirza et al., 2011) (734)	Up	Abhd4, Adssl1, Bhlhb2, Bmp7, **Casp1**, Casp4, Xcl1, Ccl5, Cxcr3, Csprs, Endod1, Esm1, Eomes, Gbp3, Hmgn3, Ier3, Klf9, Lrrk1, Lpxn, Myo1f, Nkg7, Naip2, Ryk, Serpina9, Serpina3g, Zcchc18	p < 1.866e-15
Human CD4+ (181)	Mouse Naïve (65)	Down	**Foxp1**	p < 0.387
Human CD4+ (181)	Mouse Naïve (Mirza et al., 2011) (1382)	Down	Calb2, Epb4.1, Eef1d, **Foxp1**, Gpa33, Tgfbr2	p < 0.102
Human CD4+ (181)	Mouse Memory (107)	Down	I7Rn6, Trat1, Ube2n,	p < 0.047
Mouse Naïve (65)	Mouse Naïve (Mirza et al., 2011) (1382)	Down	Actn2, Actn1, Bcl9l, Ecm1, **Foxp1**, Mid1,	p < 0.166

Rows performing comparison with data from current study include genes differentially expressed at FDR ≤0.05. Bolded terms were identified in multiple comparisons. Parenthesis indicate total number of genes used for comparison. Note that genes beginning with LOC were removed from gene lists from the current study for these comparisons, as they had been removed from the other studies, and thus the totals are slightly lower than reported in Fig. 1. P-values were calculated using the hypergeometric test

regulated genes, *Foxp1* (Forkhead box protein P1) was down-regulated with age in humans as well as both naïve mouse CD4$^+$ datasets. Foxp1 promotes T cell quiescence via suppression of both the *Il7r* gene and Erk signaling [31, 32], and is thought to antagonize the actions of Foxo1-which was also down-regulated at the transcript level in our human and naïve mouse datasets. Our comparison highlights several genes which change with age in T cells from both mice and humans, in particular up-regulation of *Casp1* and down-regulation of *Foxp1*.

Discussion

The age-related changes in functional networks we observed in both naïve and memory subsets echo previous reported as hallmarks of aging in the immune system and beyond. "Inflamm-aging" is a term used to define the well-established increase in low-grade inflammatory signaling associated with aging [33]. The increased expression of Il-2/Stat5 signaling, NF-κB target genes, IFNγ response, and inflammatory response genes with age seen in our GSEA results appear to reflect the effects of inflamm-aging. We find increased expression of cytokine and cytokine receptor genes in both naïve and memory subsets, a result previously observed in mouse and human T cells [16, 34]. Down-regulation of oxidative phosphorylation genes, which we observed in both subsets, is a common age-related phenotype for many tissues [21, 35]. In addition to increased "TNFα signaling via NF-κB" in aged cells from both subsets as indicated by GSEA, we also observed enrichment for putative NF-κB binding sites in the regulatory regions of genes up-regulated with age in both naïve and memory subsets (although this appeared to be stronger in naïve cells). Increased NF-κB signaling is another reoccurring feature of aging in the immune system [36] and other tissues [37], and has been proposed as a central cause of inflamm-aging [36]. Supporting the relevance of our findings in humans, a recent microarray study of aging human CD4$^+$ T cells found gene expression mediated by NF-κB was increased during aging [20]. This same group also found aberrant activation of NF-κB target genes in the absence of stimulation in CD4+ T cells collected from older individuals [38]. In addition, our recently published work found that aging was associated with increased expression of the *NFKB1* gene in human CD4$^+$ T cells [21]. Our findings support a major role of NF-κB in driving age-related gene expression changes in T cells.

One of the main distinguishing features we found for naïve CD4$^+$ cells was an increase in genes with a role in apoptosis. The role of apoptosis in aging T cells appears complex; some studies report an age-related increase in apoptosis [6, 39] while others report an age-related impairment of apoptosis [7, 40]. The conflicting results

may reflect differences in mice and humans. In mice, aging of naïve CD4$^+$ cells is reportedly associated with longer cellular lifespan and reduced expression of the pro-apoptotic protein Bim [7]. It has been proposed that impaired apoptosis and increased lifespan leads to the accumulation of molecular damage and functional impairment in aged cells [7, 40]. Importantly, the genes we identified with an annotated role in apoptosis appear to have both pro-and anti-apoptotic roles, indicating a complex regulation of this cellular function in aged naïve cells. We also find that the pro-apoptotic *Casp1* gene is up-regulated with age in mice in both naïve and memory CD4$^+$ cells, and also in human CD4$^+$ cells.

Although it was just above our significance threshold (FDR = 0.058), we report that GSEA indicated a decline in ribonucleoprotein (RNP) complex genes in naïve CD4$^+$ cells. The decline in RNP genes was also observed during aging in our recent study of human monocytes and CD4$^+$ T cells [21], and was previously observed in aging human leukocytes [41]. Thus, decline in RNP genes may be a hallmark of T cell aging in mice and humans. Furthermore, RNP genes are regulated by Myc [42], and we also our GSEA results also indicate a decrease in Myc target genes. Thus, the decreased expression of RNP genes with age may be due to a dysfunctional or purposeful (i.e., compensatory) decline in Myc signaling. This is especially interesting considering the recent finding that decreased expression of Myc enhances lifespan and healthspan in mice [43].

We also observed specific enrichment of enhancer marks H3K27ac and H3K4me1 (derived from 8-week old mouse thymus) near genes down-regulated in naïve cells. Although enhancers are known to play a major role in gene regulation, little is currently known about the role of enhancers in aging. A recent study of human monocytes by our lab found that age-associated DNA methylation alterations which were also associated with cis-gene expression (age-eMS), were enriched for enhancer regions, indicated by H3K27ac and H3K4me1 marks (previously mapped in a young monocyte sample by EN-CODE) [44]. Similarly, Shah et al. [45] found that H3K27me3 peaks lost during aging were strongly enriched for H3K27ac sites previously mapped in young fibroblasts. Overall, these results suggest that altered enhancer activity during aging may contribute to age-related changes in gene expression in naïve CD4$^+$ T cells. Further studies are necessary to confirm specific regulatory functions identified in the current study - e.g., ChIP-seq of enhancer histone modification in young and aged T cells-before they are pursued as potential means of therapy to reverse age-related gene expression changes in T cells. As epigenetic modifications are highly cell-type specific, future studies may also benefit from further subset purification, e.g., central vs. effector memory populations.

Class O forkhead box (Foxo) transcription factors are well known regulators of both T cell function [46] and the aging process [47]. Our findings indicate that altered activity and/or expression of several different classes of forkhead box transcription factor genes, including Foxo1 and Foxo3, may be important in T cell aging. We find *Foxo1* mRNA is down-regulated in naïve mouse cells and human CD4 cells, together with the enrichment for putative Foxo binding sites near down-regulated genes in naïve cells. Foxo1 is a positive regulator of T cell pro-liferation via activation of the *Il7r* gene [31] (although we did not observe altered expression of *Il7r* in mice or humans) and thus decline in expression/activity may cause reduced proliferation of naïve cells with age. In support of reduced Foxo1 expression/activity with age in naïve T cells, we did observe decreased expression of *Foxo1* target gene *Klf2* [46] but surprisingly Foxo1 target genes *Eomes* and *Ctla4* showed increased expression. Putative Foxd3 binding sites are enriched near genes up-regulated with age in memory cells. This gene does not have an established role in T cell biology but is thought to act as a tumor suppressor and regulator of pluripo-tency in embryonic stem cells [48]. However, *Foxd3* transcripts were not detectable in memory cells in our analysis. Although this does not preclude the possibility of *Foxd3* expression (transcription factor mRNAs are often expressed at very low levels), these results should be interpreted with caution. Finally, we find that the *Foxp1* gene is down-regulated during aging in naïve mouse CD4+ cells and human CD4+ cells. Foxp1 opposes Foxo1 function in T cells by repressing *Il7r* expression, thus promoting T cell quiescence [32]. The down-regulation of both *Foxo1* and *Foxp1* may be a result of compensatory mechanisms. Together these findings indicate potentially important subset specific roles for different Fox proteins in T cell aging.

Overlap between mouse results with our previous results from human CD4+ cells is low. This may be due to the heterogeneity of human CD4+ cells, or may reflect differences in mouse and human aging programs. How-ever, our analysis did identify several interesting genes with similar age-related changes that occur consistently in mice and humans. Among these genes were *Casp1* and *Foxp1*, which we discuss above. We also found *Dusp6* to be up-regulated in naïve and memory CD4+ cells, as well as human CD4+ cells. Dusp6 expression was previously reported to increase in naïve CD4+ T cells during aging in humans and cause functional de-fects in TCR-ERK signaling [14], although this increase was reported at the protein but not mRNA level. Our findings indicate that *Dusp6* mRNA does with age, in both mouse (naïve and memory) and human CD4+ T cells. Murine models may therefore represent a clinically relevant model to study the cause and effect of age-

related increase of Dusp6 in CD4+ cells and to test therapies to reverse this process.

One potential limitation of our study is the sole use of CD44 as a marker to distinguish naïve and memory T cells. The CD4+/CD44^{high} population is likely to be somewhat heterogeneous, containing both central and effector memory populations, as wells regulatory T cells. The use of additional markers, such as CD62 and FoxP3, in future studies would allow for isolation of more homogeneous populations. An additional limitation is the lack of validation studies-specifically qPCR to valid-ate age-related changes in expression of key candidate genes identified by microarray, and ChIP-qPCR and/or ChIP-seq to validate potential age-related changes in binding of transcription factors and histone modifica-tions in the regulatory regions of genes that show altered expression with age. Finally, we note that the microarray technology employed in this study is not as sensitive or comprehensive as RNA-seq.

Conclusions

Our findings show that naïve and memory CD4+ subsets both undergo substantial changes in gene expression during the aging process. Genes with altered expression are generally distinct; however, functional annotation analyses indicate that aging affects a number of common gene expression networks in the two subsets. These com-mon features include: increased expression of cytokine/cytokine receptor genes, decreased expression of oxidative phosphorylation and Myc target genes, up-regulation of NF-κB target genes, and increased inflammatory signaling. Our results also suggest that both subsets also exhibit unique transcriptomic alterations; specifically, genes up-regulated with age in naïve cells were specifically enriched for apoptotic signaling function, and genes down-regulated with age in naïve cells were enriched for nearby enhancer histone modifications and Foxo transcription factor binding sites. Memory cells, on the other hand, showed little specific enrichment for gene function; how-ever, the regulator regions of age-associated genes in this subset did show enrichment of specific TFBSs near genes, particularly Foxd3 and Irf-1. Lastly, we show that several well-characterized genes previously reported to be affected by age in human CD4+ T cells (e.g., DUSP6) show similar expression changes in mice. However, an important finding from our comparison with human results was the low overall overlap of genes affected by age in humans and mice.

Both naïve and memory CD4+ T cells undergo age-related functional decline. Our study highlights specific genes and gene pathways that may underlie this func-tional decline. Furthermore, we also identify upstream regulatory factors that may potentially drive these changes and provide attractive targets for future studies on T cell aging. Finally, our findings highlight the need for caution when interpreting results from murine models of T cell aging.

Acknowledgements
The MESA Epigenomics Study was funded by NHLBI grant R01HL101250 to Wake Forest University Health Sciences. The MESA Epigenomics & Transcriptomics Study was funded by NHLBI grant R01HL101250 to Wake Forest University Health Sciences. J.R.T. was supported by T32AG033534 from the National Institute of Aging.

Methods

Mice

C57BL/6 mice were used for all studies. Young mice (2–3 months) were acquired from Harlan Laboratories (Indianapolis, IN) and aged mice (28 months) were acquired from Charles River Laboratories (Wilmington, MA) via the National Institute on Aging (Bethesda, MD). Mice were sacrificed by cervical dislocation following anesthesia by isoflurane. Animal housing and procedures were approved by the Animal Care and Use Committee of Wake Forest University Health Sciences. Principles of laboratory animal care (NIH publication No. 86–23, revised 1985) were followed during euthanasia procedures.

T cell isolation

For each mouse, the spleen was removed and homogenized in ice cold RPMI medium with 2% FBS. Cell suspensions were filtered through a 40 μM filter, and red blood cells were lysed with RBC Lysis buffer (Biolegend, San Diego, CA) per the manufacturer's instructions. Cells were filtered again, then incubated with Fixable Viability Dye eFluor® 450 (eBioscience, San Diego, CA), a cocktail of FITC-conjugated lineage antibodies (CD11b, CD8a, CD49b, CD45RO, Gr-1, and Ter119), CD4-PE, and CD44-APC antibodies for 30 minutes at 4 °C, washed and resuspended in RPMI without phenol red $^+$ 2% FBS before proceeding FACS. All antibodies were purchased from eBiosciences (San Diego, CA) or BD Biosciences (San Jose, CA).

FACS

FACS was performed on a FACS Aria cell sorter (BD Biosciences, San Jose, CA). Naïve (CD44$^{low/intermediate}$) and memory (CD44^{high}) Lin$^-$/CD4$^+$ T cells were sorted into cold FBS. After sorting, cells were pelleted at 500 × g for 10 min and lysed in QIAzol (QIAGEN, Valencia, CA) reagent before storage at −80 °C. Isotype and single color controls were used for every sort.

RNA extraction

RNA extraction was performed using the miRNeasy Micro kit (QIAGEN, Valencia, CA) according to manufacturer

directions. Eluted RNA was initially quantified using a Nanodrop. RNA quality and concentration was also assessed with a RNA 6000 Pico kit (Agilent Technologies, Santa Clara, CA) on a 2100 Bioanalyzer (Agilent Technologies). All samples had RIN values > 8.0, with an average value of 9.7.

Global gene expression quantification

50 ng of total RNA from each sample was amplified and labeled using the Illumina® TotalPrep™-96 RNA Amplification Kit (Life Technologies, Carlsbad, CA). The MouseWG-6 v2.0 Expression BeadChip and Illumina Bead Array Reader were used to perform the genome-wide expression analysis, following the Illumina expression protocol. Seven hundred monogram of biotinylated cRNA was hybridized to a BeadChip at 58 °C for 16 – 17 h. To avoid potential biases due to batch, chip, and position effects, a stratified random sampling technique was used to assign individual samples to specific Bead-Chips (6 samples/chip) and chip position.

Microarray data pre-processing and differential expression analysis

Background corrected bead-level data was obtained from Illumina GenomeStudio software and subsequent pre-processing, quality control, and statistical analysis were performed in *R* using *Bioconductor* packages. Quantile normalization was performed with the *neqc* function of the *limma* package, with the addition of a small recommended offset [49]. Normalized probe values were log$_2$ transformed and control probe and outlier samples were eliminated from the expression matrix. Multidimensional scaling plots showed that naïve and memory samples clustered by cell type and age. One young naïve sample was removed due to low signal and one old memory sample was detected as an outlier by multidimensional scaling analysis and was also removed. Detection *p*-values were computed using negative controls from the beadarray. To detect differential expression between two groups with small sample sizes, the regularized *t*-test implemented in the limma R package was used [50]. The false discovery rate (FDR) using q-value method [51] was reported.

Functional annotation analysis

Functional annotation of genes differentially expressed between young and old mice was performed using DAVID Bioinformatic Resources v6.7 [52]. Lists of up- and down-regulated Illumina probe IDs (FDR ≤ 0.05 for main text table and FDR ≤ 0.1 for supplemental table) were entered into the Functional Annotation Tool web application, with lists of all detectable Illumina probe IDs for naïve or memory cells used as background. An FDR ≤ 0.05 was used to define enrichment. Broad terms such as "signal" and "disulfide bond" were excluded from results. Gene Set Enrichment Analysis [53] was performed using the Java application available from The Broad Institute (www.broadinstitute.org/gsea/). As this software incorporates all (detectable) probe values for each sample, separate results for each FDR threshold were not necessary. Gene set databases used were Hallmarks (h.all.v5.0.symbols.gmt) and Gene Ontology (c5.all.v5.0.symbols.gmt). One thousand gene set permutations were performed. An FDR cutoff of ≤ 0.05 was used for enriched terms, as is recommended when performing permutations by gene set.

Cis-regulatory analysis

i-cisTarget [25] and oPOSSUM-3 [28] web applications were used for analysis of cis-regulatory regions, defined in both programs as $^+/-$ 10 kb from the transcription start site of each gene (excluding coding regions). For i-cisTarget, ROC threshold for AUC calculation was set to 0.005. i-cisTarget uses a ranking and recovery method which produces a Normalized Enrichment Score (NES). An NES of 3 roughly corresponds to a FDR ≤ 0.05 [54] and is the default enrichment cutoff for the program. However, we found NES scores up to 5.5 for ChIP-seq (although many reflected thymic tissue) and up to 4.3 for PWM (i.e., consensus DNA binding sequence for a transcription factor) database results when running lists of all detectable T cell genes, and thus used these scores as cutoffs for enrichment in order to compensate for tissue specific gene expression. For oPOSSUM-3, mouse Single Site Analysis was used with a conservation cutoff of 0.60 and a matrix score threshold of 85%. A list of all detectable genes in naïve or memory cells was used for background. oPOSSUM analyzes TFBS enrichment through both Z-score and F-score, which is the negative log of the Fisher one-tailed exact probability. The Z-score used compare the rate of occurrence of a TFBS in the target set of genes to the expected rate estimated from the precomputed background. F-score is based on the one-tailed Fisher exact probability, which compares the proportion of co-expressed genes containing a particular TFBS to the proportion contained in the background set. Thus the F-score/p-value does not consider the number of times a TFBS appears near a gene beyond once. For enrichment of TFBSs, we employed a combined threshold of 7 for Z-score and 2 (corresponding to a p-value of 0.01) for F-score, based on available recommendations and literature [55].

Comparison with previous datasets

For comparison of mouse and human gene lists, human genes were converted to mouse orthologs using the ENSMBL Biomart tool. Analyzed data from Mirza et al. [17] was downloaded from the NCBI Gene Expression Omnibus (Accession number GSE28165). A hypergeometric test was used to compare significance of overlap between two datasets. The test was performed using a publically available calculator (http://nemates.org/MA/progs/overlap_stats.html).

Additional files

Additional file 1: Figure S1. FACS profile for sorting naïve and memory CD4+ T cells. Representative gates for FACS setup used to separate naïve and memory CD4+ T cells. Spleen cells were separated based on forward and side scatter (P1 and P2). Dead cells (violet positive) were removed (P3), as were lineage/FITC positive (see methods) (P4), before CD4+ cells (y-axis, bottom left plot) were separated based on CD44 expression (x-axis, bottom left plot) to isolate naïve (CD44 low) and memory (CD44 high) populations. Bottom right plot shows alternate representation of CD44 expression.

Additional file 2: Genes differentially expressed in young and old, memory and naïve CD4+ T cells. list of gene symbols, Illumina probe IDs, log2 fold change, p-values and FDR for all genes differentially expressed between young and old naïve (CD44 Low) and young and old memory (CD44 high) at a FDR of ≤

Additional file 3: Table S1. DAVID results from expanded gene list (FDR ≤0.1). Lists of genes differentially expressed between young and old mice at FDR ≤0.1 in naïve and memory CD4+ T cells were used as input, with all expressed genes in naïve and memory cells used as background. Broad terms such as "signal" and "disulfide bond" were excluded. A FDR of 0.05 was used as a threshold for enriched terms. No terms were

Additional file 4: Table S2. Cis-regulatory analysis of expanded gene list (FDR ≤0.1) by i-cisTarget. Table shows transcription factor binding sites and histone modifications found to be enriched in +/− 10 kb regions flanking transcription start site of target genes (excluding coding regions). Parenthesis indicate database from which enriched feature was derived. NES = Normalized Enrichment Score. PWM = Positional Weight Matrix. P-value calculated

Additional file 5: Table S3. Cis-regulatory analysis of genes differentially expressed (FDR ≤0.1) during aging by oPOSSUM-3. Table shows transcription factor binding sites found to be enriched in +/− 10 kb regions flanking transcription start site of target genes (excluding coding regions). See Methods for explanation of Z-score and Fisher p

Additional file 6: Table S4. Comparison with previous mouse and human results. Rows performing comparison with data from current study include genes differentially expressed at FDR ≤0.1. * indicates value or gene from the current study differentially expressed at FDR < 0.05; those without a * were differentially expressed at a FDR >0.05 and ≤ 0.1. Bolded terms were identified in multiple comparisons. Parenthesis indicate total number of genes used for comparison. Note that genes beginning with LOC were removed from gene lists from the current study for these comparisons, as they had been removed from the other studies, and thus the totals are slightly lower than reported in Fig. 1. P

Acknowledgements

We would like to thank Beth Holbrook, James C. Wood, and Martha Alexander-Miller in the Wake Forest Flow Cytometry core for assistance with FACS.

Funding

The MESA Epigenomics Study was funded by NHLBI grant R01HL101250 to Wake Forest University Health Sciences. The MESA Epigenomics & Transcriptomics Study was funded by NHLBI grant R01HL101250 to Wake Forest University Health Sciences. J.R.T. was supported by T32AG033534 from the National Institute of Aging.

Authors' contributions

J.R.T. designed and performed experiments, performed data analysis, and wrote the manuscript. L.R. performed data analysis and assisted with manuscript preparation. L.H. and W.C. assisted with experiments. K.L. performed data analysis. S.K., C.M., and Y.L. designed experiments, assisted with data analysis and interpretation, and assisted with manuscript preparation. All authors read and approved the final manuscript.

Competing interests

The authors declare that they have no competing interests.

Author details

[1]Department of Epidemiology & Prevention, Public Health Sciences, Wake Forest School of Medicine, Winston-Salem, NC 27157, USA. [2]Department of Internal Medicine, Wake Forest School of Medicine, Winston-Salem, NC 27157, USA. [3]Present Address: Department of Molecular Biology, Cell Biology, Biochemistry at Brown University, Providence, RI 02912, USA.

References

1. Goronzy JJ, Fang F, Cavanagh MM, Qi Q, Weyand CM. Naive T Cell Maintenance and Function in Human Aging. J Immunol. 2015;194:4073– doi:10.4049/jimmunol.1500046.
2. Nikolich-Žugich J. Aging of the T cell compartment in mice and humans: from no naive expectations to foggy memories. J Immunol. 2014;193:2622–9. doi:10.4049/jimmunol.1401174.
3. Goronzy JJ, Weyand CM. Understanding immunosenescence to improve responses to vaccines. Nat Immunol. 2013;14:428–36. doi:10.1038/ni.2588.
4. Goronzy JJ, Weyand CM. Immune aging and autoimmunity. Cell Mol Life Sci. 2012;69:1615–23.
5. Canonica GW, Ciprandi G, Caria M, Dirienzo W, Shums A, Norton-koger B, et al. Defect of autologous mixed lymphocyte reaction and interleukin-2 in aged individuals. Mech Ageing Dev. 1985;32:205–12.
6. Aggarwal S, Gupta S. Increased apoptosis of T cell subsets in aging humans: altered expression of Fas (CD95), Fas ligand, Bcl-2, and Bax. J Immunol. 1998;160:1627–37.
7. Tsukamoto H, Clise-Dwyer K, Huston GE, Duso DK, Buck AL, Johnson LL, et al. Age-associated increase in lifespan of naive CD4 T cells contributes to T-cell homeostasis but facilitates development of functional defects. Proc Natl Acad Sci U S A. 2009;106:18333–8. doi:10.1073/pnas.0910139106.
8. Goronzy JJ, Lee WW, Weyand CM. Aging and T-cell diversity. Exp Gerontol. 2007;42(5 SPEC. ISS):400–6.
9. Haynes L, Eaton SM, Burns EM, Randall TD, Swain SL. CD4 T cell memory derived from young naive cells functions well into old age, but memory generated from aged naive cells functions poorly. Proc Natl Acad Sci U S A. 2003;100:15053–8. doi:10.1073/pnas.2433717100.
10. Naylor K, Li G, Vallejo AN, Lee W-W, Koetz K, Bryl E, et al. The influence of age on T cell generation and TCR diversity. J Immunol. 2005;174:7446–52.
11. Weng NP, Levine BL, June CH, Hodes RJ. Human naive and memory T lymphocytes differ in telomeric length and replicative potential. Proc Natl Acad Sci U S A. 1995;92:11091–4.
12. Weng N, Akbar AN, Goronzy J. CD28-T cells: their role in the age-associated decline of immune function. Trends Immunol. 2009;30:306–12. doi:10.1016/j.it.2009.03.013.
13. Liu Y, Sanoff HK, Cho H, Burd CE, Torrice C, Ibrahim JG, et al. Expression of p16 [INK4a] in peripheral blood T-cells is a biomarker of human aging. Aging Cell. 2009;8:439–48. doi:10.1111/j.1474-9726.2009.00489.x.
14. Li G, Yu M, Lee W-W, Tsang M, Krishnan E, Weyand CM, et al. Decline in miR-181a expression with age impairs T cell receptor sensitivity by increasing DUSP6 activity. Nat Med. 2012;18:1518–24. doi:10.1038/nm.2963.
15. Chen G, Lustig A, Weng N. T Cell Aging: A Review of the Transcriptional Changes Determined from Genome-Wide Analysis. Front Immunol. 2013;4:121. doi:10.3389/fimmu.2013.00121.
16. Mo R, Chen J, Han Y, Bueno-Cannizares C, Misek DE, Lescure PA, et al. T cell chemokine receptor expression in aging. J Immunol. 2003;170:895–904.
17. Mirza N, Pollock K, Hoelzinger DB, Dominguez AL, Lustgarten J. Comparative kinetic analyses of gene profiles of naïve CD4 + and CD8 + T cells from young and old animals reveal novel age-related alterations. Aging Cell. 2011;10:853–67.
18. Han SN, Adolfsson O, Lee C-K, Prolla TA, Ordovas J, Meydani SN. Age and vitamin E-induced changes in gene expression profiles of T cells. J Immunol. 2006;177:6052–61. doi:10.4049/JIMMUNOL.177.9.6052.
19. Hsu HC, Scott DK, Mountz JD. Impaired apoptosis and immune senescence - Cause or effect? Immunol Rev. 2005;205:130–46.
20. Bektas A, Zhang Y, Lehmann E, Iii WHW, Becker KG, Ferrucci L, et al. Age-associated changes in basal NF-kappaB function in human CD4+ T lymphocytes via dysregulation of PI3 kinase. Aging. 2014;6:957–74.
21. Reynolds LM, Ding J, Taylor JR, Lohman K, Soranzo N, de la Fuente A, et al. Transcriptomic profiles of aging in purified human immune cells. BMC Genomics. 2015;16:333. doi:10.1186/s12864-015-1522-4.
22. Zhao C, Davies JD. A peripheral CD4+ T cell precursor for naive, memory, and regulatory T cells. J Exp Med. 2010;2010:207.
23. Puré E, Cuff CA. A crucial role for CD44 in inflammation. Trends Mol Med. 2001;7:213–21.
24. Kapasi ZF, Murali-Krishna K, McRae ML, Ahmed R. Defective generation but normal maintenance of memory T cells in old mice. Eur J Immunol. 2002;32:1567–73.
25. Imrichová H, Hulselmans G, Atak ZK, Potier D, Aerts S. I-cisTarget 2015 update: Generalized cis-regulatory enrichment analysis in human, mouse and fly. Nucleic Acids Res. 2015;43:W57–64.
26. Creyghton MP, Cheng AW, Welstead GG, Kooistra T, Carey BW, Steine EJ, et al. Histone H3K27ac separates active from poised enhancers and predicts developmental state. Proc Natl Acad Sci U S A. 2010;107:21931–6.
27. Visel A, Blow MJ, Li Z, Zhang T, Akiyama JA, Holt A, et al. ChIP-seq accurately predicts tissue-specific activity of enhancers. Nature. 2009;457:854–8. doi:10.1038/nature07730.
28. Kwon AT, Arenillas DJ, Worsley Hunt R, Wasserman WW. oPOSSUM-3: advanced analysis of regulatory motif over-representation across genes or ChIP-Seq datasets. G3 (Bethesda). 2012;2:987–1002. doi:10.1534/g3.112.003202.
29. Savitsky D, Tamura T, Yanai H, Taniguchi T. Regulation of immunity and oncogenesis by the IRF transcription factor family. Cancer Immunol Immunother. 2010;59:489–510.
30. Peters VA, Joesting JJ, Freund GG. IL-1 receptor 2 (IL-1R2) and its role in immune regulation. Brain Behav Immun. 2012;2:1–8. doi:10.1016/j.bbi.2012.11.006.
31. Skon CN, Jameson SC. Fox factors fight over T cell quiescence. Nat Immunol. 2011;12:522–4. doi:10.1038/ni.2040.
32. Feng X, Wang H, Takata H, Day TJ, Willen J, Hu H. Transcription factor Foxp1 exerts essential cell-intrinsic regulation of the quiescence of naive T cells. Nat Immunol. 2011;12:544–50. doi:10.1038/ni.2034.
33. Franceschi C, Bonafè M, Valensin S, Olivieri F, De Luca M, Ottaviani E, et al. Inflamm-aging. An evolutionary perspective on immunosenescence. Ann N Y Acad Sci. 2000;908:244–54.
34. Remondini D, Salvioli S, Francesconi M, Pierini M, Mazzatti DJ, Powell JR, et al. Complex patterns of gene expression in human T cells during in vivo aging. Mol Biosyst. 2010;6:1983–92. doi:10.1039/c004635c.
35. de Magalhães JP, Curado J, Church GM. Meta-analysis of age-related gene expression profiles identifies common signatures of aging. Bioinformatics. 2009;25:875–81.
36. Salminen A, Huuskonen J, Ojala J, Kauppinen A, Kaarniranta K, Suuronen T. Activation of innate immunity system during aging: NF-kB signaling is the molecular culprit of inflamm-aging. Ageing Res Rev. 2008;7:83–105.
37. Adler AS, Sinha S, Kawahara TLA, Zhang JY, Segal E, Chang HY. Motif module map reveals enforcement of aging by continual NF-kappaB activity. Genes Dev. 2007;21:3244–57. doi:10.1101/gad.1588507.
38. Bektas A, Zhang Y, Wood WH, Becker KG, Madara K, Ferrucci L, et al. Age-associated alterations in inducible gene transcription in human CD4+ T lymphocytes. Aging. 2013;5:18–36. doi:10.18632/aging.100522.
39. Pahlavani M, Vargas D. Aging but not dietary restriction alters the activation-induced apoptosis in rat T cells. FEBS Lett. 2001;491:114–8. doi:10.1016/S0014-5793(01)02184-6.
40. Spaulding CC, Walford RL, Effros RB. The accumulation of non-replicative, non-functional, senescent T cells with age is avoided in calorically restricted mice by an enhancement of T cell apoptosis. Mech Ageing Dev. 1997;93:25–33.
41. Harries LW, Hernandez D, Henley W, Wood AR, Holly AC, Bradley-Smith RM, et al. Human aging is characterized by focused changes in gene expression and deregulation of alternative splicing. Aging Cell. 2011;10:868–78.

42. van Riggelen J, Yetil A, Felsher DW. MYC as a regulator of ribosome biogenesis and protein synthesis. Nat Rev Cancer. 2010;10:301–9. doi:10.1038/nrc2819.

43. Hofmann JW, Zhao X, De Cecco M, Peterson AL, Pagliaroli L, Manivannan J, et al. Reduced expression of MYC increases longevity and enhances healthspan. Cell. 2015;160:477–88.

44. Reynolds LM, Taylor JR, Ding J, Lohman K, Johnson C, Siscovick D, et al. Age-related variations in the methylome associated with gene expression in human monocytes and T cells. Nat Commun. 2014;5:5366. doi:10.1038/ncomms6366.

45. Shah PP, Donahue G, Otte GL, Capell BC, Nelson DM, Cao K, et al. Lamin B1 depletion in senescent cells triggers large-scale changes in gene expression and the chromatin landscape. Genes Dev. 2013;27:1787–99.

46. Hedrick SM, Hess Michelini R, Doedens AL, Goldrath AW, Stone EL. FOXO transcription factors throughout T cell biology. Nat Rev Immunol. 2012;12:649–61. doi:10.1038/nri3278.

47. Partridge L, Brüning JC. Forkhead transcription factors and ageing. Oncogene. 2008;27:2351–63.

48. Hanna LA, Foreman RK, Tarasenko IA, Kessler DS, Labosky PA. Requirement for Foxd3 in maintaining pluripotent cells of the early mouse embryo. Genes Dev. 2002;16:2650–61.

49. Shi W, Oshlack A, Smyth GK. Optimizing the noise versus bias trade-off for Illumina whole genome expression BeadChips. Nucleic Acids Res. 2010;38:e204.

50. Smyth GK. Linear Models and Empirical Bayes Methods for Assessing Differential Expression in Microarray Experiments Linear Models and Empirical Bayes Methods for Assessing Differential Expression in Microarray Experiments. Stat Appl Genet Mol Biol. 2004;3:1–26.

51. Storey JD, Tibshirani R. Statistical significance for genomewide studies. Proc Natl Acad Sci U S A. 2003;100:9440–5. doi:10.1073/pnas.1530509100.

52. Huang DW, Lempicki RA, Sherman BT. Systematic and integrative analysis of large gene lists using DAVID bioinformatics resources. Nat Protoc. 2009;4:44–57.

53. Subramanian A, Tamayo P, Mootha VK, Mukherjee S, Ebert BL, Gillette MA, et al. Gene set enrichment analysis: a knowledge-based approach for interpreting genome-wide expression profiles. Proc Natl Acad Sci U S A. 2005;102:15545–50. doi:10.1073/pnas.0506580102.

54. Janky R, Verfaillie A, Imrichová H, van de Sande B, Standaert L, Christiaens V, et al. iRegulon: From a Gene List to a Gene Regulatory Network Using Large Motif and Track Collections. PLoS Comput Biol. 2014;10:e1003731.

55. Ho Sui SJ, Mortimer JR, Arenillas DJ, Brumm J, Walsh CJ, Kennedy BP, et al. oPOSSUM: Identification of over-represented transcription factor binding sites in co-expressed genes. Nucleic Acids Res. 2005;33:3154–64.

The insulin receptor substrate Chico regulates antibacterial immune function in *Drosophila*

Sarah McCormack[†], Shruti Yadav[†], Upasana Shokal, Eric Kenney, Dustin Cooper and Ioannis Eleftherianos[*]

Abstract

Background: Molecular and genetic studies in model organisms have recently revealed a dynamic interplay between immunity and ageing mechanisms. In the fruit fly *Drosophila melanogaster*, inhibition of the insulin/insulin-like growth factor signaling pathway prolongs lifespan, and mutations in the insulin receptor substrate Chico extend the survival of mutant flies against certain bacterial pathogens. Here we investigated the immune phenotypes, immune signaling activation and immune function of *chico* mutant adult flies against the virulent insect pathogen *Photorhabdus luminescens* as well as to non-pathogenic *Escherichia coli* bacteria.

Results: We found that *D. melanogaster chico* loss-of-function mutant flies were equally able to survive infection by *P. luminescens* or *E. coli* compared to their background controls, but they contained fewer numbers of bacterial cells at most time-points after the infection. Analysis of immune signaling pathway activation in flies infected with the pathogenic or the non-pathogenic bacteria showed reduced transcript levels of antimicrobial peptide genes in the *chico* mutants than in controls. Evaluation of immune function in infected flies revealed increased phenoloxidase activity and melanization response to *P. luminescens* and *E. coli* together with reduced phagocytosis of bacteria in the *chico* mutants. Changes in the antibacterial immune function in the *chico* mutants was not due to altered metabolic activity.

Conclusions: Our results indicate a novel role for *chico* in the regulation of the antibacterial immune function in *D. melanogaster*. Similar studies will further contribute to a better understanding of the interconnection between ageing and immunity and lead to the identification and characterization of the molecular host components that modulate both important biological processes.

Keywords: *Drosophila melanogaster*, Long-lived mutant, *Chico*, Ageing, Infection, Insect pathogen, *Photorhabdus*, Innate immunity

Background

Ageing involves a large number of complex changes in the physiology of animals. Most of these changes lead to general decline in the fitness of the animal, deterioration of many vital functions, and a subsequent exponential increase in mortality [1]. The constant threat posed by infectious microbes has made the host immune response an essential feature across phyla [2, 3]. The immune system plays a pivotal role in ageing, age-associated disorders and longevity determination. Earlier reports have also indicated that ageing is correlated with a decline in immune functions [4]. Immune deficiencies are associated with pathologies, many of which increase in frequency with age. Ageing individuals suffer increased mortality upon infection due to reduced capacity to activate immune mechanisms in response to microbial challenge [5].

Deterioration in immune function with age has been observed in both invertebrate and vertebrate organisms. Invertebrate model organisms are excellent systems for the study of complex biological processes. The common

* Correspondence: ioannise@gwu.edu
†Equal contributors
Insect Infection and Immunity Laboratory, Department of Biological Sciences, Institute for Biomedical Sciences, The George Washington University, 800 Science and Engineering Hall, 22nd Street NW, Washington, D.C. 20052, USA

fruit fly, *Drosophila melanogaster*, has emerged as the organism of choice to investigate the regulation of immunity and ageing signaling pathways that share extensive similarity to those of mammals [6–8]. In addition, *D. melanogaster* is devoid of an adaptive immune system, and thus it is an ideal model to elucidate pristine innate immune defenses [9]. The genetic tools and genomic information available in *D. melanogaster* allow the molecular and physiological dissection of the interaction between ageing and immunity [10].

The Insulin/Insulin-like Growth Factor Signaling pathway (IIS) is an evolutionary conserved pathway that regulates ageing [11]. Mutations in certain genes that decrease IIS signaling can significantly extend life span in diverse species including *D. melanogaster*. The effect of IIS on life span has been attributed to increased resistance to oxidative stress and increased activity of cellular detoxification pathways [12, 13]. Chico is the *D. melanogaster* homolog of vertebrate insulin receptor substrates that modulates IIS. Mutations in *chico* substantially affect cell growth and proliferation, but they have little effect on cell fate and differentiation and no effect on cell viability [14, 15]. Previous studies have shown increased survival of long-lived *D. melanogaster chico* mutant flies in response to bacterial infection [16]; however, enhanced survival ability was not due to significant upregulation of antimicrobial peptide (AMP) genes in the mutant flies.

Here we have expanded these studies by testing the immune response of *chico* loss-of-function mutant flies against pathogenic *Photorhabdus luminescens* and non-pathogenic *Escherichia coli* bacteria. *P. luminescens* are remarkable bacteria because they possess two contrasting lifestyles, mutualistic and pathogenic [17]. They live in mutualism with their nematode vector *Heterorhabditis bacteriophora*, however, when the nematode invades an insect host, the bacteria switch to a lethal insect pathogen. Previous research has shown that *P. luminescens* contains a large number of genes encoding toxins and virulence factors, as well as molecules that assist the bacteria in evading the insect host humoral and cellular immune response [18, 19].

In the present study, we have shown that *chico* mutants have increased resistance to bacterial infection, they differentially regulate AMP gene transcripts, they have increased phenoloxidase activity but lower phagocytic ability, and they show no changes in their metabolic function. Our findings strongly suggest that *chico* participates in the immune response of *D. melanogaster* against pathogenic and non-pathogenic bacteria.

Results

Survival of *chico* mutants is unaffected upon bacterial infection

We first investigated the survival response of *chico* mutants and their yellow white (yw) background control

flies to infection by harmless *E. coli* bacteria. We found no significant differences in survival between the *chico* flies and their background controls following injection of *E. coli* (log-rank test, $P > 0.05$; Fig. 1a). We also found that intrathoracical injection of *P. luminescens* pathogenic bacteria resulted in substantial mortality of the flies; however, again there were no significant differences in the survival ability between the infected *chico* mutants and yw control flies (log-rank test, $P > 0.05$; Fig. 1b). These results suggest that loss of chico in *D. melanogaster* does not alter the survival phenotype of the flies against infection by the specific pathogenic or non-pathogenic bacteria.

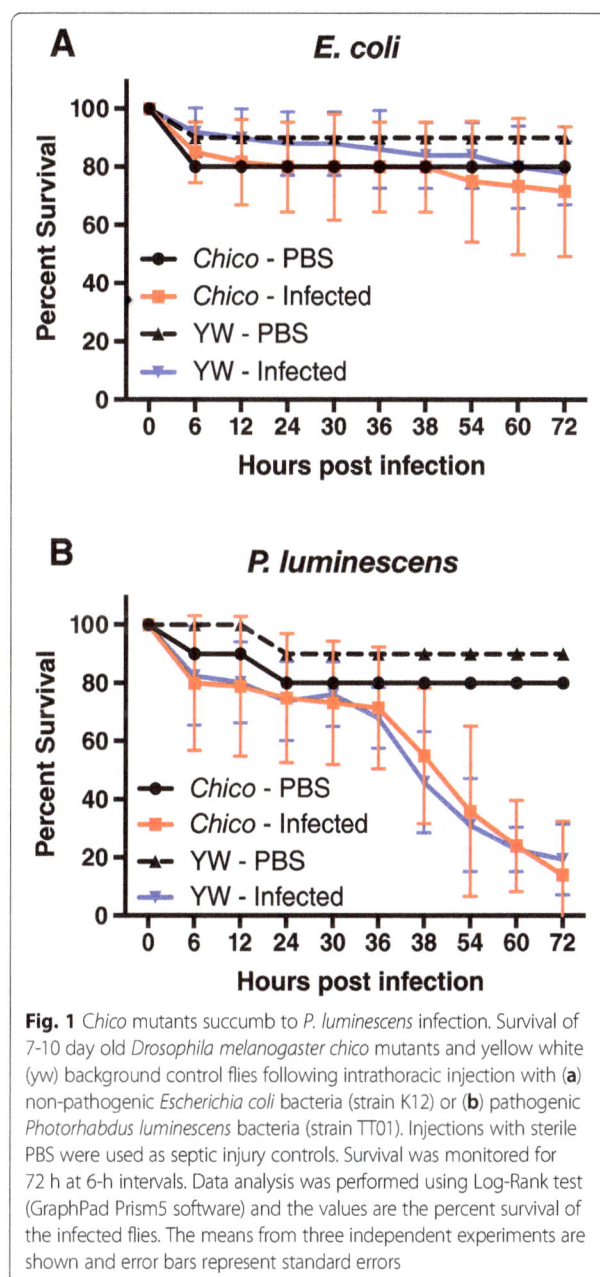

Fig. 1 *Chico* mutants succumb to *P. luminescens* infection. Survival of 7-10 day old *Drosophila melanogaster chico* mutants and yellow white (yw) background control flies following intrathoracic injection with (**a**) non-pathogenic *Escherichia coli* bacteria (strain K12) or (**b**) pathogenic *Photorhabdus luminescens* bacteria (strain TT01). Injections with sterile PBS were used as septic injury controls. Survival was monitored for 72 h at 6-h intervals. Data analysis was performed using Log-Rank test (GraphPad Prism5 software) and the values are the percent survival of the infected flies. The means from three independent experiments are shown and error bars represent standard errors

Chico mutants have increased resistance to bacterial infection

To investigate whether *chico* mutants have altered resistance or tolerance following bacterial infection [20], we injected *E. coli* or *P. luminescens* cells into adult flies and estimated bacterial load over time. We found significantly higher numbers of *E. coli* cells in yw flies compared to *chico* mutants at an early (3 h) and relatively middle (16 h) time-point post infection ($P < 0.0005$ and $P < 0.05$, respectively; Fig. 2a); however, numbers of *E. coli* cells in *chico* flies were significantly higher than in yw individuals at a later (30 h) time-point ($P < 0.0005$; Fig. 2a). These results suggest that *chico* flies have increased resistance to *E. coli* at 3 and 16 h post infection, but decreased resistance to infection by these bacteria at 30 h post infection. For infections with the pathogen *P. luminescens*, we consistently found that yw flies contained significantly higher pathogen titers than *chico* mutant flies for each time-point tested in our experiments ($P < 0.05$; Fig. 2b). These results suggest that *chico* mutants have increased resistance to infection with the pathogen *P. luminescens*. Overall, these results indicate that *chico* can control resistance to pathogenic and non-pathogenic bacterial infections in *D. melanogaster*.

Chico mutants have decreased transcript levels of AMP genes

To examine whether activation of immune deficiency (Imd) and Toll signaling is altered in *chico* mutants following infection with pathogenic or non-pathogenic bacteria [21], we estimated the transcript levels of AMP encoding genes in *D. melanogaster* flies injected by either *P. luminescens* or *E. coli* (Fig. 3). We found that *Diptericin* transcripts were significantly higher in yw than in *chico* flies at 3 h post infection with *E. coli* ($P < 0.01$; Fig. 3a), and there were no significant changes thereafter ($P > 0.05$; Fig. 3a). Infection with *P. luminescens* significantly upregulated *Diptericin* transcript levels in yw flies compared to *chico* mutants at 48 h post infection ($P < 0.001$; Fig. 3b), and there were no other significant changes at 3 and 24 h post infection with the pathogen ($P > 0.05$; Fig. 3b). Similarly, there were significantly higher mRNA levels of *Cecropin-A1* in yw controls than in *chico* mutants at 3 h post infection with *E. coli* ($P < 0.01$; Fig. 3c) and at 48 h post infection with *P. luminescens* bacteria ($P < 0.0001$; Fig. 3d), and no other significant changes in *Cecropin-A1* transcripts were observed for the rest of the time-points ($P > 0.05$; Fig. 3c and d). *Drosomycin* transcripts were significantly increased in yw compared to *chico* flies at 24 h after infection with *E. coli* or *P. luminescens* ($P < 0.01$; Fig. 3e and $P < 0.05$; Fig. 3f); however, *Drosomycin* transcripts were significantly higher in *Chico* mutants than in control individuals ($P < 0.05$; Fig. 3e). No significant changes

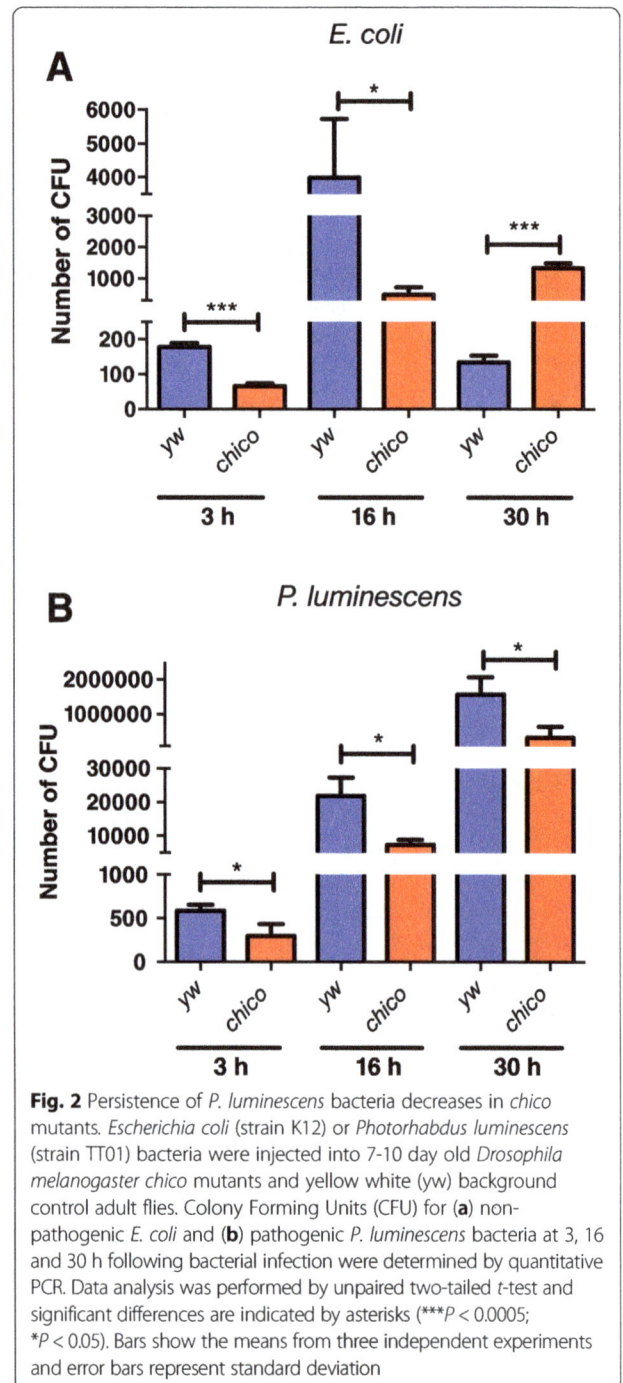

Fig. 2 Persistence of *P. luminescens* bacteria decreases in *chico* mutants. *Escherichia coli* (strain K12) or *Photorhabdus luminescens* (strain TT01) bacteria were injected into 7-10 day old *Drosophila melanogaster chico* mutants and yellow white (yw) background control adult flies. Colony Forming Units (CFU) for (**a**) non-pathogenic *E. coli* and (**b**) pathogenic *P. luminescens* bacteria at 3, 16 and 30 h following bacterial infection were determined by quantitative PCR. Data analysis was performed by unpaired two-tailed *t*-test and significant differences are indicated by asterisks (***P < 0.0005; *P < 0.05). Bars show the means from three independent experiments and error bars represent standard deviation

in *Drosomycin* transcript levels between mutants and controls were found at any time-point after infection with these bacteria ($P > 0.05$; Fig. 3e and f). These results imply that Chico can regulate the transcriptional activation of the nuclear factor kappaB (NF-κB) immune signaling pathways in *D. melanogaster* in response to infection by certain pathogenic and non-pathogenic bacteria.

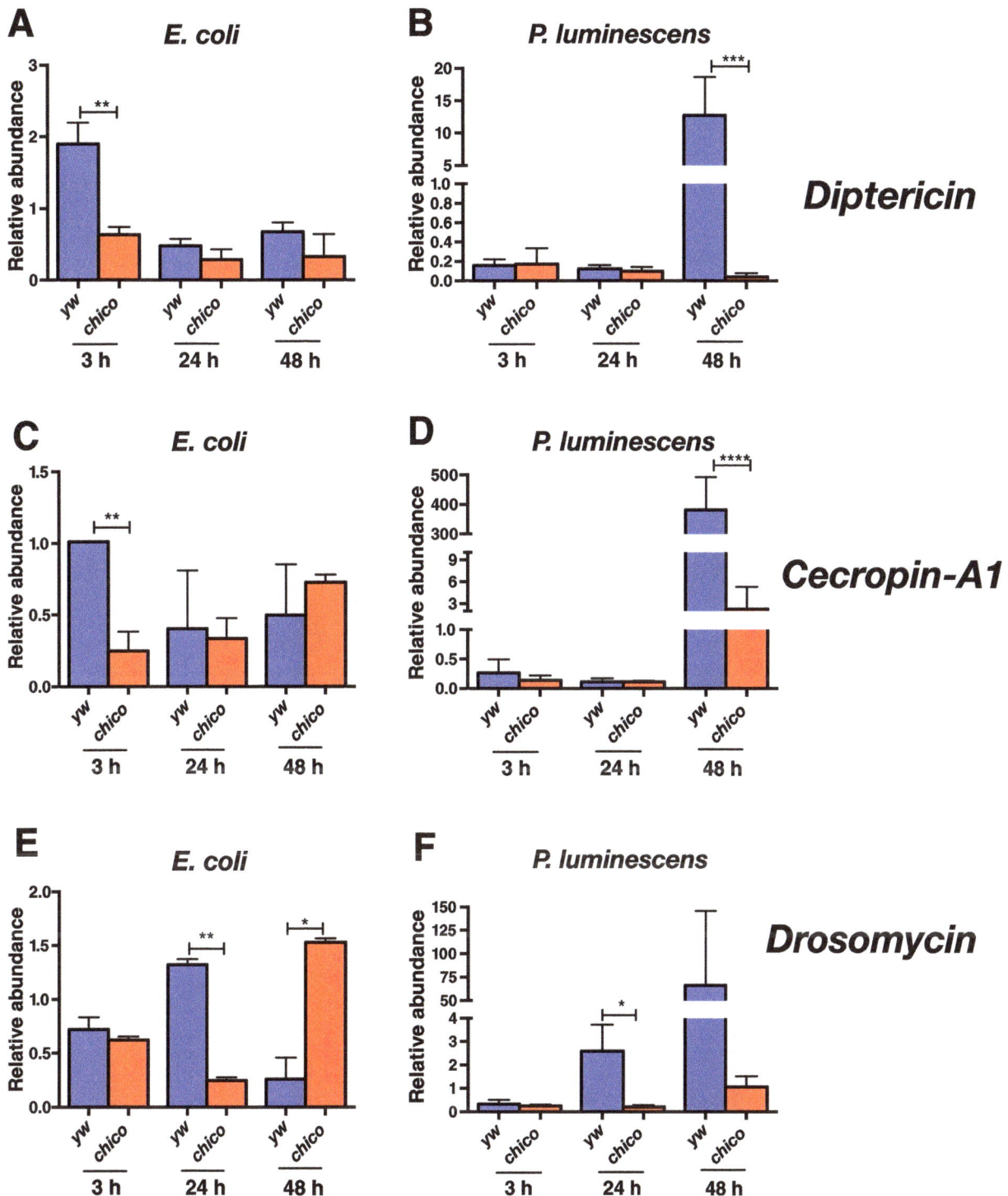

Fig. 3 Transcript levels of antimicrobial peptide encoding genes are differentially regulated in *chico* mutants following bacterial infection. Gene transcript levels for (**a**, **b**) *Diptericin*, (**c**, **d**) *Cecropin-A1*, and (**e**, **f**) *Drosomycin* in 7-10 day old *Drosophila melanogaster chico* mutants and yellow white (yw) background control flies at 3, 24 and 48 h after infection with non-pathogenic *Escherichia coli* (strain K12) or pathogenic *Photorhabdus luminescens* (strain TT01) bacteria. Gene transcript levels are shown as relative abundance of transcripts normalized to gene *RpL32* and expressed as a ratio compared to flies injected with sterile PBS (negative control). Values represent the means from three biological replicates and error bars represent standard deviations. ****P < 0.0001; ***P < 0.001; **P < 0.01; *P < 0.05 (one way analysis of variance with a Tukey *post hoc* test, GraphPad Prism5 software)

Chico mutants have increased melanization and phenoloxidase activity

The in vivo melanization response of yw control and *chico* mutant flies was examined superficially by visually inspecting the wound site 3 h after injection of bacteria or phosphate buffered saline (PBS, septic injury control). The darkness of the wound is associated with relative melanization activity and therefore phenoloxidase activity, with a darker spot indicating a higher degree of melanization. We found that melanization of the wound site following injection with bacteria or PBS was more intense in the *chico* flies compared to background controls (Fig. 4a). The degree of phenoloxidase activity in response to infection or wounding was assessed in *chico* mutants and yw flies by collecting hemolymph 3 h after infection and measuring the capacity of this extract for the oxidation of L-Dopa, which results in a color change that is quantifiable by optical density (OD) [22].

Injection with *E. coli, P. luminescens* bacteria, or PBS resulted in significantly higher phenoloxidase activity in *chico* mutants as compared to yw background flies for all three treatments ($P < 0.05$; Fig. 4b). Together, these results demonstrate a consistently higher level of phenoloxidase activity in *chico* mutant flies as compared to their yw background controls, which suggests that *chico* can act as regulator of the phenoloxidase antibacterial immune response in *D. melanogaster*.

Chico mutants have decreased phagocytosis ability

To evaluate whether absence of *chico* leads to changes in the phagocytic ability of *D. melanogaster* flies, *chico* mutants as well as background control flies were injected with inactivated unopsonized fluorogenic pHrodo *E. coli* particles. These particles are labeled with a pH sensitive dye that fluoresces in acidic environment. Thus, when pHrodo-labeled bacteria are phagocytosed by the

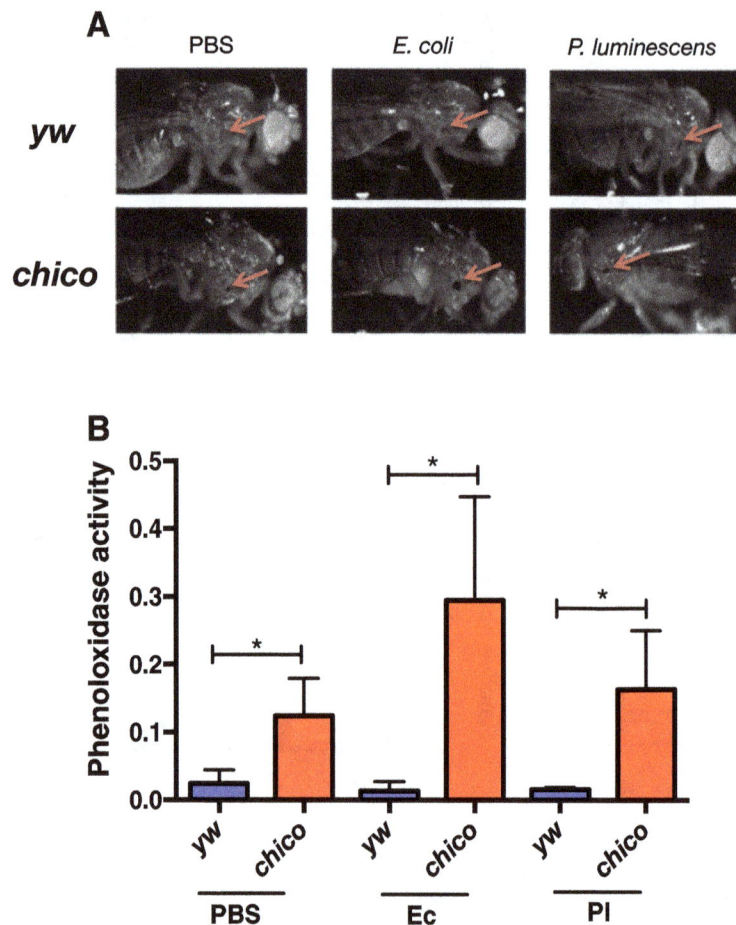

Fig. 4 Melanization and phenoloxidase activity are elevated in *chico* mutants. **a** Melanization of the wound site is shown at 40x magnification 3 h after injection with non-pathogenic *Escherichia coli* (strain K12), pathogenic *Photorhabdus luminescens* (strain TT01) bacteria, or sterile PBS in 7-10 day old *Drosophila melanogaster chico* mutants and yellow white (yw) background control flies. **b** Phenoloxidase activity in the hemolymph plasma of *chico* mutant and yw control flies injected with PBS, *E. coli* (Ec), or *P. luminescens* (Pl) as measured by the optical density at 492 nm after incubation with L-Dopa. Values are shown as the mean of three independent experiments with error bars representing standard deviations. *$P < 0.05$ (unpaired two-tailed *t*-test, GraphPad Prism5 software)

hemocytes and exposed to lysosomal acidic environment, the cells emit red fluorescence [23, 24]. Hence, phagocytosis around the periostial regions of the heart can be imaged through the dorsal surface of live flies. At 1 h post bacterial injection, we observed fewer fluorescent *E. coli* bioparticles in *chico* than in yw background control flies (Fig. 5a). Quantification of fluorescence confirmed that phagocytosis of *E. coli* particles in *chico* flies was significantly lower compared to control individuals ($P < 0.01$, Fig. 5b). These results suggest that inactivation of *chico* drastically affects phagocytosis of bacteria in *D. melanogaster*.

Chico mutants do not show changes in metabolic functions

To test whether the absence of *chico* affects the metabolic function in *D. melanogaster* adult flies in response to bacterial infection, *chico* mutants and their background

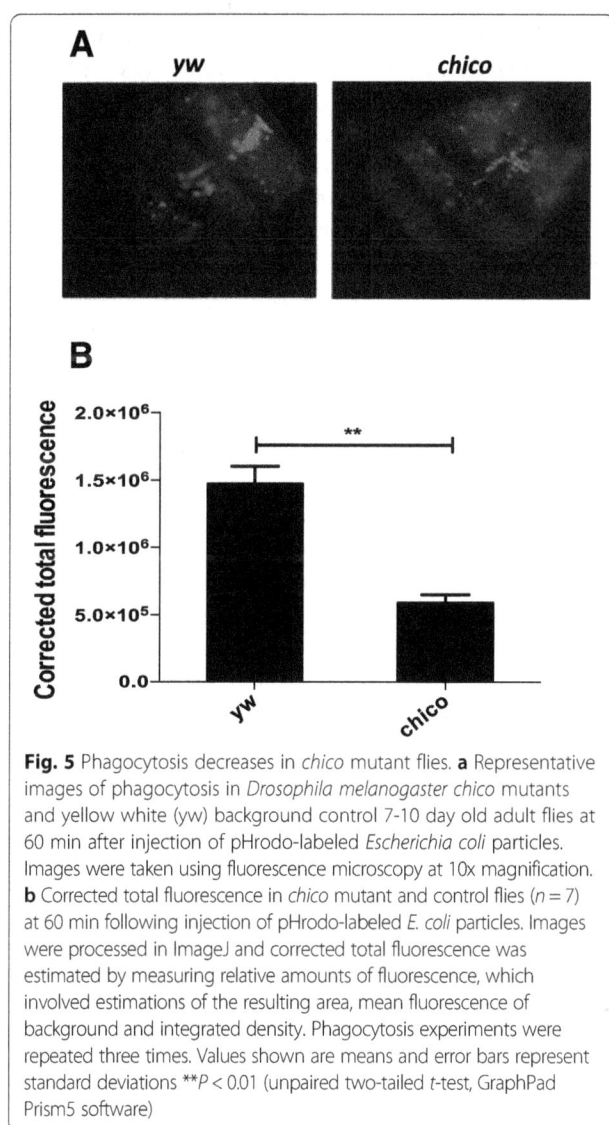

Fig. 5 Phagocytosis decreases in *chico* mutant flies. **a** Representative images of phagocytosis in *Drosophila melanogaster chico* mutants and yellow white (yw) background control 7-10 day old adult flies at 60 min after injection of pHrodo-labeled *Escherichia coli* particles. Images were taken using fluorescence microscopy at 10x magnification. **b** Corrected total fluorescence in *chico* mutant and control flies ($n = 7$) at 60 min following injection of pHrodo-labeled *E. coli* particles. Images were processed in ImageJ and corrected total fluorescence was estimated by measuring relative amounts of fluorescence, which involved estimations of the resulting area, mean fluorescence of background and integrated density. Phagocytosis experiments were repeated three times. Values shown are means and error bars represent standard deviations **$P < 0.01$ (unpaired two-tailed t-test, GraphPad Prism5 software)

control flies were injected with *E. coli*, *P. luminescens* or PBS. Total protein, triglyceride, glucose and trehalose concentrations were estimated at 3 and 18 h post-injection. We observed no significant differences in triglyceride (Fig. 6a), glucose (Fig. 6b) and trehalose (Fig. 6c) concentrations between uninfected *chico* flies and their background yw controls. Similarly, no major differences in triglyceride, glucose and trehalose amounts were found in flies previously infected with *E. coli* or *P. luminescens* bacteria (Fig. 6a-c). These results evidently demostrate that *chico* is not invloved in the control of metabolic processes in *D. melanogaster* in the absence or presence of infection with the specific bacteria.

Discussion

Here we have tested the immune response of *D. melanogaster* flies mutant for the insulin receptor substrate Chico against pathogenic and non-pathogenic bacteria. We have chosen to use a professional insect pathogen, the virulent bacterium *P. luminescens*, the genome of which contains a large number of genes coding for proteins with high insecticidal activity [25, 26]. As a direct comparison to the Gram-negative *P. luminescens*, we used a non-pathogenic strain of *E. coli* that is similar to *P. luminescens* at the genome level, but is not virulent to wild-type flies [27]. We have found that although *chico* mutants survive equally a challenge by *P. luminescens* or *E. coli* bacteria compared to controls, they contain less bacteria during the infection, they express AMP-encoding genes at low levels, they activate phenoloxidase and melanization responses at high levels, and they are less able to phagocytose bacterial bioparticles.

Current survival results demonstrate that suppression of insulin signaling in *D. melanogaster* by mutation of the insulin receptor substrate Chico does not affect the survival of the mutant flies upon bacterial infection. These findings are not in line with results from a previous study reporting nearly three-fold increased survival for *Chico* homozygous and heterozygous flies following infection with two pathogenic bacteria, the Gram-negative *Pseudomonas aeruginosa* and the Gram-positive *Enterococcus faecalis* [16]. One possibility that could explain the discrepancy between the survival results in the two studies could be the use of flies heterozygous and homozygous for the *Chico* mutation in the previous study, whereas in our study the *chico* flies have the *chico* hypomorphic but not null alleles [28]. A second possibility to take into account is that the previous study involved pathogenic bacteria that are not natural pathogens of insects [29], whereas the current study involves infection with the insect pathogenic bacterium *P. luminescens*. Therefore the responses of the *chico* mutant flies to pathogenic challenges may vary substantially. In addition, the previous study omitted an estimate of

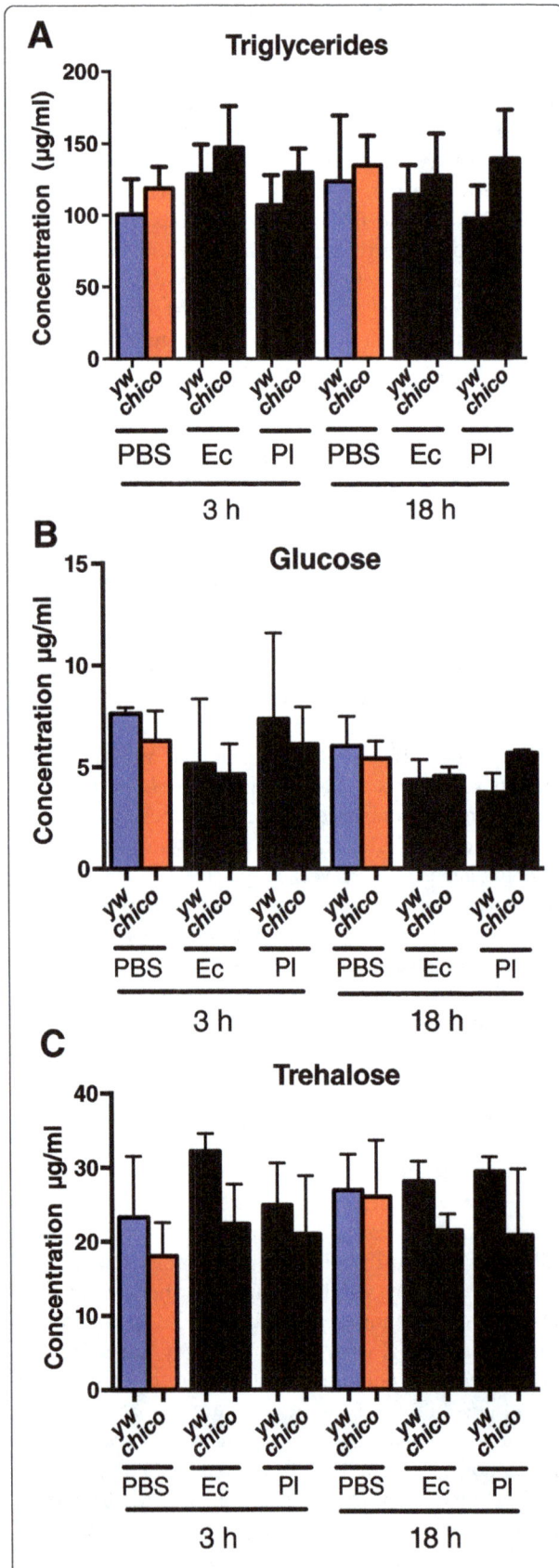

Fig. 6 Mutant flies for *chico* show no changes in metabolism upon infection with bacteria. **a** Triglyceride, (**b**) Glucose and (**c**) Trehalose concentrations in *Drosophila melanogaster chico* mutant and yellow white (yw) background control 7-10 day old adult flies at 3 and 18 h post-injection with PBS buffer, *Escherichia coli* (Ec, strain K12) or *Photorhabdus luminescens* (Pl, strain TT01) bacteria. Triglyceride, glucose and trehalose contents were estimated based on their respective standard curves. The experiment was repeated three times. Values shown are means and error bars represent standard deviations (one way analysis of variance with a Tukey *post hoc* test, GraphPad Prism5 software)

the numbers of bacterial cells in the *chico* mutants during the course of infection. Estimating the bacterial load in an infected host is important because we can distinguish between resistance (the ability of the host to control pathogen load) and tolerance (the ability of the host to withstand the damage and consequences at a given pathogen load) [30]. Here we have investigated for the first time bacterial load in the long-lived *chico* mutant flies. We have found that although both fly strains succumb similarly to infection by *P. luminescens* and they are both unaffected by infection with *E. coli*, the *chico* mutants contain fewer pathogenic or non-pathogenic bacteria than their background controls. Therefore we have concluded that inactivation of *chico* can restrain the growth of certain bacteria and confer immune resistance to *D. melanogaster*.

To understand the reduced growth of *P. luminescens* and *E. coli* in *chico* mutant flies, we first estimated the activation of the NF-κB signaling pathways Imd and Toll that regulate the expression of AMP genes in *D. melanogaster* [31, 32]. The expression of certain AMP genes in *D. melanogaster* is used as an indicator of the activation of the humoral immune response against microbial infections [33]. Therefore we analyzed the transcript levels of *Diptericin* and *Drosomycin* genes that are convenient read-outs for Imd and Toll pathway activation [34]. Although our experiments involved infections with two Gram-negative bacteria, we assessed *Drosomycin* gene transcript levels because this AMP can be reasonably stimulated from the Imd pathway in the systemic immune response of the fly [35]. We further tested *Cecropin-A1* gene transcripts because this AMP can act against different types of bacteria [36]. Here we were expecting to find increased transcriptional activation of AMP genes in *chico* infected mutants that would elucidate the decreased replication of bacteria in these flies. However, we have unexpectedly found no changes in AMP gene transcripts between *chico* mutants and controls infected with *E. coli* or *P. luminescens* or in some cases there were reduced mRNA levels of AMP genes in *chico* flies infected with either bacterial species. Interestingly, there was only one case in which *Drosomycin* transcript levels were higher in *chico* flies than in background controls following infection with the pathogen *P. luminescens*. We can conclude from these findings that inactivation of *chico* in *D. melanogaster* does not affect, or in some cases reduces, AMP transcript levels in response to *E. coli* or *P. luminescens* challenge, an outcome that does not affect the survival of the mutant flies, but it can limit the growth of these bacteria.

We then determined the melanization response and phenoloxidase activity, which overlap the humoral and cellular arms of the immune response in *D. melanogaster* and form rapid immune reactions upon invasion of foreign microbes into the hemolymph of the fly [37, 38]. A few hours after injection of the bacteria, we measured both qualitative differences in melanization at the site of injection as well as quantitative changes in phenoloxidase enzyme activity in the hemolymph of the infected flies. In all three treatments there were visibly larger size melanin spots at the site of injection on the cuticle of the *chico* flies compared to the background controls, and increased melanization was accompanied by elevated levels of phenoloxidase activity in the mutants. The fact that phenoloxidase activity levels are higher in *chico* mutants than in yw controls injected with PBS probably suggests that *chico* flies possess high amounts of endogenous enzyme in its active form, which can further increase upon bacterial infection. The molecular/biochemical basis to interpret the increased levels of phenoloxidase in *chico* mutants is currently unknown and it will form a topic for future investigation. We also noticed that phenoloxidase activity remains at low levels in control flies challenged with *P. luminescens*. This could be due to the ability of this pathogen to suppress phenoloxidase activity in *D. melanogaster*, as it was shown previously in other insects [39–41]. Interestingly, this is not the case in *P. luminescens* infected *chico* mutants where phenoloxidase activity remains at high levels. This could imply that the pathogen is unable to interfere with the activation of the prophenoloxidase cascade in the absence of *Chico*. We were not surprised to find low phenoloxidase activity in yw flies infected by *E. coli*; we have shown recently that this strain exhibits low phenoloxidase response compared to other reference laboratory fly strains [42].

We further estimated the *D. melanogaster* cellular response, which is mainly governed by the function of phagocytosis that involves the activity of circulating macrophage-like insect blood cells called plasmatocytes [43]. We avoided using stained *P. luminescens* bacteria in these experiments because this pathogen is able to suppress the insect cellular immune response by producing factors that inhibit phagocytosis; this forms a strategy for promoting pathogen persistence and replication in the host [44]. Although our expectation was that reduced bacterial persistence in the *chico* mutants would

be probably due to increased cellular immune activity in these flies, increased phagocytosis does not seem to account for the lower levels of viable cells since fewer phagocytic events were observed in the mutants.. The sharp decrease in the ability of *chico* mutants to engulf inactive *E. coli* particles implies that for a reason that is currently unkown, phagocytosis is disrupted in *chico* deficient *D. melanogaster* flies. This could be either the result of substantial reduction in the number of plasmatocytes present in the hemolymph of *chico* mutants or a decline in bacterial uptake by plasmatocyte cells, or a combination of these two possibilities. Alternatively, if the bacteria are eliminated by the phenoloxidase/melanization response, then there would be fewer cells available to be phagocytosed. Thus, the fewer phagocytic events in *chico* flies could reflect fewer available bacteria and may not mean that the mutants have a reduced phagocytic ability.

We have found increased resistance of *chico* mutants to *E. coli* and *P. luminescens* because these flies diminish the burden of bacteria during infection. Given the similarity in survival between the *chico* mutants and their background controls, the observed elevation in resistance could be possibly balanced by a reduction in tolerance that could in turn cause disease symptoms in *chico* flies. Therefore we examined the metabolic activity of *chico* infected and uninfected mutants by measuring the amount of glucose and trehalose produced in these flies. In addition, we tested triglyceride concentrations because lipid is the main component of insect fat body cells, and more than 90 % of stored lipid is triglyceride [45, 46]. Our results clearly demonstrate that *chico* flies do not exhibit metabolic changes upon infection with pathogenic *P. luminescens* or non-pathogenic *E. coli*, and the increased resistance of the mutants to infection by these bacteria is not accompanied by changes in energy stores.

Conclusions

In this study we have shown that the *D. melanogaster* long-lived *chico* mutant flies have increased resistance to infection by two bacteria; the pathogen *P. luminescens* and a non-pathogenic strain of *E. coli*. To understand the mechanism behind the increased resistance in *chico* mutant flies, we examined the three resistance mechanisms of the *D. melanogaster* innate immune response that are important for limiting microbial growth: AMP production, phenoloxidase activity/melanization, and phagocytosis [47, 48]. Although AMP gene transcripts and phagocytosis rates were unaffected or lower in *chico* flies than in controls, *chico* mutants showed elevated levels of melanization and phenoloxidase activity, which could potentially contribute to higher resistance against the two bacteria. These results reveal that *chico* plays a distinct regulatory role in the *D. melanogaster* immune response against certain bacterial infections. Taken together, the current study indicates that research in model systems, such as *D. melanogaster*, can provide critical evidence for the interaction between immunity and ageing mechanisms, and whether altering one process can affect the other. Furthermore, studies using long-lived *D. melanogaster* mutants in immunity research will significantly serve to identify key players involved in the regulation of the immune response in vertebrate animals, perhaps even in humans.

Methods

Fly and bacterial strains

Chico[KG00032] mutant strain and its background yw strain were used in all experiments. Flies were purchased from Blomington Stock Center and grown at 25 °C on standard diet, as previously described [49]. Mutant flies for *chico* were backcrossed into the yw background controls for over six generations. Equal number of young male and female 7-10 days old adult flies were used for infections with bacteria. All fly injections were perfromed during the morning hours.

The insect pathogenic bacterium *Photorhabdus luminescens* subsp. laumondii (strain TT01) and the nonpathogenic K12 strain of *Escherichia coli* were used for fly infections. Bacterial cultures were grown for 18 h at 30 °C on a rotary shaker at 210 rpm and then prepared for infections as described before [49].

Fly survival

Adult flies of the *chico* mutant and its background control were anesthetized briefly with carbon dioxide and then injected into the thorax with 18.4 nl containing approximately 100-300 colony-forming units (CFU) of *P. uminescens* or *E. coli* using a microinjector (Nanoject II, Drummond Scientific) and glass capillaries. Injection with 1x sterile PBS served as septic injury control. All flies were placed into newly prepared vials post-injection and kept in an incubator at 25 °C. Infected and uninfected flies were observed every 6 h for 72 h post injection and the number of dead individuals was recorded. Two replicates of 10 flies were used for each experimental condition and each experiment was repeated three times.

Bacterial load

Four adult flies from each strain were injected with *E. coli* or *P. luminescens* and the flies were subsequently frozen at 3, 16 and 30 h post infection. DNA was extracted using the DNeasy Blood and Tissue kit (Qiagen) following the manufacturer's instructions. DNA concentrations were measured using a NanoDrop. Each PCR reaction included 10 μl of EXPRESS SYBR® GreenER

with Premixed ROX (Invitrogen), 10 μM of each forward and reverse primer sets and 300 ng of each DNA sample. The primers used were Mcf-1 (*P. luminescens*), Forward: TTGGCGGGGTGGTAGTCG and Reverse: CAGTT CAGCTTCCTTCTCTAA; and 16S rRNA (*E. coli*), Forward: GGAAGAAGCTTGCTTCTTTGCTGAC and Reverse: AGCCCGGGGATTTCACATCTGACTTA. Cycling conditions were 50 °C for 2 min, 95 °C for 2 min, 40 cycles of 95 °C for 15 s and an annealing step of 61 °C for 15 s. All samples were run in technical duplicates and three independent experiments were carried out. Bacterial load (numbers of CFU) was estimated from the standard curves that were generated for *E. coli* and *P. luminescens*.

Gene transcript levels

Infected and PBS-injected *chico* mutant and yw background control flies were collected at 3, 24 and 48 h post infection and stored in a -80 °C freezer. Four flies were used for each experimental condition. Total RNA was extracted using the PrepEase RNA spin kit (Affymetrix USB) following the manufacturer's instructions. cDNA synthesis was carried out using a MultiScribe Reverse Transcriptase Kit (Applied Biosystems), random primers and 0.1 μg of RNA template as starting material in a total reaction volume of 20 μl following the manufacturer's protocol. Resulting cDNA samples were diluted 1:10 in nuclease-free water and 1 μl was used as template for quantitative RT-PCR experiments. These were performed using the EXPRESS SYBR® GreenER kit with Premixed ROX (Invitrogen) in twin.tec real-time PCR 96-well plates on a Mastercycler ep realplex[2] (Eppendorf). Primers were purchased from Eurofin MWG Operon. Primer sequences for *Diptericin* (CG12763) *Drosomycin* (CG10146), and *Cecropin-A1* (CG1365) have been given before [48]. The reactions were carried out in a total volume of 20 μl under the following conditions: 50 °C for 2 min, 95 °C for 2 min, 40 cycles of 95 °C for 15 s and an annealing step for 45 s. mRNA values were normalized to mRNA values of the control housekeeping gene *RpL32* (CG7939) [50]. Normalized data were used to quantify the relative level of a given mRNA as previously described [49]. Data are presented as the ratio between infected versus PBS injected flies (negative controls). Technical duplicates were run for each sample and set of primers and each experiment was replicated three times.

Phenoloxidase activity and melanization

Twenty flies were injected with bacteria or PBS as mentioned above and hemolymph samples were extracted 3 h after injection. First, the flies were placed on a 10 μM spin column (ThermoFisher Scientific) containing 30 μl of 2.5X Protease inhibitor (Sigma) and then they were covered with five 4 mm glass beads (VWR). Spin columns were centrifuged at 13,000 rpm for

20 min at 4 °C. Protein concentrations were adjusted using a Pierce™ BCA Protein assay kit (ThermoFisher Scientific) following the manufacturer's instructions. A total volume of 40 µl containing a mixture of 15 µg of protein (diluted in 2.5x protease inhibitor) with 5 mM Cacl₂ was added to 160 µl of L-DOPA solution (15 mM in phosphate buffer, pH 6.6). After 30 min of incubation in the dark at 29 °C, the OD at 492 nm was measured for each sample against a blank control. Each assay was carried out in biological duplicates and each experiment was repeated three times. Melanization spots on the thorax of the challenged flies were visualized at 3 h post injection using Nikon SMZ18 microscope with Zyla (ANDOR) 5.5 camera. Images were analyzed using Nikon Software Suite.

Phagocytosis estimation
Seven flies from each strain were injected with 50 nL of 1 mg/ml pHrodo labeled *E. coli* (Molecular Probes) and allowed to phagocytose at room temperature for 60 min. The flies were fixed ventrally on a glass slide using clear nail paint. Fluorescent images of the dorsal surface were obtained using Nikon ECLIPSE N*i* microscope (10x magnification) fitted with Zyla (ANDOR) 5.5 camera. The images were analyzed with ImageJ software. The relative amounts of fluorescence were measured by estimating the resulting area, mean fluorescence of background and integrated density. Corrected total fluorescence was determined using the following equation: Corrected total fluorescence (CTF) = Integrated Density (ID)– (Area * Mean fluorescence of background). The experiment was repeated three times on three different days.

Metabolic activity assays
Five adult flies from each strain were injected with *E. coli, P. luminsecens*, or 1x sterile PBS and samples were collected at 3 and 18 h post injection. Samples were processed using a previously published protocol [51]. Protein quantification was performed using the Pierce™ BCA Protein assay kit (ThermoFisher Scientific) following the manufacturer's instructions. The microtiter plate was covered and placed on a shaker for 30 s followed by incubation at 37 °C for 30 min. Absorbance was measured at 562 nm on a Synergy HT plate reader (BioTek). Protein concentrations of samples were calculated from the standard curve. For estimating metabolic functions in infected and PBS-injected flies, the protein concentrations of the samples were normalized. Standard curve for triglyceride estimation was made using the Glycerol Standard Solution (Sigma). Triglyceride content was measured at 37 °C and 520 nm using the Infinity™ Triglycerides Liquid Stable Reagent (ThermoFisher Scientific). Glucose standard curve was constructed using the

Glucose Standard Solution (Sigma) and the trehalose standard curve was made using Trehalose Dihydrate (Sigma). Free glucose in the samples was measured at 340 nm using the HK reagent (Sigma). Trehalose measurement was obtained by subtracting the absorbance of free glucose from samples that were digested with trehalase. Trehalose content was then calculated using the trehalose standard curve. All samples and standards were run in duplicates and three independent experiments were carried out.

Statistical analysis
Statistical analysis was performed using the GraphPad Prism5 software. Analysis of survival data was performed using Log-Rank test (Mantel-Cox). *P* values below 0.05 were considered statistically significant. For gene transcript levels and metabolic activity estimation, data were analyzed using a one-way analysis of variance (ANOVA) with a Tukey post hoc test for multiple comparisons. For bacterial load, phenoloxidase activity and phagocytosis estimation, samples were analyzed using two-tailed *t*-test.

Abbreviations
AMP: antimicrobial peptide; ANOVA: analysis of variance; CFU: colony forming units; CTF: corrected total fluorescence; ID: integrated density; IIS: insulin/insulin-like growth factor signaling pathway; Imd: immune deficiency; NF-κB: nuclear factor kappaB; OD: optical density; PBS: phosphate buffered saline; yw: yellow white.

Competing interests
The authors declare that they have no competing interests.

Authors' contributions
SMC, US, SY, EK and IE conceived and designed the experiments; SMC, US, SY, EK and DC carried out the experiments; SMC, US, SY, EK and IE analyzed the data; SMC, US, SY, EK and IE wrote the paper. All authors read and approved the final version of the manuscript.

Acknowledgements
This research was supported by a fund from the Columbian College of Arts and Sciences at GWU to IE, the GWU Luther Rice Fellowship and the Enosinian Program to SMC, and Harlan summer fellowships from the Department of Biological Sciences at GWU to SMC, US, SY and EK.

References
1. Campisi G, Chiappelli M, De Martinis M, Franco V, Ginaldi L, Guiglia R, et al. Pathophysiology of age-related diseases. Immun Ageing. 2009;6:12.
2. Brodsky IE, Medzhitov R. Targeting of immune signalling networks by bacterial pathogens. Nat Cell Biol. 2009;11:521–6.
3. Kumar H, Kawai T, Akira S. Pathogen recognition by the innate immune system. Int Rev Immunol. 2011;30:16–34.
4. Weiskopf D, Weinberger B, Grubeck-Loebenstein B. The aging of the immune system. Transpl Int. 2009;22:1041–50.
5. Dorshkind K, Montecino-Rodriguez E, Signer RA. The ageing immune system: is it ever too old to become young again? Nat Rev Immunol. 2009;9:57–62.
6. Zerofsky M, Harel E, Silverman N, Tatar M. Aging of the innate immune response in Drosophila melanogaster. Aging Cell. 2005;4:103–8.
7. Alper S. Model systems to the rescue: The relationship between aging and innate immunity. Commun Integr Biol. 2010;3:409–14.
8. Eleftherianos I, Castillo JC. Molecular mechanisms of aging and immune system regulation in Drosophila. Int J Mol Sci. 2012;13:9826–44.
9. Kounatidis I, Ligoxygakis P. Drosophila as a model system to unravel the layers of innate immunity to infection. Open Biol. 2012;2:120075.

10. Paaby AB, Schmidt PS. Dissecting the genetics of longevity in *Drosophila melanogaster*. Fly. 2009;3:29–38.

11. Barbieri M, Bonafè M, Franceschi C, Paolisso G. Insulin/IGF-I-signaling pathway: an evolutionarily conserved mechanism of longevity from yeast to humans. Am J Physiol Endocrinol Metab. 2003;285:E1064–71.

12. McElwee JJ, Schuster E, Blanc E, Piper MD, Thomas JH, Patel DS, et al. Evolutionary conservation of regulated longevity assurance mechanisms. Genome Biol. 2007;8:R132.

13. Piper MD, Selman C, McElwee JJ, Partridge L. Separating cause from effect: How does insulin/IGF signalling control lifespan in worms, flies and mice? J Intern Med. 2008;263:179–91.

14. Böhni R, Riesgo-Escovar J, Oldham S, Brogiolo W, Stocker H, Andruss BF, et al. Autonomous control of cell and organ size by CHICO, a *Drosophila* homolog of vertebrate IRS1-4. Cell. 1999;97:865–75.

15. Clancy DJ, Gems D, Harshman LG, Oldham S, Stocker H, Hafen E, Leevers SJ, Partridge L. Extension of life-span by loss of CHICO, a *Drosophila* insulin receptor substrate protein. Science. 2001;292:104–6.

16. Libert S, Chao Y, Zwiener J, Pletcher SD. Realized immune response is enhanced in long-lived puc and chico mutants but is unaffected by dietary restriction. Mol Immunol. 2008;45:810–7.

17. Waterfield NR, Ciche T, Clarke D. *Photorhabdus* and a host of hosts. Annu Rev Microbiol. 2009;63:557–74.

18. Rodou A, Ankrah DO, Stathopoulos C. Toxins and secretion systems of *Photorhabdus luminescens*. Toxins. 2010;2:1250–64.

19. Eleftherianos I, ffrench-Constant RH, Clarke DJ, Dowling AJ, Reynolds SE. Dissecting the immune response to the entomopathogen *Photorhabdus*. Trends Microbiol. 2010;18:552–60.

20. Medzhitov R, Schneider DS, Soares MP. Disease tolerance as a defense strategy. Science. 2012;335:936–41.

21. Tanji T, Hu X, Weber AN, Ip YT. Toll and IMD pathways synergistically activate an innate immune response in *Drosophila melanogaster*. Mol Cell Biol. 2007;27:4578–88.

22. Sorrentino RP, Small CN, Govind S. Quantitative analysis of phenol oxidase activity in insect hemolymph. Biotechniques. 2002;32:815–6,818,820,822–3.

23. Elrod-Erickson M, Mishra S, Schneider S. Interactions between the cellular and humoral immune responses in *Drosophila*. Curr Biol. 2000;10:781–4.

24. Miksa M, Komura H, Wu R, Shah KG, Wang P. A novel method to determine the engulfment of apoptotic cells by macrophages using pHrodo succinimidyl ester. J Immunol Methods. 2009;342(1-2):71–7.

25. ffrench-Constant R, Waterfield N, Daborn P, Joyce S, Bennett H, Au C, et al. *Photorhabdus*: towards a functional genomic analysis of a symbiont and pathogen. FEMS Microbiol Rev. 2003;26:433–56.

26. Wilkinson P, Waterfield NR, Crossman L, Corton C, Sanchez-Contreras M, Vlisidou I, et al. Comparative genomics of the emerging human pathogen *Photorhabdus asymbiotica* with the insect pathogen *Photorhabdus luminescens*. BMC Genomics. 2009;10:302.

27. Duchaud E, Rusniok C, Frangeul L, Buchrieser C, Givaudan A, Taourit S, et al. The genome sequence of the entomopathogenic bacterium *Photorhabdus luminescens*. Nat Biotechnol. 2003;21:1307–13.

28. Song W, Ren D, Li W, Jiang L, Cho KW, Huang P, et al. SH2B regulation of growth, metabolism, and longevity in both insects and mammals. Cell Metab. 2010;11:427–37.

29. Neyen C, Bretscher A, Binggeli O, Lemaitre B. Methods to study *Drosophila* immunity. Methods. 2014;68:116–28.

30. Schneider D, Ayers J. Two ways to survive infection: what resistance and tolerance can teach us about treating infectious diseases. Nat Rev Immunol. 2008;8:889–95.

31. Kleino A, Silverman N. The *Drosophila* IMD pathway in the activation of the humoral immune response. Dev Comp Immunol. 2014;42:25–35.

32. Lindsay S, Wasserman S. Conventional and non-conventional *Drosophila* Toll signaling. Dev Comp Immunol. 2014;42:16–24.

33. Ferrandon D, Imler J, Hetru C, Hoffmann J. The *Drosophila* systemic immune response: sensing and signalling during bacterial and fungal infections. Nat Rev Immunol. 2007;7:862–74.

34. Lemaitre B, Hoffmann J. The host defense of *Drosophila melanogaster*. Annu Rev Immunol. 2007;25:697–743.

35. Leulier F, Rodriguez A, Khush RS, Abrams JM, Lemaitre B. The *Drosophila* caspase Dredd is required to resist gram-negative bacterial infection. EMBO Rep. 2000;1:353–8.

36. Kylsten P, Samakovlis C, Hultmark D. The cecropin locus in *Drosophila*; a compact gene cluster involved in the response to infection. EMBO J. 1990;9:217–24.

37. Tang H. Regulation and function of the melanization reaction in *Drosophila*. Fly. 2009;3:105–11.

38. Eleftherianos I, Revenis C. Role and importance of phenoloxidase in insect hemostasis. J Innate Immun. 2011;3:28–33.

39. Eleftherianos I, Boundy S, Joyce SA, Aslam S, Marshall JW, Cox RJ, et al. An antibiotic produced by an insect-pathogenic bacterium suppresses host defenses through phenoloxidase inhibition. Proc Natl Acad Sci U S A. 2007; 104:2419–24.

40. Eleftherianos I, Waterfield NR, Bone P, Boundy S, ffrench-Constant RH, Reynolds SE. A single locus from the entomopathogenic bacterium *Photorhabdus luminescens* inhibits activated Manduca sexta phenoloxidase. FEMS Microbiol Lett. 2009;293:170–6.

41. Crawford JM, Portmann C, Zhang X, Roeffaers MB, Clardy J. Small molecule perimeter defense in entomopathogenic bacteria. Proc Natl Acad Sci U S A. 2012;109:10821–6.

42. Eleftherianos I, More K, Spivack S, Paulin E, Khojandi A, Shukla S. Nitric oxide levels regulate the immune response of *Drosophila melanogaster* reference laboratory strains to bacterial infections. Infect Immun. 2014;82:4169–81.

43. Vlisidou I, Wood W. *Drosophila* blood cells and their role in immune responses. FEBS J. 2015;282:1368–82.

44. Gatsogiannis C, Lang AE, Meusch D, Pfaumann V, Hofnagel O, Benz R, et al. A syringe-like injection mechanism in *Photorhabdus luminescens* toxins. Nature. 2013;495:520–3.

45. Canavoso LE, Jouni ZE, Karnas KJ, Pennington JE, Wells MA. Fat metabolism in insects. Annu Rev Nutr. 2001;21:23–46.

46. Arrese EL, Soulages JL. Insect fat body: energy, metabolism, and regulation. Annu Rev Entomol. 2010;55:207–25.

47. Ayres JS, Schneider DS. The role of anorexia in resistance and tolerance to infections in *Drosophila*. PLoS Biol. 2009;7:e1000150.

48. Dionne MS, Schneider DS. Host-pathogen interactions in *Drosophila*. Dis Model Mech. 2008;1:67–8.

49. Castillo JC, Shokal U, Eleftherianos I. Immune gene transcription in *Drosophila* adult flies infected by entomopathogenic nematodes and their mutualistic bacteria. J Insect Physiol. 2013;59:179–85.

50. Rugjee KN, Roy Chaudhury S, Al-Jubran K, Ramanathan P, Matina T, Wen J, et al. Fluorescent protein tagging confirms the presence of ribosomal proteins at *Drosophila* polytene chromosomes. PeerJ. 2013;1:e15.

51. Tennessen JM, Barry WE, Cox J, Thummel CS. Methods for studying metabolism in *Drosophila*. Methods. 2014;68:105–15.

4

Frailty has a stronger association with inflammation than age in older veterans

P. Van Epps[1,2*], D. Oswald[2], P. A. Higgins[1,4], T. R. Hornick[1,3], H. Aung[1,2], R. E. Banks[1], B. M. Wilson[1], C. Burant[1,4], S. Gravenstein[3] and D. H. Canaday[1,2]

Abstract

Background: Upregulation of pro-inflammatory cytokines has not only been associated with increased morbidity and mortality in older adults but also has been linked to frailty. In the current study we aimed to compare the relative relationship of age and frailty on inflammation and thrombosis in older veterans.

Results: We analyzed 117 subjects (age range 62–95 years; median 81) divided into 3 cohorts: non-frail, pre-frail and frail based on the Fried phenotype of frailty. Serum inflammatory markers were determined using commercially available ELISA kits. Frail and pre-frail (PF) subjects had higher levels than non-frail (NF) subjects of IL-6 (NF vs. PF: $p = 0.002$; NF vs. F: $p < 0.001$), TNFR1 (NF vs. F: $p = 0.012$), TNFRII (NF vs. F: 0.002; NF vs. PF: $p = 0.005$) and inflammatory index: $= 0.333*\log(IL-6) + 0.666*\log(sTNFR1)$ (NF vs. F: $p = 0.009$; NF vs. PF: $p < 0.001$). Frailty status explained a greater percent of variability in markers of inflammation than age: IL-6 (12 % vs. 0.3 %), TNFR1 (5 % vs. 4 %), TNFR2 (11 % vs. 6 %), inflammatory index (16 % vs. 8 %). Aging was significantly associated with higher fibrinogen ($p = 0.04$) and D-dimer levels ($p = 0.01$) but only among NF subjects.

Conclusion: In conclusion, these data suggest that among older veterans, frailty status has a stronger association with inflammation and the inflammatory index than age does. Larger studies, in more diverse populations are needed to confirm these findings.

Keywords: Inflammatory index, Cytokines, Functional decline and coagulation

Background

The paradoxical phenomena of decline in immune function or immunosenescence and increased inflammation are well described in aging. Immune dysregulation in older adults results in imbalance between pro and anti-inflammatory cytokines and consequently a low-grade chronic inflammatory state [1, 2]. Upregulation of cytokines such as interleukin-1 (IL-1), interleukin-6 (IL-6) and tumor necrosis factor-α (TNF-α) that contribute to systemic inflammation have been independently associated with increased morbidity and mortality in older adults [3, 4]. It is now also well accepted that aging is associated with markers of activated coagulation, contributing to an overall pro-inflammatory state [5–7]. The

term "inflammaging" refers to this inflammatory state and its association with age-associated diseases [8].

Besides the increased risk of morbidity, chronic inflammation has also been linked to functional decline in older adults and has been theorized as a potential explanation for the biologic basis of frailty [9, 10]. In this study, frailty is defined according to Linda Fried's phenotype as a biologic syndrome of decreased reserve and decreased resistance to stressors that is a strong marker for poor health outcomes including falls, disability and death [11]. There is growing link between frailty and inflammation. Elevated serum levels of IL6, TNF-α, and C-reactive protein (CRP) have been linked with poor function and mobility status [9, 12]. Elevated levels of IL-6 have been associated with slower gait velocity and are predictive of gait speed decline in community-dwelling older adults [13]. Higher plasma IL-6 levels have also been seen in older adults with performance deficits in activities of daily living (ADLs) than those without any functional deficits [14]. Similarly, markers of coagulation

* Correspondence: puja.vanepps@va.gov
[1]Geriatric Research, Education, and Clinical Center, Louis Stokes Cleveland VA Medical Center, Cleveland, OH, USA
[2]Division of Infectious Disease, Case Western Reserve University, Cleveland, OH, USA
Full list of author information is available at the end of the article

and endothelial dysfunction have been linked to frailty and associated with poorer outcomes. D-dimer and other markers of activated coagulation have been associated with limitation in a wide variety of functional domains, including independent activities of daily living [15, 16]. Frail and pre-frail subjects from the Cardiovascular Health Study had significantly higher levels of fibrinogen, factor VIII, and D-dimer compared with the non-frail group [17]. Frail adults are also at increased risk of venous thromboembolism when compared with non-frail persons of the same age [18]. Despite the mounting evidence for role of inflammation and coagulation in aging and frailty, measurements of inflammatory markers have not yet been incorporated into standard clinical practice, partly because a "gold standard" to reliably predict incident adverse outcomes in older adults is needed. More recently, inflammatory index, an additive index of serum IL-6 and soluble TNF-α receptor −1 (TNFR1) has been shown not only to best capture age-associated chronic inflammation but also predict mortality in older adults [19]. There are limited data regarding the inflammatory index in the context of frailty. For that matter, data on the relative association of age and frailty on inflammation and coagulation in older adults is also lacking. In the present study, we examined how age and frailty are related to an expanded set of inflammatory and coagulation markers.

Methods

Study subjects

We enrolled 117 veteran subjects, 60 years of age or older (age range 62–95 years; median 81), receiving care at the Louis Stokes Cleveland Veteran Affairs Medical Center (LSCVAMC) outpatient clinics for this study. We also enrolled 25 subjects, which included veteran and non-veteran subjects, younger than 60 (age range 22–54, median 39). Subjects receiving immunosuppressive medications or with immunosuppressive conditions including HIV, cancer undergoing chemotherapy, severe anemia were excluded from the study. Each subject underwent a blood draw for the measurements of inflammatory and coagulation markers. Informed consent was obtained from all participants. Human experimentation guidelines of the Department of Health and Human Services were followed in the conduct of this study. The study was reviewed and approved by Institutional Review Boards at the LSCVAMC and Case Western Reserve University.

Frailty measurement

The Fried's frailty assessment tool, a widely accepted and validated instrument of frailty measurement in older adults, was utilized for functional assessments [11]. Study staff administered the five components of Fried frailty assessment tool: weakness as assessed by grip strength (measured by Jamar dynamometer average of 3 trials with dominant hand), walking speed (15 feet, straight line, one way), unintended weight loss >= 10 pounds in the past year, self-reported exhaustion (two Likert-type questions from CES-D Depression Scale [20]), and physical activity based on the Minnesota Leisure Time activity questionnaire [21]. Grip strength was stratified by sex and body mass index, walking speed was stratified by sex and height and physical activity score was stratified by sex as suggested by Fried and colleagues. Subjects were assigned to the non-frail (NF) category if for 0 criteria met, pre-frail (PF) for 1–2 criteria and frail (F) for 3 or more criteria met on the Fried frailty instrument.

Biomarker measurements

Serum and soluble inflammatory and coagulation markers were obtained using commercially available kits. Assays were performed according to the manufacture's protocols. The following markers were measured in blood: pro-inflammatory cytokines serum IL-6 (Human IL-6 Qunatikine HS Elisa Kit), serum IL-18 (Human IL-18/IL-1 F4 ELISA), soluble TNF-α receptor-1 (TNFR1) (Human sTNF RI/TNFRSF1A Quantikine ELISA Kit), and soluble TNF-α receptor-2 (TNFR2) (Human sTNF RII/TNFRSF1B Quantikine ELISA Kit), Interferon gamma-induced protein-10 (IP-10)(Human CXCL10/IP-10 Quantikine ELISA Kit), soluble CD14 (Human CD14 Quantikine ELISA Kit) (all R&D System, Minneapolis, MN, USA) and pro-inflammatory protein C-reactive protein (CRP) (EIA kit, Cayman Chemical Company, Ann Arbor, MI, USA), Serum Amyloid A (SAA) (ELISA, Assaypro, St. Charles, MO, USA) and were also measured. Inflammatory index is a calculated parameter: $0.333*\log$ (IL-6) + $0.666*\log$ (sTNFR1). The following markers of thrombosis and coagulation were also measured: Plasminogen activator inhibitor-1 (PAI-1) (AssayMax Human PAI-1 ELISA kit, Assaypro, St. Charles, MO, USA), D-dimer (ELISA ZYMUTEST DDimer, ANIARA, West Chester, OH, USA) and Fibrinogen (immunoperoxidase assay, GenWay, San Diego, CA, USA).

Statistical analysis

Analysis was completed in SPSS; Graphpad Prism 6.0 and R 3.2.2 using the *ggplot2* packages were used to graphically represent the data. ANOVA was used to compare means of various biomarkers between frailty groups. In cases where the frailty F statistic suggested a significant overall affect, post hoc pairwise comparisons were performed with p value adjustment with Bonferroni or Tamhane, as determined by homogeneity of variance. Associations between age and each biomarker measured were examined using Spearman rank correlations. Log transformed values were used to represent correlations with frailty groups. The Spearman Rank correlation is robust to transformations and outliers. These correlations were also examined within groups of frailty. The explained variability in biomarkers, as measured by R-squared values, obtained from Pearson correlations for age and ANOVA for frailty group, was compared between age and frailty. The R-squared statistic measures the percent of variability in an outcome explained by one or more covariates. For a single continuous covariate, it can be calculated as the square of the Pearson correlation coefficient; for a single categorical variable, it can be calculated as the regression sum of squares due divided by the total sum of squares as summarized in typical ANOVA results. Thus, comparing the squared Pearson correlation coefficient to the ANOVA-based R-squared allows the percent of variability in an outcome explained by a categorical variable and a continuous variable to be identically measured [22]. For patients with available outpatient data from the two years prior to enrollment, we also obtained outpatient diagnosis codes from the electronic database and calculated the Charlson comorbidity index using a validated list of diagnosis codes [23]. The index was calculated, without the addition of points for age, for 103 subjects (mean = 2.75, range = 0 to 8). We performed regression analyses comparing the explained variability using comorbidity and age vs. comorbidity and frailty.

Results

The one hundred and seventeen subjects over age 60 were divided into 3 cohorts based on the Fried frailty measurement categories: non-frail ($N = 23$), pre-frail ($N = 50$) and frail ($N = 44$). The median age in NF group (68 years, range 62–90) was significantly lower than the PF (80 years; 62–92) and frail (82 years; 62–92) groups ($p < 0.005$ for both). As expected for an older veteran population, majority of the subjects were male (96 %). African Americans accounted for over half (54 %) of the study subjects.

Markers of inflammation and the inflammatory index among frailty groups

We compared all the markers of inflammation tested among frailty groups. Frail and pre-frail subjects had higher levels of markers incorporated into the Inflammatory Index as well as a higher calculated Inflammatory Index levels (Fig. 1). Mean IL-6 levels among frail subjects were nearly three times those found in NF subjects (1.88 pg/mL vs. 5.09 pg/mL; $p < 0.001$) and nearly twice as high among PF subjects compared with NF subjects (1.88 vs. 3.56; $p = 0.002$) than non-frail subjects. Similarly TNFR1 levels were significantly higher among frail subjects compared with NF subjects (1577 pg/mL vs.

2624 pg/mL; $p = 0.012$). Inflammatory index levels were higher in both PF and frail groups compared with NF group (NF vs. PF: $p < 0.001$; NF vs. F: $p = 0.009$). An additional marker that was significantly elevated in both the PF and frail groups was TNFRII (NF vs. F: 0.002; NF vs. PF: $p = 0.005$; Fig. 2). The mean level of SAA was significantly higher in frail group compared with NF group (2.8 vs. 4.5; $p = 0.035$). Notably there were no differences in markers of inflammation detected between PF and frail subjects. We also did not find any significant differences among frailty groups between sCD14, IP10, CRP and IL-18 levels (Fig. 2).

Frailty explains the variability in markers of inflammation not age

When all the subjects were grouped together, using Spearman Rank correlations, age was positively associated with TNFR1 ($r = 0.22$; $p = 0.02$), TNFR2 ($r = 0.25$; $p = 0.02$) and the inflammatory index ($r = 0.28$, $p = 0.008$) but not IL-6 ($r = 0.05$; $p = 0.5$) (Fig. 3). No other markers tested correlated with age in the cohort of patients over the age of 60 years (data not shown). When correlations were tested within frailty status groups however, there were no statistically significant associations between age and markers of inflammation (data not shown). In order to determine whether frailty status or age had a greater association with markers of inflammation, the R^2 values from ANOVA were compared with R^2 from spearman rank correlations. Frailty status explained a greater percent of variability in markers of inflammation than age: IL-6 (12 % vs. 0.3 %), TNFR1 (5 % vs. 4 %), TNFR2 (11 % vs. 6 %), inflammatory index (16 % vs. 8 %). We did not find any significant interactions between age and frailty among the markers of inflammation and coagulation tested. For the subset of patients for which we had data available to calculate Charlson comorbidity index, we performed regression analyses controlling for comorbidity. After controlling for comorbidity, frailty explained more of the variability compared with age in IL-6 levels (12 % vs. 1.5 %), inflammatory index (18 % vs. 15 %), CRP (8 % vs. 3 %), SAA (12 % vs. 1 %) sCD14 (8 % vs. 7 %). On the other hand, after controlling for comorbidity, age was slightly better at explaining variability in TNFR1 (18 % vs. 12 %) and TNFR2 (18 % vs. 16 %). We also examined relationship between CMV seropositivity and various inflammatory markers, however the vast majority of our subjects were CMV+ (76 %) and we did not detect such a relationship (data not shown).

Coagulation markers, frailty and age

Fibrinogen, PAI-1 and D-dimer levels were not significantly different among frailty groups. Age was positively associated with both fibrinogen ($r = 0.21$; $p = 0.04$) and

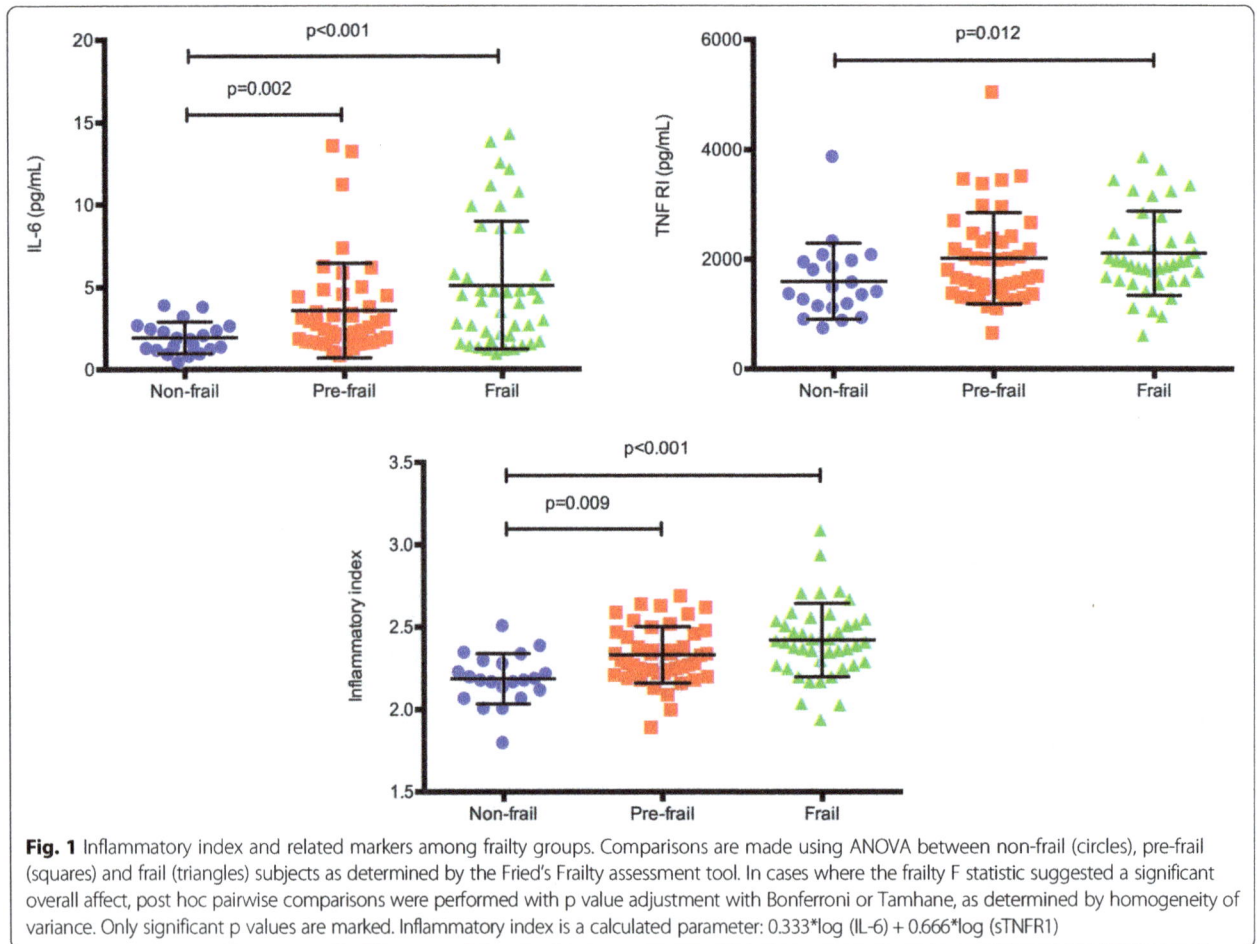

Fig. 1 Inflammatory index and related markers among frailty groups. Comparisons are made using ANOVA between non-frail (circles), pre-frail (squares) and frail (triangles) subjects as determined by the Fried's Frailty assessment tool. In cases where the frailty F statistic suggested a significant overall affect, post hoc pairwise comparisons were performed with p value adjustment with Bonferroni or Tamhane, as determined by homogeneity of variance. Only significant p values are marked. Inflammatory index is a calculated parameter: 0.333*log (IL-6) + 0.666*log (sTNFR1)

D-dimer ($r = 0.27$; $p = 0.01$) (data not shown). However, within frailty status groups, the only statistically significant associations between age and coagulation markers were seen in the NF group. Both D-dimer ($r = 0.7$, $p = 0.001$) and Fibrinogen ($r = 0.54$; $p = 0.02$) were strongly positively associated with age in this group (Fig. 4). Overall, age explained a greater percent of variability in fibrinogen (4.4 % vs. 3.9 %) and D-dimer (7 % vs. 4 %) than frailty status. After controlling for comorbidities using Charlson score in a regression analysis, age explained more variability in both D-dimer (11 % vs. 2 %) and fibrinogen (7 % vs. 6 %).

Discussion

In the present study we sought to determine the relative effect of age compared with frailty on markers of inflammation and coagulation in older adults. We observed significant elevations in pro-inflammatory cytokines as well as the inflammatory index among older adults who were pre-frail or frail. While age was associated with some of the markers studied, in particular the inflammatory index, these associations were not present within frailty groups. Additionally we also observed that the

variability in inflammatory markers was explained to a much greater extent by frailty status than age. Coagulation markers fibrinogen and D-dimer, on the other hand, were not significantly different among frailty groups but did correlate with age. These correlations persisted among those with intact functional status. Age appeared to explain the variability in coagulation markers more than frailty.

Similar to prior studies we found elevations in IL-6, SAA, TNFR1 and TNFR2 levels among those with functional decline [4, 12, 14, 24, 25]. A measure validated in older adults, the inflammatory index, which incorporates two of these markers, has recently been shown to be independently associated with frailty among aging HIV-infected and uninfected injection drug users [26]. We also found the inflammatory index scores to be significantly increased in frail and pre-frail older adults. Interestingly, unlike a previous report where the greatest differences between IL-6, TNF-α and CRP levels were seen between the pre-frail and frail adults [27], we did not see any significant differences between PF and frail subjects. In our cohort, pre-frail inflammatory profile

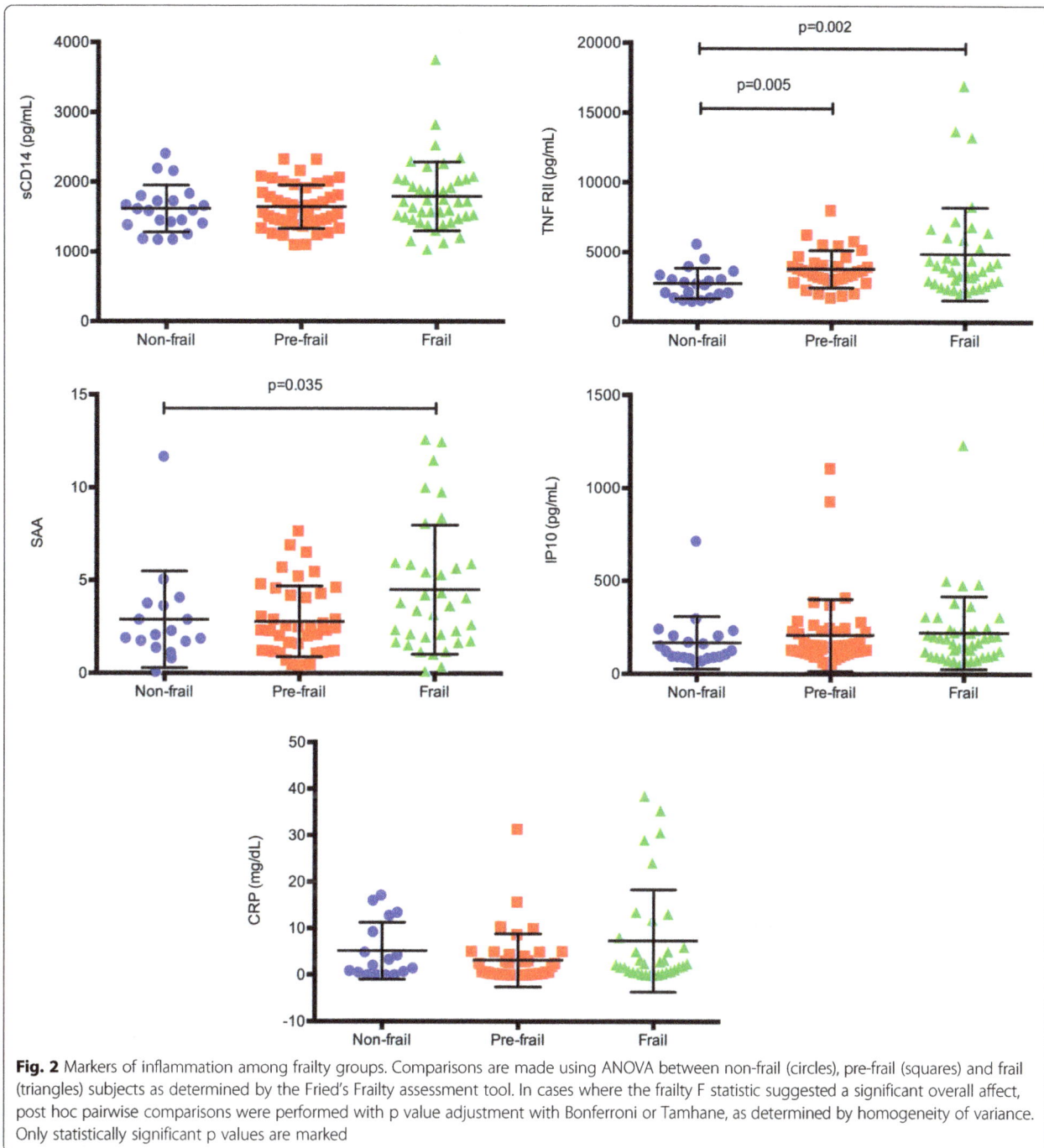

Fig. 2 Markers of inflammation among frailty groups. Comparisons are made using ANOVA between non-frail (circles), pre-frail (squares) and frail (triangles) subjects as determined by the Fried's Frailty assessment tool. In cases where the frailty F statistic suggested a significant overall affect, post hoc pairwise comparisons were performed with p value adjustment with Bonferroni or Tamhane, as determined by homogeneity of variance. Only statistically significant p values are marked

more closely resembled that of frail subjects than those that were still functionally intact. While both the PF and frail groups were significantly older than NF group, we showed that in fact age did not explain variations in inflammatory markers as much as frailty status. This finding may indicate that even before functional decline becomes clinically apparent, the pro-inflammatory phenotype has already been set in motion.

Age was associated with increased TNFR1 and TNFR2, but unlike previously cited studies we did not find IL-6 or CRP levels to be significantly associated with age in this cohort over 60 years of age. The data presented in this study focused on those over the age of 60. When subjects of all ages were included in the analysis, IL-6 did correlate with age. Aging was associated with increasing inflammatory index score in our study, as has previously been shown [19]. However, age was not associated with the inflammatory index, or any other markers, when frailty groups were examined separately. This finding was confirmed by comparing the percentage of variability in markers explained

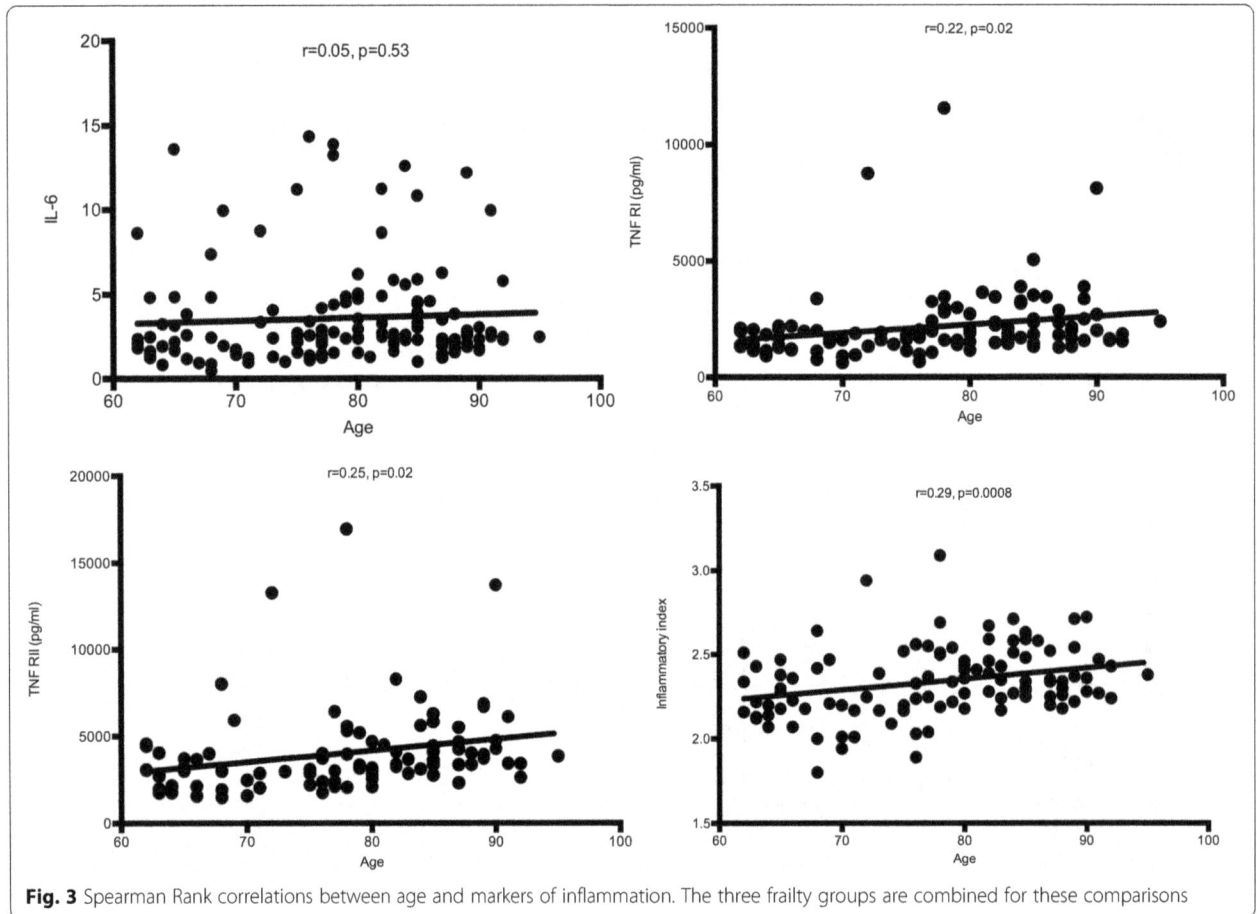

Fig. 3 Spearman Rank correlations between age and markers of inflammation. The three frailty groups are combined for these comparisons

by age vs. frailty. Frailty status had consistently greater association with inflammation than did age. Interestingly, this trend seemed to persist for most inflammatory markers, particularly IL-6, inflammatory index and CRP, even after controlling for comorbid conditions. This suggests that while chronic inflammation is a feature of aging looking over the entire age span, the inflammatory milieu is closely linked with frailty such that irrespective of chronologic age, frailty phenotype maybe a stronger predictor of chronic inflammation. However, as with other cross-sectional studies demonstrating association between frailty and inflammation, our study provides no insights into causality. It has been hypothesized that chronic inflammation may be the driving force behind functional decline and may form the biologic basis of age-associated conditions including frailty [28, 29]. Elevated levels of IL-6 have been linked to multiple age-associated conditions, such as atherosclerosis [30], dementia [31] and frailty [32], however causality and pathogenesis is yet to be proven. It is also plausible that increased levels of inflammatory cytokines maybe a compensatory mechanism in frailty and other age-associated conditions. Inflammatory response maybe triggered by chronic viral infections such as cytomegalovirus or other herpes viruses [33]. We were unable to link CMV chronic infection to inflammation due to very low numbers of seronegative subjects in our study. It is also possible that markers of inflammation are simply a byproduct of another causal mechanism of frailty such as excessive oxidative stress. Frailty in older adults has been associated with superoxide anion overproduction by nicotinamide adenine dinucleotide phosphate-oxidase (NADPH) oxidase and low-grade chronic inflammation [2]. Biomarkers of oxidative stress have also been associated with frailty in the Framingham Offspring Study, suggesting oxidative stress as the underlying mechanism contributing to frailty [34]. Whether targeted interventions at preventing functional decline may result in an improved pro and anti-inflammatory balance, regardless of age of the patient remains to be established.

We also tested the associations between frailty and age among markers of coagulation. In the present cohort there were no differences between D-dimer and fibrinogen levels among frailty groups. Prior studies have linked D-dimer and other markers of activated coagulation with limitation in functional abilities [4, 35]. It has been proposed that aging represents a pro-thrombotic state and that some of the markers of coagulation and thrombosis begin to rise early during the process of aging,

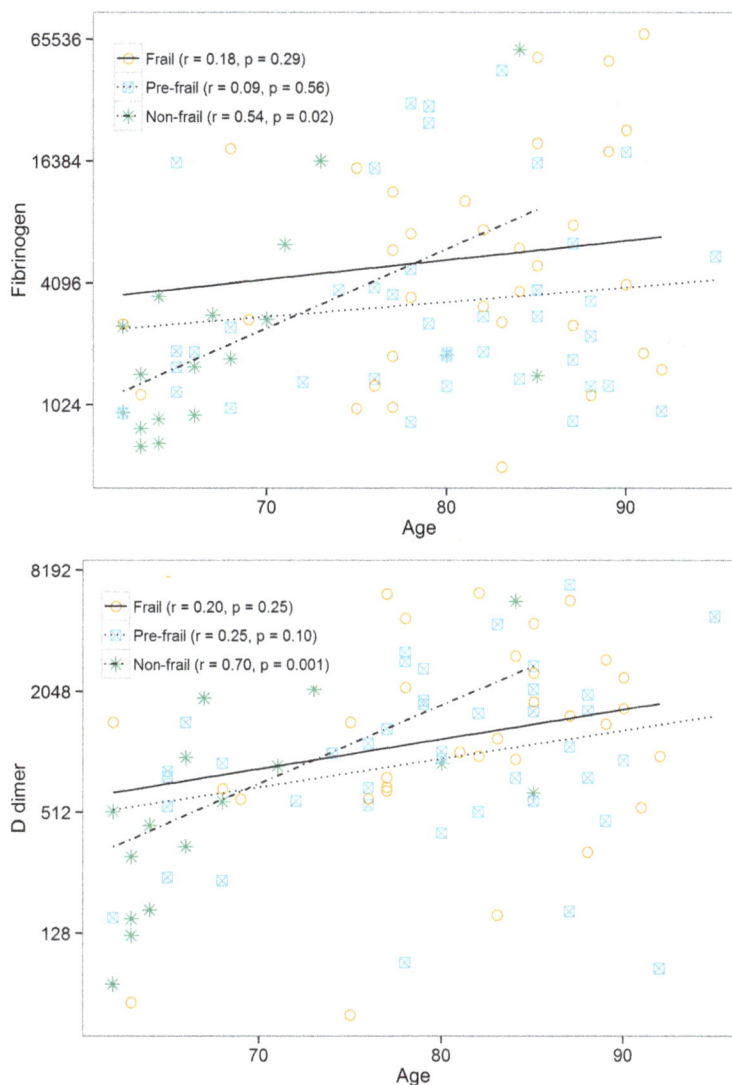

Fig. 4 Spearman Rank correlations between age and markers of coagulation within frailty groups. Corresponding r and p values are listed for each frailty group non-frail (star with dashed line), pre-frail (square with dotted line), frail (open circle with continuous line)

suggesting a potential usefulness as markers for frailty [3]. We did find aging to be not only associated with both these coagulation markers but also more strongly associated with a pro-thrombotic state than frailty status. This association was present even after controlling for comorbid conditions. Surprisingly, when age was examined within frailty groups, the association remained very strong but only among non-frail subjects. This suggests that while aging results in a pro-thrombotic state, its effect maybe less pronounced in those who already have evidence of functional decline.

This study not only provides further evidence of association between frailty and inflammation but also demonstrates that chronological age maybe less important than functional ability when it comes to chronic inflammation among older adults. Further studies are not only needed to establish the nature of this association but also to investigate the effects of interventions to prevent functional decline or modulate the inflammatory cytokines in an effort to prevent age-associated conditions.

Conclusion
In conclusion, among older adults, these data suggest that frailty may be more strongly related to inflammation and the inflammatory index than age. Coagulation factors, on the other hand appear to have a stronger association with chronological age than frailty. These findings warrant further investigation in larger, more diverse populations.

Abbreviations

ANOVA: Analysis of variance; CMV: Cytomegalovirus; CRP: C reactive protein; EIA: Enzyme immunoassay; ELISA: Enzyme-linked immunosorbent assay; IL-1: Interleukin-1; IL-6: Interleukin-6; IP-10: Interferon gamma-induced protein-10; LSCVAMC: Louis Stokes Cleveland Veteran Affairs Medical Center; NADPH: Nicotinamide adenine dinucleotide phosphate-oxidase; NF: Non-frail; PAI-1: Plasminogen activator inhibitor-1; PF: Pre-frail; SAA: Serum Amyloid A; TNFR1: Tumor necrosis factor-α receptor 1; TNFR2: Tumor necrosis factor-α receptor 2; TNF-α: Tumor necrosis factor-α

Acknowledgments

We thank all the US Veterans who participated in this study.

Funding

The work was supported by Sanofi Pasteur, VA Merit Review and National Institutes of Health (RO1 AI108972). None of the funding sources had any role in design of the study, collection, analysis and interpretation of data or writing of the manuscript. Final draft of the manuscript was shared with Sanofi Pasteur prior to submitting.

Authors' contributions

PV analyzed and interpreted the data as well as prepared the manuscript. DO performed the experiments, PA assisted in frailty assessments, TH assisted in subject recruitment and frailty assessments, HA prepared the peripheral blood mononuclear cells (PBMCs), RB was the study coordinator and responsible for subject recruitment and blood draws, BMW provided statistical analysis and graphical data representation as well as contributed to writing of the manuscript, CB performed majority of the statistical analysis and contributed to writing of the manuscript, SG designed the study and interpreted the results, DHC assisted in study design, data analysis, interpretation and contributed in writing the manuscript. All authors read and approved the final manuscript.

Competing interests

The authors declare that they have no competing interests.

Author details

[1]Geriatric Research, Education, and Clinical Center, Louis Stokes Cleveland VA Medical Center, Cleveland, OH, USA. [2]Division of Infectious Disease, Case Western Reserve University, Cleveland, OH, USA. [3]Division of Geriatrics, Department of Medicine, Case Western Reserve University, Cleveland, OH, USA. [4]School of Nursing, Case Western Reserve University, Cleveland, OH, USA.

References

1. Michaud M, Balardy L, Moulis G, Gaudin C, Peyrot C, Vellas B, Cesari M, Nourhashemi F. Proinflammatory cytokines, aging, and age-related diseases. J Am Med Dir Assoc. 2013;14:877–82.
2. Baptista G, Dupuy AM, Jaussent A, Durant R, Ventura E, Sauguet P, Picot MC, Jeandel C, Cristol JP. Low-grade chronic inflammation and superoxide anion production by NADPH oxidase are the main determinants of physical frailty in older adults. Free Radic Res. 2012;46:1108–14.
3. Schlaudecker J, Becker R. Inflammatory response and thrombosis in older individuals. Semin Thromb Hemost. 2014;40:669–74.
4. Cohen HJ, Harris T, Pieper CF. Coagulation and activation of inflammatory pathways in the development of functional decline and mortality in the elderly. Am J Med. 2003;114:180–7.
5. Deguchi K, Deguchi A, Wada H, Murashima S. Study of cardiovascular risk factors and hemostatic molecular markers in elderly persons. Semin Thromb Hemost. 2000;26:23–7.
6. Scarabin PY, Aillaud MF, Amouyel P, Evans A, Luc G, Ferrieres J, Arveiler D, Juhan-Vague I. Associations of fibrinogen, factor VII and PAI-1 with baseline findings among 10,500 male participants in a prospective study of myocardial infarction–the PRIME Study. Prospective Epidemiological Study of Myocardial Infarction. Thromb Haemost. 1998;80:749–56.
7. Pieper CF, Rao KM, Currie MS, Harris TB, Cohen HJ. Age, functional status, and racial differences in plasma D-dimer levels in community-dwelling elderly persons. J Gerontol A Biol Sci Med Sci. 2000;55:M649–657.
8. Franceschi C, Bonafe M, Valensin S, Olivieri F, De Luca M, Ottaviani E, De Benedictis G. Inflamm-aging. An evolutionary perspective on immunosenescence. Ann N Y Acad Sci. 2000;908:244–54.
9. Saum KU, Dieffenbach AK, Jansen EH, Schottker B, Holleczek B, Hauer K, Brenner H. Association between Oxidative Stress and Frailty in an Elderly German Population: Results from the ESTHER Cohort Study. Gerontology. 2015;61:407–15.
10. Kanapuru B, Ershler WB. Inflammation, coagulation, and the pathway to frailty. Am J Med. 2009;122:605–13.
11. Fried LP, Tangen CM, Walston J, Newman AB, Hirsch C, Gottdiener J, Seeman T, Tracy R, Kop WJ, Burke G, et al. Frailty in older adults: evidence for a phenotype. J Gerontol A Biol Sci Med Sci. 2001;56:M146–156.
12. Leng SX, Tian X, Matteini A, Li H, Hughes J, Jain A, Walston JD, Fedarko NS. IL-6-independent association of elevated serum neopterin levels with prevalent frailty in community-dwelling older adults. Age Ageing. 2011;40:475–81.
13. Verghese J, Holtzer R, Oh-Park M, Derby CA, Lipton RB, Wang C. Inflammatory markers and gait speed decline in older adults. J Gerontol A Biol Sci Med Sci. 2011;66:1083–9.
14. de Gonzalo-Calvo D, de Luxan-Delgado B, Rodriguez-Gonzalez S, Garcia-Macia M, Suarez FM, Solano JJ, Rodriguez-Colunga MJ, Coto-Montes A. Interleukin 6, soluble tumor necrosis factor receptor I and red blood cell distribution width as biological markers of functional dependence in an elderly population: a translational approach. Cytokine. 2012;58:193–8.
15. McDermott MM, Greenland P, Green D, Guralnik JM, Criqui MH, Liu K, Chan C, Pearce WH, Taylor L, Ridker PM, et al. D-dimer, inflammatory markers, and lower extremity functioning in patients with and without peripheral arterial disease. Circulation. 2003;107:3191–8.
16. McDermott MM, Liu K, Guralnik JM, Ferrucci L, Green D, Greenland P, Tian L, Criqui MH, Lo C, Rifai N, et al. Functional decline in patients with and without peripheral arterial disease: predictive value of annual changes in levels of C-reactive protein and D-dimer. J Gerontol A Biol Sci Med Sci. 2006;61:374–9.
17. Watson DJ, Rhodes T, Cai B, Guess HA. Lower risk of thromboembolic cardiovascular events with naproxen among patients with rheumatoid arthritis. Arch Intern Med. 2002;162:1105–10.
18. Folsom AR, Boland LL, Cushman M, Heckbert SR, Rosamond WD, Walston JD. Frailty and risk of venous thromboembolism in older adults. J Gerontol A Biol Sci Med Sci. 2007;62:79–82.
19. Varadhan R, Yao W, Matteini A, Beamer BA, Xue QL, Yang H, Manwani B, Reiner A, Jenny N, Parekh N, et al. Simple biologically informed inflammatory index of two serum cytokines predicts 10 year all-cause mortality in older adults. J Gerontol A Biol Sci Med Sci. 2014;69:165–73.
20. Orme JG, Reis J, Herz EJ. Factorial and discriminant validity of the Center for Epidemiological Studies Depression (CES-D) scale. J Clin Psychol. 1986;42:28–33.
21. Taylor HL, Jacobs Jr DR, Schucker B, Knudsen J, Leon AS, Debacker G. A questionnaire for the assessment of leisure time physical activities. J Chronic Dis. 1978;31:741–55.
22. Maindonald JH, Braun J. Data analysis and graphics using R : an example-based approach. 2nd ed. Cambridge; New York: Cambridge University Press; 2007.
23. Quan H, Sundararajan V, Halfon P, Fong A, Burnand B, Luthi JC, Saunders LD, Beck CA, Feasby TE, Ghali WA. Coding algorithms for defining comorbidities in ICD-9-CM and ICD-10 administrative data. Med Care. 2005;43:1130–9.

24. de Gonzalo-Calvo D, Fernandez-Garcia B, de Luxan-Delgado B, Rodriguez-Gonzalez S, Garcia-Macia M, Suarez FM, Solano JJ, Rodriguez-Colunga MJ, Coto-Montes A. Long-term training induces a healthy inflammatory and endocrine emergent biomarker profile in elderly men. Age (Dordr). 2012;34:761–71.

25. Ershler WB, Keller ET. Age-associated increased interleukin-6 gene expression, late-life diseases, and frailty. Annu Rev Med. 2000;51:245–70.

26. Piggott DA, Varadhan R, Mehta SH, Brown TT, Li H, Walston JD, Leng SX, Kirk GD. Frailty, Inflammation, and Mortality Among Persons Aging With HIV Infection and Injection Drug Use. J Gerontol A Biol Sci Med Sci. 2015;70:1542–7.

27. Hubbard RE, O'Mahony MS, Savva GM, Calver BL, Woodhouse KW. Inflammation and frailty measures in older people. J Cell Mol Med. 2009;13:3103–9.

28. Walston J. Frailty–the search for underlying causes. Sci Aging Knowledge Environ. 2004;2004:pe4.

29. Walston J, McBurnie MA, Newman A, Tracy RP, Kop WJ, Hirsch CH, Gottdiener J, Fried LP, Cardiovascular Health S. Frailty and activation of the inflammation and coagulation systems with and without clinical comorbidities: results from the Cardiovascular Health Study. Arch Intern Med. 2002;162:2333–41.

30. Hwang AC, Liu LK, Lee WJ, Chen LY, Peng LN, Lin MH, Chen LK. Association of Frailty and Cardiometabolic Risk Among Community-Dwelling Middle-Aged and Older People: Results from the I-Lan Longitudinal Aging Study. Rejuvenation Res. 2015;18:564–72.

31. Miwa K, Okazaki S, Sakaguchi M, Mochizuki H, Kitagawa K. Interleukin-6, interleukin-6 receptor gene variant, small-vessel disease and incident dementia. Eur J Neurol. 2016;23:656–63.

32. De Martinis M, Franceschi C, Monti D, Ginaldi L. Inflammation markers predicting frailty and mortality in the elderly. Exp Mol Pathol. 2006;80:219–27.

33. Mathei C, Vaes B, Wallemacq P, Degryse J. Associations between cytomegalovirus infection and functional impairment and frailty in the BELFRAIL Cohort. J Am Geriatr Soc. 2011;59:2201–8.

34. Liu CK, Lyass A, Larson MG, Massaro JM, Wang N, D'Agostino Sr RB, Benjamin EJ, Murabito JM. Biomarkers of oxidative stress are associated with frailty: the Framingham Offspring Study. Age (Dordr). 2016;38:1.

35. McDermott MM, Ferrucci L, Liu K, Criqui MH, Greenland P, Green D, Guralnik JM, Ridker PM, Taylor LM, Rifai N, et al. D-dimer and inflammatory markers as predictors of functional decline in men and women with and without peripheral arterial disease. J Am Geriatr Soc. 2005;53:1688–96.

The anti-ageing molecule sirt1 mediates beneficial effects of cardiac rehabilitation

Giusy Russomanno[1†], Graziamaria Corbi[2†], Valentina Manzo[1], Nicola Ferrara[3,4], Giuseppe Rengo[3,4], Annibale A. Puca[1,5], Salvatore Latte[6], Albino Carrizzo[7], Maria Consiglia Calabrese[1], Ramaroson Andriantsitohaina[8], Walter Filippelli[9], Carmine Vecchione[1,7], Amelia Filippelli[1*] and Valeria Conti[1]

Abstract

Background: An exercise-based Cardiac Rehabilitation Programme (CRP) is established as adjuvant therapy in heart failure (HF), nevertheless it is underutilized, especially in the elderly. While the functional and hemodynamic effects of CRP are well known, its underlying molecular mechanisms have not been fully clarified. The present study aims to evaluate the effects of a well-structured 4-week CRP in patients with stable HF from a molecular point of view.

Results: A prospective longitudinal observational study was conducted on patients consecutively admitted to cardiac rehabilitation. In fifty elderly HF patients with preserved ejection fraction (HFpEF), levels of sirtuin 1 (Sirt1) in peripheral blood mononuclear cells (PBMCs) and of its targets, the antioxidants catalase (Cat) and superoxide dismutase (SOD) in serum were measured before (Patients, P) and at the end of the CRP (Rehabilitated Patients, RP), showing a rise of their activities after rehabilitation.

Endothelial cells (ECs) were conditioned with serum from P and RP, and oxidative stress was induced using hydrogen peroxide. An increase of Sirt1 and Cat activity was detected in RP-conditioned ECs in both the absence and presence of oxidative stress, together with a decrease of senescence, an effect not observed during Sirt1 and Cat inhibition.

Conclusions: In addition to the improvement in functional and hemodynamic parameters, a supervised exercise-based CRP increases Sirt1 activity and stimulates a systemic antioxidant defence in elderly HFpEF patients. Moreover, CRP produces antioxidant and anti-senescent effects in human endothelial cells mediated, at least in part, by Sirt1 and its target Cat.

Keywords: Heart failure, Rehabilitation, Sirtuin, Catalase, Oxidative stress, Endothelium

Background

Despite recent advances in clinical/diagnostic tools and therapies, the incidence and prevalence of Heart Failure (HF) show a steady increase [1]. A cardiac rehabilitation programme (CRP) based on exercise training, has been recognized as a fundamental component in the continuum of care for patients with HF. Meta-analyses of randomized controlled trials on CRPs have demonstrated a significant reduction of all-cause mortality, with lower rates of re-infarction and cardiac mortality [2].

However, these studies included very few elderly or high-risk patients, and exercise is rarely viewed as a necessary prescription for these patients because they have more barriers to participation in exercise training [3].

In HF patients, exercise was shown to be associated with significant improvement in functional and hemodynamic parameters [4–7], nevertheless there are few data explaining the molecular mechanisms underlying exercise-based CRP.

It has been established both in humans and in animal models that exercise training can stimulate the natural antioxidant defences thereby contrasting reactive oxygen species (ROS) accumulation [8, 9].

The NAD^+-dependent deacetylase sirtuin 1 (Sirt1) is now recognized as a mediator of the response to

---

* Correspondence: afilippelli@unisa.it

[†]Equal contributors

[1]Department of Medicine, Surgery and Dentistry, University of Salerno, Via S. Allende 43, 84081 Baronissi, Italy

Full list of author information is available at the end of the article

oxidative stress and endothelial dysfunction, phenomena both correlated with endothelial cell pathophysiology and Cardiovascular Diseases (CVDs), including HF [10]. Evidence about the protective role of Sirt1 in vascular biology has indicated Sirt1 as a possible target in preventing CVDs and other diseases [11, 12]. Indeed, Sirt1 plays a crucial role in both cellular senescence and ageing, and it was recognized as modulator of the oxidative stress response by inducing the expression of antioxidant enzymes such as superoxide dismutase (SOD) and catalase (Cat) [13, 14]. Recently, Lu et al. [15] showed that in advanced HF, low Sirt1 expression in ageing might be a significant contributing factor in the downregulation of antioxidants and upregulation of oxidative stress and apoptosis. We previously showed that moderate exercise promoted Sirt1 activity in rats and induced increasing SOD and Cat expression. Notably, in aged sedentary rats there was lower levels of Cat comparing to young rats and exercise led to a complete recover of such antioxidant enzyme [16].

Cat, a molecular target of Sirt1, represents a primary safeguard of the antioxidant system [17], and recent studies have suggested that this enzyme might play an important role in the pathophysiology of HF [18, 19].

In humans, exercise training improves cardiovascular function and endothelial homeostasis, although the benefit achieved varies widely depending on the type and duration of exercise [20, 21].

In the present study, we aim at investigating the molecular changes possibly induced by a 4-week CRP on Sirt1 activity in peripheral blood mononuclear cells (PBMCs) and antioxidant status in serum of patients with stable HF. Moreover, we looked at changes induced by the conditioning of human endothelial cells, exposed or not to oxidative stress induced by H_2O_2, with serum isolated from patients before and at the end of the CRP.

Results

Heart failure elderly patient recruitment and characterisation

Fifty-three consecutive patients affected by HF were recruited from the Cardiac Rehabilitation Unit. All patients completed the CRP. As only three patients were women, they were excluded from the analysis. Therefore, the final study population consisted of 50 elderly male patients (mean age 68.6 ± 6.3 years). None of the patients had experienced a myocardial infarction (MI) in the 12 months preceding the study. All patients were in clinically stable condition, and classified as in NYHA II and III class with a preserved Ejection Fraction (EF) [10 patients with HF mid-range EF; 40 with HF preserved EF]. All definitions were based on the ESC and ACCF/AHA criteria, in which the term "stable" defines treated patients with symptoms

and signs that have remained generally unchanged for at least 1 month [22].

The clinical and demographic features of the study population are listed in Table 1. Information on comorbidities and concomitant medications were gathered from all patients. No racial/ethnic-based differences were present. At baseline, no differences in medical therapy were found, and no changes occurred during the study period.

Data are expressed as mean (SD) or number of subjects (%). BMI, Body Mass Index; SBP, Systolic Blood Pressure; DBP, Diastolic Blood Pressure; HR, Heart Rate; bpm, beat/minutes; CAD, Coronary Artery Disease; PTCA, Percutaneous Transluminal Coronary Angioplasty; CABG, Coronary Artery Bypass Graft; COPD, Chronic Obstructive Pulmonary Disease; ARBs, Angiotensin II Receptor Blockers.

Table 1 Study population characteristics and medication use

Age (y.o.), *mean (SD)*	68.6 (6.3)	Medications, *n (%)*	
Gender *(M/F)*	50/0	β-blockers	46 (92)
BMI (kg/m^2), *mean (SD)*	28.03 (3.17)	ACE-inhibitors	29 (58)
SBP (mmHg), *mean (SD)*	122 (6)	ARBs	9 (18)
DBP (mmHg), *mean (SD)*	80 (9)	Diuretics	8 (16)
HR (bpm), *mean (SD)*	84 (8)	Nitrates	6 (12)
CAD, *n (%)*	49 (98)	Ca^{2+}-antagonists	4 (8)
ischemic	47 (94)	α-antagonists	2 (4)
hypertrophic	1 (2)	Aspirin	46 (92)
dilatative	1 (2)	Anticoagulants	31 (62)
PTCA, *n (%)*	33 (66)	Other cardiac drugs	3 (6)
CABG, *n (%)*	9 (18)	Antiarrhythmics	2 (4)
Valvular substitution, *n (%)*	1 (2)	Statins	49 (98)
Smoking, *n (%)*	35 (70)	Gastro-protective drugs	44 (88)
Familiarity, *n (%)*	15 (30)	Polyunsaturated fats	13 (26)
Hypertension, *n (%)*	29 (58)	Oral hypoglycaemics	9 (18)
Dyslipidaemia, *n (%)*	28 (56)	Insulin	5 (10)
Diabetes, *n (%)*	13 (26)		
COPD, *n (%)*	6 (12)		
Obesity, *n (%)*	4 (8)		
Peripheral Artery Disease, *n (%)*	2 (4)		
Arrhythmias, *n (%)*	2 (4)		
Distyroidism, *n (%)*	1 (2)		
Other diseases, *n (%)*	1 (2)		

Biochemical, echocardiographic and cardiopulmonary stress test features of patients before (P) and at the end of the CRP (RP) are shown in Table 2. A CRP significantly reduced cholesterol and increased creatinine levels (both $P < 0.0001$).

Cardiopulmonary stress test revealed a reduction in maximum systolic blood pressure ($P = 0.002$), and increased maximum heart rate ($P = 0.034$), rate-pressure product ($P < 0.0001$), test duration ($P < 0.0001$), and VO2 max ($P < 0.0001$) with consequent significantly higher exercise tolerance, one of the most crucial target in the HF treatment, after CRP.

CRP-induced changes in antioxidant capacity in heart failure elderly patients

The activity of Sirt1 and of its molecular targets, Cat and SOD before and at the end of the CRP were evaluated.

The CRP enhanced Sirt1 activity measured in PBMCs from patients (RP *vs* P, $P = 0.02$) (Fig. 1, Panel a). Likewise, Cat and SOD activities measured in serum were greater in RP than in P ($P < 0.005$ and $P < 0.05$, respectively) (Fig. 1, Panels b and c).

Sirt1, Cat and SOD activities in endothelial cells conditioned with patients' sera

To investigate the possible role of Sirt1, Cat and SOD in modulating the beneficial effects of the CRP, an *in*

Table 2 Changes in biochemical, echocardiographic and cardiopulmonary stress test parameters induced by CRP

	P	RP	P value
Biochemistry			
Cholesterol (mmol/L)	157.61 ± 37.11	150.67 ± 30.37	*<0.0001*
Creatininemia (mmol/L)	0.94 ± 0.24	0.97 ± 0.20	*<0.0001*
Hemoglobin (g/dL)	13.58 ± 1.35	13.42 ± 0.53	0.494
Echocardiographic parameters			
EF (%)	53.33 ± 8.97	55.10 ± 6.79	*0.011*
LVEDD (mm)	51.37 ± 3.77	51.31 ± 3.13	0.804
Cardiopulmonary stress test			
SBP max (mmHg)	169.02 ± 15.54	165.51 ± 19.29	*0.002*
DBP max (mmHg)	81.46 ± 5.62	80.64 ± 5.15	0.077
HR max (bpm)	117.56 ± 21.55	123.13 ± 13.20	*0.034*
Rate-pressure product (mmHg x bpm)	19892.69 ± 3841.64	20261.54 ± 3743.32	*<0.0001*
Test duration (sec)	359.41 ± 112.57	451.89 ± 109.78	*<0.0001*
VO2 max (ml/kg/min)	20.30 ± 4.61	24.51 ± 5.81	*<0.0001*

P, HF patients pre-CRP; RP, the same patients post-CRP. Data are expressed as mean ± SD. *EF*, Ejection Fraction; *LVEDD*, Left Ventricle End Diastolic Diameter; *SBP*, Systolic Blood Pressure; *DBP*, Diastolic Blood Pressure; *HR*, Heart Rate; bpm, beat/minutes. A P value <0.05 was considered significant

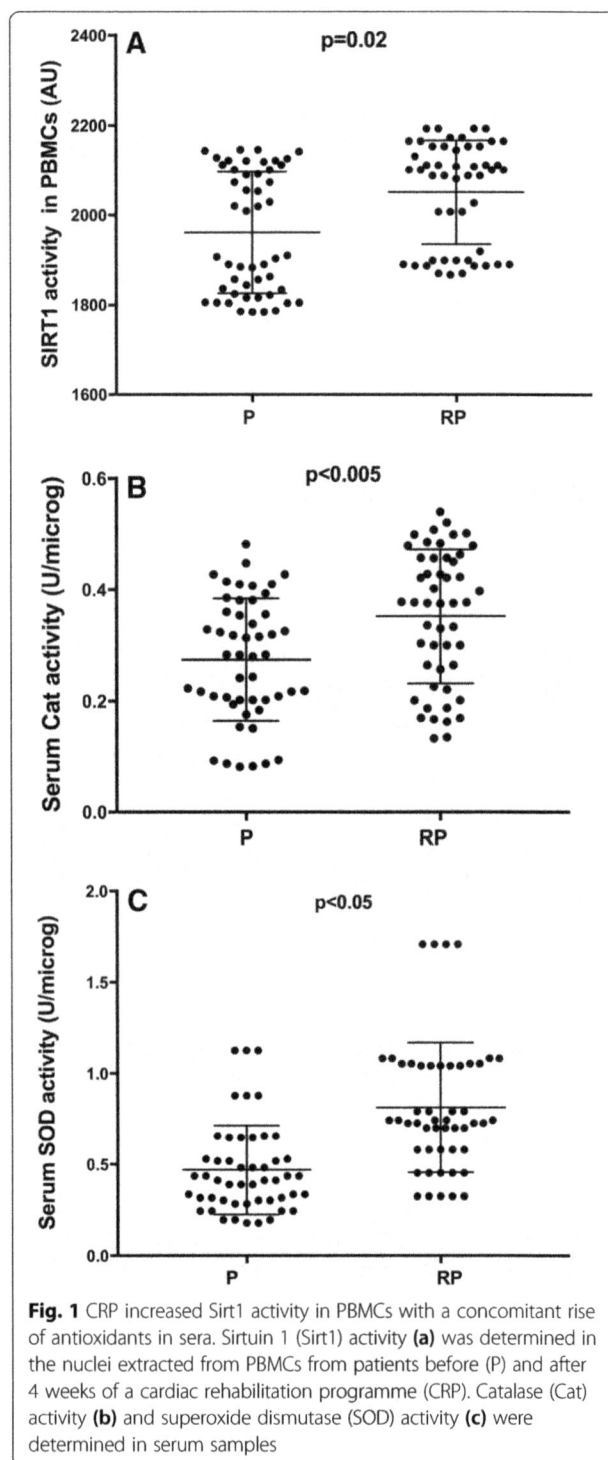

Fig. 1 CRP increased Sirt1 activity in PBMCs with a concomitant rise of antioxidants in sera. Sirtuin 1 (Sirt1) activity **(a)** was determined in the nuclei extracted from PBMCs from patients before (P) and after 4 weeks of a cardiac rehabilitation programme (CRP). Catalase (Cat) activity **(b)** and superoxide dismutase (SOD) activity **(c)** were determined in serum samples

vivo-in vitro model was set up by conditioning human endothelial cells (ECs) with sera from patients at time 0 (Patient serum-conditioned ECs, P-ECs) and at the end of the CRP (Rehabilitated Patient serum-conditioned ECs, RP-ECs). Moreover, the antioxidant response in such conditioned cells was evaluated after the induction of stress using H_2O_2.

Sirt1 and Cat activities were higher in RP-ECs than in P-ECs (both, $P < 0.0001$) (Fig. 2, Panels a and b). Conversely, SOD activity decreased in RP-ECs ($P < 0.05$) compared with P-ECs (Fig. 2, Panel c).

In the presence of H_2O_2-induced oxidative stress, Sirt1 and Cat activities were higher in RP-ECs than in P-ECs ($P < 0.0001$ and $P < 0.05$, respectively) (Fig. 2, Panels a and b), whereas SOD activity did not change (Fig. 2, Panel c).

These results showed that a CRP induced Sirt1 and Cat activation in both the absence and presence of oxidative stress, suggesting the role of Sirt1 in stimulating the antioxidant response.

Role of Sirt1 and Cat in endothelial cell senescence

The senescence in endothelial cells (ECs) conditioned with patients' sera was measured. ECs conditioned with sera from patients at the end of a 4-week CRP (RP-ECs) showed a significantly reduced senescence compared to that conditioned with sera from patients before CRP (P-ECs), in both the absence and presence of induced oxidative stress (both, $P < 0.0001$; Fig. 3).

To investigate the possible role played by Sirt1 and its molecular target Cat in the modulation of cell senescence, P-ECs and RP-ECs, either exposed or not to oxidative stress, were treated with Sirt1 and Cat pharmacological inhibitors, EX-527 and 3-amino-1,2,4-triazole (ATZ) respectively.

As shown in Fig. 3, the inhibition of Sirt1 activity by EX-527 caused an increase of senescence in RP-ECs compared with baseline ($P = 0.001$), but not in P-ECs. Interestingly, in the presence of H_2O_2 oxidative stress, EX-527 induced a rise in senescence, in both P-ECs ($P < 0.05$) and RP-ECs ($P = 0.001$). Hence, Sirt1 inhibition abolished the anti-senescent effect of a CRP, suggesting Sirt1 as a modulator of endothelial cell senescence.

Also the inhibition of Cat activity by ATZ resulted in an increased senescence, in both P-ECs and RP-ECs (both, $P < 0.0001$), compared with baseline. In the presence of H_2O_2-induced oxidative stress, ATZ treatment caused a significant increase in the senescence rate in ECs conditioned with RP sera ($P < 0.0001$) compared with basal levels. Of note, senescence become higher in stressed RP-ECs compared with stressed P-ECs when Cat was inhibited ($P = 0.001$). These data suggest that Cat is, at least in part, responsible for the reduced senescence rate observed in ECs conditioned with RP sera.

Discussion

Most of the studies in both young and older adults have been planned after considering functional and hemodynamic outcomes, without clarifying the effects of a CRP from a molecular point of view.

In this study, we showed an increase of Sirt1 activity in PBMCs alongside an increase of antioxidant capability in serum isolated from patients with HF after 4 weeks of a CRP.

In vivo-in vitro experiments performed in endothelial cells conditioned with patients before and after CRP showed that serum from the rehabilitated patients is able to stimulate Sirt1 activity and the cellular antioxidant defence by increasing activity of the Sirt1 target Cat.

Furthermore, the conditioning of human endothelial cells with serum from rehabilitated patients attenuated senescence in both the absence and presence of oxidative stress induction and such effect was eliminated by the pharmacological inhibition of Sirt1 or Cat activity.

Cellular senescence is a hallmark of ageing and a process in which competent cells are brought into a permanent form of growth arrest. If and how senescence is correlated with age-associated frailty and diseases is still one of the major unanswered questions in ageing physiology and clinical geriatrics [23]. An increase of oxidative stress-induced senescence can be dangerous to endothelial cells, resulting in impairment of endothelial structure and function. Some authors showed that cellular senescence is involved in endothelial dysfunction and atherogenesis, and this was confirmed by a histological study on atherosclerotic human plaques demonstrating morphological features of senescence [24]. As oxidative stress-induced endothelial dysfunction is strictly connected to HF, researching methods to modify this condition is certainly of clinical interest.

The role played by Sirt1 in the regulation of ageing, endothelial homeostasis and cellular senescence is now recognized. Indeed, several studies demonstrated that a H_2O_2 treatment caused a reduction of Sirt1 protein expression, and the inhibition of Sirt1 contributed to a H_2O_2-induced senescence in endothelial cells [25, 26]. Furthermore, the Sirt1 target Cat was also shown to be involved in ageing and senescence control [27, 28]. We previously demonstrated that Cat is reduced during ageing [16], and involved in the reduction of endothelial senescence during an aerobic exercise training [20, 21]. Some studies in animal models demonstrated that over-expression of Cat in heart and vessels may have a beneficial impact on HF. In particular, Cat may prevent adverse myocardial remodelling and contribute to the preservation of geometric and functional changes by alleviating stress in the endoplasmic reticulum [18, 29].

Notably, patients enrolled in the present study were HF elderly patients with preserved ejection fraction, a phenotype of HF that is attracting particular attention from both physicians and researchers. Actually, pharmacological trials performed to assess improving of outcome and symptoms, including exercise intolerance, in

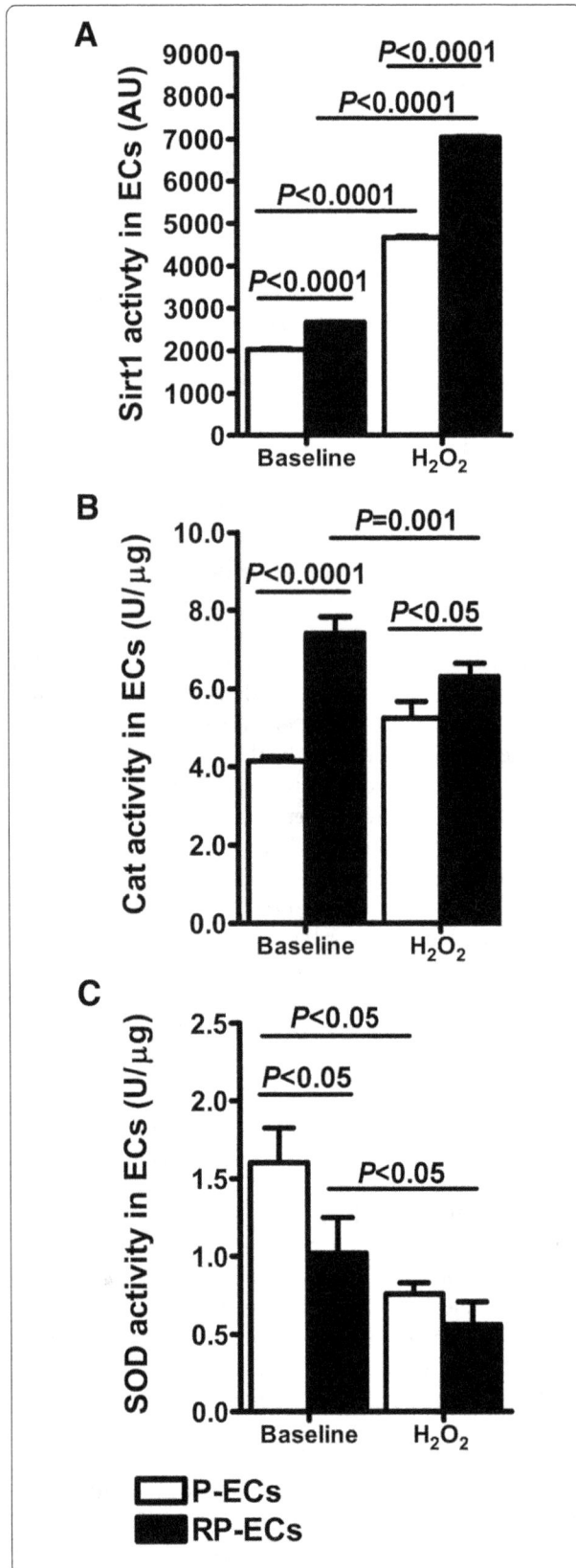

Fig. 2 Sirt1, Cat and SOD activities in conditioned endothelial cells. Sirt1 **(a)**, Cat **(b)** and SOD **(c)** activities in endothelial cells (ECs) conditioned with sera from patients before (P) and after (RP) a 4-week well-structured CRP in either the presence or absence of H_2O_2-induced oxidative stress

HFpEF patients have been shed light the absence of effective drugs [30, 31].

On the other hand, some recent studies in such patients have suggested that exercise training is a promising therapeutic strategy to improve exercise intolerance [32], increase exercise capacity, as measured objectively using peak oxygen consumption, and ameliorate quality of life and diastolic function, assessed by echocardiography [6, 7, 33].

Here we showed that, in addition to the improvement of hemodynamic parameters and exercise tolerance (assessed by cardiopulmonary stress test), an exercise-based CRP increases Sirt1 activity and stimulates a systemic antioxidant defence in HFpEF elderly patients and was able to produce antioxidant and anti-senescent effects in endothelial cells mediated, at least in part, by Sirt1 and its target Cat.

Limitations

A possible limitation of the present study could be the lack of a group of heart failing patients not undergone CR. However, the main outcome was represented by the investigation of the molecular changes occurred before and after a well-structured 4-week rehabilitation

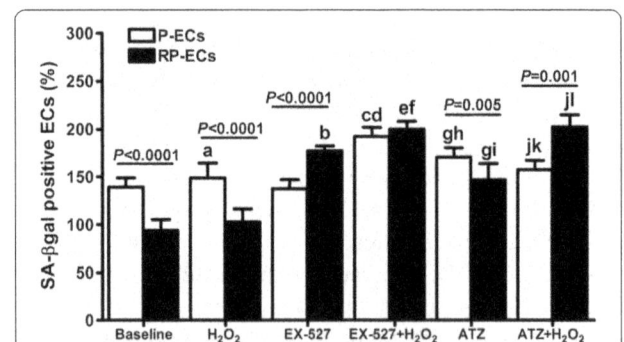

Fig. 3 Effect of the inhibition of Sirt1 and Cat activities on endothelial cell senescence. SA-β-gal staining of ECs conditioned with sera from HF patients in the presence and absence of oxidative stress. Sirt1 and Cat activities were inhibited by EX-527 and 3-amino-1,2,3-triazole (ATZ), respectively. Senescence values are shown as a percentage of the reference condition (FBS-conditioned ECs), which is 100%. a) $P < 0.05$ vs baseline; b) $P = 0.001$ vs baseline; c) $P < 0.05$ vs H_2O_2; d) $P = 0.01$ vs EX-527; e) $P = 0.001$ vs H_2O_2; f) $P < 0.02$ vs EX-527; g) $P < 0.0001$ vs baseline; h) $P < 0.01$ vs EX-527; i) $P < 0.05$ vs EX-527; j) $P < 0.05$ vs ATZ; k) $P < 0.02$ vs EX-527 + H_2O_2; l) $P < 0.0001$ vs H_2O_2. (B): a) $P = 0.001$ vs baseline; b) $P < 0.02$ vs baseline; c) $P < 0.005$ vs baseline; d) $P = 0.002$ vs H_2O_2; e) $P = 0.01$ vs EX-527; f) $P < 0.01$ vs baseline; g) $P < 0.05$ vs EX-527; h) $P < 0.05$ vs H_2O_2; i) $P = 0.002$ vs EX-527 + H_2O_2; j) $P = 0.001$ vs EX-527 + H_2O_2; k) $P < 0.005$ vs H_2O_2

program in patients affected by chronic HF, who did not change their clinical characteristics and pharmacological therapy during the study period.

Another drawback is the lack of women in the study population. Actually, we did recruit only three women, and then we decided to exclude them because of the small number. This is in line with the fact that women are less inclined to take part in cardiac rehabilitation programs [34]. Therefore, further studies are necessary to better clarify the molecular effects of CR also in female patients.

Conclusion

The ability of exercise training to regulate vascular endothelial function and oxidative stress response is an example of how lifestyle and/or tools such as exercise-based CRPs can complement both clinical and pharmacological means of managing CVDs. In particular, cardiac rehabilitation is a helpful medical practice in which several molecular factors mutually influence each other. The exercise training included in CRPs acts as a non-pharmacological inductor of antioxidant response.

To determine the molecular mechanisms underlying the beneficial effects of CRPs is an essential step in developing a strategy to facilitate the clinical practice of exercise training. Further studies should be addressed to evaluate the possibility of reducing the number and the dosage of drugs in HF patients, including those with preserved ejection fraction by implementing exercise programs, especially in high-risk elderly subjects.

Methods
Study Design and Population
A prospective longitudinal observational study was conducted on patients consecutively admitted to the Cardiac Rehabilitation Unit of "San Gennaro dei Poveri" Hospital in Naples, Italy. Patients' information and consent forms were approved by the ethical committee of ASL of Salerno Registry of Observational Studies (RSO) n.10/14.

The study was performed in accordance with the Declaration of Helsinki Seventh Revision (2013) and its amendments. This report adheres to the standards for the reporting of observational trials and was written according to the STROBE guidelines for Observational Studies in Epidemiology - Molecular Epidemiology (STROBE-ME) [35].

Exclusion criteria included unstable angina pectoris, uncompensated HF, complex ventricular arrhythmias, pacemaker implantation and orthopaedic or neurological limitations to exercise.

All enrolled patients underwent a physical examination, collection of demographic and routine blood chemistry tests, chest X-ray, blood pressure measurement, electrocardiographic and echocardiographic examinations, cardiopulmonary stress test and a 6-min walking test with Borg index evaluation. For interval training, low muscle commitment calisthenics and respiratory exercises were performed.

Training Protocol
The CRP consisted of 30-min sessions of aerobic exercise, 5 days a week. A daily training session comprised a warm-up (10 min), endurance training (15 min) and a cool-down (5 min) on a cycle ergometer at 50% of the VO2 max achieved on the cardiopulmonary stress test.

Blood Sample Collection
Overnight fasting blood samples were obtained from patients before starting and at the end of the CRP. After centrifugation at $1500 \times g$ for 10 min, serum samples were transferred to new tubes and stored at -80 °C until analysis. PBMCs were isolated from whole blood by Ficoll-Paque PLUS (GE Healthcare, Munich, Germany), according to manufacturer's procedures.

Samples isolated from patients before CR were indicated as P, while those collected from patients after CR were designated as RP.

Cell Culture and Treatments
Human Umbilical Vein Endothelial Cells (HUVECs, ECs) were purchased from Clonetics (Walkersville, MD). The cells were cultured in an endothelial growth medium, containing FBS at a concentration of 2% and bovine brain extract (with FGF-2 at a concentration of 100–500 pg/ml). The cells were subcultured by trypsinization, seeded on cell culture dishes coated with 0.1% gelatin and growth in an atmosphere of 5% CO2 at 37 °C. Pilot experiments to identify the concentration of hydrogen peroxide ($H_2O_2 = 100$–750 µM) that effectively induced a significant decrease in the survival of control cells, were conducted and a concentration of 500 µM was chosen. Moreover, we evaluated the effect of oxidative stress 12, 24, 48, and 72 h after a treatment with 500 µM H_2O_2. Finally, we chose the time of 48 h as representative of the most relevant change.

Therefore, ECs were seeded and cultured for 48 h in a medium supplemented with either the patient's serum (10%) at time 0 (Patient serum-conditioned ECs, P-ECs) and post CR (Rehabilitated Patient serum-conditioned ECs, RP-ECs), or FBS (10%) as a control and were exposed or not to oxidative stress induced by 500 µM H_2O_2. Four hours after H_2O_2 exposure, the growth medium was replaced with fresh medium containing FBS.

All experiments were performed at a population doubling level (PDL) of 8 to 12.

Sirt1 Activity

Crude nuclear samples were extracted by suspending the cells into 1 mL of lysis buffer (10 mM of Tris HCl at pH 7.5, 10 mM of NaCl, 15 mM of $MgCl_2$, 250 mM of sucrose, 0.5% NP-40, 0.1 mM of EGTA). Cells were spun through 4 ml of sucrose cushion (30% sucrose, 10 mM of Tris HCl at pH 7.5, 10 mM of NaCl, 3 mM of $MgCl_2$) at $1300 \times g$ for 10 min at 4 °C. The isolated nuclei were suspended in 50–100 µl of extraction buffer (50 mM of HEPES KOH at pH 7.5, 420 mM of NaCl, 0.5 mM of EDTA Na_2, 0.1 mM of EGTA, 10% glycerol). After centrifugation at 15,000 rpm for 10 min, the protein concentration of the crude nuclear extract without protease inhibitor was determined by the Bradford method. Sirt1 activity in the nuclei was determined using the CycLex SIRT1/Sir2 Deacetylase Fluorometric Assay Kit (Ina, Nagano, Japan). The reaction was carried out by simultaneously mixing fluorescent-labeled acetylated peptide as substrate and 10 µl of the sample, trichostatin A, NAD, and lysyl endopeptidase. The intensity of the fluorescence at 440 nm was measured 60 min after the onset of the reaction. Values are reported as relative fluorescence/µg of protein (AU). All data are the means ± standard deviation (SD) of three independent experiments.

Catalase and Superoxide Dismutase Antioxidant Activities

Catalase (Cat) and superoxide dismutase (SOD) activities were determined using the Catalase Assay Kit and the Superoxide Dismutase Assay Kit (Cayman Chemical, USA). Samples were previously diluted with buffer (1:10 for serum; 1:2 for cell lysate). The values were reported as U/µg of protein. All data are the means ± SD of three independent experiments.

Sirt1 and Catalase Activities Inhibition

To investigate if Sirt1 or Cat activity influenced changes in the senescence of the conditioned cells either exposed or not to H_2O_2, their respective activities were inhibited using EX-527 (Sigma, Milan-Italy) at a concentration of 5 µM for 1 h and 3-amino-1,2,4-triazole (ATZ) (Sigma, Milan-Italy) at a concentration of 10 mM for 3 h.

Senescence-Associated β-galactosidase (SA-β-gal) Activity

Cultured cells were washed in PBS and fixed with 2% formaldehyde and 2% glutaraldehyde for 10 min at room temperature. The cells were washed and then incubated at 37 °C in staining buffer with the following components: 40 mM citric acid/sodium phosphate (pH 6.0), 0.15 M NaCl, 2 mM $MgCl_2$, 5 mM potassium ferrocyanide, and 1 mg/mL X-gal (5-bromo-4 chloro-3-indolyl β-D-galactoside). After 4 h, the SA-β-gal rate was obtained by counting four random fields per dish and assessing the percentage of SA-β-gal-positive cells from 100 cells

per field. Senescence values are shown as a percentage of the reference condition (FBS-conditioned ECs), which is 100%.

Statistical Analysis

Continuous variables are expressed as mean ± SD and compared by paired or unpaired Student's t test (normally distributed variables) or by two or three way ANOVA when appropriate, or as median ± interquartile range value and compared by the Mann–Whitney U test (not normally distributed). Normality of data distribution was evaluated using the Kolmogorov-Smirnov test. Non-normally distributed continuous variables were converted to their natural log functions. Categorical variables are expressed as a proportion and compared by the χ^2 test, with risk ratios and 95% confidence intervals quoted.

All data were analysed using SPSS version 19.0 (SPSS, Inc., Chicago, Illinois-USA). Statistical significance was accepted at $P < 0.05$.

Abbreviations

EX-527: Sirtuin 1 inhibitor; ACCF: American College of Cardiology Foundation; AHA: American Heart Association; ARBs: Angiotensin II Receptor Blockers; ATZ: 3-amino-1,2,4-triazole; AU: Arbitrary unit; BMI: Body mass index; bpm: Beat/minutes; CABG: Coronary artery bypass graft; CAD: Coronary artery disease; Cat: Catalase; COPD: Chronic obstructive pulmonary disease; CRP: Cardiac rehabilitation programme; CVDs: Cardiovascular diseases; DBP: Diastolic blood pressure; ECs: Endothelial cells; EF: Ejection fraction; EGTA: Ethylene glycol tetraacetic acid; ESC: European Society of Cardiology; FBS: Foetal bovine serum; H_2O_2: Oxygen peroxide; HCl: Hydrogen chloride; HEPES: 4-(2-hydroxyethyl)-1-piperazineethanesulfonic acid; HF: Heart failure; HR: Heart rate; KOH: Potassium hydroxide; LVEDD: Left ventricle end diastolic diameter; $MgCl_2$: Magnesium chloride; MI: Myocardial infarction; MnSOD: Manganese-dependent superoxide dismutase; NaCl: Sodium chloride; NAD^+: Nicotinamide adenine dinucleotide coenzyme; NP-40: 4-nonylphenyl-polyethylene glycol; NYHA: New York Heart Association functional classification of heart failure; O_2: Oxygen; P: Patients before cardiac rehabilitation programme; PDL: Population doubling level; P-ECs: Patient serum-conditioned endothelial cells; PTCA: Percutaneous transluminal coronary angioplasty; ROS: Reactive oxygen species; RP: Rehabilitated patients; RP-ECs: Rehabilitated patient serum-conditioned endothelial cells; SA-β-gal: Senescence-Associated β-galactosidase; SBP: Systolic blood pressure; Sirt1: Sirtuin 1; SOD: Superoxide dismutase; VO2: Maximal oxygen consumption; X-gal: 5-bromo-4 chloro-3-indolyl β-D-galactoside.

Acknowledgements

None.

Funding

This work was supported by the Department of Medicine, Surgery and Dentistry of University of Salerno [ORSA128783 to A.F.] and the Department of Medicine and Health Sciences of the University of Molise [R-DIPA_20112013300118CORBI-GR to G.C.].

Authors' contributions

All authors read and met *Immun. Ageing* criteria for authorship. Graziamaria Corbi, Valeria Conti, Nicola Ferrara and Amelia Filippelli conceived and designed the experiments. Giusy Russomanno, Valentina Manzo, Giuseppe Rengo and Albino Carrizzo performed the experiments. Salvatore Latte and Maria Consiglia Calabrese contributed with acquisition of clinical data and human samples. Graziamaria Corbi, Valeria Conti and Giusy Russomanno performed the analysis and interpretation of the data and wrote the paper. Nicola Ferrara, Annibale A. Puca, Ramaroson Andriantsitohaina, Walter Filippelli, Carmine Vecchione, Amelia Filippelli critically revised the paper. All authors read and approved the final paper.

Competing interests
The authors have no conflicts of interest to report.

Author details
[1]Department of Medicine, Surgery and Dentistry, University of Salerno, Via S. Allende 43, 84081 Baronissi, Italy. [2]Department of Medicine and Health Sciences, University of Molise, Campobasso, Italy. [3]Department of Translational Medical Sciences, Federico II University of Naples, Naples, Italy. [4]Salvatore Maugeri Foundation, IRCCS, Scientific Institute of Telese Terme, Benevento, Italy. [5]IRCCS MultiMedica, Milan, Italy. [6]Cardiac Rehabilitation Unit of "San Gennaro dei Poveri" Hospital, Naples, Italy. [7]Vascular Physiopathology Unit, IRCCS INM Neuromed, Pozzilli, Italy. [8]INSERM U1063, Stress Oxydant et Pathologies Métaboliques, Institut de Biologie en Santé, Université d'Angers, Angers, France. [9]Department of Institutional Study and Territorial Systems, University of Naples "Parthenope", Naples, Italy.

References
1. Mozaffarian D, Benjamin EJ, Go AS, Arnett DK, Blaha MJ, Cushman M, et al. Heart disease and stroke statistics–2015 update: a report from the American Heart Association. Circulation. 2015;131:e29–322.
2. Lawler PR, Filion KB, Eisenberg MJ. Efficacy of exercise-based cardiac rehabilitation post-myocardial infarction: a systematic review and meta-analysis of randomized controlled trials. Am Heart J. 2011;162:571–84. e2.
3. Schutzer KA, Graves BS. Barriers and motivations to exercise in older adults. Prev Med. 2004;39:1056–61.
4. Rengo G, Leosco D, Zincarelli C, Marchese M, Corbi G, Liccardo D, et al. Adrenal GRK2 lowering is an underlying mechanism for the beneficial sympathetic effects of exercise training in heart failure. Am J Physiol Heart Circ Physiol. 2010;298:H2032–2038.
5. Leosco D, Rengo G, Iaccarino G, Golino L, Marchese M, Fortunato F, et al. Exercise promotes angiogenesis and improves beta-adrenergic receptor signalling in the post-ischaemic failing rat heart. Cardiovasc Res. 2008;78:385–94.
6. Nolte K, Herrmann-Lingen C, Wachter R, Gelbrich G, Düngen H-D, Duvinage A, et al. Effects of exercise training on different quality of life dimensions in heart failure with preserved ejection fraction: the Ex-DHF-P trial. Eur J Prev Cardiol. 2015;22:582–93.
7. Ismail H, McFarlane JR, Nojoumian AH, Dieberg G, Smart NA. Clinical outcomes and cardiovascular responses to different exercise training intensities in patients with heart failure: a systematic review and meta-analysis. JACC Heart Fail. 2013;1:514–22.
8. Corbi G, Conti V, Russomanno G, Rengo G, Vitulli P, Ciccarelli AL, et al. Is physical activity able to modify oxidative damage in cardiovascular aging? Oxid Med Cell Longev. 2012;2012:728547.
9. Meyer P, Gayda M, Juneau M, Nigam A. High-intensity aerobic interval exercise in chronic heart failure. Curr Heart Fail Rep. 2013;10:130–8.
10. Tanno M, Kuno A, Horio Y, Miura T. Emerging beneficial roles of sirtuins in heart failure. Basic Res Cardiol. 2012;107:273.
11. Corbi G, Conti V, Russomanno G, Longobardi G, Furgi G, Filippelli A, et al. Adrenergic signaling and oxidative stress: a role for sirtuins? Front Physiol. 2013;4:324.
12. Yu W, Fu Y-C, Chen C-J, Wang X, Wang W. SIRT1: a novel target to prevent atherosclerosis. J Cell Biochem. 2009;108:10–3.
13. Rahman M, Halade GV, Bhattacharya A, Fernandes G. The fat-1 transgene in mice increases antioxidant potential, reduces pro-inflammatory cytokine levels, and enhances PPAR-gamma and SIRT-1 expression on a calorie restricted diet. Oxid Med Cell Longev. 2009;2:307–16.
14. Conti V, Corbi G, Simeon V, Russomanno G, Manzo V, Ferrara N, et al. Aging-related changes in oxidative stress response of human endothelial cells. Aging Clin Exp Res. 2015;27:547–53.
15. Lu T-M, Tsai J-Y, Chen Y-C, Huang C-Y, Hsu H-L, Weng C-F, et al. Downregulation of Sirt1 as aging change in advanced heart failure. J Biomed Sci. 2014;21:57.

16. Ferrara N, Rinaldi B, Corbi G, Conti V, Stiuso P, Boccuti S, et al. Exercise training promotes SIRT1 activity in aged rats. Rejuvenation Res. 2008;11:139–50.
17. Leopold JA, Loscalzo J. Oxidative enzymopathies and vascular disease. Arterioscler Thromb Vasc Biol. 2005;25:1332–40.
18. Qin F, Lennon-Edwards S, Lancel S, Biolo A, Siwik DA, Pimentel DR, et al. Cardiac-specific overexpression of catalase identifies hydrogen peroxide-dependent and -independent phases of myocardial remodeling and prevents the progression to overt heart failure in G(alpha)q-overexpressing transgenic mice. Circ Heart Fail. 2010;3:306–13.
19. Conti V, Forte M, Corbi G, Russomanno G, Formisano L, Landolfi A, Izzo V, Filippelli A, Vecchione C, Carrizzo A. Sirtuins: Possible Clinical Implications in Cardio and Cerebrovascular Diseases. Curr Drug Targets. 2017;18(4):473–84.
20. Conti V, Corbi G, Russomanno G, Simeon V, Ferrara N, Filippelli W, et al. Oxidative stress effects on endothelial cells treated with different athletes' sera. Med Sci Sports Exerc. 2012;44:39–49.
21. Conti V, Russomanno G, Corbi G, Guerra G, Grasso C, Filippelli W, et al. Aerobic training workload affects human endothelial cells redox homeostasis. Med Sci Sports Exerc. 2013;45:644–53.
22. Ponikowski P, Voors AA, Anker SD, Bueno H, Cleland JGF, Coats AJS, et al. 2016 ESC Guidelines for the diagnosis and treatment of acute and chronic heart failure: The Task Force for the diagnosis and treatment of acute and chronic heart failure of the European Society of Cardiology (ESC)Developed with the special contribution of the Heart Failure Association (HFA) of the ESC. Eur Heart J. 2016;37:2129–200.
23. Campisi J. Cellular senescence: putting the paradoxes in perspective. Curr Opin Genet Dev. 2011;21:107–12.
24. Minamino T, Komuro I. Vascular cell senescence: contribution to atherosclerosis. Circ Res. 2007;100:15–26.
25. Ota H, Eto M, Kano MR, Ogawa S, Iijima K, Akishita M, et al. Cilostazol inhibits oxidative stress-induced premature senescence via upregulation of Sirt1 in human endothelial cells. Arterioscler Thromb Vasc Biol. 2008;28:1634–9.
26. Song Z, Liu Y, Hao B, Yu S, Zhang H, Liu D, et al. Ginsenoside Rb1 prevents H2O2-induced HUVEC senescence by stimulating sirtuin-1 pathway. PLoS One. 2014;9:e112699.
27. Ota H, Eto M, Kano MR, Kahyo T, Setou M, Ogawa S, et al. Induction of endothelial nitric oxide synthase, SIRT1, and catalase by statins inhibits endothelial senescence through the Akt pathway. Arterioscler Thromb Vasc Biol. 2010;30:2205–11.
28. Schriner SE, Linford NJ, Martin GM, Treuting P, Ogburn CE, Emond M, et al. Extension of murine life span by overexpression of catalase targeted to mitochondria. Science. 2005;308:1909–11.
29. Ge W, Ge W, Zhang Y, Han X, Ren J. Cardiac-specific overexpression of catalase attenuates paraquat-induced myocardial geometric and contractile alteration: role of ER stress. Free Radic Biol Med. 2010;49:2068–77.
30. Massie BM, Carson PE, McMurray JJ, Komajda M, McKelvie R, Zile MR, Anderson S, Donovan M, Iverson E, Staiger C, Ptaszynska A. I-PRESERVE Investigators. Irbesartan in patients with heart failure and preserved ejection fraction. N Engl J Med. 2008;359:2456–67.
31. Kitzman DW, Hundley WG, Brubaker PH, Morgan TM, Moore JB, Stewart KP, Little WC. A randomized double-blind trial of enalapril in older patients with heart failure and preserved ejection fraction: effects on exercise tolerance and arterial distensibility. Circ Heart Fail. 2010;3:477–85.
32. Upadhya B, Haykowsky MJ, Eggebeen J, Kitzman DW. Exercise intolerance in heart failure with preserved ejection fraction: more than a heart problem. J Geriatr Cardiol. 2015;12:294–304.
33. Ponikowski P, Voors AA, Anker SD, Bueno H, Cleland JGF, Coats AJS, et al. 2016 ESC Guidelines for the diagnosis and treatment of acute and chronic heart failure: The Task Force for the diagnosis and treatment of acute and chronic heart failure of the European Society of Cardiology (ESC). Developed with the special contribution of the Heart Failure Association (HFA) of the ESC. Eur J Heart Fail. 2016;18:891–975.
34. Grace SL, Racco C, Chessex C, Rivera T, Oh P. A narrative review on women and cardiac rehabilitation: program adherence and preferences for alternative models of care. Maturitas. 2010;67(3):203–8. doi:10.1016/j.maturitas.2010.07.001.
35. Gallo V, Egger M, McCormack V, Farmer PB, Ioannidis JPA, Kirsch-Volders M, et al. STrengthening the Reporting of OBservational studies in Epidemiology–Molecular Epidemiology (STROBE-ME): an extension of the STROBE Statement. PLoS Med. 2011;8:e1001117.

HCV monoinfection and HIV/HCV coinfection enhance T-cell immune senescence in injecting drug users early during infection

Bart P. X. Grady[1,2], Nening M. Nanlohy[3] and Debbie van Baarle[3,4,5*]

Abstract

Background: Injecting drug users (IDU) are at premature risk of developing multimorbidity and mortality from causes commonly observed in the elderly. Ageing of the immune system (immune-senescence) can lead to premature morbidity and mortality and can be accelerated by chronic viral infections. Here we investigated the impact of HCV monoinfection and HIV/HCV coinfection on immune parameters in (ex-) IDU. We analyzed telomere length and expression of activation, differentiation and exhaustion markers on T cells *at baseline (t = 1) and at follow-up (t = 2)* (median interval 16.9 years) in IDU who were: HCV mono-infected (*n* = 21); HIV/HCV coinfected (*n* = 23) or multiple exposed but uninfected (MEU) (*n* = 8).

Results: The median time interval between t = 1 and t = 2 was 16.9 years. Telomere length within $CD4^+$ and $CD8^+$ T cells decreased significantly over time in all IDU groups (*p* ≤ 0.012). $CD4^+$ T-cell telomere length in HCV mono-infected IDU was significantly reduced compared to healthy donors at t = 1 (*p* < 0.008). HIV/HCV coinfected IDU had reduced $CD4^+$ and $CD8^+$ T-cell telomere lengths (*p* ≤ 0.002) to healthy donors *i* at t = 1. This was related to persistent levels of immune activation but not due to increased differentiation of T cells over time. Telomere length decrease was observed within all T-cell subsets, but mainly found in immature T cells ($CD27^+CD57^+$) (*p* ≤ 0.015).

Conclusions: HCV mono-infection and HIV/HCV coinfection enhance T-cell immune-senescence. Our data suggest that this occurred early during infection, which warrants early treatment for both HCV and HIV to reduce immune senescence in later life.

Keywords: Substance abuse, People who inject drugs, Frailty, Immunosenescence, Longitudinal

Background

As people age, the immune system exhibits age-associated changes resulting in impaired immunity. This so-called immune senescence is a complex multifactorial phenomenon characterized by a number of features including: i) reduced number of naïve T cells; ii) increased frequencies of differentiated $CD28^-CD57^+$ T cells that have a reduced proliferative capacity; iii) reduced CD4/CD8 ratio; oligoclonal expansion of CD8 T cells, and iv) progressive shortening of telomeres [1–3]. Telomeres are repetitive $(TTAGGG)_n$ nucleotide sequences that shorten with each cell division [4]. Among people aged over 60 years, short leukocyte telomere length has been associated with higher mortality rates from infectious diseases [5].

People who inject drugs (injecting drug users, IDU) are at increased risk of contracting both acute and chronic infections [6, 7]. The prevalence of HCV antibodies in IDU ranges from 15–98 % [8, 9]. Upon HCV infection, 75 % of individuals progress to chronic infection and are at risk for progressive liver disease, liver cirrhosis and hepatocellular carcinoma [10]. The worldwide prevalence of HIV infection among IDU is

* Correspondence: Debbie.van.baarle@rivm.nl
[3]Department of Immunology, University Medical Center Utrecht, Utrecht, The Netherlands
[4]Department of Internal Medicine, University Medical Center Utrecht, Utrecht, The Netherlands
Full list of author information is available at the end of the article

estimated to be 18 % [11]. With the advent of combination antiretroviral therapy (cART) and decline in drug-related causes of death, the mean age of IDU is increasing [12, 13] and IDU are at premature risk of developing multimorbidity and mortality from causes commonly observed in the elderly [14, 15].

Immunological changes and increased levels of inflammation could form the basis of this premature burden of morbidity and mortality among ageing DU. Progression of immune senescence was shown to be accelerated by chronic viral infections such as HIV through (long-term) continuous immune activation [16, 17]. Despite adequate combination antiretroviral therapy (cART), HIV infected individuals have increased risk for non-AIDS morbidity as compared to age-matched controls [18, 19]. There is a growing body of literature that suggests that HCV has a role in extrahepatic morbidity and mortality likely through a similar mechanism of immune activation [20, 21]. Indeed, like HIV, HCV infection also leads to PD-1^{high} and TIM-3^{high} T cells, a phenotype associated with exhaustion due to persistent antigenic pressure [22]. In addition to HIV and HCV monoinfection, HIV/HCV

coinfected individuals do not only seem to have increased risk for liver disease progression [23] but also progression to AIDS [24], which suggests that both viruses could enhance each other's disease progression [25].

To assess the impact of an infection with HCV and HIV/HCV specifically, we studied parameters associated with immune senescence. To this end, we included IDU with HCV mono- or HIV/HCV coinfection. As a control group to control for use of cocaine, opioid and social practices connected with drug use, we studied IDU with similar injecting risk behavior that where multiple exposed but uninfected (MEU) from the Amsterdam Cohort Studies (ACS) among drug users, at two time-points during follow-up >15 years apart. To address the severity of immune senescence parameters, we compared these between the specific IDU groups and healthy individuals.

Results

Study population

We included 23 HIV/HCV coinfected, 21 HCV infected and 8 MEU DU (Table 1) who all injected

Table 1 Baseline and follow-up characteristics of the study population

	HD#	MEU	HCV	HIV/HCV	P-value
Number	22	8	21	23	
General characteristics					
Gender, n male (%)	*	7 (87.5)	15 (71.4)	14 (60.9)	0.36
Western ethnicity, n (%)	*	8 (100.0)	21 (100.0)	19 (82.6)	0.13
Ever injected drugs, n (%)	*	8 (100.0)	21 (100.0)	23 (100.0)	1.00
Years of injecting (IQR)	*	6.7 (6.1–13.6)	13.4 (5.4–19.6)	9.0 (6.4–14.6)	0.20
Baseline (T = 1)					
Age, median (IQR)	36.4 (31.5–40.1)	32.8 (28.7–35.2)	34.4 (30.7–37.5)	35.2 (32.6–39.8)	0.30
Sample since study entry (months), median (IQR)	*	12.7 (0–47.6)	12.6 (1.7–31.7)	14.7 (0–25.8)	0.98
Year of sample, median (IQR)	*	1992 (1989–1994)	1992 (1990–1994)	1991 (1989–1993)	0.43
Injecting past 6 months(%)	*	1 (12.5)	14 (66.7)	16 (73.9)	0.07
CD 4 cell counts 10^6 cells/L, median (IQR)	*	*	*	590 (470–742)	*
cART, n (%)	*	*	*	1 (4.5)	*
Follow-up (T = 2)					
Age, median (IQR)	52.7 (48.3–57.6)	51.7 (49.2–54.8)	51.7 (47.4–55.5)	50.4 (47.7–54.2)	0.97
Injecting past 6 months (%)	*	1 (12.5)	4 (19.0)	4 (17.9)	0.92
CD 4 cell counts 10^6 cells/L, median (IQR)	*	*	*	341 (233–663)	*
cART, n (%)	*	*	*	20 (87.0)	*
Years on cART, median (IQR)	*	*	*	7.1 (2.1–10.7)	*

cART combination anti-retroviral therapy, HCV Hepatitis C virus, HD Healthy donor, IQR Interquartile range, MEU Multiple exposed but uninfected with HCV or HIV
#HD at T = 1 and T = 2 are not the same individuals; * Data unavailable

drugs for at least 2 years. The number of years of injecting risk behavior was comparable between groups, although MEU IDU reported less injecting in the past 6 months prior to the baseline time point ($p = 0.07$). At baseline, 1 out of 23 (4.5 %) HIV/HCV IDU was on combination antiretroviral therapy (cART) and this number increased to 20 out of 23 (87.0 %) at follow-up. The remaining three HIV/ HCV cases never received cART. For those who received cART the median time since start cART was 7.1 years (IQR 2.1–10.7). Median nadir CD4 count was 130 cells/mm^3 (IQR 90–210).

Flowcytometric analyses of telomere length

Using flow-FISH, telomere length can be measured in distinct cell populations without prior cell sorts [26]. Here we extended the flow-FISH protocol [27, 28] to a 5 color- flow-FISH (incorporating the phenotypic markers CD3, CD8, CD27 and CD57) enabling us to investigate CD4 and CD8 phenotypic T cell subsets in one sample. The assay has been shown to be sensitive enough to detect significant decreases in telomere length [28].

During ageing the relative telomere length (RTL) decreases, as shown in Fig. 1a in CD8$^+$ T cells over a period of 17 years. Using CD27/CD57 expression for

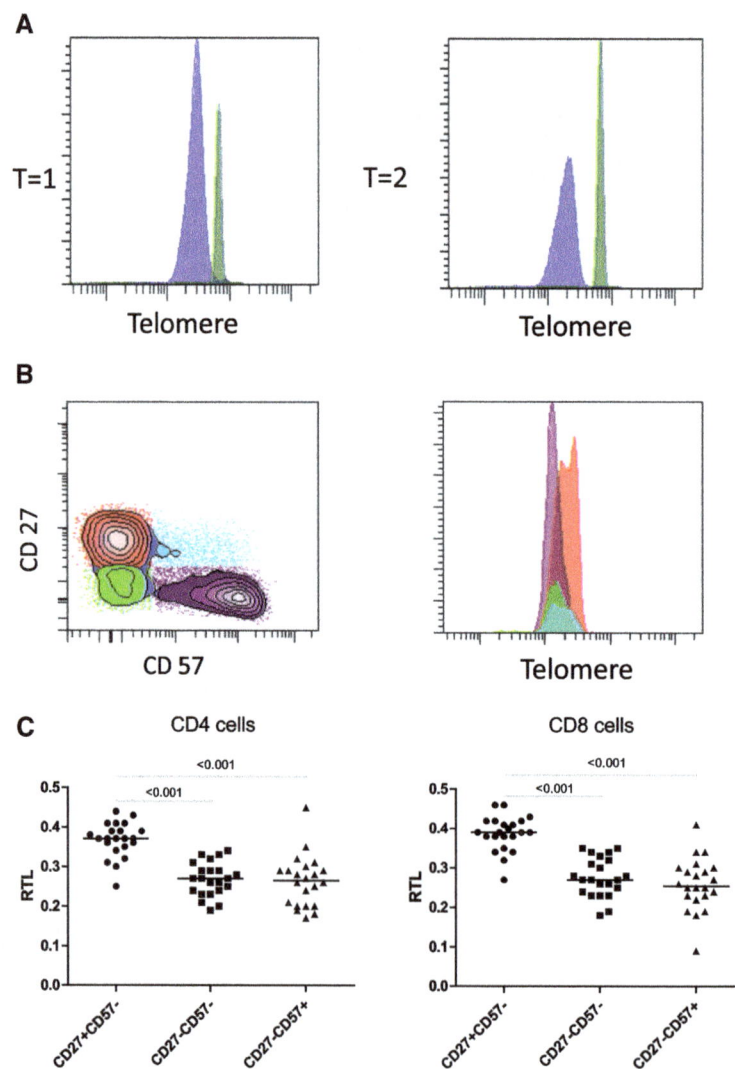

Fig. 1 Flowcytometric analysis of telomere length within T-cell subsets. **a** Representative histograms of CD8+ telomere length (blue) and calf thymocytes (green) at the baseline timepoint (t = 1) and a follow-up timepoint more than 15 years later (t = 2). **b** Telomere length analysis (or relative Telomere lengths) within T-cell subsets defined by CD27 and CD57-expression (*left panel*) as CD27$^+$CD57$^-$ (red), CD27$^-$CD57$^-$ (green) and CD27$^-$CD57$^+$ (purple). **c** Differences in relative telomere length (RTL) in healthy donors between immature (CD27$^+$CD57$^-$), mature (CD27$^-$CD57$^-$) and mature differentiated (CD27$^-$CD57$^+$) T cells stratified for CD4 (*left panel*) and CD8 T cells (*right panel*). The black lines represent median values. Statistical analyses were performed using Kruskal-Wallis and post hoc Mann-Whitney *U* test, a two sided *p*-value <0.05 was considered statistically significant

defining immature (CD27$^+$CD57$^-$), mature (CD27$^-$CD57$^-$) and mature differentiated (CD27$^-$CD57$^+$) phenotypes [29, 30] (Fig. 1b), we were also able to show differences in telomere length between these subsets (Fig. 1c). In both CD4$^+$ and CD8$^+$ T cells, immature cells had significantly longer RTL compared to mature and mature differentiated cells ($p < 0.001$). Shortened telomeres have been associated with CD57 expression on the surface of T-cells [31]. Here we show that loss of CD27 expression is already associated with reduced RTL in CD4$^+$ and CD8$^+$ T cells. Mature and mature differentiated cells have similar RTL, indicating that they have undergone comparable rounds of proliferation (Fig. 1c).

Telomere length decreases over time in CD4$^+$ and CD8$^+$ T cells and is mostly affected by HIV/HCV coinfection

We investigated whether there was a decrease in RTL among CD4$^+$ and CD8$^+$ T cells over time (Fig. 2a). The RTL of CD4$^+$ T cells decreased significantly over time in all IDU groups ($p \leq 0.012$). An impact at baseline of HCV monoinfection and HIV/HCV coinfection was observed among the RTL in CD4$^+$ T cells compared to healthy donors ($p = 0.008$ and $p = 0.002$ respectively). Among CD8$^+$ T cells the RTL also decreased in all IDU

groups ($p \leq 0.017$). The median RTL of CD8$^+$ T cells from HIV/HCV coinfected IDU at baseline was significantly lower than in healthy donors ($p = 0.0015$) and comparable to the median RTL of healthy donors, HCV and MEU at follow-up (T = 2). In a sensitivity analysis, using a linear regression model with age included as a fixed variable, we demonstrated that the observed difference as mentioned above were independent of age (Additional file 1: Table S1). To analyse the decline in RTL per individual, the 10 year RTL decline was calculated. With increasing age, the RTL decline rate did not statistically differ between the study groups (Fig. 2b). Taken together, these results suggest The effect of these infections occurred before the first time point of the study of HIV/HCV coinfection on immune senescence.

Lower telomere lengths in immature T cells in HIV/HCV coinfected IDU coincides with increased numbers of differentiated cells

Persistent antigenic stimulation leads to linear differentiation of naïve cells losing CD27 [32, 33] and gradually gaining CD57 [30], resulting in a decreased capacity to proliferate [34]. Therefore long-term effects of persistent antigenic stimulation could be reflected in the percentage

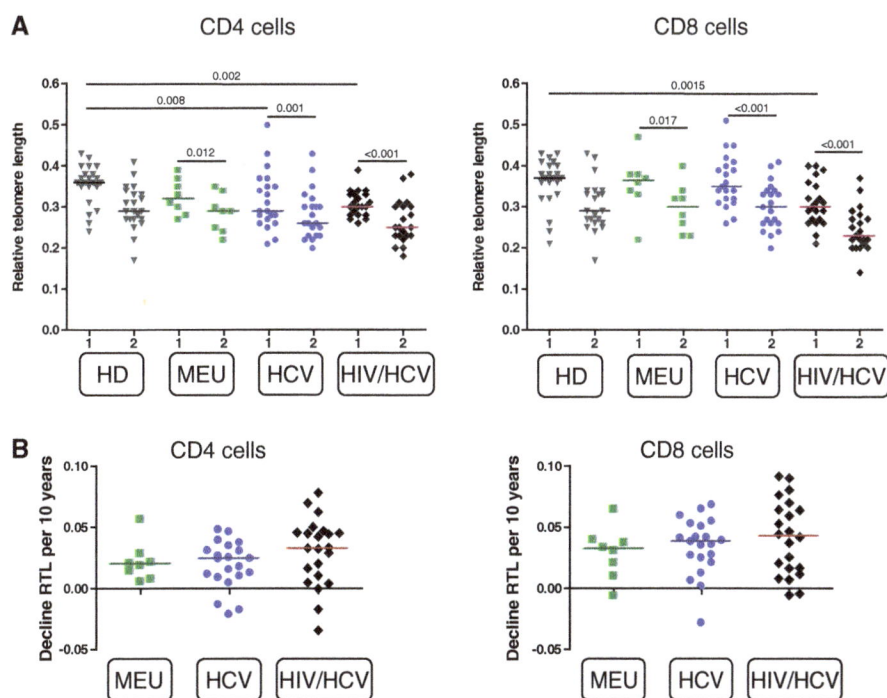

Fig. 2 Telomere length decreases over time in CD4$^+$ and CD8$^+$ T cells. **a** RTL of peripheral CD4 T cells (*left panel*) and CD8 T cells (*right panel*) over time of: healthy donors (HD); multiple exposed uninfected (MEU) injecting drug users (IDU); HCV monoinfected IDU and HIV/HCV coinfected DU. RTL was measured in the first available sample since study entry (t = 1) and the most recent sample (t = 2) of MEU, HCV monoinfected and HIV/HCV coinfected DU. HD at time point 1 and 2 are not the same individuals. The median time interval for all groups between time point 1 and 2 was 16.9 years. Medians are depicted in the scatterplots. Wilcoxon-signed rank test was used for comparison within groups with the same individuals (MEU, HCV and HIV/HCV). Kruskall-Wallis test were used to compare between groups followed by post hoc Mann-Withney U tests. **b** Median levels of RTL decrease over time calculated per individual per 10 years for CD4 T cells (*left panel*) and CD8 T cells (*right panel*)

of immature, mature and mature differentiated T-cell subsets. As shown in Fig. 3a the proportion of immature CD4$^+$ and CD8$^+$ T cells was significantly lower among HIV/HCV coinfected IDU than healthy donors at both baseline and follow-upt ($p < 0.01$) (Fig. 3c) fitting with the lower telomere lengths in this patient group. However, we did not observe a significant increase in the percentage of differentiation over time within each of the study groups, indicating that loss of telomere length over time is not simply due to increased T-cell differentiation. Even more, the RTL significantly decreased over time in all T-cell subsets for all IDU groups (≤ 0.027, Fig. 3b and c). In addition, in immature CD8$^+$ T cells, the RTL in HIV/HCV infected IDU was significantly lower compared to healthy donors ($p = 0.015$). The CD27$^+$CD57$^-$ immature CD4$^+$ T cells from young IDU with HCV or HIV/HCV also had a lower RTL than healthy donors ($p = 0.056$ and $p < 0.001$ respectively). Thus, the decrease in telomere length over time does not seem to be due to enhanced differentiation of T cells, but affects all T-cell subsets.

Increased levels of activation and exhaustion in peripheral T cells of HCV monoinfected and HIV/HCV coinfected DU

To investigate whether the observed decrease in RTL over time could be due to enhanced immune activation, we analyzed the expression of HLA-DR and CD38 on T cells. IDU with HIV/HCV coinfection had a significantly higher frequency of CD4$^+$ and CD8$^+$ T-cell activation (HLADR$^+$CD38$^+$) compared to healthy donors at both baseline and follow-up ($p < 0.004$, Fig. 4). IDU with HCV monoinfection had higher levels of CD8$^+$ T cell activation at baseline compared to healthy donors ($p < 0.001$), but this effect diminished over time. The level of CD4$^+$ and CD8$^+$ T cell activation declined over time in HIV/HCV infected DU, but was still higher than in healthy donors ($p < 0.001$). The expression of activation markers was also significantly higher in HCV and HIV/HCV infected IDU compared to MEU DU. Interestingly, young MEU IDU were comparable to young healthy donors with respect to immune activation, which suggests there was no impact of drug use or social practices on immune activation. However, the levels of CD38 and HLA-DR among MEU IDU remained stable over time, suggesting that MEU IDU may actively suppress immune activation.

Persistent antigen exposure does not only lead to a rapid turnover and telomere erosion but can also lead to a subset of T cells that become functionally exhausted. To investigate whether T-cell exhaustion is upregulated by HIV and/or HCV we evaluated programmed death factor 1 (PD-1) expression levels, shown to be marker of exhaustion in chronic viral diseases but increasingly also considered as activation marker after acute infection (to

control T-cell activity). At baseline both CD4$^+$ and CD8$^+$ T cells of HIV/HCV infected IDU expressed higher levels of PD-1 than healthy donors. Over time, the CD8 PD-1 expression of HIV/HCV infected IDU declined significantly ($p = 0.014$) to a level comparable to healthy donors, most likely due to cART. Among HCV monoinfected IDU the expression of PD-1 in CD4$^+$ T cells was higher compared to healthy donors ($p = 0.023$). Even though PD-1 expression in these cells significantly increased over time ($p = 0.005$) the expression level was comparable to older healthy donors, MEU and HIV/HCV coinfected DU. Thus HIV/HCV coinfection leads to both general increased immune activation and increased PD-1 expression.

Methods
Study population

Study subjects were recruited from the ACS among DU, an open, prospective cohort study to investigate the prevalence, incidence, and risk factors of HIV infections and other blood-borne diseases [35]. Enrollment is voluntary, anonymous, and written informed consent is obtained from each participant at the intake visit. The medical ethics committee of the Academic Medical Center approved this observational study. Blood is drawn each visit for laboratory testing and storage of peripheral blood mononuclear cells (PBMC) and serum. HIV testing and HCV testing have been described before [36]. In short, all participants were prospectively tested for HIV antibodies and were confirmed by Western blot. Chronic HCV infection was defined by the presence of positive anti-HCV tests and the presence of HCV RNA at multiple time-points during follow up, without evidence for spontaneous clearance of HCV. None of HCV-infected participants received HCV-treatment.

For this study we included three groups of DU, namely: IDU who had an HIV/HCV coinfection ($n = 23$), IDU who had a chronic HCV infection ($n = 21$) and as a control for a drug using career IDU who were multiple exposed but uninfected (MEU) ($n = 8$) (Table 1). Subjects were included if they had an injecting drug use career greater than 2 years, were aged between 43 and 60 years and had PBMCs available. In addition to these follow-up samples we also included the first available PBMCs sample since study entry in the ACS for each subject. Unfortunately we were unable to include healthy donors with stored PBMC over the same time period. Therefore, to compare the study groups to healthy donors we recruited 2 groups of anonymous healthy donors from the blood bank, one aged between 43–60 years and one aged between 23–43 years, in order to match the ages of our study groups. In order to donate blood, voluntary participating individuals are tested for HIV, HBV, HCV and

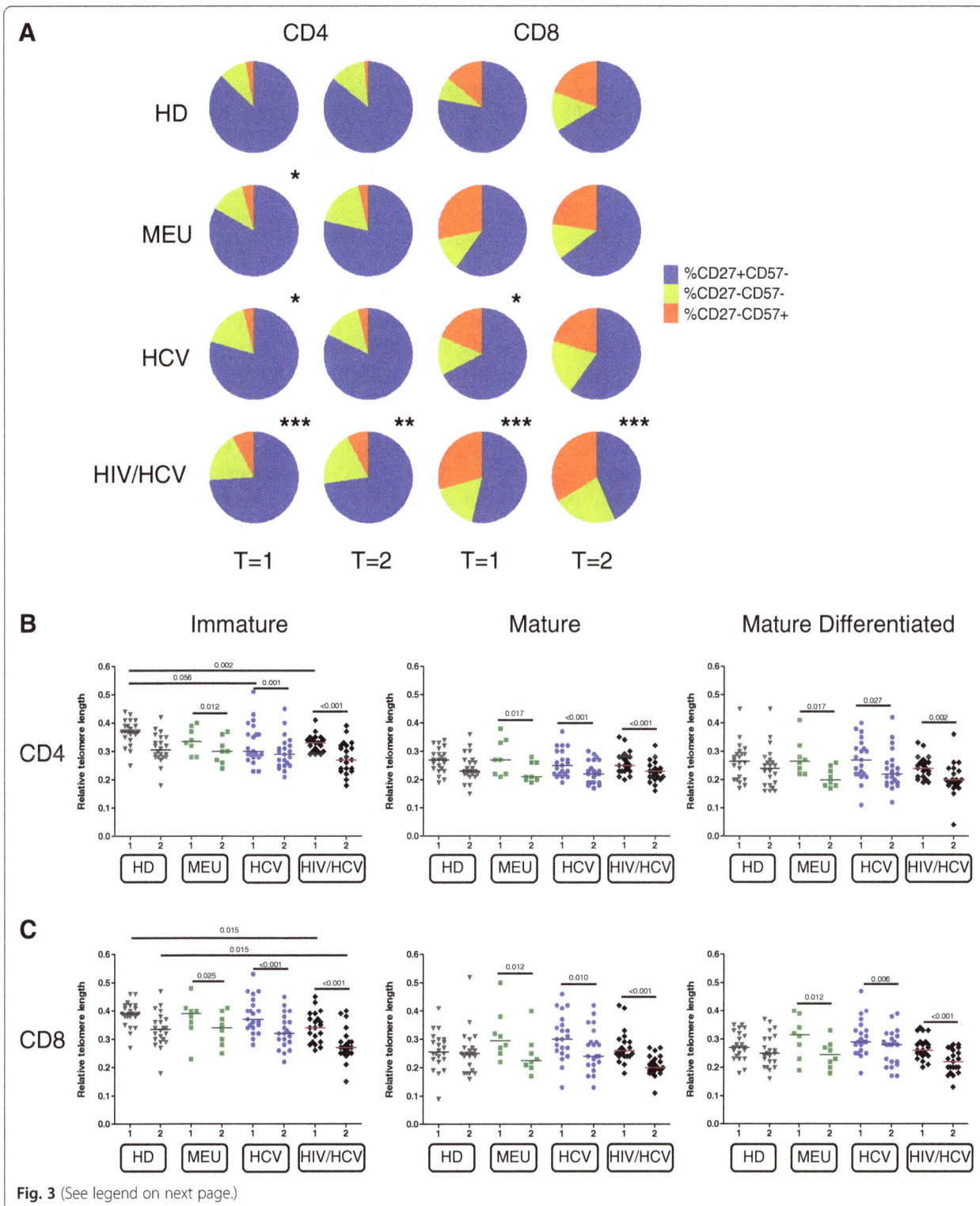

Fig. 3 (See legend on next page.)

(See figure on previous page.)
Fig. 3 No enhanced T-cell differentiation in time and lower relative telomere lengths (RTL) in immature CD4+ and CD8+ T cells. **a** Pie charts of normalised median frequencies of immature (blue), mature (green) and mature differentiated (red) CD4+ (*left panels*) and CD8+ T cells (*right panels*). Frequencies of immature cells were compared with HD for CD4+ and CD8+ T cells for time-point 1 and for time-point 2. *P*-values were calculated using the Mann- Whitney *U* test. *$p < 0.05$; **$p < 0.01$; *** < 0.001. **b** Relative telomere length (RTL) of peripheral CD4 T cell subsets (**b**) and CD8 T cell subsets (**c**) of: healthy donors (HD); multiple exposed uninfected (MEU) drug users (DU); HCV monoinfected IDU and HIV/HCV coinfected DU. RTL was measured in the first available sample since study entry (t = 1) and the most recent sample (t = 2) of MEU, HCV monoinfected and HIV/HCV coinfected DU. Subsets are depicted as follows: immature (CD27+CD57-), mature (CD27-CD57-) and mature differentiated (CD27-CD57+). HD at time point 1 and 2 are not the same individuals. The median time interval for all groups between time point 1 and 2 was 16.9 years. Medians are depicted in the plots. Wilcoxon-signed rank test was used for comparison within groups with the same individuals (MEU, HCV and HIV/HCV). Kruskall-Wallis test were used to compare between groups followed by post hoc Mann-Withney U tests

HEV. The blood bank actively screens for IDU and men who have sex with men or a history of IDU or men who have sex with men. These individuals were excluded from blood donation.

PBMC storage
From all study participants, PBMCs were isolated from heparinized blood using a Ficoll-Hypaque density gradient centrifugation and cryopreserved using a computerized freezing system in liquid nitrogen within 24 h of collection.

Flow cytometric analyses
Stored PBMCs were rapidly thawed and $1*10^6$ cells were stained in PBS with 0.5 % bovine serum albumin (BSA) and 0.1 % sodium azide using combinations of the following antibodies: CD4 Pacific Blue, CD3 AlexaFluor700, HLA-DR PerCP (Biolegend), CD8 Horizon V500, CD27 APC-eFluor780 (eBioscience), CD38 PE (Caltag) and PD-1 PerCP-Cy5.5. Cells were incubated with the antibodies for 20 min at 4 °C. After washing with PBS/0.5 % BSA, cells were fixed with Cellfix (BD) and directly analyzed by flow cytometry. For each sample a minimum of 100,000

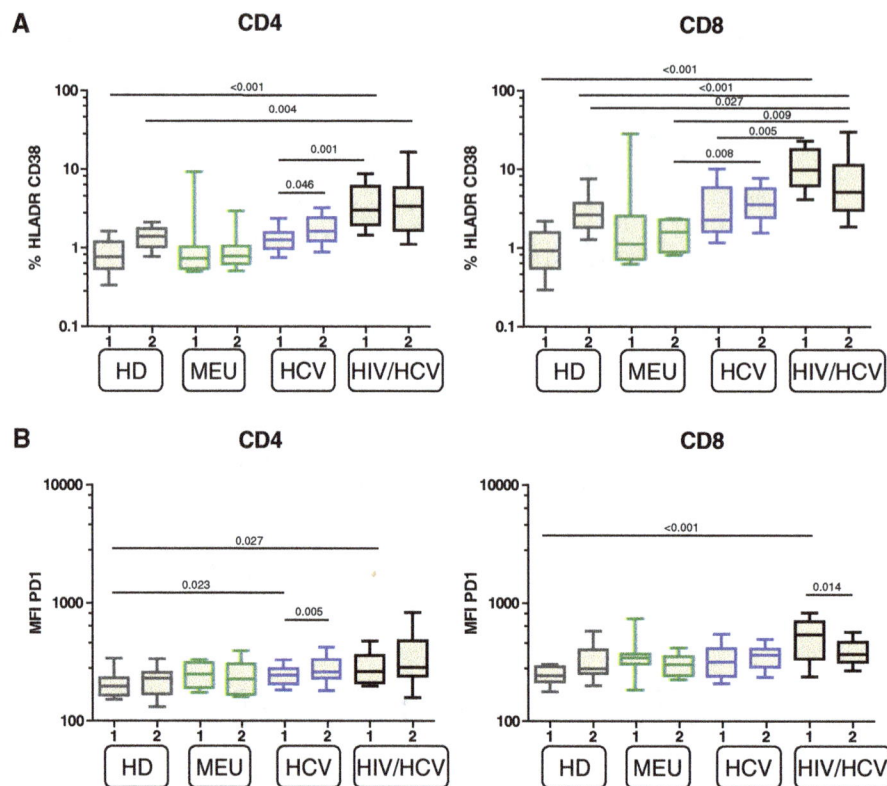

Fig. 4 Levels of immune activation and exhaustion are increased in HCV/HIV coinfected injecting drug users (IDU). Percentages of HLA-DR/CD38 positive peripheral CD4+ T cells and CD8+ T cells (**a**) of: healthy donors (HD); MEU IDU; HCV monoinfected IDU and HIV/HCV coinfected DU. RTL was measured in the first available sample since study entry (t = 2) and the most recent sample (t = 2) of MEU, HCV monoinfected and HIV/HCV coinfected DU. **b** Median fluorescent intensity (MFI) of PD1 in peripheral CD4+ T cells and CD8+ T cells. Box and whisker plots show the median and 10–90 percentiles. The Wilcoxon-signed rank test was used for comparison within groups with the same individuals (MEU, HCV and HIV/HCV). Kruskall-Wallis test were used to compare between groups followed by post hoc Mann-Withney U tests

cells were acquired using a LSRII FACS (BD) and data were processed using FACSDiva 6.0 software (BD).

Flowcytometric analysis of telomere length in T cell subsets

Telomere length of PBMCs was assessed using a five color flow cytometry fluorescent in situ hybridization (flow-FISH) protocol, adapted from Baerlocher et al. [27] Here, telomeres are hybridized to an AlexaFluor488 labeled peptide nucleic acid (PNA) telomeric $(C3TA2)^3$ probe and subsequently analyzed by flow cytometry. In short, stored PBMCs were rapidly thawed and $2*10^6$ cells were stained with heat-stable fluorochrome-labeled antibodies for CD3 Pacific Blue (eBioscience), CD8 V500 (BD), CD27 Alexa fluor 647 (BD) and CD57-biotin (Biolegend), followed by streptavidin-Cy3 (Sigma). After washing, the cells were fixed with bis(sulfosuccinimidyl)-suberate (BS^3, Pierce) for 30 min at 4 °C in the dark. Cells were washed with PBS and incubated for 10 min with an hybridization solution, with and without the PNA probe and 15 min at 82 °C to denature the DNA. After 1 h of hybridization at room temperature and in the dark, cells were washed and analyzed immediately by flow cytometry. Samples were gated on live, singlet CD3 $^+$ T cells. Calf thymocytes were included in each experiment as an internal control. The gating strategy is shown in Additional file 2: Figure S1. Relative telomere length (RTL) of each sample was calculated as the ratio between the median fluorescent intensity (MFI) of the T cell subset of interest with probe (minus the MFI without probe) divided by the MFI of the calf thymocytes with probe (minus the MFI without probe). All experiments were performed in duplo and RTLs were averaged per sample.

Statistical analyses

To test for statistical significance between groups we used the Kruskall-Wallis test and if significant followed by post-hoc Mann-Whitney U test. Comparisons within groups (related samples) were made using the paired Wilcoxon signed rank test, otherwise the Mann-Whitney U test was used. A two sided p-value <0.05 was considered statistically significant. To investigate whether the decline in RTL could be confounded by age we performed a sensitivity analysis using a linear regression model with age as a fixed variable. All analyses were performed using SPSS (version 20.0; SPSS Inc.) statistical software. Graphs were made using Graphpad (version 6.1; GraphPad Software, Inc.)

Discussion

In this longitudinal study we observed significantly decreased telomere lengths among ageing HIV/HCV coinfected IDU as compared to healthy donors. In the period in which IDU had no access to cART, the impact of HIV/HCV on telomere length was noticeable already at the first timepoint in infection that we analysed, in both the CD4 and CD8 T-cell compartment with significantly reduced telomere lengths. During a period of 16 years we observed no increased decline of telomere length between the study groups. These data suggest that the lower telomere lengths were induced earlier in infection. HCV monoinfected IDU had significantly decreased telomere lengths in their CD4$^+$ T cells, but CD8$^+$ T cells were not affected by increased telomere erosion. Over time we observed no increase in the percentage of differentiated cells in each study group, but we did observe a continued decline of telomere erosion. Therefore it is unlikely that T-cell differentiation alone explains the continued telomere erosion. Telomere decline could be explained by increased peripheral levels of activation (HLA-DR$^+$CD38$^+$), mature differentiated (CD27$^-$CD57$^+$) cells and exhaustion (PD-1) in peripheral T cells of HCV monoinfected and HIV/HCV coinfected IDU which indicates a state of chronic immune activation.

As expected, we observed that telomere length decreased over time in all IDU groups. However this was independent of viral coinfections (HCV or HIV/HCV). Interestingly, at a relatively young age the telomere length of predominantly CD8$^+$ T cells, but also CD4$^+$ T cells, was markedly decreased in HIV/HCV coinfected individuals and was comparable to more than 15 year older healthy donors. As most HIV/HCV coinfected individuals were cART naïve early during infection, the immune system responds to HIV with high levels of activation and proliferation rates [37]. Consequently HIV drives T cells to increasingly differentiated phenotypes that are oligoclonally expanded, less functional and more prone to apoptosis [38]. We demonstrated that loss of telomere length is not simply due to increased differentiation but mainly to continued immune activation. Importantly, this study demonstrates that the loss in telomere length mainly occurred at the first time-point in infection that we analysed and was not restored to the level of healthy individuals with the initiation of cART. We could not rule out that cART, via telomerase inhibition [39], negatively affects telomere length. However a recent cross-sectional study by Zanet et al. demonstrated no association between low telomere length and cART exposure [40].

Here we found that HCV monoinfected IDU had lower CD4$^+$ T cell telomere lengths than healthy donors at the first timepoint in infection that we analysed, suggesting that HCV on its own may have an effect on immune senescence. However, CD8$^+$ T cell telomere length was not affected. Unfortunately we had no clinical outcomes to relate to, but a hospital-based study found that, independent of age, decreased CD4$^+$

memory telomere length was associated with increased liver fibrosis [41]. In addition, longer CD4[+] and CD8[+] T cell telomere lengths were both associated with a sustained virological response following HCV treatment. We demonstrated that in HCV monoinfected IDU the decreased telomere length in CD4[+] T cells occurred mainly in the immature T cells. Although this population consists of both naïve and central memory cells [42], reduced numbers of CD4 naïve T cells and reduced recent thymic emigrants have been associated with HCV infection, especially if fibrosis is present [43, 44]. This fits with a model in which CD4[+] T cells are continuously activated during persistent HCV infection, especially when the infection aggravates.. However, due to a lack of samples we were unable to investigate the specific responses of HIV/HCV coinfected DU.

The exact mechanisms through which HIV, HCV and natural ageing collectively affect disease progression remains to be resolved. Accumulating evidence points towards a role for systemic immune senescence affecting multiple organs/tissues. Data from a recent study among IDU demonstrated that higher levels of interleukin 6, a proinflammmatory cytokine, were independently associated with HCV monoinfection, HIV/HCV coinfection and increasing age [45]. Decreased telomere length has also been associated with atherosclerosis and cardiovascular disease, and is likely to be correlated with interleukin 6 levels [46].

Of interest, MEU IDU tended to have lower levels of immune activation compared to healthy donors. This special group of IDU has been shown to have detectable HIV-specific [47] and HCV-specific T-cell responses [48], indicating their exposure to both infections. The notion of a naturally occurring resistance to certain viral pathogens has major implications for T-cell vaccine development. In a recent study though, robust activation of natural killer cells, but not HCV-specific adaptive immune responses, was associated with protection against infection with HCV among MEU DU [49].

There were several limitations in this study. Due to instability to heat we were unable to use CD45RA and CCR7 as markers of memory and differentiation in our assay. Interestingly, it did enable us to demonstrate that loss of CD27 was significantly associated with telomere loss in both CD4[+] and CD8[+] T cell, which occurred before the upregulation of CD57 [31].

This study is limited by the unknown duration of HIV and HCV infection. However, as the observed peak incidence of HIV in Amsterdam occurred during the 80's [50] we assumed that our first time point of analysis was close to the actual infection time point. For HCV the observed peak prevalence also occurred during the 80's. We demonstrated that the reduction in telomere length

already occurred at the first time-point and that we did not find any difference in the rate of telomere length decline over a period of almost 17 years between MEU, HCV monoinfected and HIV coinfected IDU. This suggests that the telomere decline occurred earlier during infection. But, we can not rule out that the HIV or HCV infected IDU had lower telomere lengths pre-acquisition of HIV or HCV. To prove our hypothesis it would be of future interest to investigate telomere decline in HIV and HCV seroconverters. Unfortunately we had no access to bloodsamples of healthy donors followed over time. Because we used different healthy donors for the two time-points the decline in RTL could be biased by inter-individual variations.

Conclusions
We found increased levels of immune senescence at the first timepoint that we analysed in HCV mono- and HIV/HCV coinfected DU. This suggests that HCV mono-infection and HIV/HCV coinfection enhance T-cell immune-senescence probably early during infection. As both viruses have detrimental long-term effects on morbidity and mortality, these data express the need for early treatment, both for HCV and HIV infection.

Competing interests
The authors who have taken part in this study declare they do not have anything to disclose regarding funding from industry or conflict of interest with respect to this manuscript.

Authors' contributions
BG and DB participated in the design of the study. BG and NN performed the research and analysed the data. BG was responsible for the statistical analyses. BG drafted the manuscript. DB critically revised the manuscript. All authors have read and approved the final manuscript.

Acknowledgments
The authors would like to thank all subjects for study participation; research nurses L.C. del Grande and W.M. van der Veldt for coordination, data collection and blood sampling; Dr. I. Schellens and Dr. J.A.M. Borghans for their critical appraisal on this manuscript.

Funding
This work supported by the Amsterdam Cohort Studies (ACS) on HIV infection and AIDS, a collaboration between the Amsterdam Public Health Service, the Academic Medical Center of the University of Amsterdam, Sanquin Blood Supply Foundation, and the University Medical Center Utrecht. The ACS is part of the Netherlands HIV Monitoring Foundation and

is financially supported by the Netherlands National Institute for Public Health and the Environment. Website: http://www.amsterdamcohortstudies.org/. The funders had no role in study design, data collection and analyses, decision to publish, or preparation of the manuscript.

Author details
[1]Department of Research, Cluster Infectious Diseases, Public Health Service, Amsterdam, The Netherlands. [2]Center for Infection and Immunity Amsterdam (CINIMA), Academic Medical Center, Amsterdam, The Netherlands. [3]Department of Immunology, University Medical Center Utrecht, Utrecht, The Netherlands. [4]Department of Internal Medicine, University Medical Center Utrecht, Utrecht, The Netherlands. [5]Present address: Department of Immune Mechanisms, Center for Infectious Disease Control, National Institute for Public Health and the Environment (RIVM), Bilthoven, The Netherlands.

References

1. Pawelec G, Effros RB, Caruso C, Remarque E, Barnett Y, Solana R. T cells and aging (update February 1999). Front Biosci. 1999;4:D216–69.
2. Lynch HE, Goldberg GL, Chidgey A, Van den Brink MR, Boyd R, Sempowski GD. Thymic involution and immune reconstitution. Trends Immunol. 2009; 30(7):366–73. doi:10.1016/j.it.2009.04.003.
3. Deeks SG. HIV infection, inflammation, immunosenescence, and aging. Annu Rev Med. 2011;62:141–55. doi:10.1146/annurev-med-042909-093756.
4. Harley CB, Futcher AB, Greider CW. Telomeres shorten during ageing of human fibroblasts. Nature. 1990;345(6274):458–60. doi:10.1038/345458a0.
5. Cawthon RM, Smith KR, O'Brien E, Sivatchenko A, Kerber RA. Association between telomere length in blood and mortality in people aged 60 years or older. Lancet. 2003;361(9355):393–5. doi:10.1016/S0140-6736(03)12384-7.
6. Dwyer R, Topp L, Maher L, Power R, Hellard M, Walsh N, et al. Prevalences and correlates of non-viral injecting-related injuries and diseases in a convenience sample of Australian injecting drug users. Drug Alcohol Depend. 2009;100(1–2):9–16. doi:10.1016/j.drugalcdep.2008.08.016.
7. Crofts N, Aitken CK. Incidence of bloodborne virus infection and risk behaviours in a cohort of injecting drug users in Victoria, 1990–1995. Med J Aust. 1997;167(1):17–20.
8. Memon MI, Memon MA. Hepatitis C: an epidemiological review. J Viral Hepat. 2002;9(2):84–100.
9. Vickerman P, Hickman M, May M, Kretzschmar M, Wiessing L. Can hepatitis C virus prevalence be used as a measure of injection-related human immunodeficiency virus risk in populations of injecting drug users? An ecological analysis. Addiction. 2010;105(2):311–8. doi:10.1111/j.1360-0443.2009.02759.x.
10. Seeff LB. The history of the "natural history" of hepatitis C (1968–2009). Liver Int. 2009;29 Suppl 1:89–99. doi:10.1111/j.1478-3231.2008.01927.x.
11. Mathers BM, Degenhardt L, Phillips B, Wiessing L, Hickman M, Strathdee SA, et al. Global epidemiology of injecting drug use and HIV among people who inject drugs: a systematic review. Lancet. 2008;372(9651):1733–45. doi:10.1016/S0140-6736(08)61311-2.
12. Armstrong GL. Injection drug users in the United States, 1979-2002: an aging population. Arch Intern Med. 2007;167(2):166–73. doi:10.1001/archinte.167.2.166.
13. Grebely J, Dore GJ. What is killing people with hepatitis C virus infection? Semin Liver Dis. 2011;31(4):331–9. doi:10.1055/s-0031-1297922.
14. Klein RS. Trends related to aging and co-occurring disorders in HIV-infected drug users. Subst Use Misuse. 2011;46(2-3):233–44. doi:10.3109/10826084.2011.522843.
15. Salter ML, Lau B, Go VF, Mehta SH, Kirk GD. HIV infection, immune suppression, and uncontrolled viremia are associated with increased multimorbidity among aging injection drug users. Clin Infect Dis. 2011; 53(12):1256–64. doi:10.1093/cid/cir673.
16. Ferrando-Martinez S, Ruiz-Mateos E, Romero-Sanchez MC, Munoz-Fernandez MA, Viciana P, Genebat M, et al. HIV infection-related premature immunosenescence: high rates of immune exhaustion after short time of infection. Curr HIV Res. 2011;9(5):289–94.
17. Effros RB. Genetic alterations in the ageing immune system: impact on infection and cancer. Mech Ageing Dev. 2003;124(1):71–7.
18. Losina E, Schackman BR, Sadownik SN, Gebo KA, Walensky RP, Chiosi JJ, et al. Racial and sex disparities in life expectancy losses among HIV-infected persons in the united states: impact of risk behavior, late initiation, and early discontinuation of antiretroviral therapy. Clin Infect Dis. 2009;49(10):1570–8. doi:10.1086/644772.
19. Antiretroviral Therapy Cohort C. Life expectancy of individuals on combination antiretroviral therapy in high-income countries: a collaborative analysis of 14 cohort studies. Lancet. 2008;372(9635):293–9. doi:10.1016/S0140-6736(08)61113-7.
20. Jacobson IM, Cacoub P, Dal Maso L, Harrison SA, Younossi ZM. Manifestations of chronic hepatitis C virus infection beyond the liver. Clin Gastroenterol Hepatol. 2010;8(12):1017–29. doi:10.1016/j.cgh.2010.08.026.
21. Negro F. Hepatitis C, in 2013: HCV causes systemic disorders that can be cured. Nat Rev Gastroenterol Hepatol. 2014;11(2):77–8. doi:10.1038/nrgastro.2013.222.
22. Thimme R, Binder M, Bartenschlager R. Failure of innate and adaptive immune responses in controlling hepatitis C virus infection. FEMS Microbiol Rev. 2012;36(3):663–83. doi:10.1111/j.1574-6976.2011.00319.x.
23. Sulkowski MS, Mehta SH, Torbenson MS, Higgins Y, Brinkley SC, de Oca RM, et al. Rapid fibrosis progression among HIV/hepatitis C virus-co-infected adults. Aids. 2007;21(16):2209–16. doi:10.1097/QAD.0b013e3282f10de9.
24. Kovacs A, Karim R, Mack WJ, Xu J, Chen Z, Operskalski E, et al. Activation of CD8 T cells predicts progression of HIV infection in women coinfected with hepatitis C virus. J Infect Dis. 2010;201(6):823–34. doi:10.1086/650997.
25. van der Helm J, Geskus R, Sabin C, Meyer L, Del Amo J, Chene G, et al. Effect of HCV infection on cause-specific mortality after HIV seroconversion, before and after 1997. Gastroenterology. 2013;144(4):751–60. doi:10.1053/j.gastro.2012.12.026. e2.
26. Aubert G, Hills M, Lansdorp PM. Telomere length measurement-caveats and a critical assessment of the available technologies and tools. Mutat Res. 2012;730(1–2):59–67. doi:10.1016/j.mrfmmm.2011.04.003.
27. Baerlocher GM, Vulto I, de Jong G, Lansdorp PM. Flow cytometry and FISH to measure the average length of telomeres (flow FISH). Nat Protoc. 2006; 1(5):2365–76. doi:10.1038/nprot.2006.263.
28. van Baarle D, Nanlohy NM, Otto S, Plunkett FJ, Fletcher JM, Akbar AN. Progressive telomere shortening of Epstein-Barr virus-specific memory T cells during HIV infection: contributor to exhaustion? J infect Dis. 2008; 198(9):1353–7. doi:10.1086/592170.
29. Hoare M, Shankar A, Shah M, Rushbrook S, Gelson W, Davies S, et al. gamma-H2AX + CD8+ T lymphocytes cannot respond to IFN-alpha, IL-2 or IL-6 in chronic hepatitis C virus infection. J Hepatol. 2013;58(5):868–74. doi:10.1016/j.jhep.2012.12.009.
30. Papagno L, Spina CA, Marchant A, Salio M, Rufer N, Little S, et al. Immune activation and CD8+ T-cell differentiation towards senescence in HIV-1 infection. PLoS Biol. 2004;2(2):E20. doi:10.1371/journal.pbio.0020020.
31. Brenchley JM, Karandikar NJ, Betts MR, Ambrozak DR, Hill BJ, Crotty LE, et al. Expression of CD57 defines replicative senescence and antigen-induced apoptotic death of CD8+ T cells. Blood. 2003;101(7):2711–20. doi:10.1182/blood-2002-07-2103.
32. Plunkett FJ, Franzese O, Finney HM, Fletcher JM, Belaramani LL, Salmon M, et al. The loss of telomerase activity in highly differentiated CD8 + CD28-CD27- T cells is associated with decreased Akt (Ser473) phosphorylation. J Immunol. 2007;178(12):7710–9.
33. Appay V, Papagno L, Spina CA, Hansasuta P, King A, Jones L, et al. Dynamics of T cell responses in HIV infection. J Immunol. 2002;168(7):3660–6.
34. Henson SM, Franzese O, Macaulay R, Libri V, Azevedo RI, Kiani-Alikhan S, et al. KLRG1 signaling induces defective Akt (ser473) phosphorylation and proliferative dysfunction of highly differentiated CD8+ T cells. Blood. 2009; 113(26):6619–28. doi:10.1182/blood-2009-01-199588.
35. van den Hoek JA, Coutinho RA, van Haastrecht HJ, van Zadelhoff AW, Goudsmit J. Prevalence and risk factors of HIV infections among drug users and drug-using prostitutes in Amsterdam. Aids. 1988;2(1):55–60.
36. van den Berg CH, Grady BP, Schinkel J, van de Laar T, Molenkamp R, van Houdt R, et al. Female sex and IL28B, a synergism for spontaneous viral clearance in hepatitis C virus (HCV) seroconverters from a community-based cohort. PLoS One. 2011;6(11):e27555. doi:10.1371/journal.pone.0027555.
37. Srinivasula S, Lempicki RA, Adelsberger JW, Huang CY, Roark J, Lee PI, et al. Differential effects of HIV viral load and CD4 count on proliferation of naive and memory CD4 and CD8 T lymphocytes. Blood. 2011;118(2):262–70. doi:10.1182/blood-2011-02-335174.

38. Desai S, Landay A. Early immune senescence in HIV disease. Curr HIV/AIDS
     Rep. 2010;7(1):4–10. doi:10.1007/s11904-009-0038-4.

39. Leeansyah E, Cameron PU, Solomon A, Tennakoon S, Velayudham P,
     Gouillou M, et al. Inhibition of telomerase activity by human
     immunodeficiency virus (HIV) nucleos(t)ide reverse transcriptase inhibitors: a
     potential factor contributing to HIV-associated accelerated aging. J Infect
     Dis. 2013;207(7):1157–65. doi:10.1093/infdis/jit006.

40. Zanet DL, Thorne A, Singer J, Maan EJ, Sattha B, Le Campion A, et al.
     Association between short leukocyte telomere length and HIV infection in a
     cohort study: No evidence of a relationship with antiretroviral therapy. Clin
     Infect Dis. 2014;58(9):1322–32. doi:10.1093/cid/ciu051.

41. Hoare M, Gelson WT, Das A, Fletcher JM, Davies SE, Curran MD, et al.
     CD4+ T-lymphocyte telomere length is related to fibrosis stage, clinical
     outcome and treatment response in chronic hepatitis C virus infection.
     J Hepatol. 2010;53(2):252–60. doi:10.1016/j.jhep.2010.03.005.

42. De Jong R, Brouwer M, Hooibrink B, Van der Pouw-Kraan T, Miedema F, Van
     Lier RA. The CD27- subset of peripheral blood memory CD4+ lymphocytes
     contains functionally differentiated T lymphocytes that develop by
     persistent antigenic stimulation in vivo. Eur J Immunol. 1992;22(4):993–9.
     doi:10.1002/eji.1830220418.

43. Hartling HJ, Gaardbo JC, Ronit A, Salem M, Laye M, Clausen MR, et al.
     Impaired thymic output in patients with chronic hepatitis C virus infection.
     Scand J Immunol. 2013. doi:10.1111/sji.12096.

44. Yonkers NL, Sieg S, Rodriguez B, Anthony DD. Reduced naive CD4 T cell
     numbers and impaired induction of CD27 in response to T cell receptor
     stimulation reflect a state of immune activation in chronic hepatitis C virus
     infection. J Infect Dis. 2011;203(5):635–45. doi:10.1093/infdis/jiq101.

45. Salter ML, Lau B, Mehta SH, Go VF, Leng S, Kirk GD. Correlates of elevated
     interleukin-6 and C-reactive protein in persons with or at high-risk for HCV
     and HIV infections. J Acquir Immune Defic Syndr. 2013. doi:10.1097/QAI.
     0b013e3182a7ee2e.

46. Savale L, Chaouat A, Bastuji-Garin S, Marcos E, Boyer L, Maitre B, et al.
     Shortened telomeres in circulating leukocytes of patients with chronic
     obstructive pulmonary disease. Am J Respir Crit Care Med. 2009;179(7):
     566–71. doi:10.1164/rccm.200809-1398OC.

47. Makedonas G, Bruneau J, Lin H, Sekaly RP, Lamothe F, Bernard NF. HIV-specific
     CD8 T-cell activity in uninfected injection drug users is associated with
     maintenance of seronegativity. Aids. 2002;16(12):1595–602.

48. Ruys TA, Nanlohy NM, van den Berg CH, Hassink E, Beld M, van de Laar T, et
     al. HCV-specific T-cell responses in injecting drug users: evidence for
     previous exposure to HCV and a role for CD4+ T cells focussing on
     nonstructural proteins in viral clearance. J Viral Hepat. 2008;15(6):409–20.
     doi:10.1111/j.1365-2893.2007.00963.x.

49. Sugden PB, Cameron B, Mina M, Lloyd AR, on behalf of the Hi. Protection
     against hepatitis C infection via NK cells in highly-exposed uninfected
     injecting drug users. J Hepatol. 2014. doi:10.1016/j.jhep.2014.05.013.

50. de Vos AS, van der Helm JJ, Matser A, Prins M, Kretzschmar ME. Decline
     in incidence of HIV and hepatitis C virus infection among injecting
     drug users in Amsterdam; evidence for harm reduction? Addiction.
     2013;108(6):1070–81. doi:10.1111/add.12125.

Herpes virus seroepidemiology in the adult Swedish population

Jan Olsson[1*], Eloise Kok[2], Rolf Adolfsson[3], Hugo Lövheim[4] and Fredrik Elgh[1]

Abstract

Background: Herpes viruses establish a life-long latency and can cause symptoms during both first-time infection and later reactivation. The aim of the present study was to describe the seroepidemiology of Herpes simplex type 1 (HSV1), Herpes simplex type 2 (HSV2), Cytomegalovirus (CMV), Varicella Zoster virus (VZV) and Human herpes virus type 6 (HHV6) in an adult Swedish population (35–95 years of age).

Methods: Presence of antibodies against the respective viruses in serum from individuals in the Betula study was determined with an enzyme-linked immunosorbent assay (ELISA). Singular samples from 535 persons (53.9% women, mean age at inclusion 62.7 ± 14.4 years) collected 2003-2005 were analyzed for the five HHVs mentioned above. In addition, samples including follow-up samples collected 1988–2010 from 3,444 persons were analyzed for HSV.

Results: Prevalence of HSV1 was 79.4%, HSV2 12.9%, CMV 83.2%, VZV 97.9%, and HHV6 97.5%. Herpes virus infections were more common among women ($p = 0.010$) and a lower age-adjusted HSV seroprevalence was found in later birth cohorts ($p < 0.001$). The yearly incidence of HSV infection was estimated at 14.0/1000.

Conclusion: Women are more often seropositive for HHV, especially HSV2. Age-adjusted seroprevalence for HSV was lower in later birth cohorts indicating a decreasing childhood and adolescent risk of infection.

Keywords: Herpes, Herpes simplex, Cytomegalovirus, Varicella zoster virus, Seroprevalence, Epidemiology

Introduction

Human herpesviruses (HHV1-8) are ubiquitous human pathogens with a global distribution. Epidemiological studies have identified geographic location, socioeconomic status, and age as primary factors for acquisition of HHV infection [1]. The infection cycle involves a primary infection, followed by a latency phase that may be interrupted by episodes of reactivated infection [1]. Although this pattern of infection is shared by all HHVs, variation among the included viral species exists e.g. concerning the tissue involved in the latency phase of the infection. HHV1-3 (HSV1, HSV2 and VZV) establish latency in sensory ganglia, while the other HHVs (EBV, CMV, HHV6-8) employ lymphocytes, monocytes, and sometimes also epithelium for latency. When reactivated, HHV1-3 spread along nerves, HHV4 (EBV), HHV7 and HHV8 expand in lymphocyte populations, while HHV5 (CMV) and HHV6 often spread systemically [1]. HHVs have been attributed a role in the development of chronic disorders, such as Alzheimer's disease [2–6], cardiovascular disease [7–9], cognitive impairment [10, 11], and depression [12–14]. We, and others researching the field of late neurological sequela from HHV infections have had great use of serological screening in cohorts of adult and elderly individuals [5, 6, 15–18]. Although literature on the seroepidemiology of HHV infections is extensive, most studies focus on young individuals or selected populations posing already known risks from HHV infections [19–22]. We therefore performed the present study with the aim to estimate the prevalence of HHV1 (HSV1), HHV2 (HSV2), HHV3 (VZV), HHV5 (CMV), and HHV6 in serum samples retrieved from individuals in the Betula study [23], reflecting a population of adults, including the elderly, in Sweden. For HSV1&2 combined, we further analyzed a larger cohort with longitudinal samples allowing for estimation on the trend in yearly incidence.

* Correspondence: jan.l.olsson@umu.se
[1]Department of Clinical Microbiology, Virology, Umeå University, Umeå, Sweden
Full list of author information is available at the end of the article

Methods

Participants

The Betula study is an ongoing longitudinal, prospective cohort study with the overall aim of investigating how memory function and health develop across the adult life span [23]. The study is designed as a mixed cohort and cross-sectional study, modeled after Schaie [24, 25], to enable the separation of age, cohort and time of measurement effects.

The Betula study started in 1988 by recruiting 1,000 persons from the municipality of Umeå – a municipality of about 120,000 inhabitants located in Northern Sweden. The participants were randomly selected from the Swedish Population Registry, and were invited to participate via an introductory letter and a follow-up telephone call. Recruitment continued until participants within all age groups were fully enrolled. In the first wave, 1,976 persons were contacted to obtain 1,000 participants. To fulfill the primary study aims, persons with severe visual or auditory deficits, cognitive deficits due to intellectual disability, severe psychiatric illness, suspected dementia, and those who did not speak and understand the Swedish language were excluded.

The first cohort (sample 1; S1) of 1,000 persons was investigated in 1988 – 1990 (time-point 1; T1), and was followed-up every five years thereafter until 2008 – 2010 (T2 to T5). Additional cohorts, from the same geographical region were included at each subsequent wave of investigation (T2 to T5). At T2 (1993 – 1995) two cohorts (S2, $n = 997$, and S3, $n = 966$) were enrolled, at T3 (1998 – 2000) one cohort of 563 persons (S4), and T4 (2003 – 2005) another cohort of 562 persons (S5) was enrolled.

S1 and S2 comprised persons aged 35, 40, 45, 50, 55, 60, 65, 70, 75 and 80 years at inclusion, with up to 100 individuals in each age group. The S3 cohort comprised persons aged 40 to 85 at inclusion, up to 100 in each age group, and the S4 and S5 cohorts comprised people in 12 different age groups from 35 to 95 years old at inclusion, with up to 50 in each group. The proportion of men and women in each cohort and age group was equal, roughly corresponding to the gender distribution in the general population.

The S3 cohort, like S1, was followed with repeated examinations every five years until T5. A part of the S2 cohort was re-examined at T3 but not thereafter, whereas S4 (1998 – 2000) and S5 (2004 – 2006) were examined only at the time of inclusion.

Samples included for the cross-sectional analysis of anti-HSV1, anti-HSV2, anti-VZV, anti-CMV and anti-HHV6 were all stored serum samples available from S5T4 ($n = 535$, age 35-95, sampling timepoint 2003-2005). One sub-cohort, sampled once, was selected from the Betula study to make assessment of the five HHVs seroprevalence affordable, and this particular cohort (S5T4) was found suitable because its samples are relatively recent, and it contains participants of a wide age-distribution. Samples included in the additional cross-sectional and longitudinal analysis of anti-HSV were all stored serum samples available from S1-5 T1-5. The total number of participants was 3,444, from which 2,213 contributed one sample, and 1,231 provided two or more samples from different sampling timepoints (1988 – 1990, 1993 – 1995, 1998 – 2000, 2003 – 2005, and 2008 – 2010).

Serum analyses

Frozen serum samples were thawed and analyzed for anti-HSV, anti-VZV, anti-CMV, and anti-HHV6 IgG antibodies using Enzyme-linked immunosorbent assays (ELISA). In a procedure to separate anti-HSV positive samples into anti-HSV1, anti-HSV2, or anti-HSV1 + 2 positive, anti- HSV positive samples were further analyzed for presence of anti-HSV2 IgG, afterwhich anti-HSV2 positive samples were analyzed for presence of anti-HSV1 IgG. For anti-HSV, anti-VZV, and anti-CMV, ELISA assays developed in-house were used [26–28], for anti-HSV1 and anti-HSV2 HerpeSelect®-assays (Focus diagnostics) were utilised, and for anti-HHV6 the HHV-6 IgG Antibody ELISA Kit (Advanced biotechnologies inc.) was used. For the in-house methods, antigens against HSV, VZV, and CMV were acquired by growth of HSV1 Umeå clinical isolate 3458-13 on GMK cells, VZV strain SMI 1197 on VeroE6 cells, and CMV strain Ad169 on HumB cells, respectively. Plasma incubation on antigen-coated ELISA plates was performed at 4 °C overnight. Analyses were performed in duplicate using uninfected cell extract as a negative control. In each ELISA run, high and low positive controls and a negative control were included to monitor the quality of individual runs and inter-assay variation. Plasma were diluted 1/420 in phosphate buffered saline supplemented with 0.05% (v/v) Tween-20 and 1% dried milk. IgG antibodies were identified using goat F(ab)2 anti-human IgG, alkaline phosphatase conjugate (Invitrogen) diluted 1/6000, and developed using p-nitrophenyl phosphate disodium substrate (Sigma-Aldrich). The IgG antibody activity of the individual sample was expressed in arbitrary units (AU) as a percentage of the net-absorbance at 405 nm (absorbance of virus-coated well minus absorbance of control antigen well) of the positive control. Samples with IgG values of 5 AU or above were regarded as positive for HHV IgG antibody content.

All serological methods were run according to routine analyses performed in the clinical diagnostics lab, which is a part of Norrlands Universitetssjukhus (NUS). The methods are accredited by Swedac according to ISO 17025 standards.

Statistics

Chi-2 test, independent sample t-test, and Pearson correlation were used for univariate analyses as appropriate. A multiple logistic regression model was used to differentiate between the effect of the variables age, sex, and birth year of HSV IgG seroprevalence. To plot HSV seroprevalence in relation to age, a linear regression model was used to fit regression lines.

The HSV incidence was calculated by dividing the number of new cases with the total follow-up time (person-years) among HSV negative participants. New cases were calculated as the number of seroconvertants subtracted by the number of serorevertants.

$P < 0.05$ was regarded as statistically significant. The SPSS 20.0 software for Mac was used for statistical calculations.

Results

The seroprevalence of IgG antibodies towards five common human herpes viruses was cross-sectionally investigated in a representative sample (T5 S4) from an adult Swedish population. The sample included 535 people (274 women and 261 men) aged 35 to 95 years (mean age 60.7 ± 16.2 years). The seroprevalence of IgG antibodies against HSV1, HSV2, VZV, CMV and HHV6 are presented in Table 1.

The relationship between age and sex, and the presence of herpes virus antibodies was investigated (Table 2). Women were seropositive for on average 3.8 $\pm 0.7/5$ of the analyzed antibodies, compared to 3.6 $\pm 0.7/5$ for men, $p = 0.010$. Women were more likely to be HSV2- positive compared to men ($p = 0.013$). Age correlated positively with CMV- and HSV1-IgG presence ($p < 0.001$ and $p < 0.001$ respectively), but negatively with HHV6-IgG presence ($p = 0.034$). A relationship between the presence of anti-HSV1 IgG and anti-CMV IgG was found (Pearson's r 0.167, $p < 0.001$), but not between any other combination.

Table 1 Herpes virus seroprevalence, $N = 535$

Virus IgG antibodies	$N_{positive}/N_{total}$	%	95% confidence interval
Herpes simplex type 1	425/535	79.4	76.0 – 82.9
Herpes simplex type 2	69[a]/535	12.9	10.1 – 15.8
Varicella zoster virus	524/535	97.9	96.7 – 99.1
Cytomegalovirus	445/535	83.2	80.0 – 86.4
Human herpes virus type 6	517/530[b]	97.5	96.2 – 98.9

Note: [a]Among the 69 HSV2 positive, 50 were HSV1 positive and 16 were HSV1 negative
[b]Five samples were unavailable for HHV-6 analysis

A larger sample of 3,444 participants from all five cohorts (S1-5 T1-5) (sampled 1988-2010) was investigated for HSV IgG seroprevalence with an ELISA developed in-house. The 535 people in the analyses above were a subsample of the 3,444. All singular samples and the first sample from persons that contributed multiple samples were included. The age ranged between 35 and 95 years, and the mean age was 62.7 ± 14.4. There were 1,860 (54%) women. The anti-HSV IgG seroprevalence was 3,038/3,444 = 88.2%. In this sample HSV was significantly more common among women (1,671 (89.8%) versus 1,367 men (86.3%), p = 0.001), and the mean age of HSV positive individuals was higher, when compared to HSV negative (63.9 ± 14.0 years versus 53.6 ± 14.0 years, $p < 0.001$).

In a multiple linear regression model with age and sex as independent variables, and anti-HSV IgG seropositivity as the outcome variable, the calculated increase in anti-HSV seroprevalence for each subsequent year of age was 0.0051. This value thus corresponds to 0.0051 x 3,444 = 17.6 estimated new cases each year.

The age, sex, and year of birth of the participants were included in a logistic regression model to individually investigate the effects of these three variables on the outcome variable anti-HSV IgG seropositivity (Table 3). Female sex and earlier year of birth was associated with a higher anti-HSV IgG prevalence, while increasing age was not. The birth cohort effect, giving lower age-specific anti-HSV IgG prevalence in later birth cohorts, is illustrated in Fig. 1 showing HSV IgG seroprevalence in relation to age in two temporally separated study cohorts (S1T1: 1988-1990 and S5T4: 2003-2005).

Samples from 1,231 people who contributed one or several follow-up sample(s) were included in a longitudinal analysis. These people contributed in total 14,089.83 person-years (PY) of follow-up time, defined as the timespan from first sample until the last sample, of which participants who were anti-HSV IgG free at the beginning of each period contributed 1,289.83 PY follow-up time. During the follow-up period, 28 people seroconverted while 10 people seroreverted, hence 28 – 10 = 18 was regarded as the number of incident HSV cases. We treated serorevertants as false negatives and assumed a similar frequency of false-positives. HSV incidence was hence calculated as 18/1,289.83 = 14.0/1000 PY.

In order to discriminate the incidence rate from birth cohort effects, the calculated incidence, 14.0/1000 PY, was compared to the figure of yearly increase for the whole study cohort (17.6).

The 14.0/1000 PY incidence multiplied with 406 anti-HSV IgG negative participants at baseline would predict 5.7 new anti-HSV IgG positive cases during the forthcoming year. New incident cases hence would account for

Table 2 Relationship between presence of Herpes virus IgG antibodies, and age and sex

	HSV1	HSV2	VZV	CMV	HHV6
IgG positive$_{women}$, n (%)	218 (79.6)	45 (16.4)	269 (98.2)	234 (85.4)	266 (98.9)
IgG positive$_{men}$, n (%)	207 (79.3)	24 (9.2)	255 (97.7)	211 (80.8)	251 (96.2)
p-value men vs. women	0.943	0.013	0.699	0.159	0.143
Age$_{IgG\ positive}$, mean ± SD	62.9 ± 16.0	61.5 ± 15.3	60.7 ± 16.1	62.2 ± 16.0	60.3 ± 16.1
Age$_{IgG\ negative}$, mean ± SD	52.2 ± 14.0	60.6 ± 16.3	61.3 ± 20.1	53.2 ± 15.4	69.9 ± 12.4
p-value for difference in mean age	<0.001	0.638	0.902	<0.001	0.034

$5.7/17.6 = 32.2\%$ of the observed effect of age to anti-HSV IgG seroprevalence, with the remaining being the birth cohort effect.

Discussion

We report seroprevalence estimates of five common human herpes viruses in the general adult population in Sweden. The most frequent species, VZV and HHV6, both showed more than 97% prevalence. Studies from USA report similar figures for VZV (99%) [29]. Even HHV6 is reported to be prevalent almost ubiquitously in the adult population [30–33]. We noted a lower prevalence for anti-HHV6 antibodies with increasing age, in line with earlier reports [34, 35]. The prevailing explanation is that the primary infection, and corresponding humoral immunity, almost exclusively occurs in early childhood, and that antibody titers decline with age and thus in some patients goes below our assay's detection limit [34]. The seroprevalence for CMV was 83%, confirming the high prevalence figures earlier reported from Sweden, regardless of region studied or urbanization status [36–38]. Reports from USA have shown 67%, for a younger cohort [39, 40] and 87% for a cohort of women aged 70––79 [41]. Increasing age is associated with increased seroprevalence for CMV, in line with reports of a significant rate of seroconversion in adults [42]. Seroprevalence for HSV1 was 79%, in good agreement with comparable studies from Switzerland (80%) [43], Sweden (88%) [44] and Finland (86%) [18]. The HSV2 seroprevalence was 13%, placing our cohort in the lower range of comparable earlier studies from Sweden, (16%) [44], or USA, (17%) [45]. The prevalence was significantly higher in women (16%), confirming other cited studies.

Table 3 Multiple binary logistic regression model of HSV positivity, $N = 3,444$

	Odds ratio	95% confidence interval	p-value
Age (years)	1.009	0.989 – 1.030	0.370
Female sex	1.332	1.075 – 1.651	0.009
Year of birth (four digits)	0.958	0.939 – 0.978	<0.001

Year of birth affected HSV seroprevalence significantly. As illustrated in Fig. 1, the age-specific HSV prevalence is shifted downward in subjects sampled 2003–2005 compared to subjects sampled 1988–1990. When investigated in a logistic regression model, age per se had no significant effect on anti-HSV IgG seropositivity. This surprising outcome should be interpreted in the way that in this study cohort - designed to allow separation of the two connected variables age and year of birth - the latter dominates over the former. By analysis of longitudinal samples, the HSV incidence was calculated at 14.0/1000 PY in this population and this incidence rate explains approximately one third of the increase in prevalence by age. The remaining increase can be attributed to year of birth differences in the sub-cohorts, in that later sub-cohorts have a lower prevalence. The year of birth differences could be explained by a decreasing childhood and adolescent risk of HSV, especially HSV1, infection in the population [46, 47]. Changing lifestyle may also influence HSV spread, given its routes of transmission. The lack of analysis on the impact of socio-demographic factors such as level of education and overcrowding, is a limitation of the present study. Further studies and the inclusion of younger participants would be needed to confirm the observation of a

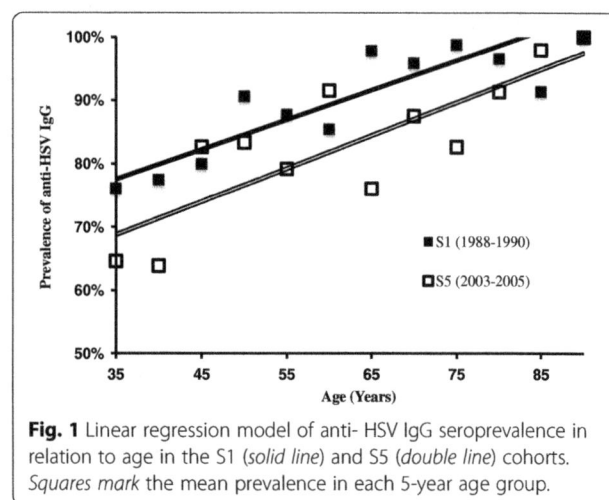

Fig. 1 Linear regression model of anti- HSV IgG seroprevalence in relation to age in the S1 (*solid line*) and S5 (*double line*) cohorts. *Squares mark* the mean prevalence in each 5-year age group.

decreasing prevalence and could possibly also provide insights on the underlying causes. In light of the accumulating evidence for a role of HSV1 infection in Alzheimer's disease development [3, 5, 6, 48], it is also worth mentioning that the incidence of dementia is declining in both USA and Sweden [49, 50]. Well-designed comparative studies of age-weighted trajectories will hopefully shed further light on the impact of HHV infectious burden and neuronal damage, leading to sequela such as Alzheimer's disease.

Conclusion
Prevalence of HSV1 was 79.4%, HSV2 12.9%, CMV 83.2%, VZV 97.9%, and HHV6 97.5%. Women were more often found to be seropositive for HHV, especially HSV2. Age-adjusted seroprevalence for HSV was lower in later birth cohorts indicating a decreasing childhood and adolescent risk of infection.

Acknowledgements
The authors would like to acknowledge Dr. Per Juto for the original development of ELISA methods used in this study, and Emma Honkala, Julia Wigren and Ingrid Marklund for skillful technical assistance.

Funding
This study was supported financially by grants from Västerbotten County Council, Kempe foundations, Swedish Medical Association, the Swedish Dementia Association, Trolle-Wachtmeister foundation, The Northland Dementia Fund, Swedish Alzheimer Fund, Stohne foundation, and Umeå University Foundation for Medical Research. The funders had no role in study design, data collection and analysis, decision to publish, or preparation of the manuscript.

Authors' contributions
HL and FE initialized the study and outlined the manuscript. RA designed the sample cohort. JO and FE supervised the serological analyses. HL, JO EK and FE analyzed the material. All authors contributed to the manuscript and approved the final version.

Competing interest
The authors have no conflicts of interest to declare.

Author details
[1]Department of Clinical Microbiology, Virology, Umeå University, Umeå, Sweden. [2]Department of Forensic Medicine, University of Tampere, Tampere 33520, Finland. [3]Department of Clinical Sciences, Psychiatry, Umeå University, Umeå, Sweden. [4]Department of Community Medicine and Rehabilitation, Geriatric Medicine, Umeå University, Umeå, Sweden.

References
1. Arvin A, et al. Human Herpesviruses Biology, Therapy, and Immunoprophylaxis. Cambridge: Cambridge University Press; 2007. p. 1. online resource (1408 p.).
2. Ball MJ. Limbic predilection in Alzheimer dementia: is reactivated herpesvirus involved? Can J Neurol Sci. 1982;9(3):303–6.
3. Steel AJ, Eslick GD. Herpes viruses increase the risk of Alzheimer's disease: a meta-analysis. J Alzheimers Dis. 2015;47(2):351–64.
4. Itzhaki RF, et al. Microbes and Alzheimer's disease. J Alzheimers Dis. 2016; 51(4):979–84.
5. Lovheim H, et al. Reactivated herpes simplex infection increases the risk of Alzheimer's disease. Alzheimers Dement. 2015;11(6):593–9.
6. Lovheim H, et al. Herpes simplex infection and the risk of Alzheimer's disease: A nested case-control study. Alzheimers Dement. 2015;11(6):587–92.
7. Ji YN, et al. Cytomegalovirus infection and coronary heart disease risk: a meta-analysis. Mol Biol Rep. 2012;39(6):6537–46.
8. Marra F, Ruckenstein J, Richardson K. A meta-analysis of stroke risk following herpes zoster infection. BMC Infect Dis. 2017;17(1):198.
9. Wu YP, et al. Herpes simplex virus type 1 and type 2 infection increases atherosclerosis risk: evidence based on a meta-analysis. Biomed Res Int. 2016;2016:2630865.
10. Tarter KD, et al. Persistent viral pathogens and cognitive impairment across the life course in the third national health and nutrition examination survey. J Infect Dis. 2014;209(6):837–44.
11. Watson AM, et al. Persistent infection with neurotropic herpes viruses and cognitive impairment. Psychol Med. 2013;43(5):1023–31.
12. Chen MH, et al. Risk of depressive disorder among patients with herpes zoster: a nationwide population-based prospective study. Psychosom Med. 2014;76(4):285–91.
13. Liao CH, et al. High prevalence of herpes zoster in patients with depression. J Clin Psychiatry. 2015;76(9):e1099–104.
14. Wang X, et al. Meta-analysis of infectious agents and depression. Sci Rep. 2014;4:4530.
15. Kobayashi N, et al. Increase in the IgG avidity index due to herpes simplex virus type 1 reactivation and its relationship with cognitive function in amnestic mild cognitive impairment and Alzheimer's disease. Biochem Biophys Res Commun. 2013;430(3):907–11.
16. Agostini S, et al. Lack of evidence for a role of HHV-6 in the pathogenesis of Alzheimer's disease. J Alzheimers Dis. 2015;49(1):229–35.
17. Shim SM, et al., Elevated Epstein-Barr Virus Antibody Level is Associated with Cognitive Decline in the Korean Elderly. J Alzheimers Dis. 2017;55(1): 293-301.
18. Olsson J, et al., HSV presence in brains of individuals without dementia: the TASTY brain series. Dis Model Mech. 2016;9(11):1349-55.
19. Cohen JA, et al. Herpes simplex virus seroprevalence and seroconversion among active duty US air force members with HIV infection. J Clin Virol. 2016;74:4–7.
20. Delaney S, et al. Seroprevalence of herpes simplex virus type 1 and 2 among pregnant women, 1989-2010. JAMA. 2014;312(7):746–8.
21. Saadatian-Elahi M, et al. Seroprevalence of varicella antibodies among pregnant women in Lyon-France. Eur J Epidemiol. 2007;22(6):405–9.
22. Politou M, et al. Seroprevalence of HHV-6 and HHV-8 among blood donors in Greece. Virol J. 2014;11:153.
23. Nilsson LG, et al. The Betula prospective cohort study: Memory, health and aging. Aging Neuropsychol Cognit. 1997;4(1):1–32.
24. Schaie KW. A general model for the study of developmental problems. Psychol Bull. 1965;64:92–107.
25. Schaie KW. Quasi-experimental research designs in the psychology of aging. In: Birren JE, editor. Handbook of the psychology of aging. New York: Van Nostrand; 1977. p. 39–58.
26. Juto P, Settergren B. Specific serum IgA, IgG and IgM antibody determination by a modified indirect ELISA-technique in primary and recurrent herpes simplex virus infection. J Virol Methods. 1988;20(1):45–55.
27. Sundstrom P, et al. An altered immune response to Epstein-Barr virus in multiple sclerosis: a prospective study. Neurology. 2004;62(12):2277–82.
28. Sjostrom S, et al. Human immunoglobulin G levels of viruses and associated glioma risk. Cancer Causes Control. 2011;22(9):1259–66.
29. Kilgore PE, et al. Varicella in Americans from NHANES III: implications for control through routine immunization. J Med Virol. 2003;70 Suppl 1:S111–8.
30. Nielsen L, Vestergaard BF. Competitive ELISA for detection of HHV-6 antibody: seroprevalence in a danish population. J Virol Methods. 1996; 56(2):221–30.
31. Baillargeon J, Piper J, Leach CT. Epidemiology of human herpesvirus 6 (HHV-6) infection in pregnant and nonpregnant women. J Clin Virol. 2000;16(3):149–57.
32. Saxinger C, et al. Antibody reactivity with HBLV (HHV-6) in U.S. populations. J Virol Methods. 1988;21(1-4):199–208.
33. Ihira M, et al. Serological examination of human herpesvirus 6 and 7 in patients with coronary artery disease. J Med Virol. 2002;67(4):534–7.
34. Parker CA, Weber JM. An enzyme-linked immunosorbent assay for the detection of IgG and IgM antibodies to human herpesvirus type 6. J Virol Methods. 1993;41(3):265–75.
35. Brown NA, et al. Fall in human herpesvirus 6 seropositivity with age. Lancet. 1988;2(8607):396.

36. Ahlfors K. IgG antibodies to cytomegalovirus in a normal urban Swedish population. Scand J Infect Dis. 1984;16(4):335–7.

37. Manicklal S, et al. The "silent" global burden of congenital cytomegalovirus. Clin Microbiol Rev. 2013;26(1):86–102.

38. Nilsson BO, et al. Antinuclear antibodies in the oldest-old women and men. J Autoimmun. 2006;27(4):281–8.

39. Bate SL, Dollard SC, Cannon MJ. Cytomegalovirus seroprevalence in the United States: the national health and nutrition examination surveys, 1988-2004. Clin Infect Dis. 2010;50(11):1439–47.

40. Simanek AM, et al. Seropositivity to cytomegalovirus, inflammation, all-cause and cardiovascular disease-related mortality in the United States. PLoS One. 2011;6(2):e16103.

41. Schmaltz HN, et al. Chronic cytomegalovirus infection and inflammation are associated with prevalent frailty in community-dwelling older women. J Am Geriatr Soc. 2005;53(5):747–54.

42. Hecker M, et al. Continuous cytomegalovirus seroconversion in a large group of healthy blood donors. Vox Sang. 2004;86(1):41–4.

43. Bunzli D, et al. Seroepidemiology of Herpes Simplex virus type 1 and 2 in Western and Southern Switzerland in adults aged 25–74 in 1992–93: a population-based study. BMC Infect Dis. 2004;4:10.

44. Jonsson MK, et al. Minimal change in HSV-2 seroreactivity: a cross-sectional Swedish population study. Scand J Infect Dis. 2006;38(5):357–65.

45. Xu F, et al. Trends in herpes simplex virus type 1 and type 2 seroprevalence in the United States. JAMA. 2006;296(8):964–73.

46. Bradley H, et al. Seroprevalence of herpes simplex virus types 1 and 2–United States, 1999–2010. J Infect Dis. 2014;209(3):325–33.

47. Woestenberg PJ, et al. Herpes simplex virus type 1 and type 2 in the Netherlands: seroprevalence, risk factors and changes during a 12-year period. BMC Infect Dis. 2016;16:364.

48. Itzhaki RF, et al., Microbes and Alzheimer's Disease. J Alzheimers Dis. 2016; 51(4):979-84.

49. Langa KM, et al., A Comparison of the Prevalence of Dementia in the United States in 2000 and 2012. JAMA Intern Med. 2017;177(1):51-58.

50. Qiu C, et al. Twenty-year changes in dementia occurrence suggest decreasing incidence in central Stockholm. Sweden Neurology. 2013;80(20):1888–94.

Changes in peripheral immune cell numbers and functions in octogenarian walkers – an acute exercise study

Kornelis S. M. van der Geest[1], Qi Wang[1], Thijs M. H. Eijsvogels[2], Hans J. P. Koenen[3], Irma Joosten[3], Elisabeth Brouwer[1], Maria T. E. Hopman[2], Joannes F. M. Jacobs[3] and Annemieke M. H. Boots[1*]

Abstract

Background: Age-related changes of the immune system, termed immunosenescence, may underlie the increased risk of infections and morbidity in the elderly. Little is known about the effects of acute exercise on peripheral immune parameters in octogenarians. Therefore, we investigated acute exercise-induced changes in phenotype and function of the immune system in octogenarians participating in the 2013 edition of the Nijmegen Four Days Marches. Blood sampling was performed at baseline and immediately after 4 days of the walking exercise (30 km/day). A comprehensive set of adaptive and innate immune traits were enumerated and analyzed by flow-cytometry. Peripheral blood mononuclear cells, isolated before and after walking were stimulated with LPS and supernatants were analysed for IL-1β, IL-6, IL-8 and TNF-α concentrations by ELISA. CMV serostatus was determined by ELISA.

Results: The walking exercise induced a clear leucocytosis with numerical increases of granulocytes, monocytes and lymphocytes. These exercise-induced changes were most profound in CMV seropositive subjects. Within lymphocytes, numerical increases of particularly CD4+ T cells were noted. Further T cell differentiation analysis revealed profound increases of naïve CD4+ T cells, including naïve Treg. Significant increases were also noted for CD4+ memory T cell subsets. In contrast, only slight increases in naïve and memory CD8+ T cell subsets were detected. Exercise did not affect markers of immune exhaustion in memory T cell subsets. NK cells demonstrated a numerical decline and a change in cellular composition with a selective decrease of the mature CD56[dim] NK cells. The latter was seen in CMV seronegative subjects only. Also, a higher IL-6 and IL-8 production capacity of LPS-stimulated PBMC was seen after walking.

Conclusion: In this exceptional cohort of octogenarian walkers, acute exercise induced changes in immune cell numbers and functions. A clear response of CD4+ T cells, rather than CD8+ T cells or NK cells was noted. Remarkably, the response to exercise within the CD4+ T cell compartment was dominated by naïve CD4+ subsets.

Keywords: T cells, Recent thymic emigrants, NK cells, Monocytes, Ageing, Immune System

Background

Age-related changes of the immune system may contribute to increased vulnerability for infectious disease, impaired responses to vaccination and the development of late-onset chronic inflammatory diseases [1–3]. This process, termed immunosenescence, is caused by changes in both the adaptive and innate immune system. The causes underlying immunosenescence may be largely environmental as a recent systems level analysis in healthy twins revealed that non-heritable (environmental) factors rather than heritable factors shape the immune system over time [4]. In particular, the broad impact of human Cytomegalovirus (CMV) infection, a non-heritable factor, on the phenotype of the immune system was demonstrated, thereby confirming previous findings [5, 6]. The effects of exercise as another non-heritable (behavioural) factor on the phenotype of the ageing immune system has been less well studied.

The development of immunosenescence includes the decline of naïve T cells due to thymus involution,

* Correspondence: m.boots@umcg.nl
[1]Departments of Rheumatology and Clinical Immunology and Translational Immunology Groningen (TRIGR), University of Groningen, University Medical Center Groningen, Hanzeplein 1, 9700RB Groningen, The Netherlands
Full list of author information is available at the end of the article

increases in late-stage effector memory T cells, decreased CD4/CD8 ratio's and the development of immune exhaustion [7, 8]. These changes result in inadequate T cell help to B cells, thereby affecting the development of productive immune responses. CMV infection is known to accelerate immune ageing through oligoclonal expansion of CMV-specific CD8 effector memory T cells [5, 6]. In addition, several studies report on increases in T regulatory cells (Treg) leading to increased Treg/Teffector ratio's in healthy elderly which may further add to the development of immunosenescence [9–11].

Whilst adaptive immune responses decline with age, the activity of the innate immune system appears to increase with age. This is evidenced by numerical increases in natural killer (NK) cells and monocytes and by increased serum levels of acute phase proteins and inflammatory cytokines such as interleukin-1 β (IL-1β), Interleukin-6 (IL-6), interleukin-8 (IL-8) and Tumor Necrosis Factor-α (TNFα) [12, 13]. The molecular mechanisms underlying this chronic, low grade inflammation (coined inflamm-ageing) are currently unknown but may be associated with an altered innate response to an altered gut microbiota [12, 14].

NK cells are key in the protection against infection and cancer. Ageing-associated alterations have shown an increase in the more mature CD56^{dim} subset and a decline of the immature, CD56^{bright} NK subset, irrespective of CMV infection [15]. CD56^{dim} NK cells are the most abundant subset in the blood, and demonstrate a higher cytotoxicity, whereas the CD56^{bright} NK cells demonstrate higher cytokine production. CMV chronic infection is associated with an expansion of a "memory-like" (CD56^{dim}) NK cell subset characterized by NKG2C expression and lack of NKG2A [15].

Physical activity and exercise have profound effects on the immune system and contribute to health, well-being and longevity [16, 17]. Single bouts of exercise induce a prominent leukocytosis followed by a redistribution of immune effector cells to the tissue compartments [18]. This biphasic response to exercise may enhance the immune response against pathogens in the lymph nodes and in peripheral tissues (e.g. skin, mucosa, lungs). In adult individuals, exercise-induced lymphocytosis is largely attributed to NK cells and CD8 effector memory T cells [19, 20]. Interestingly, these subsets share functional characteristics such as cytotoxicity and tissue migration, which are important in immunosurveillance. Notably, CMV serostatus was found to influence the magnitude and the kinetics of the NK and CD8+ memory T cell responses to exercise [21, 22]. To our knowledge, the effects of acute exercise on the phenotype and function of the immune system in octogenarians have not yet been documented.

In the current study we thus investigated the effects of acute exercise on a comprehensive set of adaptive and innate immune traits in a small cohort of 20 elderly octogenarian walkers participating in the 2013 Nijmegen Four Days Marches. All participants walked a total 120 km in four consecutive days (4 x 30 km) at a self-selected pace. Blood samples were drawn at baseline and immediately after completion of the march at day 4. A post hoc analysis was performed on the contribution of CMV serostatus to exercise-induced immune changes.

Methods

Participants

Twenty elderly male and female participants (mean age 81.3 ± 1.9 years) of the 2013 Nijmegen Four Days Marches volunteered to participate in our study. The Nijmegen Four Days Marches represents the largest mass participation walking event in the world with approximately 45,000 participants annually. Based on sex and age, individuals walk 30, 40 or 50 km per day for 4 consecutive days. Blood samples were drawn before and after (within 10 min after exercise cessation) the 4 day walking event.

Experimental design

Blood sampling logistics were performed as described previously [23]. In brief, all participants reported twice to our laboratory, which was located at the start/finish area of the event. Baseline measurements were performed 12–36 h preceding the start (Table 1). Thereafter, the participants walked 30 km a day, for four consecutive days at a self-selected pace. Exercise was performed under temperate ambient conditions with daily maximum wet bulb globe temperatures ranging between 24–27 °C. The recovery phase (fluid intake, food intake, sleep) between walking stages was uncontrolled and not monitored. Walking duration was recorded every day, while speed was calculated accordingly. Immediately (within 10 min) after finishing on the fourth day, all baseline measurements were repeated. Heart rate, as part of exercise intensity, was measured during day 1 as described previously [24]. Mean heart rate during exercise was presented in absolute values (beats per minute, (bpm)) and as a percentage of the predicted maximal heart rate. Predicted maximal heart rate (HRmax) was calculated using the Tanaka's formula: HRmax = 208 - 0.7*age [25]. During the experiment, dry bulb, wet bulb and globe temperatures were measured every 30 min using a portable climate monitoring device (Davis instruments Inc., Hayward, USA), which was positioned at the start/finish area. The wet bulb globe temperature index (WBGT) was calculated using the formula: WBGT = 0.1 (Tdry bulb) + 0.7 (Twet bulb) + 0.2 (Tglobe).

Subject characteristics

Body mass (Seca 888 scale, Hamburg, Germany) and body height were measured and body mass index (BMI) was calculated. A four-point skin fold thickness measurement

Table 1 Demographics, health status and exercise characteristics of volunteers

	Men ($n = 11$)	Women ($n = 9$)
Demographic characteristics		
Age (yr)	81.0 ± 1.2	81.6 ± 2.7
Height (cm)	174 ± 5.2	159 ± 6.7
Weight (kg)	75.8 ± 6.6	55.5 ± 6.6
Body-mass index (kg/m^2)	25.0 ± 1.6	21.8 ± 1.9
Lean body mass (kg)	57.2 ± 4.7	37.8 ± 5.2
Health status		
Physical activity (hrs/week)	8.5 ± 8.0	5.8 ± 5.9
≥ 5 times/week ≥30 min exercise (%)	73	56
Blood pressure		
Systolic (mmHg)	140 ± 18	146 ± 17
Diastolic (mmHg)	81 ± 11	82 ± 10
Resting heart rate (bpm)	64 ± 20	63 ± 14
Gait speed (km/h)	4.8 ± 0.7	4.5 ± 0.7
Grip strength (kg)	41 ± 8.0	25 ± 4.5
CMV seropositive	6 (55%)	7 (78%)
Use of prescribed medicine		
Anti-hypertensive drugs	2 (18%)	3 (33%)
Statins	2 (18%)	1 (11%)
Analgesics	3 (27%)	0 (0%)
Anti-diabetics	0 (0%)	0 (0%)
Other[a]	2 (18%)	1 (11%)
Pathology		
Hypertension	2 (18%)	3 (33%)
Cardiovascular disease	2 (18%)	0 (0%)
Hypercholestorolemia[b]	2 (18%)	1 (11%)
Diabetes	0 (0%)	0 (0%)
Cancer (not further differentiated)	2 (18%)	1 (11%)
Other[a]	1 (9%)	2 (22%)
Exercise characteristics		
Exercise duration per day (hh:mm)	7:28 ± 1:10	8:07 ± 0:52
Speed (km/h)	4.2 ± 0.1	3.7 ± 0.1
Average heart rate day 1 (bpm)	99.5 ± 11.9	113.6 ± 14.3
Peak heart rate day 1 (bpm)	112.5 ± 13.1	125.0 ± 14.1
Exercise intensity day 1 (% of age-adjusted max. heart rate)	65.7 ± 7.7	75.4 ± 9.6
Fluid balance		
Fluid intake (L)[c]	1.88 ± 0.8	1.98 ± 0.8
Change in body mass (absolute kg)[c]	-0.80 ± 0.9	-0.19 ± 0.6
Change in body mass (relative %)[c]	-1.04 ± 1.1	-0.38 ± 1.0
Change in plasma volume (relative %)[d]	+3.1 ± 3.2	+4.5 ± 3.5

[a]Volunteers who were diagnosed and treated for cancer, rheumatoid arthritis, allergy and glaucoma. [b]Hypercholesterolemia is defined as total cholesterol levels of >6.5 mmol, as previously diagnosed by a physician. [c]Daily fluid intake and changes in body mass during walking. [d]Changes in plasma volume during walking estimated according to Dill and Costill [27]. Data are presented as mean ± standard deviation

(biceps, triceps, sub-scapular, supra-iliac) was obtained in order to calculate the lean body mass [26]. Resting heart rate and blood pressure were measured twice using an automated sphygmomanometer (M5-1 intellisense, Omron Healthcare, Hoofddorp, the Netherlands) after 5 min supine rest. Finally, all subjects completed a questionnaire about their physical activity and health status.

Blood analyses

White blood cell differential counts, hemoglobin and hematocrit levels were directly analyzed on a Sysmex XE-5000 system (Sysmex Corporation, Kobe, Japan). Relative changes in plasma volume were calculated from blood hematocrit and hemoglobin concentrations using Dill and Costill's equation [27]. C-reactive protein (CRP) and creatinine measurements were measured in batches of frozen sera. Sera aliquots were stored at -20 °C directly after collection and thawed directly before analysis. All analyses were coded and anonymized. Serum CRP and creatinine were both measured on the c16000 Architect (Abbott Diagnostics, Abbott Park, IL).

Detection of CMV-specific IgG

Serum levels of CMV-specific IgG was essentially done as previously described [7]. In brief, 96-well ELISA plates (Greiner) were coated with lysates of CMV-infected fibroblasts overnight. Lysates of non-infected fibroblasts were used as negative controls. Following coating, dilutions of serum samples were incubated for 1 h. Goat-anti-human IgG was added and incubated for 1 h. Samples were incubated with phosphatase for 15 min, and the reaction was stopped with NaOH. The plates were scanned on a Versamax reader (Molecular Devices). A pool of sera from 3 seropositive individuals with known titers of CMV-specific IgG was used to quantify CMV IgG titers in the test samples.

Flowcytometry

Peripheral blood mononuclear cells (PBMC) were isolated by density gradient centrifugation with Lymphoprep (Axis-Shield) and stored in -180 °C until staining. PBMCs (10^6 cells) were stained simultaneously employing 4 different staining panels to asses markers of T cell differentiation, Treg and proliferation, NK cell inhibitory receptors and NK cell activating receptors (Table 2). All cell subsets are expressed as cell counts per liter unless indicated otherwise. Cell counts of these subsets were based on data from the full leucocyte differential in combination with the flowcytometry data. As an example, we used the absolute lymphocyte count from the full leucocyte differential and the percentage of CD3 T cells in the lymphocyte gate as assessed by flowcytometry for calculation of the T cell count. To perform intracellular staining with monoclonal antibodies to Cytotoxic T-lymphocyte-associated protein-

4 (CTLA-4), forkhead box P3 (FoxP3) and the proliferation marker ki-67, the cells were first fixed and permeabilized with a FoxP3 staining buffer set (eBioscience). Samples were measured on a LSR-II (BD) and data were analyzed with Kaluza software (Beckman Coulter).

Lipopolysacharide (LPS)-stimulated PBMC cytokine production

PBMCs at 1 x 10^6 cells/mL were stimulated with 1 μg/mL LPS (Sigma-Aldrich, St. Louis, MO, USA) or left unstimulated. Cells were cultured in polypropylene tubes (BD bioscience) in RPMI with 10% FCS for 24 h. After 24 h, supernatants were collected and stored at -20 °C. Culture supernatants were analyzed for production of the cytokines IL-1β, IL-6, IL-8 and TNF-α by enzyme-linked immunosorbent assay (ELISA, Duoset, R&D system, Minneapolis, MN, USA) according to the manufacturer's instructions, and read with a Versamax reader (Molecular Devices, Sunnyvale, CA, USA). The assay sensitivity was 8 pg/mL for IL-1β, 31 pg/mL for IL-6 and TNF-α, and 312 pg/mL for IL-8. The net cytokine production was calculated as cytokine production of the stimulated sample minus the cytokine production of the non-stimulated sample.

Statistical analyses

Statistical analysis of data was carried out using IBM SPSS Statistics 20 (IBM, Chicago, IL, USA) and Graphpad Prism 5 (Graph Pad Software, San Diego, CA, USA). Wilcoxon Signed Rank test, unless indicated otherwise, was used to compare the same volunteers before and after walking. Two-tailed p-values of less than 0.05 were considered statistically significant.

Results
Subject characteristics

All study participants ($n = 20$) successfully completed the Four Days Marches at a self selected pace (4.0 ± 0.7 km/h). On average the participants walked 7 h and 47 min daily and had an average heart rate during the first day of 106 ± 15 bpm, representing an average exercise intensity of $70 \pm 10\%$. Thus, the walking exercise in these elderly is qualified as a daily bout of moderate intensity exercise for 4 consecutive days. An overview of all subject characteristics is presented in Table 1. An exercise-induced plasma volume expansion of $3.7 \pm 3.3\%$ was observed over the 4 days, which coincided with a small, but significant decrease of hematocrit from 0.40 L/L at baseline to 0.38 L/L directly after 4 days of exercise ($p < 0.0001$).

Effects of acute exercise on the peripheral blood cellular composition

When examining the composition of the peripheral blood compartment, our data show that the walking

Table 2 Overview of staining panels and reagents for flowcytometry

Panel	Mab reagent	Clone	Provider
T cell differentiation	CD3-Efluor 605	okt-03	Ebioscience, San Diego, CA, USA
	CD8-APC-H7	RPA-T8	Ebioscience, San Diego, CA, USA
	CD45RO-FITC	UCHL-1	BD bioscience, San Jose, CA, USA
	CCR7-PE-Cy7	3D12	BD bioscience, San Jose, CA, USA
	CD31-AF647	WM-59	BD bioscience, San Jose, CA, USA
	CD28-AF700	28.2	Biolegend, San Diego, CA, USA
	PD1-PE	EH12.2H7	Biolegend, San Diego, CA, USA
	CD4-PcP	SK3	BD bioscience, San Jose, CA, USA
	CTLA-4-BV421	BNI3	BD bioscience, San Jose, CA, USA
Treg/Proliferation	CD8-PE-Cy7	RPA-T8	BD bioscience, San Jose, CA, USA
	CD25-APC	BC96	Ebioscience, San Diego, CA, USA
	CD45RA-Efluor605	HI100	Ebioscience, San Diego, CA, USA
	CD19-FITC	HD37	Dako, Santa Clara, CA, USA
	CD4-APC-H7	RPA-T4	BD bioscience, San Jose, CA, USA
	FOXP3-PE	PCH101	BD bioscience, San Jose, CA, USA
	Ki-67-PcP-Cy5.5	B56	BD bioscience, San Jose, CA, USA
NK cell	CD16-FITC	3G8	Beckman Coulter, Brea, CA, USA
Inhibitory receptors	CD56-ECD	N901	Beckman Coulter, Brea, CA, USA
	CD3-APC-AF750	UCHT1	Beckman Coulter, Brea, CA, USA
	CD45-KO	J.33	Beckman Coulter, Brea, CA, USA
	CD159c (NKG2C)-PE	134591	R&D Systems, Minneapolis, MN, USA
	CD158b (KIR2DL2/3)-PE-Cy7	GL183	Beckman Coulter, Brea, CA, USA
	CD158e1 (KIR3DL1)-APC	Z27.3.7	Beckman Coulter, Brea, CA, USA
	CD158a (KIR2DL1)-APC-AF700	EB6B	Beckman Coulter, Brea, CA, USA
	CD159a (NKG2A)-PB	Z199	Beckman Coulter, Brea, CA, USA
NK cell	CD16-FITC	3G8	Beckman Coulter, Brea, CA, USA
Activating receptors	CD56-ECD	N901	Beckman Coulter, Brea, CA, USA
	CD3-APC-AF750	UCHT1	Beckman Coulter, Brea, CA, USA
	CD45-KO	J.33	Beckman Coulter, Brea, CA, USA
	CD336 (NKp44)-PE	Z231	Beckman Coulter, Brea, CA, USA
	CD337 (NKp30)-PE-Cy5.5	Z25	Beckman Coulter, Brea, CA, USA
	CD335 (NKp46)-PE-Cy7	BAB281	Beckman Coulter, Brea, CA, USA
	CD314 (NKG2D)-APC	ON72	Beckman Coulter, Brea, CA, USA
	CD244 (2B4) -APC-AF700	C1.7.1	Beckman Coulter, Brea, CA, USA
	CD161-PB	191B8	Beckman Coulter, Brea, CA, USA

exercise resulted in a clear leucocytosis with numerical increases of granulocytes, monocytes and lymphocytes (Table 3). When analyzing the lymphocyte compartment, clear numerical increases were noted for T cells and to a lesser extent B cells. In contrast, a decline in the number of NK cells was detected. The numerical increase in T cells was largely due to an increase in CD4+ T cells (Table 3). Although CD8+ T cell numbers showed a statistical significant increase after exercise, the absolute increase was very limited. The

mean CD4/CD8 ratio, an age-appropriate value of 3 [9], was not significantly increased by the walking exercise (data not shown).

As carriage of CMV has pronounced effects on the immune system, we compared the effects of the walking exercise between CMV seropositive ($n = 13$) and CMV seronegative subjects ($n = 7$). Although an exercise induced leucocytosis was seen in both CMV seropositive and seronegative individuals, increases in granulocytes, monocytes and lymphocytes were statistically significant

Table 3 General and Immune parameters before and after walking

	Pre-Walking	Post-Walking	P-value
Hemoglobin (mmol/L)	8.7 (7.7–9.4)	8.2 (7.3–9.1)	0.0009
Thrombocytes (10^9/L)	233 (157–318)	234 (160–349)	ns
CRP (mg/L)	1 (1–9)	1 (1–47)	0.0078
Creatinin (μmol/L)	86 (47–147)	100 (54–207)	0.0008
ASAT (U/L)	28 (14–39)	(-)	(-)
ALAT (U/L)	28 (21–46)	(-)	(-)
Leukocytes (10^9/L)	6.6 (4.6–11.0)	7.7 (5.7–14.3)	0.0002
Neutrophils (10^9/L)	4.1 (2.4–8.3)	5.1 (2.9–10.4)	0.0008
Eosinophils (10^9/L)	0.15 (0.03–0.68)	0.18 (0.06–0.78)	0.0166
Basophils (10^9/L)	0.04 (0.01–0.07)	0.03 (0.02–0.05)	ns
Monocytes (10^9/L)	0.49 (0.29–0.90)	0.67 (0.40–1.21)	0.0005
Lymphocytes (10^9/L)	1.57 (1.00–2.21)	1.82 (1.07–2.97)	0.0045
CD3+ T cells (10^9/L)	0.75 (0.20–1.36)	1.11 (0.48–1.98)	0.0005
CD4+ T cells (10^9/L)	0.46 (0.06–0.99)	0.59 (0.37–1.62)	0.0007
CD8+ T cells (10^9/L)	0.15 (0.03–0.45)	0.15 (0.05–0.71)	0.0061
CD19+ B cells (10^9/L)	0.23 (0.05–0.40)	0.30 (0.09–0.51)	0.0023
CD16 + CD56+ NK cells (10^9/L)	0.40 (0.21–0.87)	0.31 (0.13–0.70)	0.0178

Medians + range are indicated (n = 20). The minimal increase in exercise-induced plasma volume (3.7%) did not influence any of the significant differences found

in CMV seropositive subjects but did not reach significance in CMV seronegative subjects (Table 4). Lymphocytosis in CMV seropositive subjects was largely caused by T cells, rather CD4 than CD8, and to a lesser extent B cells, whereas NK cell numbers remained unchanged. B cell numbers increased irrespective of CMV serostatus. Interestingly, a decrease of NK cells was seen only in CMV seronegative subjects. Thus, acute exercise

induced responses were more clear in CMV seropositive octogenarians.

Effect of acute exercise on T cells

We next examined the proliferative properties of circulating immune cells as measured by Ki-67 expression. Post walking, both CD4+ and CD8+ T cells demonstrated reduced percentages of proliferating cells (Fig. 1a).

Table 4 Immune parameters before and after walking in CMV seropositive and seronegative participants

	CMV+		CMV-	
	Before	After	Before	After
Hemoglobin[a] (mmol/L)	8.4 (7.7–9.4)	7.9 (7.3–8.7)**	8.9 (7.9–9.0)	8.7 (7.5–9.1)
CRP (mg/L)	1 (1–9)	1 (1–10)	1 (1–6)	9 (1–47)
Leukocytes (10^9/L)	6.6 (4.6–11.0)	7.9 (5.7–14.3)**	6.6 (4.8–9.1)	7.2 (6.3–12.3)*
Neutrophils (10^9/L)	3.8 (2.4–8.3)	5.0 (2.9–10.4)*	4.2 (3.2–6.6)	5.1 (4.2–9.2)*
Eosinophils (10^9/L)	0.12 (0.03–0.68)	0.19 (0.06–0.78)**	0.17 (0.08–0.28)	0.15 (0.08–0.33)
Basophils (10^9/L)	0.03 (0.01–0.06)	0.03 (0.02–0.05)	0.05 (0.02–0.07)	0.04 (0.03–0.05)
Monocytes (10^9/L)	0.48 (0.29–0.69)	0.68 (0.40–1.05)**	0.57 (0.32–0.90)	0.66 (0.42–1.21)
Lymphocytes (10^9/L)	1.65 (1.45–2.21)	2.19 (1.33–2.97)**	1.37 (1.00–1.92)	1.40 (1.07–2.08)
CD3+ T cells (10^9/L)	0.77 (0.49–1.36)	1.19 (0.73–1.98)**	0.63 (0.20–1.00)	0.76 (0.48–1.45)
CD4+ T cells (10^9/L)	0.52 (0.17–0.99)	0.73 (0.40–1.62)**	0.40 (−0.06–0.69)	0.57 (0.37–0.87)
CD8+ T cells (10^9/L)	0.21 (0.04–0.45)	0.21 (0.06–0.72)*	0.08 (0.04–0.17)	0.10 (0.05–0.19)
CD19+ B cells (10^9/L)	0.26 (0.09–0.40)	0.35 (0.11–0.51)*	0.10 (0.05–0.40)	0.16 (0.09–0.45)*
CD16 + CD56+ NK cells (10^9/L)	0.32 (0.21–0.87)	0.31 (0.13–0.70)	0.43 (0.38–0.52)	0.29 (0.22–0.43)*

CMV+ subjects (n = 13) and CMV- subjects (n = 7). Medians and range are shown. Paired analysis was peformed separately for CMV+ and CMV- subjects before and after excersise. Statistical significance by Wilcoxon signed rank test is indicated as *p < 0.05 or **p < 0.01
[a]Changes in plasma volumes estimated according to Dill and Costill were not significantly different between CMV+ and CMV- subjects

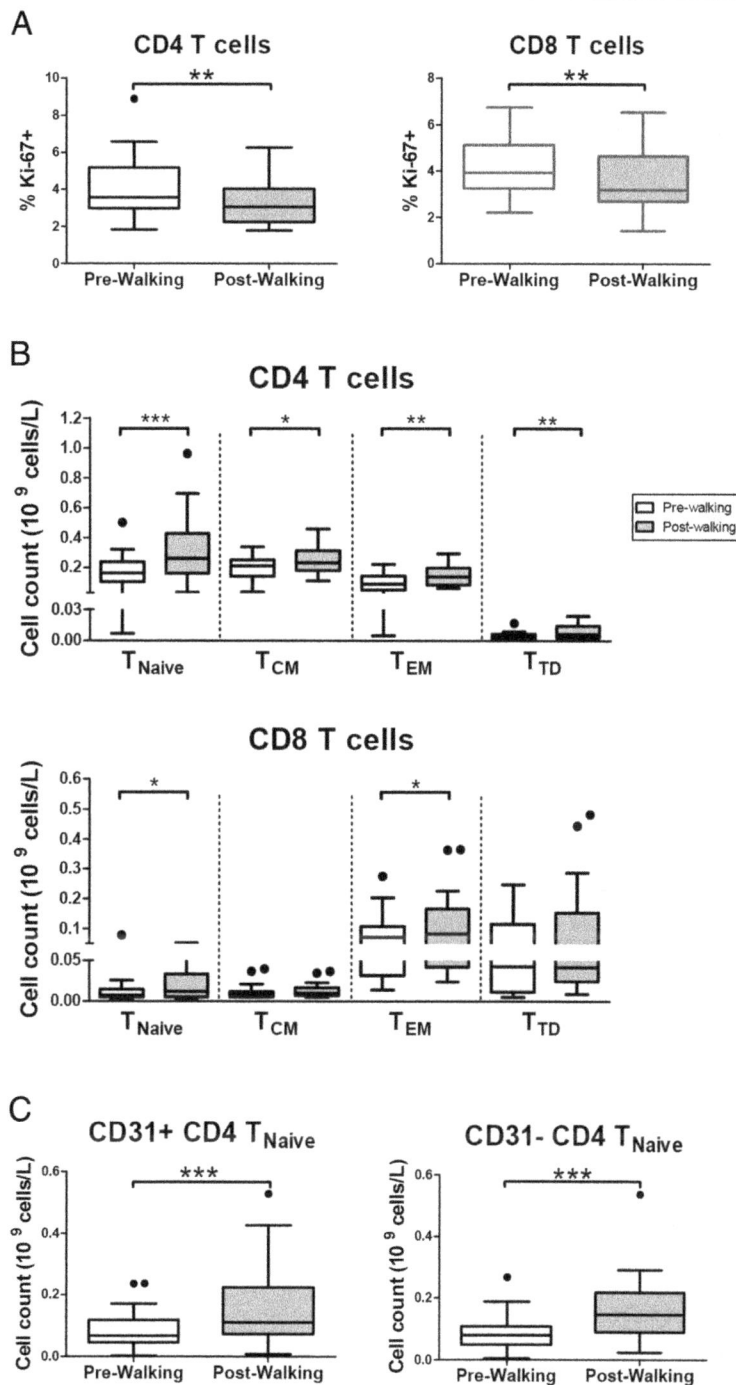

Fig. 1 Exercise reduces rates of T cell proliferation and leads to redistribution of T cell subsets. **a** Rates of CD4 (left panel) and CD8 (*right panel*) proliferation before (Pre-Walking) and after exercise (Post-Walking) assessed by Ki-67 expression using flow-cytometry. Percentages of Ki-67 expressing cells within the CD4 and CD8 populations are shown. **b** Enumeration of CD4 (upper panel) and CD8 (lower panel) T cell differentiation subsets based on CD45RO and CCR7 expression Pre- and Post-Walking. Mean (+/- SEM) numbers (10^9 cells/L) of naïve T cells ($T_{Naïve}$), central memory T cells (T_{CM}), effector memory T cells (T_{EM}) and terminally differentiated T cells (T_{TD}) are shown. **c** Mean (+/- SEM) numbers (10^9 cells/L) of recent thymic emigrants defined as CD31 + CD4 + $T_{Naïve}$ and the central naïve CD31-CD4+ $T_{Naïve}$ subsets. Statistical significance by Wilcoxon signed rank test is indicated as *$p < 0.05$, **$p < 0.01$, ***$p < 0.001$

Similar observations were seen in CMV seropositive and seronegative subjects (Additional file 1: Figure S1a). Thus, the data suggest an exercise-induced increase of T cells with low proliferative capacity [20].

To determine if certain T cell populations respond differently, we next investigated exercise-induced changes in CD4+ and CD8+ differentiation subsets. A flow-cytometric analysis employing CD45RO and CCR7 was applied to identify naïve T cells ($T_{Naïve}$), central memory T cells (T_{CM}), effector memory T cells (T_{EM}) and terminally differentiated T cells (T_{TD}) [28]. Numerical changes of differentiation subsets were most profound in the CD4+ compartment (Fig. 1b) and appeared to be linked to CMV carriage (Additional file 1: Figure S1b). Although significant increases were noted for all four differentiation subsets, the most profound increase was noted in the CD4+ $T_{Naïve}$ subset (Fig 1b). Interestingly, we also noted a significant increase of CD4+ $T_{Naïve}$ in CMV seronegative subjects (Additional file 1: Figure S1b). When analysed for the contribution of recent thymic emigrants (RTE), defined as $CD31^{pos}$ CD4 + $T_{Naïve}$ and the central naïve $CD31^{neg}$ CD4 + $T_{Naïve}$ subsets, we found both subsets significantly increased [29] (Fig. 1c). In CMV seronegative subjects the rise in CD4+ $T_{Naïve}$ appeared due to the $CD31^{neg}$ CD4 + $T_{Naïve}$ subset (Additional file 1: Figure S1c). Moreover, the naïve CD4 + $CD25^{dim}$ subset, recently described to develop in secondary lymphoid organs upon TCR priming, was found significantly increased ([30], data not shown). The combined data suggest the exercise-induced response of CD4 + $T_{Naïve}$ and CD4+ memory subsets (T_{EM} > T_{TD} > T_{CM}).

In the CD8+ compartment, slight but significant numerical increases were noted for both the CD8 T_{EM} and the CD8 + $T_{Naïve}$ subsets, whereas the T_{CM} and the T_{TD} subsets were not changed (Fig. 1b). These changes appeared associated with CMV carriage (Additional file 1: Figure S1b). Taken together, our findings show an increase of peripheral naive CD4+ T cells particularly in response to exercise. Carriage of CMV is largely associated with enhanced numbers of both CD4 and CD8 subsets.

No effect of acute exercise on markers of T cell exhaustion

As we noted numerical increases in particularly the CD4 + T_{EM} and the T_{TD} subsets and to a lesser extent the CD8 T_{EM}, but not the CD8 T_{TD} subset, we examined these subsets for expression of the exhaustion markers CTLA-4 and PD-1 [8]. Frequencies of CTLA-4 and PD-1 in the CD4+ T_{EM} and the T_{TD} subsets were largely comparable before and after the walking exercise; although a slight decrease of PD-1 expressing cells in the T_{EM} subset was detected (Additional file 2: Figure S2). In the CD8+ T_{EM} and the T_{TD} subsets, where only modest or no numerical increases were noted, respectively, only slight increases in the frequencies of CTLA4-, but

not PD1-expressing cells were observed. Expression of these markers was generally lacking on $T_{Naïve}$ and T_{CM} (data not shown). Thus, the walking exercise does not affect markers of immune exhaustion of either CD4 or CD8 T_{EM} and T_{TD} subsets.

Acute exercise-induced changes in nTreg but not memory Treg subsets

Based on CD45RA and FoxP3 expression [31], CD45RA + $FoxP3^{low}$ naïve (resting) Treg cells (nTreg) and CD45RA- $FoxP3^{high}$- memory (activated) Treg cells (memTreg) were identified in the peripheral blood of elderly walkers (Fig. 2a). Post exercise, a clear numerical increase of nTreg was observed whereas the numbers of memTreg remained stable (Fig. 2b). The increase in nTreg was seen irrespective of CMV serostatus, although the increase was more clear in CMV seropositive subjects (Additional File 3, Figure S3). Thus, as seen with the conventional CD4+ $T_{Naïve}$ cells, the peripheral numbers of nTregs in elderly walkers also increased in response to acute exercise. In contrast, whereas exercise led to increases in conventional CD4+ memory T cells (Fig. 1b), exercise did not induce numerical increases of memTreg (Fig 2b).

Effects of acute exercise on NK cells

Peripheral NK cell numbers were found reduced after exercise which was caused by a numerical decline of $CD56^{dim}$ but not $CD56^{bright}$ NK cells [15] (Table 3 and Fig. 3a). Notably, the decrease in $CD56^{dim}$ NK cells was seen in CMV seronegative donors only (Fig 3a). As $CD56^{dim}$ NK cells are most frequent in the blood (90% of total NK cells), we next investigated exercise-induced changes in the expression of inhibitory and activating NK receptors by this subset. In CMV seronegative subjects, we found comparable frequencies of cells positive for inhibitory receptors (KIR2DL1, KIR2DL2/3, KIR3DL1, NKG2A and NKG2C) and activating receptors (NKp30, NKp44, NKp46, 2B4 and NKG2D) within $CD56^{dim}$ NK cells before and after walking (Fig. 3bc). However, in CMV seropositive subjects, exercise did modulate frequencies of NK cells with inhibitory and activating receptors. More specifically, KIR2DL1-, KIR2DL2/3- and KIR3DL1-positive cells decreased with exercise, but frequencies of NKG2C-positive cells were increased (Fig. 3b). Also, frequencies of activating receptor NKG2D+ cells were found increased (Fig. 3c). Thus, the walking exercise led to a numerical decline of $CD56^{dim}$ NK cells in CMV seronegative subjects. In CMV seropositive subjects the walking exercise did not seem to affect the numbers of NK cells but down-modulated expression of most inhibitory receptors whereas the expression of activating receptors was largely unchanged, suggesting a less inhibited phenotype as a net result.

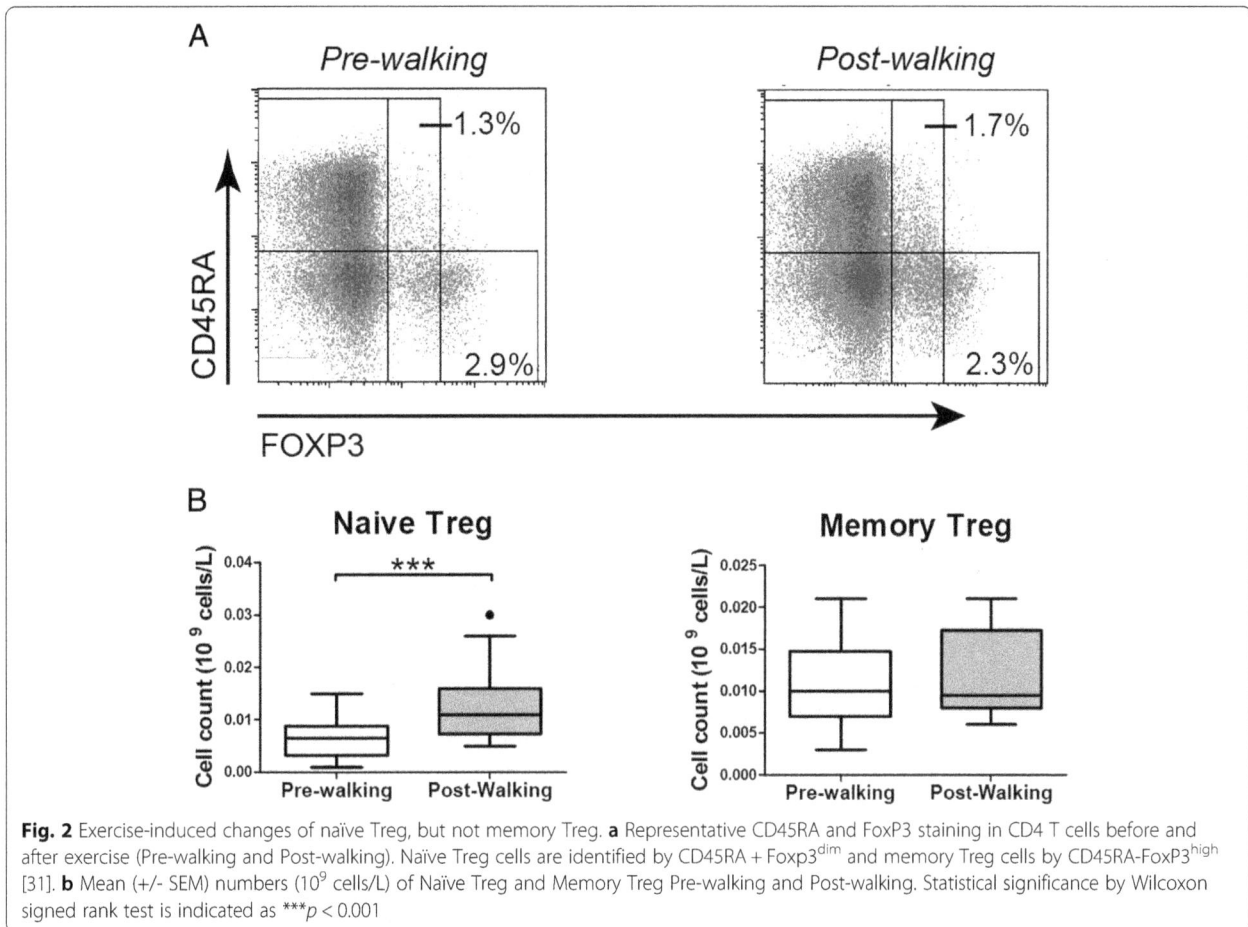

Fig. 2 Exercise-induced changes of naïve Treg, but not memory Treg. **a** Representative CD45RA and FoxP3 staining in CD4 T cells before and after exercise (Pre-walking and Post-walking). Naïve Treg cells are identified by CD45RA + Foxp3^{dim} and memory Treg cells by CD45RA-FoxP3^{high} [31]. **b** Mean (+/- SEM) numbers (10^9 cells/L) of Naïve Treg and Memory Treg Pre-walking and Post-walking. Statistical significance by Wilcoxon signed rank test is indicated as ***$p < 0.001$

Exercise leads to higher LPS-stimulated cytokine production by PBMC

We next investigated the effects of exercise on PBMC function. Hereto, we analysed the LPS stimulated production of IL-1β, TNFα, IL-6 and IL-8 by PBMC before and after walking. The data show increases in production of IL-6 and IL-8, but not IL-1β and TNFα (Fig. 4). Similar data were obtained in CMV seropositive and seronegative subjects (data not shown).

Discussion

Our main finding is that acute exercise induced changes in immune cell numbers and functions in an exceptional cohort of octogenarian walkers. A clear response of CD4 + T cells, rather than CD8+ T cells or NK cells to exercise was noted. Moreover, the response was dominated by numerical increases of naïve CD4+ subsets.

Effects of exercise were evaluated in a paired sample design study enumerating a comprehensive set of peripheral cellular traits, before and directly after the walking event. As it is known that most exercise-induced changes in immune cell counts return to pre-exercise levels within a few hours, we emphasise that our data likely reflect the effect of the final day of exercise. We

report on clear exercise-induced numerical increases of granulocytes, monocytes and lymphocytes. A retrospective analysis showed that these changes were associated with CMV carriage, thereby confirming the notion that infection history not only impacts the composition of the peripheral blood compartment but also the response to exercise, as recently suggested [21, 22].

Previous studies in adult subjects show that CD8 effector memory T cells and NK cells are the most exercise responsive lymphocytes [19, 20]. Preferential mobilization of these cells from the marginal pool is caused by increases in haemodynamic shear forces and by the relatively high expression of β-adrenergic receptors on these cells, leading to detachment of lymphocytes from endothelial cells upon catecholamine stimulation [22]. Following exercise cessation, both NK cells and CD8+ memory T cells quickly reallocate to the tissues. Only recently, it was documented that CMV latency enhances the exercise-induced mobilization of CD8 effector memory T cells in adult and middle aged (50–64 years old) subjects [21, 22, 32]. Interestingly, mobilization of NK cells was less pronounced in both adult and middle aged CMV carriers, suggesting that CMV infection may impair their mobilization [22, 33].

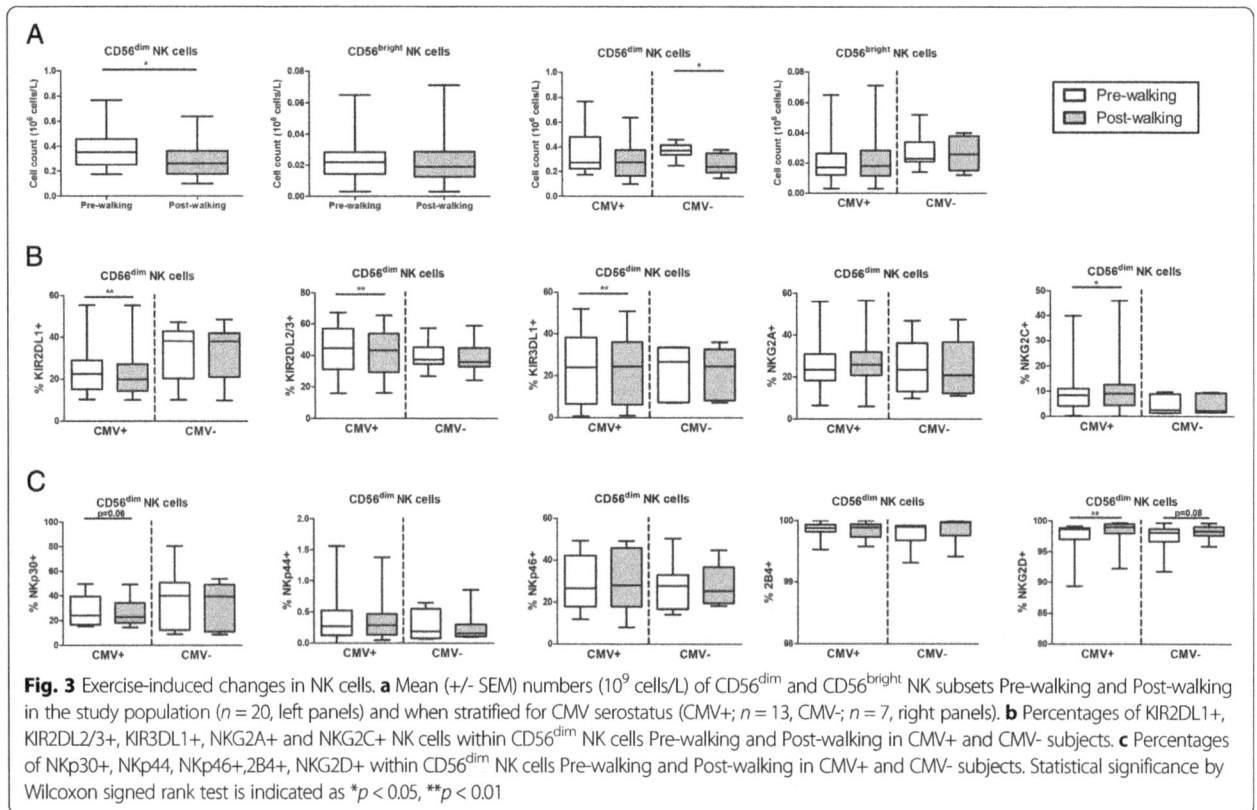

Fig. 3 Exercise-induced changes in NK cells. **a** Mean (+/- SEM) numbers (10^9 cells/L) of CD56^dim and CD56^bright NK subsets Pre-walking and Post-walking in the study population (n = 20, left panels) and when stratified for CMV serostatus (CMV+; n = 13, CMV-; n = 7, right panels). **b** Percentages of KIR2DL1+, KIR2DL2/3+, KIR3DL1+, NKG2A+ and NKG2C+ NK cells within CD56^dim NK cells Pre-walking and Post-walking in CMV+ and CMV- subjects. **c** Percentages of NKp30+, NKp44, NKp46+,2B4+, NKG2D+ within CD56^dim NK cells Pre-walking and Post-walking in CMV+ and CMV- subjects. Statistical significance by Wilcoxon signed rank test is indicated as *$p < 0.05$, **$p < 0.01$

Moreover, CMV carriage delayed the egress of both CD8 T_{EM} cells and NK cells to the tissues. The latter may be due to impaired β-adrenergic receptor signalling in CMV carriers [34].

Our study revealed a very modest increase of CD8 T_{EM} cells in CMV carriers and a decrease of CD56^dim NK cells in CMV non-carriers. This may be explained by the timing of the blood sampling, which was done within 10 min after exercise cessation, in the early recovery phase. The selective decrease of CD56^dim NK cells may indeed suggest a rapid distribution of these cells to the tissues. In contrast, we found proportions of NKG2C+ CD56^dim NK cells increased after exercise in CMV seropositive subjects, which would be in line with their delayed egress due to catecholamine insensitivity [22, 34]. Thus, also in octogenarians, CMV carriage may delay the egress of CD8 T_{EM} cells and 'memory-like' NK cells to the tissues.

Latent CMV infection may also increase the mobilization of CD4+ effector memory T cells, albeit to a lesser extent than CD8 T cells [21, 32]. Our octogenarian walkers showed limited increases in CD4+ effector memory and in terminally differentiated effector memory T cells in response to exercise. This may be explained by the notion that most memory T cells are retained in peripheral tissues as tissue resident memory T cells [35]. In line with this, markers of immune

exhaustion, such as PD-1 and CTLA-4, on memory subsets were unchanged.

Previously, the exercise induced mobilization of CD8+ naïve/early differentiated cells was found to be impaired in middle aged adults, irrespective of CMV serostatus [32]. Data on naïve CD4+ T cell mobilization in middle aged and elderly individuals are scarce. We here report on a robust response of naïve CD4+ T cells in our octogenarian cohort of habitual walkers. Numerical increases of naïve CD4+ T cells were seen irrespective of CMV status. In contrast, the response of naïve CD8 T cells was very limited and is in line with the higher turn-over rate of naïve CD8 T cells as a consequence of ageing and or frequent environmental challenges [7, 36–39]. Conversely, human CD4 naïve T cells are better maintained with age due to peripheral homeostatic proliferation mechanisms involving IL-2, a phenomenon not seen with naïve CD8 T cells [30, 40, 41]. The exercise-induced increases of CD4+ naïve T cells suggests that these cells are retained in the marginal pool and/or lymphoid tissues on to high age.

Few studies have investigated effects of exercise on diverse Treg subsets in elderly cohorts. We here report on exercise-induced changes of naïve/resting regulatory T cells but not activated/memory Treg. The increase in naïve Treg suggests, similar to the RTE and central naïve CD4+ T cells, the maintenance of these subsets on to

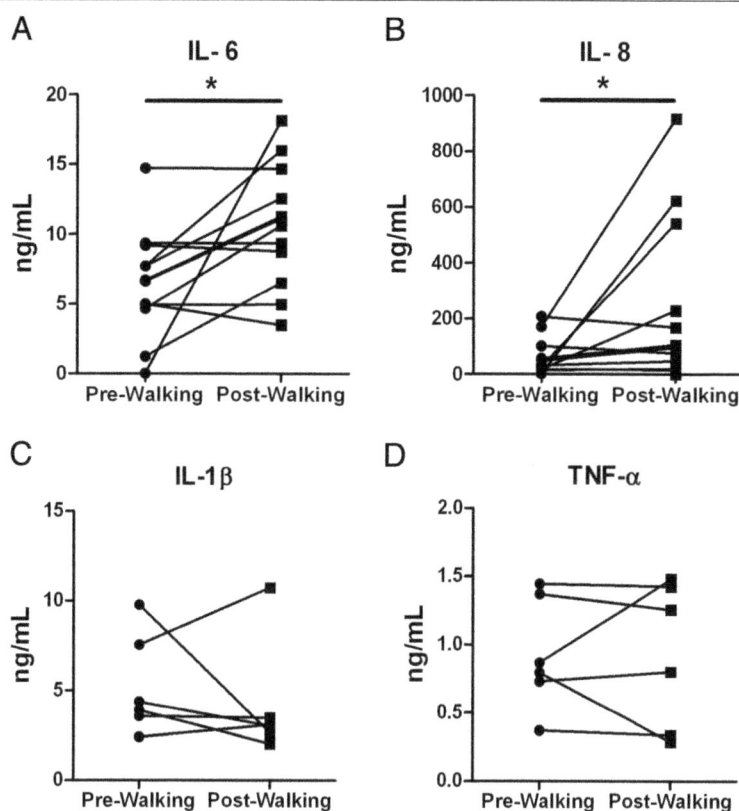

Fig. 4 LPS-stimulated PBMC cytokine production before and after walking. Cytokines (**a**) IL-6, (**b**) IL-8, (**c**) IL-1β and (**d**) TNFα in the 24 h supernatant of LPS-stimulated PBMC isolated pre and post walking. Individual pre- and post- samples are connected by lines. Cytokines in supernatants were assessed with ELISA and expressed as ng/mL. The assay sensitivity was 8 pg/mL for IL-1β, 31 pg/mL for IL-6 and TNF-α, and 312 pg/mL for IL-8. The net cytokine production was calculated as cytokine production of the stimulated sample minus the cytokine production of the non-stimulated sample. IL-6 and IL-8 were assessed in 12 walkers (8 males and 4 females). IL-1β and TNF-α were assessed in 6 walkers (4 males and 2 females). Statistical significance by Wilcoxon signed rank test is indicated as *$p < 0.05$

high age in niches of the primary and secondary lymphoid organs. In contrast, memory Treg, even more so than conventional memory T cells, appear to be retained in the tissues [42].

We found serum CRP levels elevated in response to exercise. This is likely the result of higher levels of systemic IL-6. Indeed, a higher IL-6 and IL-8 production capacity upon LPS-stimulation of PBMC was seen after walking. Yet, production levels of IL-1β and TNFα were unaltered. The higher production levels of IL-6 and IL-8 may reflect the higher number of monocytes in the PBMC fraction after exercise but do not explain why the production capacity of IL-1β and TNFα were not elevated. An age-associated reduced inflammasome activation may underlie the reduced IL-1β and TNFα production capacity of elderly monocytes; a notion that would merit further investigation.

Our study cohort was obviously biased for physical fitness, as the participants were able to complete 4 consecutive days of moderate intensity exercise. The participants, however, were not selected as healthy

individuals and 14 out of the 20 participants had at least one disease for which they were treated. Our cohort thus represents a selection of habitual elderly walkers who exercise in spite of having a disease. Yet, baseline values of both innate and adaptive immune cells compare well to values obtained in a healthy elderly cohort who were selected for their health ([9], data not shown).

Importantly, although our study was not designed and powered to definitely conclude on the effects of CMV carriage on the response to exercise, a retrospective analysis already revealed clear effects of CMV carriage on amplitude and/or kinetics of peripheral immune markers in this small cohort of octogenarians. Clearly, further studies in independent elderly cohorts are required to assess the effects of CMV carriage on acute exercise induced immune cell changes.

Conclusion

Acute exercise induced changes in immune cell numbers and functions in a group of octogenarian walkers. The massive exercise-induced response of naïve CD4+ T cells was most remarkable and adds to the notion of naïve CD4+ maintenance on to high age. The functional consequences of these changes for mobilization of immune responses to novel (and previously encountered) antigens remain to be established.

Additional files

Additional file 1: Figure S1. Exercise-induced T cell proliferation rates and T cell subset redistribution in CMV+ and CMV- subjects. (a) Rates of CD4 (left panel) and CD8 (right panel) proliferation before (Pre-Walking) and after exercise (Post-Walking) assessed by Ki-67 expression using flow-cytometry. Percentages of Ki-67 expressing cells within the CD4 and CD8 populations are shown. (b) Enumeration of CD4 and CD8 T cell differentiation subsets based on CD45RO and CCR7 expression Pre- and Post-Walking in CMV seropositive subjects (upper panel, $n = 13$) and CMV seronegative subjects (lower panel, $n = 7$). Mean (+/- SEM) numbers (10^9 cells/L) of naïve T cells ($T_{Naïve}$), central memory T cells (T_{CM}), effector memory T cells (T_{EM}) and terminally differentiated T cells (T_{TD}) are shown. (c) Mean (+/- SEM) numbers (10^9 cells/L) of recent thymic emigrants defined as CD31 + CD4 + $T_{Naïve}$ and the central naïve CD31-CD4+ $T_{Naïve}$ subsets in CMV+ and CMV- subjects. Statistical significance by Wilcoxon signed rank test is indicated as *$p < 0.05$, **p

Additional file 2: Figure S2. Exercise does not induce PD-1 and CTLA-4 on CD4 and CD8 memory T cells. (a) Percentages of PD-1 expressing cells in CD4 (left panel) and CD8 (right panel) effector memory T cells (T_{EM}) and terminally differentiated T cells (T_{TD}) pre- (white) and post-walking (grey). (b) Percentages of CTLA-4-expressing cells in CD4 (left panel) and CD8 (right panel) effector memory T cells (T_{EM}) and terminally differentiated T cells (T_{TD}

Additional file 3 Figure S3. Exercise-induced changes of naïve Treg, but not memory Treg. (a) Mean (+/- SEM) numbers (10^9 cells/L) of Naïve Treg and Memory Treg Pre-walking and Post-walking in CMV+ ($n = 13$) and CMV- ($n = 7$) subjects. Statistical significance by Wilcoxon signed rank test is indicated as *$p < 0.05$ and **p

Abbreviations
BMI: Body mass index; bpm: Beats per minute; CCR7: C-C chemokine receptor type 7; CRP: C-reactive protein; CTLA-4: Cytotoxic T-lymphocyte-associated protein 4; ELISA: Enzyme-linked immunosorbent assay; Foxp3: Forkhead box P3; HRmax: Maximal heart rate; IL-1β: Interleukin-1β; IL-6: Interleukin-6; IL-8: Interleukin-8; LPS: Lipopolysacharide; NK: Natural killer; PBMC: Peripheral blood mononuclear cells; PD-1: Programmed cell death protein 1; RTE: Recent thymic emigrants; T_{CM}: Central memory T cells; TCR: T cell receptor; T_{EM}: Effector memory T cells; $T_{Naïve}$: Naïve T cells; TNF-α: Tumor necrosis factor-α; Treg: Regulatory T cell; T_{TD}: Terminally differentiated T cells; WBGT: Wet bulb globe temperature

Acknowledgements
We are grateful to Bram van Cranenbroek (Dept Lab. Med. at Radboud university medical centre) for optimising the NK cell flow-cytometry panels. We also recognize the excellent help of the organization of the Nijmegen Four Days Marches. Above all we would like to thank our volunteers ('The Golden Oldies') for their endurance, wonderful spirits and their participation in this study.

Funding
This work was supported by the Netherlands Organization for Scientific Research (Veni Grant 016.136.101 for JFMJ and Rubicon Grant 825.12.016 for TMHE). The funding agencies had no role in design of the study, collection, analysis and interpretation of the data nor the writing of the manuscript.

Authors' contributions
KSMvdG, TMHE, HJPK, IJ, EB, MTEH, JFMJ and AMHB designed and organised the study. KSMvdG, QW, TMHE and JFMJ performed the study. KSMvdG, QW, TMHE, JFMJ and AMHB analyzed the data. KSMvdG and AMHB wrote the first draft of the paper. KSMvdG, TMHE, JFMJ and AMHB are responsible for the final content. All authors read and approved the final manuscript.

Competing interests
The authors declare that they have no competing interests.

Author details
[1]Departments of Rheumatology and Clinical Immunology and Translational Immunology Groningen (TRIGR), University of Groningen, University Medical Center Groningen, Hanzeplein 1, 9700RB Groningen, The Netherlands. [2]Department of Physiology, Radboud University Medical Centre, Nijmegen, The Netherlands. [3]Department of Laboratory Medicine, Laboratory Medical Immunology, Radboud University Medical Centre, Nijmegen, The Netherlands.

References
1. Fulop T, Kotb R, Fortin CF, Pawelec G, de Angelis F, Larbi A. Potential role of immunosenescence in cancer development. Ann N Y Acad Sci. 2010; 1197(1):158.
2. Poland GA, Ovsyannikova IG, Kennedy RB, Lambert ND, Kirkland JL. A systems biology approach to the effect of aging, immunosenescence and vaccine response. Curr Opin Immunol. 2014;29:62.
3. Yoshikawa TT. Epidemiology and unique aspects of aging and infectious diseases. Clin Infect Dis. 2000;30(6):931.
4. Brodin P, Jojic V, Gao T, et al. Variation in the human immune system is largely driven by non-heritable influences. Cell. 2015;160(1-2):37–47.
5. Fülöp T, Larbi A, Pawelec G. Human T cell aging and the impact of persistent viral infections. Front Immunol. 2013;4:271. doi:10.3389/fimmu. 2013.00271.
6. Weltevrede M, Eilers R, de Melker HE, van Baarle D. Cytomegalovirus persistence and T-cell immunosenescence in people aged fifty and older: A systematic review. Exp Gerontol. 2016;77:87–95.
7. van der Geest KS, Abdulahad WH, Horst G, et al. Quantifying Distribution of Flow Cytometric TCR-Vbeta Usage with Economic Statistics. PloS One. 2015a;10(4):e0125373.
8. Akbar AN, Henson SM. Are senescence and exhaustion intertwined or unrelated processes that compromise immunity? Nat Rev Immunol. 2011;11(4):289.
9. van der Geest KSM, Abdulahad WH, Tete SM, et al. Ageing disturbs the balance between effector and regulatory CD4+ T cells. Exp Gerontol. 2014;60:190.
10. Booth NJ, McQuaid AJ, Sobande T, et al. Different proliferative potential and migratory characteristics of human CD4+ regulatory T cells that express either CD45RA or CD45RO. J Immunol. 2010;184:4317.
11. Fessler J, Ficjan A, Duftner C, Dejaco C. The impact of aging on regulatory T-cells. Front Immunol. 2013;4:231.
12. Wang Q, Westra J, van der Geest KSM, et al. Reduced levels of cytosolic DNA sensor AIM2 are associated with impaired cytokine responses in healthy elderly. Exp Gerontol. 2016;2(78):39. doi:10.1016/j.exger.2016.02.016.
13. Franceschi C, Capri M, Monti D, et al. Inflammaging and anti-inflammaging: a systemic perspective on aging and longevity emerged from studies in humans. Mech Ageing Dev. 2007;128(1):92.
14. Biagi E, Nylund L, Candela M, et al. Through ageing, and beyond: gut microbiota and inflammatory status in seniors and centenarians. PLoS One. 2010;5(5):e10667.
15. Solana R, Campos C, Pera A, Tarazona R. Shaping of NK cell subsets by aging. Curr Opin Immunol. 2014;29:56.

16. Walsh NP, Gleeson M, Shephard RJ, et al. Position Statement. Part one: Immune function and exercise. Exerc Immunol Rev. 2011;17:6–63.

17. Eijsvogels TM, Thompson PD. Exercise Is Medicine: At Any Dose? JAMA. 2015;314(18):1915.

18. Simpson RJ, Bosch JA. Special issue on exercise immunology: current perspectives on aging, health and extreme performance. Brain Behav Immun. 2014;39:1.

19. Bigley AB, Rezvani K, Chew C, et al. Acute exercise preferentially redeploys NK-cells with a highly-differentiated phenotype and augments cytotoxicity against lymphoma and multiple myeloma target cells. Brain Behav Immun. 2014;39:160.

20. Campbell JP, Riddell NE, Burns VE, et al. Acute exercise mobilises CD8+ T lymphocytes exhibiting an effector-memory phenotype. Brain Behav Immun. 2009;6:767.

21. Turner JE, Aldred S, Witard OC. Latent Cytomegalovirus infection amplifies CD8 T-lymphocyte mobilisation and egress in response to exercise. Brain Behav Immun. 2010;24:1362.

22. Simpson RJ, Bigley AB, Spielmann G, et al. Human cytomegalovirus infection and the immune response to exercise. Exerc Immunol Rev. 2016;22:8.

23. Jacobs JF, Eijsvogels TM, van der Geest KS, et al. The impact of exercise on the variation of serum free light chains. Clin Chem Lab Med. 2014;52(11):e239.

24. Eijsvogels TM, Veltmeijer MT, George K, Hopman MT, Thijssen DH. The impact of obesity on cardiac troponin levels after prolonged exercise in humans. Eur J Appl Physiol. 2012;112(5):1725.

25. Tanaka H, Monahan KD, Seals DR. Age-predicted maximal heart rate revisited. J Am Coll Cardiol. 2001;37:153.

26. Durnin JV, Womersley J. Body fat assessed from total body density and its estimation from skinfold thickness: measurements on 481 men and women aged from 16 to 72 years. Br J Nutr. 1974;32(1):77.

27. Dill DB, Costill DL. Calculation of percentage changes in volumes of blood, plasma, and red cells in dehydration. J Appl Physiol. 1974;37(2):247.

28. Sallusto F, Geginat J, Lanzavecchia A. Central memory and effector memory T cell subsets: function, generation, and maintenance. Annu Rev Immunol. 2004;22:745.

29. Kimmig S, Przybylski GK, Schmidt CA, et al. Two subsets of naive T helper cells with distinct T cell receptor excision circle content in human adult peripheral blood. J Exp Med. 2002;195:789.

30. van der Geest KS, Abdulahad WH, Teteloshvili N, et al. Low-affinity TCR engagement drives IL-2-dependent post-thymic maintenance of naive CD4 + T cells in aged humans. Aging Cell. 2015;14(5):744.

31. Miyara M, Yoshioka Y, Kitoh A, et al. Functional delineation and differentiation dynamics of human CD4+ T cells expressing the FoxP3 transcription factor. Immunity. 2009;30:899.

32. Spielmann G, Bollard CM, Bigley AB, et al. The effects of age and latent cytomegalovirus infection on the redeployment of CD8+ T cell subsets in response to acute exercise in humans. Brain Behav Immun. 2014;39:142.

33. Bigley AB, Spielmann G, Agha N, Simpson RJ. The effects of age and latent Cytomegalovirus infection on NK-cell phenotype and exercise responsiveness in man. Oxid Med Cell Longev. 2015;2015:979645.

34. Bigley AB, Rezvani K, Pistillo M, et al. Acute exercise preferentially redeploys NK-cells with a highly-differentiated phenotype and augments cytotoxicity against lymphoma and multiple myeloma target cells. Part II: impact of latent cytomegalovirus infection and catecholamine sensitivity. Brain Behav Immun. 2015;49:59.

35. Thome JJ, Farber DL. Emerging concepts in tissue-resident T cells: lessons from humans. Trends Immunol. 2015;36(7):428.

36. Nikolich-Zugich J, Slifka MK, Messaoudi I. The many important facets of T-cell repertoire diversity. Nat Rev Immunol. 2004;4(2):123.

37. Goronzy JJ, Lee WW, Weyand CM. Aging and T-cell diversity. Exp Gerontol. 2007;42:400.

38. Blackman MA, Woodland DL. The narrowing of the CD8 T cell repertoire in old age. Curr Opin Immunol. 2011;23:537.

39. Wertheimer AM, Bennett MS, Park B, et al. Aging and cytomegalovirus infection differentially and jointly affect distinct circulating T cell subsets in humans. J Immunol. 2014;192:2143.

40. den Braber I, Mugwagwa T, Vrisekoop N, et al. Maintenance of peripheral naive T cells is sustained by thymus output in mice but not humans. Immunity. 2012;36:288.

41. Pekalski ML, Ferreira RC, Coulson RM, et al. Postthymic Expansion in Human CD4 Naive T Cells Defined by Expression of Functional High-Affinity IL-2 Receptors. J Immunol. 2013;190:2554.

42. Thome JJ, Bickham KL, Ohmura Y, et al. Early-life compartmentalization of human T cell differentiation and regulatory function in mucosal and lymphoid tissues. Nat Med. 2016;22(1):72.

Age dependent accumulation patterns of advanced glycation end product receptor (RAGE) ligands and binding intensities between RAGE and its ligands differ in the liver, kidney, and skeletal muscle

Myeongjoo Son[1,2†], Wook-Jin Chung[3,4†], Seyeon Oh[2], Hyosang Ahn[1,2], Chang Hu Choi[5], Suntaek Hong[6], Kook Yang Park[5], Kuk Hui Son[5*†] and Kyunghee Byun[1,2*†]

Abstract

Background: Much evidence indicates receptor for advanced glycation end products (RAGE) related inflammation play essential roles during aging. However, the majority of studies have focused on advanced glycation end products (AGEs) and not on other RAGE ligands. In the present study, the authors evaluated whether the accumulation of RAGE ligands and binding intensities between RAGE and its ligands differ in kidney, liver, and skeletal muscle during aging.

Results: In C57BL/6 N mice aged 12 weeks, 12 months, and 22 months, ligands accumulation, binding intensities between RAGE and its ligands, activated macrophage infiltration, M1/M2 macrophage expression, glyoxalase-1 expression, and signal pathways related to inflammation were evaluated. The RAGE ligands age-associated accumulation patterns were found to be organ dependent. Binding intensities between RAGE and its ligands in kidney and liver increased with age, but those in skeletal muscle were unchanged. Infiltration of activated macrophages in kidney and liver increased with age, but infiltration in the skeletal muscle was unchanged. M1 expression increased and M2 and glyoxalase-1 expression decreased with age in kidney and liver, but their expressions in skeletal muscle were not changed.

Conclusion: These findings indicate patterns of RAGE ligands accumulation, RAGE/ligands binding intensities, or inflammation markers changes during aging are organs dependent.

Keywords: RAGE, RAGE ligands, AGEs, Aging, Macrophage activation

Background

The aging process can be described as a universal, intrinsic, progressive accumulation of deleterious changes in cells and tissues that increase morbidity and lead to death [1]. According to the recent theory of oxidation-inflammation, chronic oxidative and inflammatory stress conditions explain the aging process [2].

Several studies have focused on the role played by receptor for advanced glycation end products (RAGE) on aging, because RAGE is known inducer of inflammation and oxidative stress.

RAGE belongs to the immunoglobulin superfamily of cell surface molecules and has an extracellular region containing one V-type immunoglobulin domain and two C-type immunoglobulin domains [3, 4]. The extracellular portion of the receptor is followed by a hydrophobic transmembrane-spanning domain and then by a highly charged, short cytoplasmic domain that is essential for intracellular RAGE signaling [3, 4].

* Correspondence: dr632@gilhospital.com; khbyun1@gachon.ac.kr
†Equal contributors
5Department of Thoracic and Cardiovascular Surgery, Gachon University Gil Medical Center, Gachon University, Incheon 21565, Republic of Korea
1Department of Anatomy and Cell Biology, Graduate School of Medicine, Gachon University, Incheon 21936, Republic of Korea
Full list of author information is available at the end of the article

RAGE has several ligands, such as, advanced glycation end products (AGEs), proinflammatory S100/calgranulin family members, and high motility group box 1 protein (HMGB1) [5, 6]. RAGE is also a signal transduction receptor for amyloid β [7] and endogenous phospholipids such as lysophosphatidic acid [8].

After binding these ligands, RAGE activates an inflammation-related signaling cascade involving nuclear factor-(NF)κB, ERK (extracellular signal-regulated kinase) 1/2, p38 MAPK (mitogen-activated protein kinases), JNK (c-Jun N terminal kinases), PKC (protein kinase C), Rac/Cdc42, and TIRAP and MyD88 (adaptor proteins for TLR 2 and 4) [5, 6].

Because AGEs accumulates in organs, such as, kidney [9], liver [10], brain [11], and skeletal muscle during aging [12], researches have tended to investigate the role played by the AGEs-RAGE pathway during aging. The AGEs-RAGE pathway is a primary contributor to kidney aging [13]. The accumulation of AGEs and a progressive decline in renal function during aging may induce the release of inflammatory mediators and the generation of reactive oxygen species (ROS) [10, 11]. Furthermore, this accumulation starts before a clinical decrease in kidney function is evident, and is one of the characteristic features of kidney aging [14, 15].

Although much evidence indicates that RAGE-related inflammation and oxidative stress participate in the aging process, the majority of studies on the topic have been focused only AGEs and not on other RAGE ligands [13–15]. In fact, few studies have addressed the roles of these other RAGE ligands in different organs in same animals.

Therefore, we sought to determine whether the accumulation patterns of the RAGE ligands which are AGEs, HMGB1, and S100β and the binding intensities between RAGE and its ligands in kidney, liver, and skeletal muscle are age-dependent.

Methods

Animals

A total of 18 male C57BL/6 N mice were used and kidney, liver, and skeletal muscle were extracted from young (12 weeks old, $n = 6$), middle-aged (12 months old, $n = 6$), and old (22 months old, $n = 6$) mice. The skeletal muscle was collected from adductor profundus of mouse hind limb. All animals were examined daily for signs of injury or illness by trained persons. When tissue samples were collected no abnormality was evident. This study was approved by Lee Gil Ya Cancer and Diabetes Institute of Gachon University, and conducted in strict accordance with the guidelines issued by our Institutional Animal Care and Use Committee (Approval number; LCDI–2015–0080).

Sample preparation

Protein preparation

Kidney, liver, and skeletal muscle proteins were extracted using the EzRIPA lysis kit (ATTO, Tokyo). All tissues were homogenized with lysis buffer plus proteinase inhibitor and phosphatase inhibitor and briefly sonicated 10 times for 10 s in a cold bath sonicator. After centrifuging at 14,000 x g for 20 mins at 4 °C, supernatant phases were collected and protein concentrations were determined using a Bicinchoninic acid assay kit (Thermo Scientific, IL, USA).

RNA isolation and cDNA synthesis

Total RNA in kidney, liver, and skeletal muscle from young, middle-aged, and old mice were isolated using a Trizol reagent (Invitrogen, CA, USA) according to the manufacturer's instructions. All tissues were homogenized in ice using a disposable pestle in 1 ml of Trizol reagent. Homogenized tissues were added to 0.2 ml of chloroform (Amresco, OH, USA), mixed, and centrifuged at 12,000 x g for 15 mins at 4 °C. Aqueous phases were collected, placed in cleaned tubes, mixed with 0.5 ml of isopropanol, and centrifuged using the same conditions. Isolated RNA was then washed with 70% ethanol, and dissolved in 30 μl of DEPC treated water. To perform quantitative real time polymerase chain reaction (qRT-PCR), 1 μg of total RNA was subjected to complementary DNA (cDNA) synthesis using the PrimeScript 1st strand cDNA Synthesis Kit (TAKARA, Japan).

Paraffin block tissue slides

Mice were anesthetized with Rumpun (2.5 mg/kg) and Zoletil (500 mg/kg). Kidney, liver, and skeletal muscle tissues from young, middle-aged, and old mice were fixed in 4% paraformaldehyde (Sigma-Aldrich, MO, USA) overnight and placed in an automatic dehydration machine (Leica ASP-300 S). Tissues were dehydrated in a series of steps, that is, with 90% ethanol for 3 × 1 h, followed by 100% ethanol for 2 × 2 h. Tissues were then cleared with 100% xylene for 3 × 1.5 h, embedded in warmed paraffin, and paraffin embedded tissue blocks were sectioned at 10 μm.

Immunohistochemistry

Macrophage infiltration was identified by the expression of Iba1 in kidney, liver and skeletal muscles. Paraffin was removed by zylene and washed three times for 10 mins each in phosphate-buffered saline (PBS). Endogenous peroxidase was blocked by 0.3% hydrogen peroxide in PBS, followed by three times rinses with PBS and we then blocked for 1 h with normal serum. The tissues sections were incubated with anti-Iba1 antibody (see in Additional file 1: Table S1) overnight at 4 °C and allowed to react with 3,3′-diaminobenzidine (DAB) from standard ABC kit (Vector Laboratories).

Enzyme-linked Immunosorbent assay (ELISA) assay

Indirect ELISA assay

AGE, HMGB1, and S100β levels in kidney, liver and skeletal muscle tissues in young, middle-aged and old mice were measured by an Indirect ELISA. Coating solution mixture (0.6% sodium bicarbonate and 0.3% sodium carbonate in distilled water) were incubated onto 96-well plates overnight at 4 °C. Protein samples were mixed with 5% skim milk containing 0.1% Triton x-100 in phosphate-buffered saline (TPBS) and then incubated overnight at 4 °C. Unbound proteins were removed by washing with TPBS and incubated with anti-AGE, anti-HMGB1, and anti-S100β antibodies for 6 h at room temperature (see in Additional file 1: Table S1). Unbound antibodies were removed by washing with TPBS, and then incubated with horseradish peroxidase (HRP) conjugated anti-rabbit antibody for 2 h at room temperature. After washing out unbound HRP conjugated antibody, color was developed by incubating samples with 3,3′,5,5′-tetramethylbenzidine (TMB) for 15 mins. The reaction was stopped by adding 100 µl of 2 M H_2SO_4 to each well, and absorbance was then measured at 450 nm using an ELISA plate reader (VERSA Max, Molecular Devices).

Sandwich ELISA assay

RAGE-RAGE ligand bindings in kidney, liver, and skeletal muscle in young, middle-aged and old mice were determined by sandwich ELISA. A 96-well plate was coated by anti-RAGE antibody with coating solution mixture overnight at 4 °C. Unbound anti-RAGE antibody was removed with washing with TPBS. To reduce non-specific binding, proteins were mixed with 5% skim milk containing TPBS and incubated overnight at 4 °C. Unbound proteins were removed by washing repeatedly with TPBS. Anti-RAGE antibody binding samples were treated with anti-AGE, anti-HMGB1, and anti-S100β antibodies for 2 h at room temperature (Additional file 1: Table S1). After washing with TPBS, bound proteins were incubated with HRP conjugated anti-rabbit secondary antibody for 2 h at room temperature. After washing off unbound HRP conjugated secondary antibody, color was developed by incubating samples with TMB for 15 mins. Reactions were terminated by adding same volumes of H_2SO_4 and absorbance was measured using the ELISA plate reader.

Quantitative real time polymerase chain reaction (qRT-PCR) analysis

To quantify genesglyoxalase 1 (GLO-1) level, we used quantitative real time polymerase chain reaction (qRT-PCR). Briefly, 300 ng cDNA, 5 µl ROX plus SYBR green premix (TAKARA) and 0.4 µM forward and 0.4 µM reverse primers (Additional file 1: Table S2) were mixed for each gene, and levels of gene expression were then determined using a CFX384 Touch™ Real-Time PCR Detection System (Bio-Rad).

Immunoblotting analysis

To estimate the M1/M2 macrophage infiltration and levels of inflammatory proteins including NFκB and interleukin-1β (IL-1β), 30 µg of proteins per lane were separated by 4–12% NuPAGE Bis-Tris gel (Thermo Scientific) electrophoresis. Proteins were then transferred to polyvinylidene fluoride (PVDF) membranes at 200 mA for 2 h. Non-specific binding was blotted with 5% skim milk. Membranes were then treated with primary antibodies (Additional file 1: Table S1), washed with Tris-buffered saline containing 0.1% Tween 20 (TTBS) three times and incubated with secondary antibodies (Additional file 1: Table S1). Membranes were developed by enhanced chemiluminescence (Thermo Scientific) on a LAS-4000 analyzer (GE healthcare).

Statistical analysis

Given the small sample size, non-parametric analysis was used. Statistical analyses were performed using SPSS version 22 (IBM Corporation, NY, USA). The Kruskal-Wallis test was used to compare groups, and the Mann-Whitney U test was used for multiple comparison.

P values of <0.05 were deemed significant. All results are expressed as means ± standard deviations.

Results

Age increased RAGE ligands levels in kidney and liver but not in skeletal muscle

The AGEs accumulation in the kidney of young group was significantly lower than in the middle-aged group, and there was difference between middle-aged and old group in the kidney. The accumulation of HMGB1 and S100β in kidney of the three age groups was significantly increased with age (Fig. 1a). In liver, AGEs accumulation was increased by aging. HMGB1 and S100β accumulations in liver were significantly lower in the young group than in the middle-aged group, and HMGB1 and S100β levels in liver were different between the middle-aged and old groups (Fig. 1b). No difference in skeletal muscle levels was found between the three age groups (Fig. 1c).

Binding intensities between RAGE and its ligands increased with age in kidney and liver but not in skeletal muscle

In kidney, binding intensities between RAGE and AGEs significantly increased with age and the RAGE/HMGB1

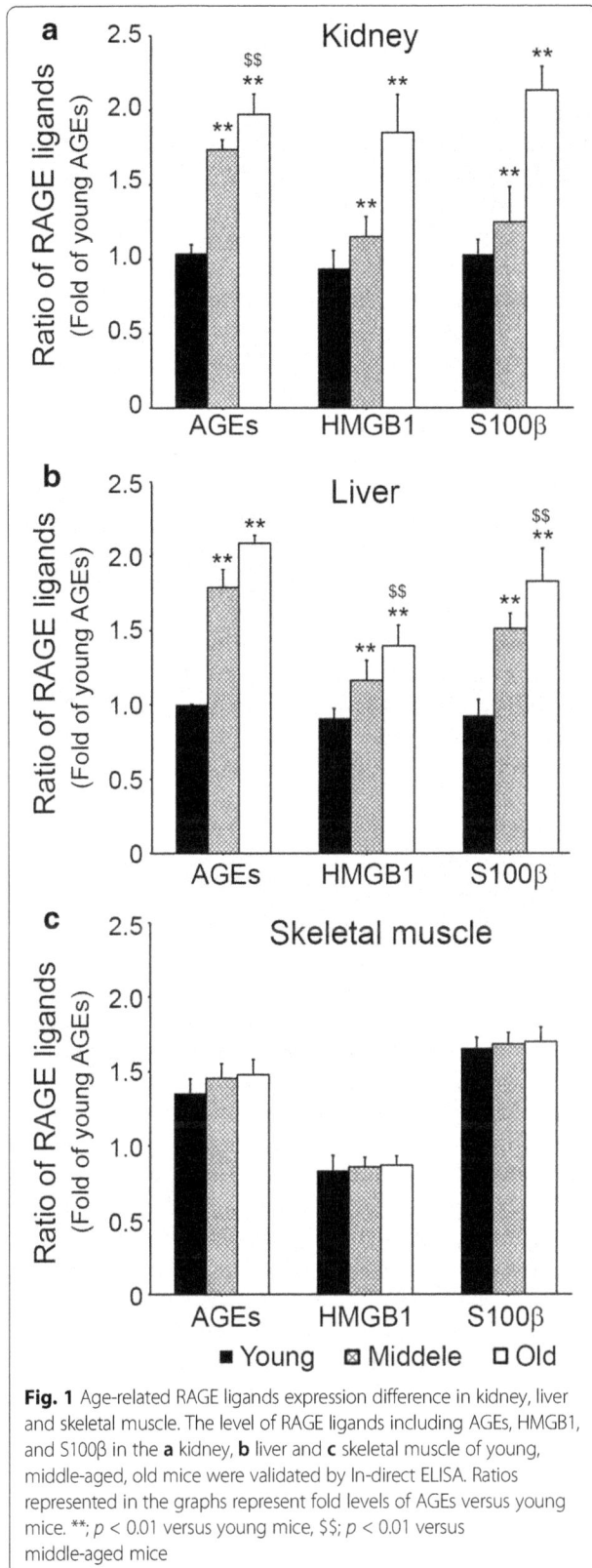

Fig. 1 Age-related RAGE ligands expression difference in kidney, liver and skeletal muscle. The level of RAGE ligands including AGEs, HMGB1, and S100β in the **a** kidney, **b** liver and **c** skeletal muscle of young, middle-aged, old mice were validated by In-direct ELISA. Ratios represented in the graphs represent fold levels of AGEs versus young mice. **; $p < 0.01$ versus young mice, $$; $p < 0.01$ versus middle-aged mice

and RAGE/S100β binding intensities increased with age (Fig. 2a). In additional, RAGE/AGEs, RAGE/HMGB1, and RAGE/S100β binding intensities were increased with aging in liver (Fig. 2b). However, in skeletal muscle, no intergroup difference was observed for any of binding intensities between the three ligands (Fig. 2c).

Increased infiltration of activated macrophages and expressions of M1 and M2 in tissues by age

In kidney and liver, infiltrations of activated macrophage (Iba1) into tissues increased significantly with age (Fig. 3a, b). However, no intergroup difference was found for activated macrophage infiltration into skeletal muscle (Fig. 3c). In kidney and liver, the expressions of M1 (iNOS) significantly increased with age (Fig. 3d, e). However, the expression of M1 in skeletal muscle was similar in the three groups (Fig. 3f). In kidney and liver, the expression of M2 (Arg1) in all three groups significantly decreases with age (Fig. 3d, e). However, the expression of M2 in skeletal muscle was similar in the three groups (Fig. 3f).

Glyoxalase-1 levels decreased and inflammatory protein levels increased in kidney and liver but not in skeletal muscle with age

In kidney and liver, GLO-1 levels were significantly different in the three groups decreased with age. In addition, there was statistical difference middle-aged and old group (Fig. 4a, b). However, in skeletal muscle no age-related differences were observed (Fig. 4c).

In kidney and liver, NFκB and IL-1β levels increased with age (Fig. 4d, e), but in skeletal muscle, no differences were observed (Fig. 4f).

Discussion

The present study shows; (1) the age-related accumulation patterns of RAGE ligands (AGEs, HMGB1, and S100β) are organ dependent; (2) binding intensities between RAGE and its ligands in kidney and liver increased with age, but binding intensities in skeletal muscle were not changed by aging; (3) infiltrations of activated macrophage into kidney and liver were increased with age, but infiltrations into skeletal muscle were not changed; (4) M1 expression was increased and M2 expression was decreased by age in kidney and liver, but M1 expression in skeletal muscle was unchanged; (5) GLO-1 expressions in kidney and liver were decreased by age, but unchanged in skeletal muscle; and (6) the activation of inflammation related signal pathway in kidney and liver increased with age, but in skeletal muscle they remained unchanged.

Several studies have shown that the AGEs-RAGE pathway is related to aging of humans and animals [16, 17]. In addition, many studies have shown AGEs

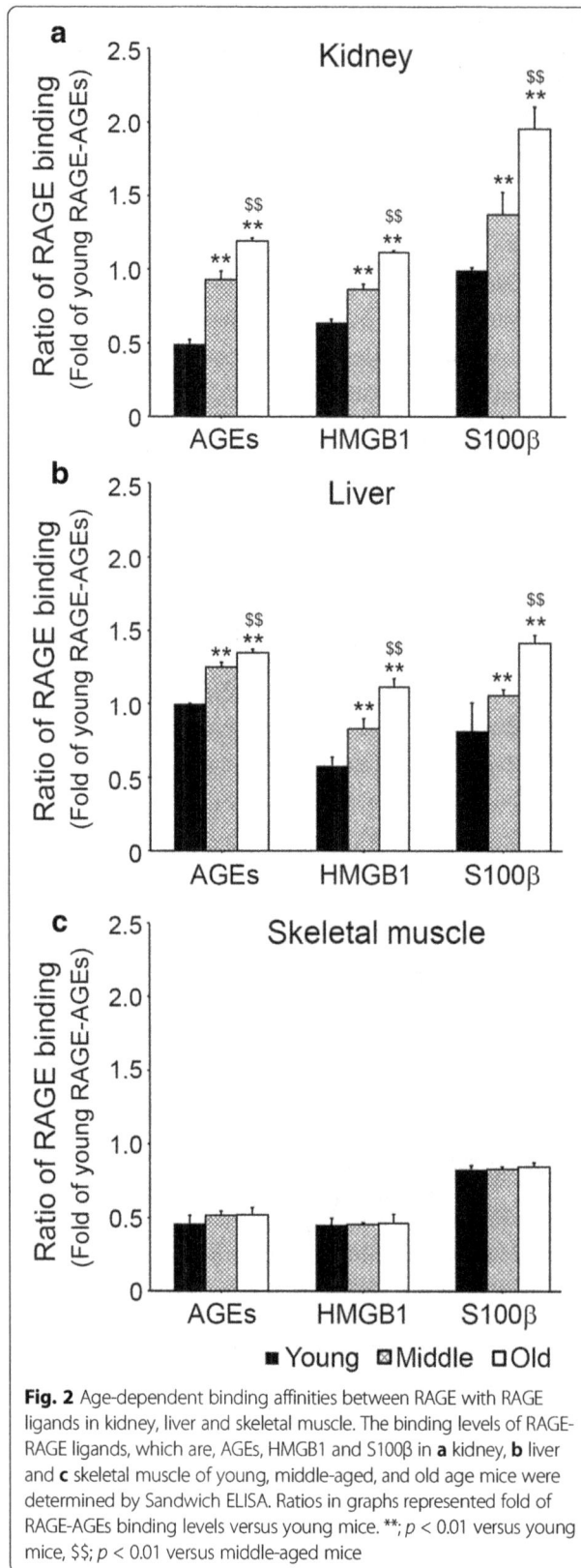

Fig. 2 Age-dependent binding affinities between RAGE with RAGE ligands in kidney, liver and skeletal muscle. The binding levels of RAGE-RAGE ligands, which are, AGEs, HMGB1 and S100β in **a** kidney, **b** liver and **c** skeletal muscle of young, middle-aged, and old age mice were determined by Sandwich ELISA. Ratios in graphs represented fold of RAGE-AGEs binding levels versus young mice. $**$; $p < 0.01$ versus young mice, $$$; $p < 0.01$ versus middle-aged mice

accumulates in tissues during aging. The liver is a site for clearance and catabolism of circulating AGEs but can also be a target organ for AGEs [10, 18]. AGEs are removed and metabolized by the kidney, but the kidney is also a site for AGEs accumulation and AGEs-associated damage [19]. It is well known that older adults exhibit increased collagen cross-linking and AGEs deposition in skeletal muscle [12]. Thus, we considered that accumulation of AGEs in liver, kidney, and skeletal muscle would be more prominent than in other tissues during aging.

In the present study, AGEs accumulations in kidney in the middle-aged and old groups were significantly higher than in the young group, however no difference was observed between the middle-aged and old groups. These results suggest AGEs accumulation in kidney reaches a maximum level even in middle-age. AGEs are generated endogenously by glycation, and this process is enhanced by ROS or hyperglycemic conditions or by ingestion of exogenous AGEs in food [13]. Physiological glycation state is regulated by a balance between the formation and clearance of AGEs [20], and this balance is maintained in part by glycation state, host defense machinery, including anti-glycation enzymes (e.g., glyoxalase), and kidney filtration function (glomerular filtration rate), which excretes AGEs and AGEs precursors from the body [13, 20].

The glomerular changes in C57B6 mice begin at 18 to 20 months of age, before recognizable tubulointerstitial changes, and these progressively increase to death at ~30 months [21, 22]. Although glomerular function might be preserved until 20 months [21, 22], it is known that GLO-1 levels in kidney decrease with age [23]. Many previous studies have shown AGEs accumulation in kidney linearly increases with age. The present study shows that AGEs accumulation peaked during middle-age in our animal model. Though we did not check glomerular function in the present study, we did observe GLO-1 expression decreased with aging, which concurs with other studies [23]. We speculate that decreasing GLO-1 activity by aging plays an important role in the renal accumulation of AGEs, because AGEs accumulation in kidney might accelerate before middle-age when glomerular filtration function is preserved [21, 22].

We found that AGEs accumulation in liver was significantly increased by aging, whereas GLO-1activity decreased, which agrees with other studies [24]. Age-related AGEs accumulation in skeletal muscle has been previously reported in an animal model [25], but in the present study, AGEs accumulation was unchanged by aging. Even GLO-1 levels were not changed in skeletal muscle. Other studies have shown an increasing pattern of AGEs accumulation in skeletal muscle by aging used 33-month rats as the old groups [25]. In the present

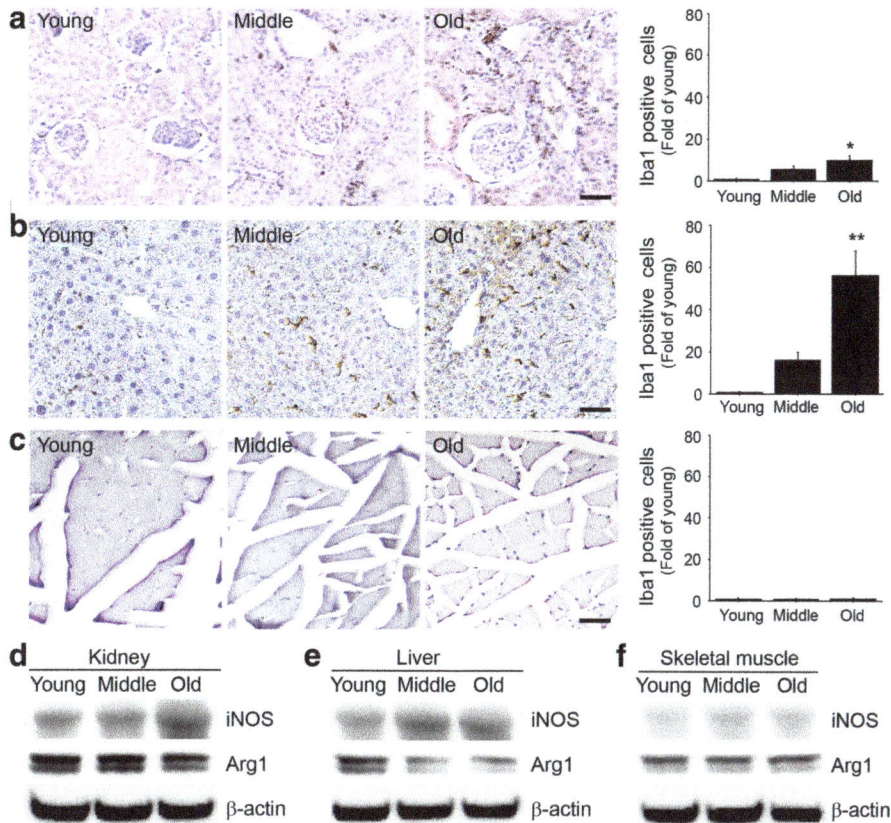

Fig. 3 Age-related expressions of total, M1, and M2 macrophages in kidney, liver and skeletal muscle. The Expression of total, M1 and M2 macrophages were determined by Immunohistochemistry and Immunoblotting. The level of Iba1 represented total macrophage expression in **a** kidney, **b** liver and **c** skeletal muscle. The level of iNOS represented M1 macrophage expression in **d** kidney, **e** liver and **f** skeletal kidney. The level of arginase 1 (Arg 1) represented M2 macrophage expression in **d** kidney, **e** liver and **f** skeletal kidney. Ratios in graphs are folds levels versus young mice. Scale bar = 100 um, *; $p < 0.05$ and **; $p < 0.01$ versus young mice

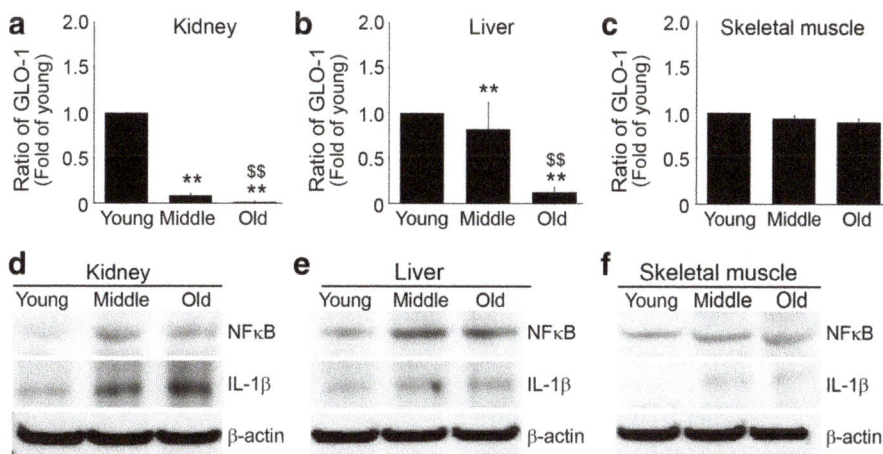

Fig. 4 Age-related changes in the levels of GLO-1 in kidney, liver and skeletal muscle. Levels of Glo-1 in **a** kidney, **b** liver and **c** skeletal muscle of the young, middle-aged, and old groups were validated by qRT-PCR. Ratios in graphs represented fold levels versus young mice. Expressions of NFκB and IL-1β were determined by immunoblotting in **d** kidney, **e** liver and **f** skeletal muscle. **; $p < 0.01$ versus young mice, $$; $p < 0.01$ versus middle-aged mice

study, we used 22-month mice, which could explain the discrepancy between results, and suggests AGEs accumulation in the skeletal muscle might accelerate after 22 months in mice.

Unlike AGEs, the age-related accumulation patterns of other RAGE ligands, such as, HMGB1 and S100β, have not been in different organs. However, the effects of the accumulations of HMGB1 and S100β during aging have been in the context of brain aging. In particular, the expression of S100 protein is increased in the aging brain [26]. It has also been reported that the distribution of HMGB1 appears to be altered in the aged brain [27]. More specifically, HMGB1 is downregulated in neurons in the aged brain, but it is upregulated in astrocytes, which suggests HMGB1 plays different roles in different types of brain cells and structures [27].

In the present study, HMGB1 and S100 β accumulation in kidney increased with age. In liver, there was no difference between the middle-aged and old groups in HMGB1 and S100β accumulation. In skeletal muscle, the accumulations of both ligands were not changed by aging.

Although RAGE ligand age-related accumulation patterns differed in kidney, liver, and skeletal muscle, binding intensities between RAGE ligands and RAGE increased with age in kidney and liver. These patterns paralleled age-related inflammation signal pathway activation, activated macrophage infiltration, M1 increases, and M2 decreases.

Ligand binding with RAGE triggers ROS increases, activates NADPH oxidase, increases the expressions of adhesion molecules, and upregulates inflammation through NFκB and other signaling pathways [18, 28]. Furthermore, activation of NFκB results in increased RAGE expression, thereby prolonging NFκB activation [29]. In addition, RAGE expression occurs in an inducible manner and is upregulated at sites where its ligands accumulate [29].

In the present study, we measured binding intensities between RAGE and its ligands rather than RAGE expression. Binding intensities between RAGE and its ligands in the liver and kidney were increased by aging, regardless of age-related ligand accumulation. The patterns of binding intensities between RAGE and its ligands in the liver and kidney matched NFκB and IL-1β activations, which suggests that binding intensity between RAGE and its ligands in the liver and kidney is a more important factor of age-related inflammation and oxidative stress than absolute ligand accumulations.

A previous study showed that the RAGE pathway can enhance macrophage migration [30] and promote proinflammatory mediator production, such as, those of IL-1β, IL-6, and TNF-α [31]. The RAGE/NF-κB pathway not only predominantly induces macrophages to secrete inflammatory cytokines but also induces M1 polarization [32], and M1 macrophages are Th1-biased and considered to be pro-inflammatory and most notably express TNFα and IL-6 [33]. The majority of the macrophages found in sites of inflammation in inflammatory diseases are considered to be M1 macrophages [33]. By contrast, M2 macrophages are Th2-biased and are thought to play more diverse roles, namely in anti-inflammatory pathways, tissue remodeling and wound healing [33].

The patterns of binding intensities between RAGE and its ligands in liver and kidney were similar to patterns of M1 expression increase and M2 expression decrease with age in liver and kidney, which suggests local tissue inflammation was increased by aging in liver and kidney and that the RAGE pathway plays an important role in the aging process. On the contrary, the aging process of skeletal muscle appears to be different from those of liver or kidney. The binding intensity between RAGE and its ligands, activation of inflammatory signal pathways, macrophage activation, and M1 polarization were not changed by aging in skeletal muscle, which suggests the RAGE pathway and inflammation induced by RAGE pathway do not play a main role in skeletal muscle aging. In aged animal skeletal muscle, AGEs cross-linking collagen was increased and those collagen made muscle stiff [11, 25]. Taken together, we speculate that mechanical property changes, such as, increased muscle stiffness caused by collagen fiber cross linking by AGEs might be more important than RAGE induced inflammation during skeletal muscle aging.

The main limitation of this study was that we did not measure ROS levels in tissues directly, however many studies have been shown that ROS levels increase during aging in many tissues. Our study shows NFκB increased with age in kidney and liver, and the NFκB signal pathway is known to be importantly related to ROS generation.

Conclusion

Our study shows binding intensities between RAGE and its ligands increased during aging and that these increases occur in parallel with activated macrophage infiltration, macrophage polarization, and inflammation signal pathway activation in the kidney and liver. However, skeletal muscle did not show any age-related changes in RAGE ligands accumulation, binding intensities, or inflammation marker changes, which suggest aging processes differ in different organs.

Abbreviations
AGEs: Advanced glycated endproducts; GLO-1: Glyoxalase-1; HMGB1: High-mobility group box 1; RAGE: Receptor of AGE; ROS: Reactive oxygen species

Acknowledgements
Not applicable.

Funding
This work was supported by Samsung Science and Technology Foundation (grant no. SSTF-BA1402–15, KB) and Korea Health Industry Development Institute (KHIDI) (grant no. HI13C-1602-010015, KHS).

Author's contributions
MS and WC analyzed and interpreted the data and they are major contributors in writing the manuscript. SH performed the experiments in revised manuscript and SO, HA and CHC performed the experiments in text. KYP provided statistical analysis and graphical data representation as well as contributed to writing of the manuscript, KHS and KB performed majority of the statistical analysis and contributed to writing of the manuscript, designed the study and interpreted the results. All authors read and approved the final manuscript.

Competing interests
The authors declare that they have no competing interests.

Ethics approval
This animal study was approved by Lee Gil Ya Cancer and Diabetes Institute of Gachon University, and conducted in strict accordance with the guidelines issued by our Institutional Animal Care and Use Committee (Approval no.; LCDI–2015–0080).

Author details
[1]Department of Anatomy and Cell Biology, Graduate School of Medicine, Gachon University, Incheon 21936, Republic of Korea. [2]Functional Cellular Networks Laboratory, Lee Gil Ya Cancer and Diabetes Institute, Gachon University, Incheon 21999, Republic of Korea. [3]Department of Cardiovascular Medicine, Gachon University, Incheon 21999, Republic of Korea. [4]Gachon Cardiovascular Research Institute, Gachon University, Incheon 21999, Republic of Korea. [5]Department of Thoracic and Cardiovascular Surgery, Gachon University Gil Medical Center, Gachon University, Incheon 21565, Republic of Korea. [6]Laboratory of Cancer Cell Biology, Department of Biochemistry, School of Medicine, Gachon University, Incheon 21999, Republic of Korea.

References
1. Falcone C, Bozzini S, Colonna A, Matrone B, Paganini EM, Falcone R, et al. Possible role of– 374T/a polymorphism of RAGE gene in longevity. Int J Mol Sci. 2013;14:23203–11.
2. Alonso-Fernández P, De la Fuente M. Role of the immune system in aging and longevity. Curr Aging Sci. 2011;4:78–100.
3. Schmidt AM, Vianna M, Gerlach M, et al. Isolation and characterization of two binding protein for advanced glycosylation end products from bovine lung which are present on the endothelial cell surface. J Biol Chem. 1992;267:14987–97.
4. Neeper M, Schmidt AM, Brett J, et al. Cloning and expression of a cell surface receptor for advanced glycosylation end products of proteins. J Biol Chem. 1992;267:14998–5004.
5. Donato R. S100: a multigenic family of calcium-modulated proteins of the EF-hand type with intracellular and extracellular functional roles. Int J Biochem Cell Biol. 2001;33:637–68.
6. Yamamoto Y, Yamamoto H. RAGE-mediated inflammation, type 2 diabetes, and diabetic vascular complication. Front Endocrinol (Lausanne). 2013;21:21–2.
7. Yan SD, Zhu H, Zhu A, et al. Receptor-dependent cell stress and amyloid accumulation in systemic amyloidosis. Nat med. 2000;6:643–51.
8. Rai V, Touré F, Chitayat S, Pei R, et al. Lysophosphatidic acid targets vascular and oncogenic pathways via RAGE signaling. J exp med. 2012;209(13):2339–50.
9. Brownlee M. Advanced protein glycosylation in diabetes and aging. Annu rev med. 1995;46:223–34.
10. Hyogo H, Yamagishi S. Advanced glycation end products (AGEs) and their involvement in liver disease. Curr Pharm des. 2008;14:969–72.
11. Kimura T, Takamatsu J, Ikeda K, Kondo A, Miyakawa T, Horiuchi S. Accumulation of advanced glycation end products of the Maillard reaction with age in human hippocampal neurons. Neurosci Lett. 1996;208:53–6.
12. Haus JM, Carrithers JA, Trappe SW, Trappe TA. Collagen, cross-linking, and advanced glycation end products in aging human skeletal muscle. J Appl Physiol. 2007;103:2068–76.
13. Vlassara H, Uribarri J, Ferrucci L, Cai W, Torreggiani M, Post JB, et al. Identifying advanced glycation end products as a major source of oxidants in aging: implications for the management and/or prevention of reduced renal function in elderly persons. Semin Nephrol. 2009;29:594–603.
14. Koschinsky T, He CJ, Mitsuhashi T, Bucala R, Liu C, Buenting C, et al. Orally absorbed reactive glycation products (glycotoxins): an environmental risk factor in diabetic nephropathy. Proc Natl Acad Sci U S a. 1997;94:6474–9.
15. Oberg BP, McMenamin E, Lucas FL, McMonagle E, Morrow J, Ikizler TA, et al. Increased prevalence of oxidant stress and inflammation in patients with moderate to severe chronic kidney disease. Kidney Int. 2004;65:1009–16.
16. Sandu O, Song K, Cai W, Zheng F, Uribarri J, Vlassara H. Insulin resistance and type 2 diabetes in high-fat–fed mice are linked to high glycotoxin intake. Diabetes. 2005;54:2314–9.
17. Kawabata K, Yoshikawa H, Saruwatari K, Akazawa Y, Inoue T, Kuze T, et al. The presence of N ε-(Carboxymethyl) lysine in the human epidermis. Biochim Biophys Acta. 1814;2011:1246–52.
18. Semba RD, Nicklett EJ, Ferrucci L. Does accumulation of advanced glycation end products contribute to the aging phenotype ? J Gerontol a Biol Sci med Sci. 2010;65:963–75.
19. Schinzel R, Münch G, Heidland A, Sebekova K. Advanced glycation end products in end-stage renal disease and their removal. Nephron. 2001;87:295–303.
20. Inagi R. RAGE and glyoxalase in kidney disease. Glycoconj J. 2016;33:619–26.
21. Zheng F, Plati AR, Potier M, Schulman Y, Berho M, Banerjee A, et al. Resistance to glomerulosclerosis in B6 mice disappears after menopause. Am J Pathol. 2003;162:1339–48.
22. Feng Z, Plati AR, Cheng QL, Berho M, Banerjee A, Potier M, et al. Glomerular aging in females is a multi-stage reversible process mediated by phenotypic changes in progenitors. Am J Pathol. 2005; 162:355–63.
23. Ikeda Y, Inagi R, Miyata T, Nagai R, Arai M, Miyashita M, et al. Glyoxalase I retards renal senescence. Am J Pathol. 2011;179:2810–21.
24. Kuhla A, Trieglaff C, Vollmar B. Role of age and uncoupling protein-2 in oxidative stress, RAGE/AGE interaction and inflammatory liver injury. Exp Gerontol. 2011;46:868–76.
25. Snow LM, Fugere NA, Thompson LV. Advanced glycation end-product accumulation and associated protein modification in type II skeletal muscle with aging. J Gerontol a Biol Sci med Sci. 2007;62:1204–10.
26. Tiu SC, Chan WY, Heizmann CW, Schäfer BW, Shu SY, Yew DT. Differential expression of S100B and S100A6 1 in the human fetal and aged cerebral cortex. Brain res dev Brain res. 2000;119:159–68.
27. Enokido Y, Yoshitake A, Ito H, Okazawa H. Age-dependent change of HMGB1 and DNA double-strand break accumulation in mouse brain. Biochem Biophys res Commun. 2008;376:128–33.
28. Bierhaus A, Schiekofer S, Schwaninger M, Andrassy M, Humpert PM, Chen J, et al. Diabetes-associated sustained activation of the transcription factor nuclear factor-κB. Diabetes. 2001;50:2792–808.
29. Basta G. Receptor for advanced glycation endproducts and atherosclerosis: from basic mechanisms to clinical implications. Atherosclerosis. 2008;196:9–21.
30. Qin Q, Niu J, Wang Z, Xu W, Qiao Z, Gu Y. Heparanase induced by advanced glycation end products (AGEs) promotes macrophage migration involving RAGE and PI3K/AKT pathway. Cardiovasc Diabetol. 2013;12:1–9.
31. Shim E, Babu JP. Glycated albumin produced in diabetic hyperglycemia promotes monocyte secretion of inflammatory cytokines and bacterial adherence to epithelial cells. J Periodontal res. 2015;50:197–204.
32. Jin X, Yao T, Zhou Z, Zhu J, Zhang S, Hu W, et al. Advanced glycation end products enhance macrophages polarization into M1 phenotype through activating RAGE/NF-κB pathway. Biomed res Int. 2015;2015:732450.

Interleukin-6 and C-reactive protein, successful aging, and mortality: the PolSenior study

Monika Puzianowska-Kuźnicka[1,2*], Magdalena Owczarz[1,3], Katarzyna Wieczorowska-Tobis[4], Pawel Nadrowski[5], Jerzy Chudek[6,7], Przemyslaw Slusarczyk[3], Anna Skalska[8], Marta Jonas[1], Edward Franek[1] and Malgorzata Mossakowska[3]

Abstract

Background: In the elderly, chronic low-grade inflammation (inflammaging) is a risk factor for the development of aging-related diseases and frailty. Using data from several thousand Eastern Europeans aged 65 years and older, we investigated whether the serum levels of two proinflammatory factors, interleukin-6 (IL-6) and C-reactive protein (CRP), were associated with physical and cognitive performance, and could predict mortality in successfully aging elderly.

Results: IL-6 and CRP levels systematically increased in an age-dependent manner in the entire study group (IL-6: $n = 3496$ individuals, $p < 0.001$ and CRP: $n = 3632$, $p = 0.003$), and in the subgroup of successfully aging individuals who had never been diagnosed with cardiovascular disease, myocardial infarction, stroke, type 2 diabetes, or cancer, and had a Mini Mental State Examination (MMSE) score ≥24 and a Katz Activities of Daily Living (ADL) score ≥5 (IL-6: $n = 1258$, $p < 0.001$ and CRP: $n = 1312$, $p < 0.001$). In the subgroup of individuals suffering from aging-related diseases/disability, only IL-6 increased with age (IL-6: $n = 2238$, $p < 0.001$ and CRP: $n = 2320$, $p = 0.249$). IL-6 and CRP levels were lower in successfully aging individuals than in the remaining study participants (both $p < 0.001$). Higher IL-6 and CRP levels were associated with poorer physical performance (lower ADL score) and poorer cognitive performance (lower MMSE score) (both $p < 0.001$). This association remained significant after adjusting for age, gender, BMI, lipids, estimated glomerular filtration rate, and smoking status. Longer survival was associated with lower concentrations of IL-6 and CRP not only in individuals with aging-related diseases/disability (HR = 1.063 per each pg/mL, 95 % CI: 1.052-1.074, $p < 0.001$ and HR = 1.020 per each mg/L, 95 % CI: 1.015-1.025, $p < 0.001$, respectively) but also in the successfully aging subgroup (HR = 1.163 per each pg/mL, 95 % CI: 1.128-1.199, $p < 0.001$ and HR = 1.074 per each mg/L, 95 % CI: 1.047-1.100, $p < 0.001$, respectively). These associations remained significant after adjusting for age, gender, BMI, lipids and smoking status. The Kaplan-Meier survival curves showed similar results (all $p < 0.001$).

Conclusions: Both IL-6 and CRP levels were good predictors of physical and cognitive performance and the risk of mortality in both the entire elderly population and in successfully aging individuals.

Keywords: Aging, Successful aging, Low-grade inflammation, Inflammaging, Interleukin 6 (IL-6), High sensitivity C-reactive protein (CRP), The Mini Mental State Examination (MMSE), The Katz Activity of Daily Living (ADL), Mortality

* Correspondence: mpuzianowska@imdik.pan.pl
[1]Department of Human Epigenetics, Mossakowski Medical Research Centre PAS, 5 Pawinskiego Street, 02-106 Warsaw, Poland
[2]Department of Geriatrics and Gerontology, Medical Centre of Postgraduate Education, 01-826 Warsaw, Poland
Full list of author information is available at the end of the article

Background

Immunosenescence is an integral part of human aging that results in a decrease in the number of naive T and B lymphocytes, the accumulation of memory and effector T and B cells, the production of defective antibodies, an increase in the production of autoantibodies, and in chronic low-grade inflammation (inflammaging) [1, 2]. Among the probable triggers of inflammaging are chronic viral infections, an aging-related increase in adiposity, dietary habits and aging-related changes in the composition of the gut microbiota [3–5]. Among its most important features are slight elevations of the concentrations of proinflammatory cytokines, chemokines, and adipokines, such as interleukin-1ß (IL-1ß), interleukin-6 (IL-6), tumor necrosis factor-α (TNF-α), and monocyte chemoattractant protein-1 (chemokine (C-C motif) ligand 2, CCL2) [6–8]. Proinflammatory cytokines stimulate the synthesis of C-reactive protein (CRP) in the liver, the level of which has been shown to increase in elderly individuals [9]. While clinical signs and symptoms of inflammaging are minimal or absent, this condition contributes to various molecular pathologies, leading to vascular damage and insulin resistance [10–12] and, therefore, increases the risk of developing type 2 diabetes, cardiovascular disease, stroke, cancer, sarcopenia, neurodegeneration, and frailty [13–22]. Furthermore, low-grade inflammation predicts mortality in elderly individuals who are affected by various pathologies [15, 17, 23–25].

IL-6 and CRP are among the most commonly used indicators of inflammation. However, while some published data suggest their causal or predictive roles in morbidity or mortality in the elderly, other studies do not support such views [26–29]. Moreover, the literature on the effects of inflammaging on mortality in successfully aging individuals is not extensive. Therefore, the main objective of the present work was to investigate whether the results of a single measurement of IL-6 and CRP levels were associated with mortality in elderly participants of the PolSenior study who were followed for an average of 4.3 years, with a particular emphasis on individuals who had never been diagnosed with aging-related diseases and remained in good physical and cognitive health. Another aim of this study was to determine possible associations between the concentrations of these factors and cognitive and physical functioning, which were assessed at the same time. Finally, we evaluated whether low-dose acetylsalicylic acid, which is frequently prescribed to seniors for the prevention of cardiovascular disease, affects IL-6 and CRP concentrations.

Methods
Material
The study group consisted of ≥65 year old seniors ($n =$ 4979 individuals) who participated in the PolSenior study. The participants were randomly recruited in bundles in a stratified, proportional draw. The response rate was 42.6 %. The recruitment details are described elsewhere [30]. The respondents belonged to similarly-sized age groups (65–69, 70–74, 75–79, 80–84, 85–89 and ≥90 years old), each containing a similar number of males and females. A detailed questionnaire was used to obtain medical histories, current health status, socioeconomic status, demographic status, and lifestyle habits for all of the study participants. The participants also underwent a detailed examination, including elements of comprehensive geriatric assessment [30]. Individuals who had never been diagnosed with cardiovascular disease, myocardial infarction, stroke, type 2 diabetes, or cancer, and had a Mini Mental State Examination (MMSE) score ≥24 and Katz Activities of Daily Living (ADL) score ≥5 were classified as successfully aging. Of the entire group, blood samples were provided by 4101 individuals. Blood collection, surveys, and physical examinations were performed either on the same day or within a few days of each other. The survival of the study subjects was taken from the Population Register. This database was accessed in 2015, indicating that 1734 PolSenior participants (1318 of those who donated blood) had died. The total number of person-years of observation was 14,535.

The PolSenior project was approved by the Bioethics Commission of the Medical University of Silesia in Katowice. Each participant gave written, informed consent to participate in the study.

Blood analysis
Venous blood was collected using a vacuum system and delivered in a cooler to local laboratories within 2 h, where serum and plasma samples were separated and frozen. All samples were then delivered to the Department of Human Epigenetics, Mossakowski Medical Research Centre in Warsaw. All of the IL-6 and CRP measurements were performed in the same laboratory. Interleukin-6 levels were measured in serum using ELISA (R&D System, Minneapolis, MN, USA, sensitivity 0.04 pg/mL) in 3895 individuals and CRP (high sensitivity CRP) levels were measured using a high-sensitivity immunoturbidimetric method (Modular PPE, Roche Diagnostics GmBH, Mannheim, Germany, sensitivity 0.11 mg/L) in 4093 individuals. In the other PolSenior participants, these measurements were not performed mostly because of refusal to provide blood or because an insufficient amount of serum was collected. Other biochemical parameters were assessed using routine techniques [30]. Study subjects with leukocyte counts >10,000/μL (indicating a considerable risk of ongoing infection) and/or who were being treated with glucocorticoids were excluded from further analyses. Therefore, analyses of IL-6 were performed in 3496 subjects, and of CRP were performed in 3632 subjects. In some of the study subjects, only IL-6 or only CRP

was measured. The results were presented as median [1st quartile, 3rd quartile] values.

Mini mental state examination and activities of daily living

Cognitive function was assessed using the MMSE [31] which was translated into Polish. The study participants were divided into five groups: normal cognition (MMSE score 28–30), minimal cognitive impairment (MMSE score 24–27), mild (MMSE score 20–23), moderate (MMSE score 10–19), or severe (MMSE score <10) cognitive impairment [32].

Physical performance was assessed using the ADL scale [33]. Based on the six domains of the ADL (transferring, feeding, bathing, dressing, personal hygiene and grooming, toileting), the study participants were divided into independent (ADL score 5–6), partially dependent (ADL score 3–4) and totally dependent (ADL score 0–2) [34].

Statistical analysis

The statistical analyses were performed using Statistica 10 software (Statsoft Inc., Tulsa, OK, USA) and R software (R Foundation for Statistical Computing, Vienna, Austria) programs. Because of the skewed distribution of the IL-6 and CRP values, the variables were presented as median [1st quartile, 3rd quartile] values. Before the analyses, the IL-6 and CRP values were log-transformed. The significance of associations between the analyzed factors was tested using analysis of variance (ANOVA), and analysis of co-variance (ANCOVA) for multifactorial analyses. Pearson's r was used as a measure of correlations between IL-6 and CRP levels.

A Kaplan-Meier plots were used to present survival curves, which were compared using the log-rank test. The Cox proportional hazards model was used for univariate survival analyses. In the multivariate survival analyses, age and body mass index (BMI) did not meet the assumption of proportional hazards. Therefore, the Cox proportional hazards model with time-dependent covariates was used. The hazard ratio (HR) of death and the 95 % confidence interval (CI) were calculated for associations between the analyzed variables and survival time.

For all of the statistical analyses, the level of significance was established at 0.05.

Results

Aging-associated changes in serum IL-6 and CRP levels

The mean age of all the study participants who met the inclusion criteria (3750 individuals, 47.8 % women, 52.2 % men) was 78.9 ± 8.6 years. The mean age of the successfully aging subgroup (35.4 % of the study population; 47.4 % women, 52.6 % men) was 76.3 ± 7.9 years, while in the remaining study participants who did not meet our definition of successful aging (64.6 % of the study population;

48 % women, 52 % men) was 80.3 ± 8.6 years. The age difference between the successfully aging participants and the remaining study participants was significant ($p < 0.001$).

Low-dose acetylsalicylic acid is commonly prescribed to seniors for the prevention of cardiovascular disease. We initially determined whether this medication affects IL-6 or CRP concentrations and whether individuals who received it should be included in the analysis or analyzed separately. The comparison between individuals who were not currently treated with low-dose acetylsalicylic acid vs. individuals who took this medication showed that the median concentrations of IL-6 were similar in both groups (2321 individuals, 2.3 pg/mL [1.5, 3.8] vs. 1175 individuals, 2.4 pg/mL [1.6, 3.8], respectively, $p = 0.22$), as were the median CRP values (2410 individuals, 2.3 mg/L [1.1, 4.8] vs. 1222 individuals, 2.3 mg/L [1.1, 4.7], respectively, $p = 0.73$). Therefore, all of the subsequent analyses were performed without considering whether the participants were treated with low-dose acetylsalicylic acid.

The median concentration of IL-6 in the entire study group (3496 individuals) was 2.3 pg/mL [1.5, 3.8]. In successfully aging study participants (1258 individuals) it was 2.0 pg/mL [1.3, 3.3], while in participants who suffered from aging-related diseases/disability (2238 individuals) it was 2.5 pg/mL [1.6, 4.2]. This difference was significant ($p < 0.001$). We also found that the older the age group, the higher was the median concentration of IL-6 not only in the entire study group and in individuals with aging-related diseases/disability, but also in the subgroup of successfully aging individuals (all $p < 0.001$, Table 1).

The median CRP concentration in the entire study group (3632 individuals) was 2.3 mg/L [1.1, 4.7]. The subgroups of successfully aging participants (1312 individuals) and those who did not meet the definition of successful aging (2320 individuals) had median concentrations 2.1 mg/L [1.0, 4.3] and 2.5 mg/L [1.1, 5.1], respectively. This difference that was significant ($p < 0.001$). In the entire study group, we observed a significant increase in the median CRP concentration as age increased ($p = 0.003$). Notably, the median CRP concentration was higher in ≥80 year old study participants than in younger age groups. In the study participants with aging-related diseases/disability, the median CRP level was not associated with age ($p = 0.25$). In the successfully aging subgroup, the median CRP levels were also higher in the older age groups, but the level of significance has not been reached ($p = 0.09$) (Table 1).

IL-6 and CRP levels were correlated with each other in the entire study group (r = 0.502, $p < 0.001$), the successfully aging subgroup (r = 0.538, $p < 0.001$), and study participants with aging-related diseases/disability (r = 0.504, $p < 0.001$).

Table 1 IL-6 and CRP concentrations in ≥65 year-old seniors

Age (years)	All[a]		Successfully aging[b]		Others[c]	
	n	Concentration[d]	n	Concentration[d]	n	Concentration[d]
	IL-6 [pg/mL]					
65–69	588	1.8 [1.2, 2.9]	296	1.8 [1.1, 3.0]	292	1.9 [1.3, 2.9]
70–74	681	1.9 [1.3, 3.1]	308	1.7 [1.1, 2.8]	373	2.2 [1.4, 3.3]
75–79	596	2.1 [1.4, 3.4]	231	1.9 [1.3, 2.8]	365	2.4 [1.6, 3.6]
80–84	557	2.5 [1.7, 3.7]	163	2.4 [1.5, 3.5]	394	2.5 [1.7, 3.8]
85–89	598	2.8 [1.8, 4.9]	173	2.7 [1.8, 4.3]	425	2.8 [1.8, 5.1]
90+	476	3.5 [2.1, 5.5]	87	3.3 [2.3, 5.1]	389	3.5 [2.1, 5.6]
	CRP [mg/L]					
65–69	614	2.2 [1.1, 4.6]	311	2.0 [1.0, 4.1]	303	2.6 [1.2, 5.5]
70–74	706	2.1 [1.1, 4.1]	321	1.9 [1.0, 3.9]	385	2.2 [1.1, 4.4]
75–79	627	2.2 [1.1, 4.4]	245	1.9 [1.0, 3.8]	382	2.6 [1.2, 4.8]
80–84	572	2.4 [1.1, 5.2]	169	2.4 [1.0, 5.3]	403	2.3 [1.1, 5.2]
85–89	621	2.5 [1.1, 5.1]	177	2.8 [1.2, 4.6]	444	2.4 [1.1, 5.2]
90+	492	2.7 [1.1, 5.5]	89	2.6 [1.3, 5.3]	403	2.7 [1.1, 5.7]

[a]: Excluded are individuals with leukocytosis exceeding 10,000/μL or treated with glucocorticoids
[b]: Only individuals without past or current cancer, type 2 diabetes, cardiovascular disease/myocardial infarction/stroke, and with the MMSE score ≥24 and the ADL score 5–6
[c]: Individuals who did not meet the definition of successful aging
[d]: Concentrations of IL-6 and CRP are shown as median [1st quartile, 3rd quartile]
n number of individuals

We also evaluated whether IL-6 and CRP concentrations differed in women and men and found that the median IL-6 concentrations were higher in men (1673 women, 2.2 pg/mL [1.5, 3.6] *vs.* 1823 men, 2.4 pg/mL [1.6, 4.0], $p = 0.006$), whereas the median CRP concentrations were not significantly different (1735 women, 2.4 mg/L [1.2, 4.7] *vs.* 1897 men, 2.2 mg/L [1.0, 4.9], $p = 0.25$).

Association between the IL-6 and CRP levels and other biochemical parameters and functional and cognitive performance

IL-6 concentrations were significantly associated with BMI ($p < 0.001$ for the entire study group, $p = 0.015$ for the successfully aging subgroup, and $p = 0.007$ for study participants with aging-related diseases/disability). Notably, in individuals with a BMI <18.5 kg/m^2, the median IL-6 value was the highest, while in overweight individuals it was the lowest, and again increased in the obese. In addition, the median IL-6 value was associated with estimated glomerular filtration rate (eGFR) ($p < 0.001$ for the entire study group, $p < 0.001$ for the successfully aging subgroup, and $p < 0.001$ for study participants with aging-related diseases/disability) and was the highest in individuals with the lowest eGFR, as well as with heart rate ($p < 0.001$, $p < 0.001$ and $p < 0.001$) where it was the highest in individuals with a heart rate >80/min. It was also associated with smoking status ($p = 0.02$ for the entire study group and $p = 0.016$ for participants with aging-related diseases/disability); it was the highest in current

smokers. No association with smoking status was found in the successfully aging subgroup. Of note, the IL-6 concentration was negatively associated with total cholesterol levels ($p < 0.001$ for the entire study group, $p < 0.001$ for the successfully aging subgroup, and $p < 0.001$ for study participants with aging-related diseases/disability), LDL cholesterol ($p < 0.001$, $p = 0.007$ and $p < 0.001$), and HDL cholesterol ($p < 0.001$, $p < 0.001$ and $p < 0.001$) (Table 2). The multifactorial analysis including age, gender, BMI, HDL, LDL, eGFR and smoking status, showed that only gender lost its significant association with IL-6 in the entire study group. In the successfully aging subgroup, gender and LDL lost their associations with IL-6, while in participants with aging-related diseases/disability the association was lost for gender and eGFR. The other factors remained significantly associated with IL-6.

We also evaluated whether IL-6 concentrations were related to functional and cognitive performance. We found that higher IL-6 levels were associated with poorer physical performance (lower ADL score) and poorer cognitive performance (lower MMSE score) (all $p < 0.001$ for the entire study group as well as for both subgroups) (Table 2). He multifactorial analyses that were adjusted for age, gender, BMI, HDL, LDL, eGFR and smoking status revealed that ADL and MMSE scores in the entire studied group remained associated with IL-6 ($p = 0.006$ and $p = 0.007$, respectively). Such an analysis was not performed separately in the successfully aging subgroup because only individuals with the highest ADL and MMSE scores,

Table 2 IL-6 and CRP concentration in ≥65 year-old seniors in relation to select clinical and biochemical parameters, and functional status

| | IL-6 [pg/mL] | | | | | | CRP [mg/L] | | | | | |
| | All[a] | | Successfully aging[b] | | Others[c] | | All[a] | | Successfully aging[b] | | Others[c] | |
	n	Concentration[d]	n	Concentration[d]	n	Concentration[d]	n	Concentration[d]	n	Concentration[d]	n	Concentration[d]
BMI [kg/m²] <18.5	60	3.2 [1.8, 5.4]	21	3.2 [1.7, 4.8]	39	3.2 [1.9, 5.7]	64	2.3 [1.0, 7.4]	21	1.8 [0.7, 7.5]	43	2.5 [1.0, 7.2]
18.5–24.9	814	2.3 [1.4, 3.9]	315	1.9 [1.2, 3.2]	499	2.5 [1.6, 4.5]	865	1.7 [0.8, 3.8]	336	1.5 [0.8, 3.0]	529	1.8 [0.9, 4.3]
25–29.9	1381	2.2 [1.4, 3.5]	548	1.9 [1.3, 3.2]	833	2.3 [1.5, 3.8]	1425	2.1 [1.0, 4.2]	569	2.0 [1.0, 4.0]	856	2.2 [1.0, 4.3]
30–39.9	997	2.3 [1.6, 3.6]	343	2.2 [1.4, 3.6]	654	2.4 [1.7, 3.6]	1025	2.8 [1.5, 5.2]	354	2.9 [1.6, 5.4]	671	2.7 [1.4, 5.1]
≥40	69	2.8 [2.1, 4.1]	17	2.5 [1.9, 3.4]	52	2.9 [2.1, 4.9]	69	4.2 [2.2, 8.8]	17	4.3 [2.5, 7.8]	52	4.1 [2.1, 9.1]
Cholesterol [mg/dL] <175	1029	2.7 [1.7, 4.8]	256	2.4 [1.5, 4.4]	773	2.8 [1.8, 5.1]	1085	2.3 [1.0, 5.3]	267	2.2 [1.0, 5.0]	818	2.4 [1.0, 5.3]
175–189	452	2.3 [1.6, 3.8]	178	2.2 [1.4, 3.7]	274	2.4 [1.7, 3.8]	478	2.4 [1.1, 5.1]	184	1.9 [1.0, 4.2]	294	2.6 [1.1, 5.7]
190–239	1302	2.2 [1.5, 3.5]	512	2.0 [1.3, 3.1]	790	2.4 [1.6, 3.8]	1375	2.2 [1.1, 4.4]	543	2.2 [1.0, 4.1]	832	2.3 [1.1, 4.7]
240–309	593	2.0 [1.4, 3.1]	275	1.8 [1.2, 2.7]	318	2.2 [1.5, 3.4]	627	2.3 [1.2, 4.5]	291	2.1 [1.2, 4.0]	336	2.7 [1.4, 5.2]
≥310	65	2.2 [1.4, 3.6]	27	2.4 [1.4, 3.7]	38	2.2 [1.5, 3.6]	67	3.3 [1.5, 5.2]	27	2.1 [1.0, 5.0]	40	3.6 [1.7, 5.3]
HDL [mg/dL] <40	774	3.0 [1.8, 4.9]	199	2.7 [1.6, 3.9]	575	3.1 [1.9, 5.3]	822	2.9 [1.4, 6.2]	211	2.6 [1.3, 5.4]	611	3.0 [1.5, 6.5]
40–44	525	2.6 [1.7, 4.4]	168	2.4 [1.6, 4.0]	357	2.7 [1.8, 4.5]	549	2.4 [1.2, 5.0]	176	2.3 [1.3, 4.7]	373	2.4 [1.2, 5.1]
45–49	528	2.4 [1.6, 4.0]	190	2.1 [1.3, 3.5]	338	2.6 [1.8, 4.2]	549	2.5 [1.1, 5.3]	201	2.5 [1.1, 4.8]	348	2.4 [1.2, 5.9]
50–59	851	2.1 [1.4, 3.4]	362	1.9 [1.3, 3.2]	489	2.2 [1.5, 3.4]	900	2.2 [1.1, 4.2]	370	2.1 [1.0, 3.9]	530	2.3 [1.1, 4.3]
≥60	760	1.8 [1.2, 3.0]	328	1.7 [1.1, 2.6]	432	2.0 [1.3, 3.3]	810	1.8 [0.8, 3.6]	353	1.6 [0.8, 3.1]	457	1.9 [0.9, 4.1]
LDL [mg/dL] <70	329	2.8 [1.8, 5.1]	53	2.2 [1.6, 3.6]	276	2.9 [1.9, 5.5]	347	2.4 [0.9, 4.9]	55	2.4 [0.7, 5.0]	292	2.4 [1.0, 4.9]
71–99	809	2.5 [1.6, 4.2]	234	2.2 [1.5, 4.1]	575	2.6 [1.6, 4.2]	860	2.3 [1.0, 4.7]	249	1.9 [1.0, 4.3]	611	2.4 [1.0, 5.0]
100–114	506	2.3 [1.6, 4.0]	204	2.1 [1.3, 3.6]	302	2.5 [1.7, 4.3]	530	2.1 [1.0, 4.8]	214	2.1 [1.0, 4.2]	316	2.1 [1.0, 5.1]
115–154	1168	2.2 [1.4, 3.5]	463	1.9 [1.3, 3.1]	705	2.4 [1.6, 3.7]	1234	2.2 [1.1, 4.6]	485	2.1 [1.0, 4.0]	749	2.5 [1.2, 5.1]
155–189	468	2.1 [1.5, 3.3]	218	1.9 [1.3, 2.9]	250	2.2 [1.6, 3.8]	494	2.5 [1.4, 4.6]	230	2.3 [1.2, 4.1]	264	2.7 [1.5, 5.5]
≥190	159	2.1 [1.3, 3.2]	75	1.8 [1.2, 3.0]	84	2.2 [1.5, 3.4]	166	2.7 [1.2, 5.4]	78	2.3 [1.2, 5.4]	88	3.0 [1.3, 5.4]
Glucose [mg/dL] <100	2133	2.3 [1.5, 3.8]	924	2.0 [1.3, 3.3]	1209	2.5 [1.7, 4.4]	2261	2.2 [1.0, 4.6]	966	2.1 [1.0, 4.1]	1295	2.4 [1.1, 5.0]
100–139.9	1042	2.4 [1.6, 3.7]	324	2.1 [1.4, 3.4]	718	2.5 [1.6, 3.8]	1089	2.3 [1.1, 4.8]	346	2.2 [1.1, 4.8]	743	2.4 [1.1, 4.9]
≥140	256	2.5 [1.7, 4.1]	na	na	256	2.5 [1.7, 4.1]	272	3.0 [1.4, 6.8]	na	na	272	3.0 [1.4, 6.8]
eGFR [mL/min/ 1.73 m²] <45	359	3.2 [2.1, 5.3]	70	3.8 [2.6, 6.7]	289	3.0 [2.0, 5.2]	378	3.2 [1.5, 6.3]	77	3.5 [1.9, 6.3]	301	3.0 [1.5, 6.3]
45–60	639	2.7 [1.7, 4.1]	187	2.4 [1.5, 3.6]	452	2.8 [1.8, 4.5]	668	2.5 [1.1, 5.4]	192	2.2 [1.1, 4.4]	476	2.7 [1.2, 6.2]
>60	2421	2.1 [1.4, 3.5]	977	1.9 [1.3, 3.1]	1444	2.3 [1.6, 3.8]	2531	2.2 [1.0, 4.4]	1019	2.0 [1.0, 4.1]	1512	2.3 [1.0, 4.7]
Heart rate [per min] <60	341	2.2 [1.5, 3.6]	126	1.8 [1.2, 2.9]	215	2.6 [1.6, 4.0]	354	1.6 [0.9, 3.6]	131	1.8 [1.0, 3.6]	223	1.5 [0.9, 3.6]
60-80	2374	2.2 [1.5, 3.6]	893	2.0 [1.3, 3.2]	1481	2.3 [1.6, 3.8]	2463	2.3 [1.0, 4.5]	929	2.1 [1.0, 4.0]	1534	2.4 [1.1, 4.9]
>80	768	2.7 [1.7, 4.8]	239	2.4 [1.5, 4.0]	529	2.8 [1.8, 5.1]	801	3.0 [1.4, 6.2]	252	2.7 [1.3, 5.6]	549	3.1 [1.4, 6.3]
Smoking Never	1968	2.3 [1.5, 3.7]	689	1.9 [1.3, 3.1]	1279	2.4 [1.6, 4.1]	2035	2.3 [1.1, 4.5]	710	2.1 [1.0, 3.9]	1325	2.4 [1.1, 4.9]

Table 2 IL-6 and CRP concentration in ≥65 year-old seniors in relation to select clinical and biochemical parameters, and functional status *(Continued)*

		n		n		n		n		n		n	
	Past	1196	2.4 [1.5, 3.8]	424	2.0 [1.4, 3.3]	772	2.5 [1.6, 4.0]	1250	2.2 [1.0, 4.8]	450	2.1 [1.0, 4.5]	800	2.3 [1.0, 5.0]
	Current	304	2.7 [1.7, 4.5]	140	2.4 [1.4, 3.7]	164	3.0 [1.8, 5.2]	319	3.1 [1.3, 6.2]	147	2.4 [1.1, 5.1]	172	3.4 [1.5, 7.7]
MMSE [points]	28–30	1121	1.9 [1.3, 3.1]	606	1.9 [1.2, 3.0]	515	2.0 [1.4, 3.1]	1153	2.0 [1.0, 4.1]	629	1.9 [1.0, 4.1]	524	2.1 [1.0, 4.1]
	24–27	1245	2.3 [1.5, 3.7]	637	2.2 [1.4, 3.6]	608	2.4 [1.6, 4.0]	1302	2.3 [1.1, 4.6]	668	2.3 [1.1, 4.4]	634	2.5 [1.1, 5.1]
	20–23	593	2.6 [1.7, 4.3]	na	na	593	2.6 [1.7, 4.3]	617	2.4 [1.2, 5.2]	na	na	617	2.4 [1.2, 5.2]
	10–19	324	3.0 [2.0, 5.5]	na	na	324	3.0 [2.0, 5.5]	348	2.5 [1.0, 5.4]	na	na	348	2.5 [1.0, 5.4]
	<10	111	3.3 [2.1, 6.0]	na	na	111	3.3 [2.1, 6.0]	114	3.7 [1.5, 8.3]	na	na	114	3.7 [1.5, 8.3]
ADL [points]	5–6	3112	2.2 [1.5, 3.6]	1258	2.0 [1.3, 3.3]	1854	2.3 [1.6, 3.7]	3220	2.2 [1.0, 4.4]	1312	2.1 [1.0, 4.3]	1908	2.2 [1.0, 4.5]
	3–4	205	3.2 [2.2, 6.2]	na	na	205	3.2 [2.2, 6.2]	220	3.4 [1.7, 9.3]	na	na	220	3.4 [1.7, 9.3]
	0–2	165	4.2 [2.6, 7.4]	na	na	165	4.2 [2.6, 7.4]	178	3.9 [1.9, 9.4]	na	na	178	3.9 [1.9, 9.4]

[a]: Excluded are individuals with leukocytosis exceeding 10,000/mm³ or treated with glucocorticoids
[b]: Only individuals without past or current cancer, type 2 diabetes, cardiovascular disease/myocardial infarction/stroke, and with the MMSE score ≥24 and the ADL score 5–6
[c]: Individuals who did not meet the definition of successful aging
[d]: Concentrations of IL-6 and CRP are shown as median [1st quartile, 3rd quartile]
n Number of individuals
na Not applicable

reflecting good physical and cognitive performance, were included in this subgroup.

The CRP concentration was significantly associated with BMI ($p < 0.001$ for the entire study group, $p < 0.001$ for the successfully aging subgroup, and $p < 0.001$ for study participants with aging-related diseases/disability). The CRP concentration was the lowest in the group of normal-weight individuals and then systematically increased as BMI increased. Notably, it was also higher in individuals with a BMI <18.5 kg/m^2 compared with normal-weight study subjects. Additionally, the CRP concentration was associated with fasting glucose in the entire study group ($p = 0.003$) and individuals with aging-related diseases/disability ($p = 0.006$) and was the highest in individuals with a glucose level ≥140 mg/dL. Notably, in the successfully aging subgroup no association was found. The CRP concentration was also associated with eGFR ($p < 0.001$ for the entire study group, $p < 0.001$ for the successfully aging subgroup, and $p < 0.001$ for participants with aging-related diseases/disability) and was the highest in individuals with the lowest eGFR, as well as with heart rate ($p < 0.001$, $p < 0.001$ and $p < 0.001$) where it was the highest in individuals with a heart rate >80/min. Furthermore, the CRP concentration was also associated with smoking status in the entire study group ($p = 0.005$) and in individuals with aging-related diseases/disability ($p = 0.002$) where it was the highest in current smokers; however, no association with smoking status was found in the successfully aging subgroup. Finally, The CRP concentration was negatively associated with the level of HDL cholesterol ($p < 0.001$, $p < 0.001$ and $p < 0.001$) (Table 2). The multifactorial analysis including age, gender, BMI, HDL, eGFR and smoking status revealed that all of the factors remained significantly associated with CRP in the entire study group and successfully aging subgroup, whereas age lost its significant association in the subgroup of participants with aging-related diseases/disability.

We also found that higher CRP levels were associated with poorer physical performance (lower ADL score) and poorer cognitive performance (lower MMSE score) (all $p < 0.001$ for the entire study group as well as for both subgroups, Table 2). The multifactorial analyses that were adjusted for age, gender, BMI, HDL, eGFR and smoking status revealed that in the entire studied group the ADL and MMSE scores remained related to CRP at statistically significant level ($p = 0.019$ and $p < 0.001$ respectively). We did not perform such an analysis in the successfully aging subgroup because only individuals with the highest ADL and MMSE scores were included in this subgroup.

Association between IL-6 and CRP levels and survival

The 1-year mortality rate was 6.6 %, 2.6 %, and 8.8 % for the entire study group, the successfully aging subgroup,

and study participants with aging-related diseases/disability, respectively. In the univariate analysis, longer survival was associated with a lower IL-6 concentration: HR = 1.077 per each pg/mL (95 % CI: 1.068–1.086, $p < 0.001$) in the entire study group, HR = 1.163 per each pg/mL (95 % CI: 1.128–1.199, $p < 0.001$) in the successfully aging subgroup, and HR = 1.063 per each pg/mL (95 % CI: 1.052–1.074, $p < 0.001$) in individuals with aging-related diseases/disability. Longer survival was also associated with a lower CRP concentration: HR = 1.025 per each mg/L (95 % CI: 1.020–1.029, $p < 0.001$) in the entire study group, HR = 1.074 per each mg/L (95 % CI: 1.047–1.100, $p < 0.001$) in successfully aging study participants, and HR = 1.020 per each pg/mL (95 % CI: 1.015–1.025, $p < 0.001$) in the remaining participants.

The results of the univariate analysis were consistent with the Kaplan-Meier survival curves, in which higher concentrations of IL-6 and CRP were associated with a lower probability of survival in the entire group of seniors, in successfully aging ones, as well as in individuals with aging-related diseases/disability (all $p < 0.001$) (Figs. 1, 2).

A statistical model was applied that included IL-6 value, gender, age, BMI, HDL, LDL, eGFR and smoking status. We found that longer survival was associated with a lower IL-6 concentration, even after adjusting for these covariates, in the entire study group: HR = 1.042 per each pg/mL (95 % CI: 1.029–1.055, $p < 0.001$), the successfully aging subgroup: HR = 1.112 per each pg/mL (95 % CI: 1.069–1.155, $p < 0.001$), as well as in study participants with aging-related diseases/disability: HR = 1.031 per each pg/mL (95 % CI: 1.018–1.045, $p < 0.001$).

We also tested a model that included CRP value, gender, age, BMI, HDL, eGFR and smoking status, and found that longer survival was associated with a lower CRP concentration after adjusting for these factors in the entire group of seniors: HR = 1.017 per each mg/L (95 % CI: 1.012–1.023, $p < 0.001$), in the successfully aging subgroup: HR = 1.035 per each mg/L (95 % CI: 1.021–1.050, $p < 0.001$), and in the remaining study participants with aging-related diseases/disability: HR = 1.013 per each pg/mL (95 % CI: 1.007–1.019, $p < 0.001$).

Discussion

It is well documented that chronic inflammation is associated with aging-related morbidity [13–22], and with mortality in affected individuals [15, 17, 23–25]. Therefore, the present study evaluated a large group of Eastern European Caucasian seniors to determine whether results of a single measurement of the levels of two proinflammatory factors, IL-6 and CRP, were associated with biochemical and functional parameters and whether they were predictors of mortality. We performed this analysis for the entire study group of ≥65 year-old seniors who were not preselected on the basis of their health and functional status, as

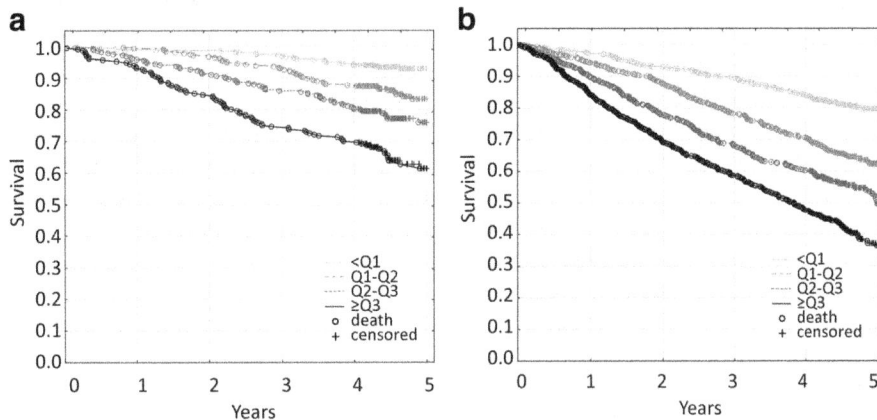

Fig. 1 Kaplan-Meier survival curves for the elderly population that was classified according to quartiles of IL-6 concentrations. **a**. In the successfully aging subgroup, the 1-year mortality rates were 1.0 % for the <1st quartile, 0.6 % for the 1st-2nd quartile, 4.1 % for the 2nd-3rd quartile, and 6.8 % for the >3rd quartile. The differences between the <1st quartile and all of the other quartiles were significant (all $p < 0.001$). **b**. In the subgroup of individuals who suffered from aging-related diseases/disability, the 1-year mortality rates were 2.9 % for the <1st quartile, 5.7 % for the 1st-2nd quartile, 10.0 % for the 2nd-3rd quartile, and 15.8 % for the >3rd quartile. The differences between the <1st quartile and all of the other quartiles were significant (all $p < 0.001$)

well as for subgroups of successfully aging individuals and individuals with aging-related chronic diseases/disability.

There is no single generally agreed upon definition of successful aging. It is usually defined as survival to an older age while being free of aging-associated diseases, such as cardiovascular disease, cancer, neurodegeneration, and type 2 diabetes, with good physical and cognitive functioning [35]. This "biological" definition is sometimes augmented by a requirement to have good social functioning and high life satisfaction [35]. However, for the purpose of this study, in which we analyzed biological factors associated with aging, we used the most common definition that is limited to the biology of aging. An additional

reason for such limitation was that social functioning and life satisfaction might be significantly influenced by non-biological factors such as income, family situation, or place of residence. We found that IL-6 and CRP levels were good predictors of physical and cognitive performance and mortality not only in the entire aging study group and in individuals with aging-related diseases/disability, but also in individuals who were aging successfully.

IL-6 is known to induce the production of CRP in the liver [36]. Therefore, as expected, the levels of IL-6 and CRP were correlated in the elderly subjects in this study. However, aging-related changes in CRP did not accurately reflect changes in IL-6. Impaired liver function, which

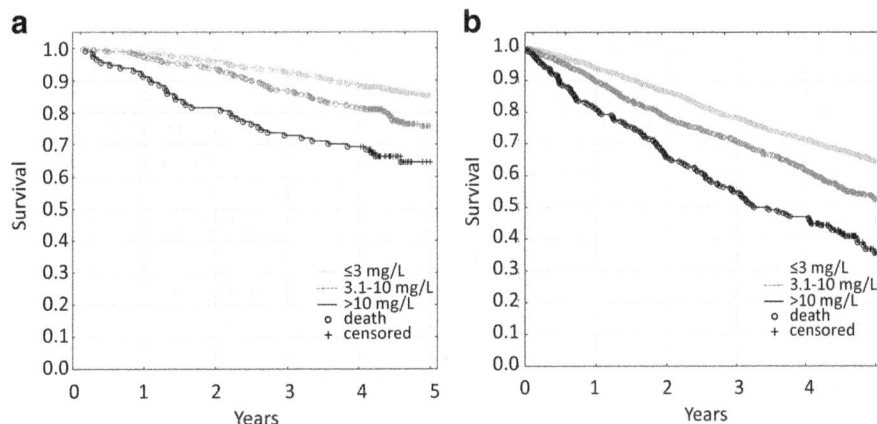

Fig. 2 Kaplan-Meier survival curves for the elderly population that was classified according to CRP concentrations. **a**. In the successfully aging subgroup, the 1-year mortality rates were 1.6 % for ≤3 mg/L, 2.8 % for 3.1–10 mg/L, and 8.8 % for >10 mg/L. The differences between ≤3 mg/L and the other concentration ranges were significant (all $p < 0.001$). **b**. In the subgroup of individuals who suffered from aging-related diseases/disability, the 1-year mortality rates were 6.3 % for ≤3 mg/L, 10.3 % for 3.1–10 mg/L, and 19.2 % for >10 mg/L. The differences between ≤3 mg/L and other concentration ranges were significant (all $p < 0.001$)

could be expected mainly in the subgroup of individuals who did not age successfully, might affect CRP production. We tested this hypothesis by correlating aspartate transaminase (AST) and alanine transaminase (ALT) levels with the CRP level and found that some negative correlations were significant, but all of the correlation coefficients were extremely low (data not shown). Therefore, we conclude that liver function had no significant influence on CRP production in our study group. Another plausible explanation for the lack of complete correspondence between IL-6 and CRP concentrations is that CRP production is affected by other cytokines, such as IL-1 and IL-17 [36], which were not measured in the present study.

Notably, although statistically significant, the differences between mean IL-6 and CRP concentrations in the successfully aging participants and remaining study participants who suffered form from aging-related diseases/disability were only approximately 20 % (2 pg/mL *vs.* 2.5 pg/mL and 2.1 mg/L *vs.* 2.5 mg/L, respectively). Therefore, the question arises as to the reason why, despite such a small differences, some individuals experienced healthy aging, while others suffered from aging-related diseases. The most likely explanation for this phenomenon is that the phenotype of aging results not only from the amount of the examined proinflammatory factors, but also from a balance between numerous proinflammatory and antiinflammatory agents (inflammaging *vs.* anti-inflammaging) [37, 38]. Moreover, the effect of such a balance might be modified by other conditions, such as diet, body fat content, level of physical activity, smoking, and other disease risk factors, including genetic background [39–42].

Another important finding of this study was that the lowest IL-6 levels were found in normal-weight and overweight individuals, and the lowest CRP levels were found in normal-weight individuals. Such a U-shaped relationship between BMI and proinflammatory factors supports the theory of the "obesity paradox" stating that in the elderly, lower morbidity and mortality are associated with a normal body weight or being overweight [43–46], whereas being underweight or obese (especially morbidly obese) poses a high risk of mortality. Based on the present results, we speculate that this phenomenon might be, at least partially, attributable to an increase in systemic inflammation in extreme weight groups. Notably, in our study participants, a BMI <18.5 kg/m^2 was associated with the highest IL-6 level and, to a lesser extent, an increase in CRP level. Data that were obtained from the revised Mini Nutritional Assessment Short Form and serum biochemical parameters indicated that these individuals were undernourished and vitamin D-deficient (even though, some of them were still able to meet our phenotypic criteria for successful aging). The available data suggest that poor nutritional status and vitamin D deficiency might be associated with increased levels of proinflammatory factors, such as TNF-α, IL-6,

and CRP [47–49]. Therefore, in our underweight elderly patients, high levels of IL-6 and CRP might result from a cumulative action of immunoaging and undernutrition/malnutrition.

We also found that the IL-6 concentration was negatively associated with concentrations of total cholesterol and its high- and low-density fractions in the entire studied population and in its subgroups, while CRP was negatively associated only with HDL. Such findings indicate that low cholesterol levels in the elderly might have adverse effects, such as the increased level of IL-6 that we detected in the present study. Our results are partially consistent with previous studies that reported the existence of similar correlations in oldest-old group of ≥85 year-old individuals [50, 51]. However, we found that such relationships were also true for seniors who were ≥65 years old. Longitudinal studies indicate that aging might be associated with a decrease in total cholesterol and LDL levels and an increase in HDL levels, which is mostly a result of decreasing weight [52]. On the other hand, increased levels of proinflammatory factors are attributable to a higher body weight [53, 54]. Therefore, an inverse relationship between lipids and proinflammatory factors in seniors might be unrelated to total adipose tissue content but may be related to the abdominal localization of adipose tissue [55, 56]. Alternatively, adipose tissue might not be a key factor in the interplay between lipids and inflammation in older age groups.

Consistent with previous findings [23, 57], we found that higher IL-6 and CRP levels were associated with poorer cognitive and/or functional performance, as well as with a higher risk of mortality. This could be explained by the fact that aging-associated chronic inflammation is one of the major causes of aging-related diseases, that might negatively affect the aging phenotype and shorten one's lifespan [13–22]. However, we found that higher levels of IL-6 and CRP posed an even higher risk of all-cause mortality in physically and cognitively healthy, successfully aging individuals who did not suffer from major aging-related diseases, reflected by 1-year mortality rates (see Figs. 1 and 2 legends), and confirmed by 3-year mortality rates (IL-6: 2.9 % for <1st quartile, 6.9 % for 1st-2nd quartile, 14.0 % for 2nd-3rd quartile and 25.3 % for >3rd quartile of IL-6 concentration; because there is no established "normal" IL-6 concentration range, we divided the study subjects into IL-6 concentration quartiles; CRP: 7.3 % for ≤3 mg/L, 13.2 % for 3.1-10 mg/L, and 27.2 % for >10 mg/L). Although these deaths could be partially attributed to newly diagnosed aging-associated diseases [21], we speculate that in the individuals who met our criteria of successful aging, elevated levels of proinflammatory factors may serve as an indicator of the increased risk of death or may actually be associated with such risk through the activation of as-yet unidentified pathological mechanisms other than those that lead to cardiovascular disease, diabetes, cancer, or neurodegeneration.

Finally, we found that low-dose acetylsalicylic acid, which is very commonly administered in the elderly population for prevention of cardiovascular events, did not affect IL-6 or CRP levels, which was consistent with recently published results regarding 35 to 75-year-old participants of the Swiss CoLaus Study [58]. This previous study and our present results suggest that the well-studied cardioprotective action of low-dose acetylsalicylic acid may not be attributable to the lowering of IL-6 or CRP levels but rather other mechanisms, such as the modification of other cytokine concentrations.

The strengths of this study reside in the large size of the study group, the mode of recruitment (from urban and rural municipalities), the equally-sized 5-year age cohorts, the equal representation of both sexes, and detailed baseline clinical and biochemical data that allowed us to identify the group of successfully aging individuals based on various parameters [30]. On the other hand, one limitation of the present study was that not all of the study participants had their blood drawn. However, those who did not provide blood were not preselected on the basis of any condition, and we believe that the chance of bias for this reason is relatively low. Another limitation is that the lack of data regarding morbidity after the baseline interview prevented us from determining whether or not and to what extent new cases of aging-related diseases might explain associations between IL-6 and CRP levels and mortality in successfully aging individuals.

Conclusions

In the present study, IL-6 and CRP levels in the elderly systematically increased in an age-dependent manner in the entire study group, the successfully aging subgroup, and in individuals who suffered from aging-related diseases/disability. Higher IL-6 and CRP levels were associated with poorer cognitive and/or functional performance, and a higher risk of mortality also in successfully aging individuals. Our data support the notion that a single measurement of IL-6 and/or CRP concentrations in elderly individuals is a good predictor of physical and cognitive performance and mortality in the entire elderly population, including successfully aging individuals.

Abbreviations

ADL, katz activities of daily living scale; BMI, body mass index; CCL2, monocyte chemoattractant protein-1 (chemokine (C-C motif) ligand 2); CRP, C-reactive protein; eGFR, estimated glomerular filtration rate; HDL, high-density cholesterol; HR, hazard ratio; IL-1ß, interleukin-1ß; IL-6, interleukin-6; LDL, low-density cholesterol; MMSE, mini mental state examination; TNF-α, tumor necrosis factor-α.

Acknowledgements

This work was supported by the Polish Ministry of Science and Higher Education grant PBZ-MEiN-9/2/2006 – K143/P01/2007/1 ("PolSenior").

Authors' contributions

MPK conceived the project, analyzed and interpreted the data and wrote the paper, MO performed the experiments and analyzed the data, JC, KWT and AS acquired and analyzed the data and revised the manuscript, EF analyzed the data and revised the manuscript, MJ and PN acquired and analyzed the data, PS performed the statistical analysis and analyzed the data, MM participated in project development, analyzed and interpreted the data, as well as revised the manuscript. All of the authors approved the final version of the manuscript.

Competing interests

The authors declare that they have no competing interests.

Author details

[1]Department of Human Epigenetics, Mossakowski Medical Research Centre PAS, 5 Pawinskiego Street, 02-106 Warsaw, Poland. [2]Department of Geriatrics and Gerontology, Medical Centre of Postgraduate Education, 01-826 Warsaw, Poland. [3]PolSenior Project, International Institute of Molecular and Cell Biology, 02-109 Warsaw, Poland. [4]Department of Palliative Medicine, Poznan University of Medical Sciences, 61-245 Poznan, Poland. [5]Third Department of Cardiology, Medical University of Silesia in Katowice, 40-635 Katowice, Poland. [6]Department of Pathophysiology, Faculty of Medicine, Medical University of Silesia in Katowice, 40-752 Katowice, Poland. [7]Deparment of Internal Medicine and Oncological Chemotherapy, Faculty of Medicine, Medical University of Silesia in Katowice, 40-027 Katowice, Poland. [8]Department of Internal Medicine and Geriatrics, Jagiellonian University Medical College, 31-351 Cracow, Poland.

References

1. Ponnappan S, Ponnappan U. Aging and immune function: molecular mechanisms to interventions. Antioxid Redox Signal. 2011;14:1551–85.
2. Cevenini E, Monti D, Franceschi C. Inflamm-ageing. Curr Opin Clin Nutr Metab Care. 2013;16:14–20.
3. Biagi E, Nylund L, Candela M, Ostan R, Bucci L, Pini E, et al. Through ageing, and beyond: gut microbiota and inflammatory status in seniors and centenarians. PLoS One. 2010; doi: 10.1371/journal.pone.0010667.
4. Simanek AM, Dowd JB, Pawelec G, Melzer D, Dutta A, Aiello AE. Seropositivity to cytomegalovirus, inflammation, all-cause and cardiovascular disease-related mortality in the United States. PLoS One. 2011; doi:10.1371/journal.pone.0016103.
5. Brinkley TE, Hsu FC, Beavers KM, Church TS, Goodpaster BH, Stafford RS, et al. Total and abdominal adiposity are associated with inflammation in older adults using a factor analysis approach. J Gerontol A Biol Sci Med Sci. 2012;67:1099–106.
6. Hager K, Machein U, Krieger S, Platt D, Seefried G, Bauer J. Interleukin-6 and selected plasma proteins in healthy persons of different ages. Neurobiol Aging. 1994;15:771–2.
7. Roubenoff R, Harris TB, Abad LW, Wilson PW, Dallal GE, Dinarello CA. Monocyte cytokine production in an elderly population: effect of age and inflammation. J Gerontol A Biol Sci Med Sci. 1998;53:M20–6.
8. Seidler S, Zimmermann HW, Bartneck M, Trautwein C, Tacke F. Age-dependent alterations of monocyte subsets and monocyte-related chemokine pathways in healthy adults. BMC Immunol. 2010; doi: 10.1186/1471-2172-11-30.
9. Ahmadi-Abhari S, Luben RN, Wareham NJ, Khaw KT. Distribution and determinants of C-reactive protein in the older adult population: European Prospective Investigation into Cancer-Norfolk study. Eur J Clin Invest. 2013; 43:899–911.
10. Xu H, Barnes GT, Yang Q, Tan G, Yang D, Chou CJ, et al. Chronic inflammation in fat plays a crucial role in the development of obesity-related insulin resistance. J Clin Invest. 2003;112:1821–30.
11. Candore G, Vasto S, Colonna-Romano G, Lio D, Caruso M, Rea IM, et al. Cytokine gene polymorphisms and atherosclerosis. In: Vandenbroeck K, editor. Cytokine gene polymorphisms in multifactorial conditions. Boca Raton: CRC Press; 2006. p. 363–78.
12. Wen H, Gris D, Lei Y, Jha S, Zhang L, Huang MT, et al. Fatty acid-induced NLRP3-ASC inflammasome activation interferes with insulin signaling. Nat Immunol. 2011;12:408–15.
13. Vasan RS, Sullivan LM, Roubenoff R, Dinarello CA, Harris T, Benjamin EJ, et al. Inflammatory markers and risk of heart failure in elderly subjects without

prior myocardial infarction: the Framingham Heart Study. Circulation. 2003; 107:1486–91.

14. Payette H, Roubenoff R, Jacques PF, Dinarello CA, Wilson PW, Abad LW, et al. Insulin-like growth factor-1 and interleukin 6 predict sarcopenia in very old community-living men and women: the Framingham Heart Study. J Am Geriatr Soc. 2003;51:1237–43.

15. Bruunsgaard H, Ladelund S, Pedersen AN, Schroll M, Jørgensen T, Pedersen BK. Predicting death from tumour necrosis factor-α and interleukin-6 in 80-year-old people. Clin Exp Immunol. 2003;132:24–31.

16. Trichopoulos D, Psaltopoulou T, Orfanos P, Trichopoulou A, Boffetta P. Plasma C-reactive protein and risk of cancer: a prospective study from Greece. Cancer Epidemiol Biomarkers Prev. 2006;15:381–4.

17. Bruunsgaard H. The clinical impact of systemic low-level inflammation in elderly populations. With special reference to cardiovascular disease, dementia and mortality. Dan Med Bull. 2006;53:285–309.

18. Tan ZS, Beiser AS, Vasan RS, Roubenoff R, Dinarello CA, Harris TB, et al. Inflammatory markers and the risk of Alzheimer disease: the Framingham Study. Neurology. 2007;68:1902–8.

19. Beyer I, Njemini R, Bautmans I, Demanet C, Bergmann P, Mets T. Inflammation-related muscle weakness and fatigue in geriatric patients. Exp Gerontol. 2012;47:52–9.

20. Collerton J, Martin-Ruiz C, Davies K, Hilkens CM, Isaacs J, Kolenda C, et al. Frailty and the role of inflammation, immunosenescence and cellular ageing in the very old: cross-sectional findings from the Newcastle 85+ Study. Mech Ageing Dev. 2012;133:456–66.

21. Jenny NS, French B, Arnold AM, Strotmeyer ES, Cushman M, Chaves PH, et al. Long-term assessment of inflammation and healthy aging in late life: the Cardiovascular Health Study All Stars. J Gerontol A Biol Sci Med Sci. 2012;67:970–6.

22. Quaglia LA, Freitas W, Soares AA, Santos RA, Nadruz Jr W, Blaha M, et al. C-reactive protein is independently associated with coronary atherosclerosis burden among octogenarians. Aging Clin Exp Res. 2014;26:19–23.

23. Wassel CL, Barrett-Connor E, Laughlin GA. Association of circulating C-reactive protein and interleukin-6 with longevity into the 80s and 90s: The Rancho Bernardo Study. J Clin Endocrinol Metab. 2010;95:4748–55.

24. Giovannini S, Onder G, Liperoti R, Russo A, Carter C, Capoluongo E, et al. Interleukin-6, C-reactive protein, and tumor necrosis factor-α as predictors of mortality in frail, community-living elderly individuals. J Am Geriatr Soc. 2011;59:1679–85.

25. Ferrando-Martínez S, Romero-Sánchez MC, Solana R, Delgado J, de la Rosa R, Muñoz-Fernández MA, et al. Thymic function failure and C-reactive protein levels are independent predictors of all-cause mortality in healthy elderly humans. Age (Dordr). 2013;35:251–9.

26. Jylhä M, Paavilainen P, Lehtimäki T, Goebeler S, Karhunen PJ, Hervonen A, et al. Interleukin-1 receptor antagonist, interleukin-6, and C-reactive protein as predictors of mortality in nonagenarians: the vitality 90+ study. J Gerontol A Biol Sci Med Sci. 2007;62:1016–21.

27. Alley DE, Crimmins EM, Karlamangla A, Hu P, Seeman TE. Inflammation and rate of cognitive change in high-functioning older adults. J Gerontol A Biol Sci Med Sci. 2008;63:50–5.

28. Beleigoli AM, Boersma E, Diniz Mde F, Vidigal PG, Lima-Costa MF, Ribeiro AL. C-reactive protein and B-type natriuretic peptide yield either a non-significant or a modest incremental value to traditional risk factors in predicting long-term overall mortality in older adults. PLoS One. 2013; doi: 10.1371/journal. pone.0075809

29. Matsushima J, Kawashima T, Nabeta H, Imamura Y, Watanabe I, Mizoguchi Y, et al. Association of inflammatory biomarkers with depressive symptoms and cognitive decline in a community-dwelling healthy older sample: a 3-year follow-up study. J Affect Disord. 2015;173:9–14.

30. Bledowski P, Mossakowska M, Chudek J, Grodzicki T, Milewicz A, Szybalska A, et al. Medical, psychological and socioeconomic aspects of aging in Poland: assumptions and objectives of the PolSenior project. Exp Gerontol. 2011;46: 1003–9.

31. Folstein MF, Folstein SE, McHugh PR. "Mini-mental state". A practical method for grading the cognitive state of patients for the clinician. J Psychiatr Res. 1975;12:189–98.

32. Klich-Rączka A, Piotrowicz K, Mossakowska M, Skalska A, Wizner B, Broczek K, et al. The assessment of cognitive impairment suspected of dementia in Polish elderly people: results of the population-based PolSenior Study. Exp Gerontol. 2014;57:233–42.

33. Katz S, Ford AB, Moskowitz RW, Jackson BA, Jaffe MW. Studies of illness in the aged: The index of ADL: A standardized measure of biological and psychosocial function. JAMA. 1963;185:94–9.

34. Skalska A, Wizner B, Więcek A, Zdrojewski T, Chudek J, Klich-Rączka A, et al. Reduced functionality in everyday activities of patients with self-reported heart failure hospitalization–population-based study results. Int J Cardiol. 2014;176:423–9.

35. Bowling A. Aspirations for older age in the 21st century: what is successful aging? Int J Aging Hum Dev. 2007;64:263–97.

36. Eklund CM. Proinflammatory cytokines in CRP baseline regulation. Adv Clin Chem. 2009;48:111–36.

37. Salvioli S, Monti D, Lanzarini C, Conte M, Pirazzini C, Bacalini MG, et al. Immune system, cell senescence, aging and longevity – inflamm-aging reappraised. Curr Pharm Des. 2013;19:1675–9.

38. Minciullo PL, Catalano A, Mandraffino G, Casciaro M, Crucitti A, Maltese G, et al. Inflammaging and anti-inflammaging: the role of cytokines in extreme longevity. Arch Immunol Ther Exp (Warsz). 2016;64:111–26.

39. Baylis D, Bartlett DB, Patel HP, Roberts HC. Understanding how we age: insights into inflammaging. Longev Healthspan. 2013;2:8. doi:10.1186/2046-2395-2-8.

40. Deelen J, Beekman M, Capri M, Franceschi C, Slagboom PE. Identifying the genomic determinants of aging and longevity in human population studies: progress and challenges. Bioessays. 2013;35:386–96.

41. Mekli K, Nazroo JY, Marshall AD, Kumari M, Pendleton N. Proinflammatory genotype is associated with the frailty phenotype in the English Longitudinal Study of Ageing. Aging Clin Exp Res. 2015 Aug 7. [Epub ahead of print] doi: 10.1007/s40520-015-0419-z.

42. Dato S, Bellizzi D, Rose G, Passarino G. The impact of nutrients on the aging rate: A complex interaction of demographic, environmental and genetic factors. Mech Ageing Dev. 2016;154:49–61.

43. Akin I, Nienaber CA. "Obesity paradox" in coronary artery disease. World J Cardiol. 2015;7:603–8.

44. Brzecka A, Ejma M. Obesity paradox in the course of cerebrovascular diseases. Adv Clin Exp Med. 2015;24:379–83.

45. Kim NH, Lee J, Kim TJ, Kim NH, Choi KM, Baik SH, et al. Body Mass Index and Mortality in the General Population and in Subjects with Chronic Disease in Korea: A Nationwide Cohort Study (2002–2010). PLoS One. 2015; doi: 10.1371/journal.pone.0139924

46. Costanzo P, Cleland JG, Pellicori P, Clark AL, Hepburn D, Kilpatrick ES, et al. The obesity paradox in type 2 diabetes mellitus: relationship of body mass index to prognosis: a cohort study. Ann Intern Med. 2015;162:610–8.

47. Laird E, McNulty H, Ward M, Hoey L, McSorley E, Wallace JM, et al. Vitamin D deficiency is associated with inflammation in older Irish adults. J Clin Endocrinol Metab. 2014;99:1807–15.

48. Wood AD, Strachan AA, Thies F, Aucott LS, Reid DM, Hardcastle AC, et al. Patterns of dietary intake and serum carotenoid and tocopherol status are associated with biomarkers of chronic low-grade systemic inflammation and cardiovascular risk. Br J Nutr. 2014;112:1341–52.

49. Oe Y, Mochizuki K, Miyauchi R, Misaki Y, Kasezawa N, Tohyama K, et al. Plasma TNF-α is associated with inflammation and nutrition status in community-dwelling Japanese elderly. J Nutr Sci Vitaminol. 2015;61:263–9.

50. Lehtimäki T, Ojala P, Rontu R, Goebeler S, Karhunen PJ, Jylhä M, et al. Interleukin-6 modulates plasma cholesterol and C-reactive protein concentrations in nonagenarians. J Am Geriatr Soc. 2005;53:1552–8.

51. Cesari M, Onder G, Zamboni V, Capoluongo E, Russo A, Bernabei R, et al. C-reactive protein and lipid parameters in older persons aged 80 years and older. J Nutr Health Aging. 2009;13:587–93.

52. Ferrara A, Barrett-Connor E, Shan J. Total, LDL, and HDL cholesterol decrease with age in older men and women. The Rancho Bernardo Study 1984–1994. Circulation. 1997;96:37–43.

53. Olszanecka-Glinianowicz M, Chudek J, Szromek A, Zahorska-Markiewicz B. Changes of systemic microinflammation after weight loss and regain - a five-year follow up study. Endokrynol Pol. 2012;63:432–8.

54. Dahlén EM, Tengblad A, Länne T, Clinchy B, Ernerudh J, Nystrom FH, et al. Abdominal obesity and low-grade systemic inflammation as markers of subclinical organ damage in type 2 diabetes. Diabetes Metab. 2014;40:76–81.

55. Valentine RJ, Vieira VJ, Woods JA, Evans EM. Stronger relationship between central adiposity and C-reactive protein in older women than men. Menopause. 2009;16:84–9.

56. Beavers KM, Beavers DP, Newman JJ, Anderson AM, Loeser Jr RF, Nicklas BJ, et al. Effects of total and regional fat loss on plasma CRP and IL-6 in overweight and obese, older adults with knee osteoarthritis. Osteoarthritis Cartilage. 2015;23:249–56.

57. Varadhan R, Yao W, Matteini A, Beamer BA, Xue QL, Yang H, et al. Simple biologically informed inflammatory index of two serum cytokines predicts 10 year all-cause mortality in older adults. J Gerontol A Biol Sci Med Sci. 2014;69:165–73.

58. Vaucher J, Marques-Vidal P, Waeber G, Vollenweider P. Cytokines and hs-CRP levels in individuals treated with low-dose aspirin for cardiovascular prevention: a population-based study (CoLaus Study). Cytokine. 2014;66:95–100.

Effect of a synbiotic on the response to seasonal influenza vaccination is strongly influenced by degree of immunosenescence

Agnieszka Przemska-Kosicka[1], Caroline E. Childs[1], Sumia Enani[1], Catherine Maidens[1], Honglin Dong[1], Iman Bin Dayel[1], Kieran Tuohy[3], Susan Todd[2], Margot A. Gosney[1] and Parveen Yaqoob[1*]

Abstract

Background: Ageing increases risk of respiratory infections and impairs the response to influenza vaccination. Pre- and probiotics offer an opportunity to modulate anti-viral defenses and the response to vaccination via alteration of the gut microbiota. This study investigated the effect of a novel probiotic, *Bifidobacterium longum bv. infantis* CCUG 52,486, combined with a prebiotic, gluco-oligosaccharide (*B. longum* + Gl-OS), on the response to seasonal influenza vaccination in young and older subjects in a double-blind, randomized controlled trial, taking into account the influence of immunosenescence markers at baseline.

Results: Vaccination resulted in a significant increase in total antibody titres, vaccine-specific IgA, IgM and IgG and seroprotection to all three subunits of the vaccine in both young and older subjects, and in general, the increases in young subjects were greater. There was little effect of the synbiotic, although it tended to reduce seroconversion to the Brisbane subunit of the vaccine and the vaccine-specific IgG response in older subjects. Immunological characterization revealed that older subjects randomized to the synbiotic had a significantly higher number of senescent (CD28−CD57+) helper T cells at baseline compared with those randomized to the placebo, and they also had significantly higher plasma levels of anti-CMV IgG and a greater tendency for CMV seropositivity. Moreover, higher numbers of CD28−CD57+ helper T cells were associated with failure to seroconvert to Brisbane, strongly suggesting that the subjects randomized to the synbiotic were already at a significant disadvantage in terms of likely ability to respond to the vaccine compared with those randomized to the placebo.

Conclusions: Ageing was associated with marked impairment of the antibody response to influenza vaccination in older subjects and the synbiotic failed to reverse this impairment. However, the older subjects randomized to the synbiotic were at a significant disadvantage due to a greater degree of immunosenscence at baseline compared with those randomized to the placebo. Thus, baseline differences in immunosenescence between the randomized groups are likely to have influenced the outcome of the intervention, highlighting the need for detailed immunological characterization of subjects prior to interventions.

Keywords: Ageing, Influenza, Prebiotic, Probiotic, Vaccination

* Correspondence: P.Yaqoob@reading.ac.uk
[1]Department of Food and Nutritional Sciences, University of Reading, PO Box 226Whiteknights, Reading, Berkshire RG6 6AP, UK
Full list of author information is available at the end of the article

Background

Influenza is a major cause of death in older people and while vaccination offers a prophylactic solution for preventing infection and associated complications, immunosenescence significantly impairs vaccine efficacy [1]. Potential adjuvants and dietary strategies to improve the immune response to influenza vaccines are therefore of interest, particularly in older people. Emerging evidence suggests that the resident gut microbiota plays an influential role in shaping antiviral defenses and modulating the outcome of viral infections [2], and this forms the basis for the hypothesis that pre- and probiotics may modulate responses to infection or vaccination.

Trials investigating the use of probiotics in prevention of common respiratory illnesses have produced mixed results [3], although a recent systematic review concluded that they significantly reduce episodes of acute URTI and antibiotic usage in infants and young to middle-aged adults [4]. Response to vaccination is increasingly being used as a surrogate for the response to infection [5]. The majority of studies investigating the impact of probiotics on responses to vaccination have been conducted in healthy adults, and some show borderline effects of probiotics on serum or salivary IgA titres, although the clinical relevance is not clear [6]. Studies in infants and in elderly subjects, particularly those examining the response to influenza vaccination, are very limited, as are studies on the effects of prebiotics on immune function [7] and vaccination [6]. Since ageing is associated with reduced biodiversity and compromised stability of the gut microbiota [8], as well as immunosenescence, older individuals may derive particular benefit from intervention with pre- and/or probiotics.

In selecting probiotics specifically for older individuals, Dominguez-Bello et al. [9] suggest that "the healthy old, rather than the healthy young, are the best donors of probiotic species for old individuals", because they may be better suited to colonization and establishment of a new equilibrium within an aged microbial community. The strain *Bifidobacterium longum bv. infantis* CCUG 52,486 fits this brief because it was originally isolated from a cohort of very healthy elderly subjects (independent life-style, free of chronic disease, and aged 90 years or over) in Italy as part of the CROWNALIFE EU FP5 project [10], it has been demonstrated to have particular ecological fitness and anti-pathogenic effects in vitro [11], and it has immunomodulatory effects which are strongly influenced by the age of the host [12]. Furthermore, this strain has been fully genome sequenced so that genetic traits can potentially be related to biological effects. In this study, we examine the ability of *Bifidobacterium longum bv. infantis* CCUG 52,486, combined with a gluco-oligosaccharide prebiotic (Gl-OS), to modulate the response to seasonal influenza vaccination in a cohort of healthy young and older subjects. We also examine the extent to which baseline markers of immunosenescence influenced the outcome of the intervention.

Results
Subject characteristics

The characteristics of the subjects recruited to the study are described in Table 1. Of the 125 volunteers who started the trial, 112 completed (Fig. 1). There were no differences in baseline characteristics between treatment groups within the young or older cohorts (data not shown).

Effect of *B. longum* + Gl-OS on vaccine subunit-specific total antibody responses to seasonal influenza vaccination
Total antibody response to the H1N1 strain

Vaccination resulted in a significant increase in antibodies to H1N1 in both young and older subjects, but the increase was greater in the young subjects (Fig. 2a). When the young and older cohorts were combined, there was a trend for a treatment effect ($p < 0.02$; Fig. 2a), but this did not remain when the cohorts were analysed separately.

Total antibody response to the H3N2 strain

Vaccination resulted in a significant increase in mean antibody titres to the H3N2 subunit of the vaccine (Fig. 2b). However, there was a significant age*time interaction ($p < 0.01$) reflecting the greater increase in antibody titres in response to vaccination in young subjects compared to

Table 1 Baseline characteristics of subjects recruited to a double-blind, placebo-controlled, randomised study of *Bifidobacterium longum bv. infantis* CCUG 52,486 combined with gluco-oligosaccharide

	Older cohort	Younger cohort
	(n = 63)	(n = 62)
Gender	18♂45♀	23♂39♀
Smoker	4/63	13/62
	mean (SD)	
Age	69 (5)	26 (4)
BMI (kg/m²)	27 (3)	23 (3)
Waist (cm)	94 (16)	80 (9)
Weight (kg)	74 (13)	68 (13)
Height (m)	1.7 (0.1)	1.7 (0.1)
BP systolic (mmHg)	138 (17)	122 (11)
BP diastolic (mmHg)	78 (9)	74 (8)
Pulse (bpm)	70 (11)	76 (10)

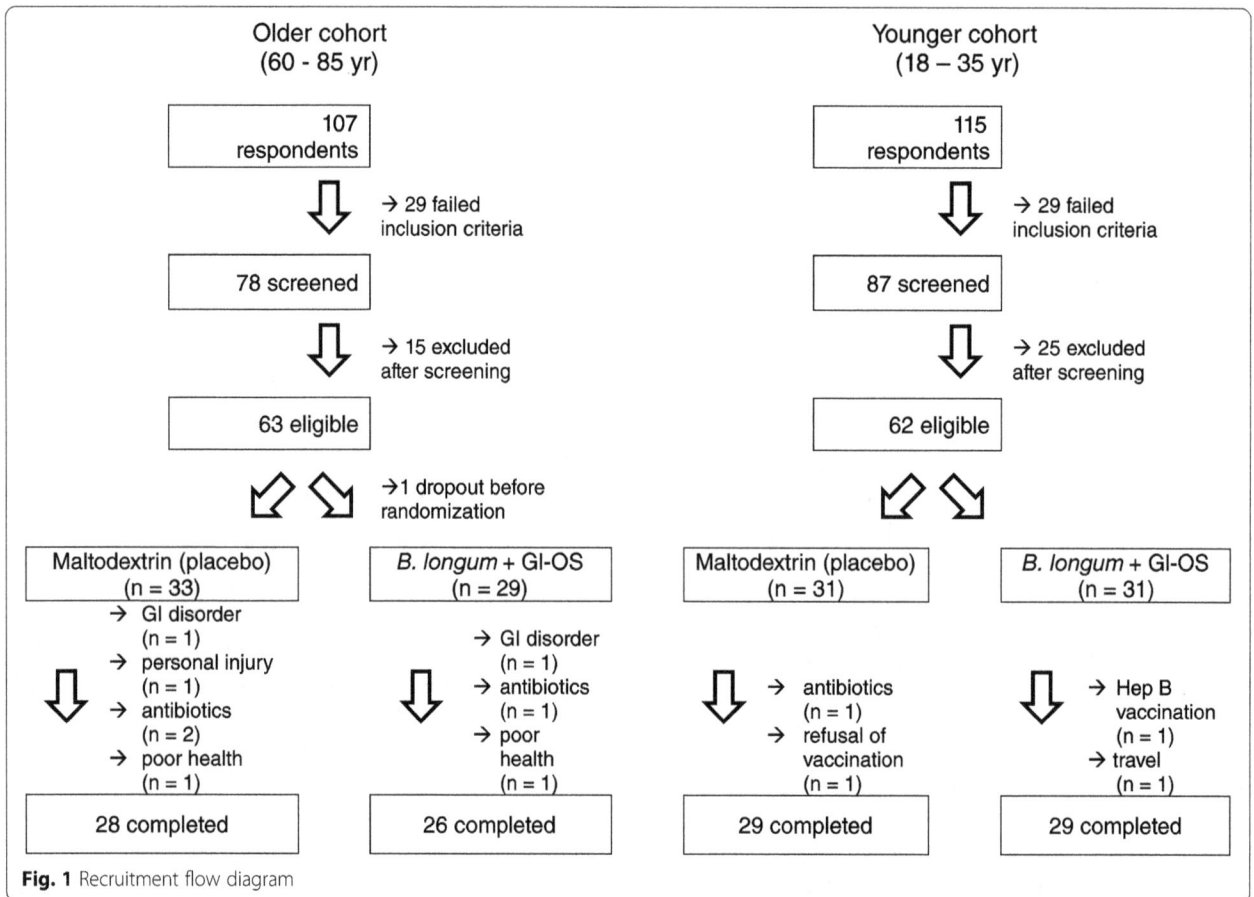

Fig. 1 Recruitment flow diagram

older subjects. There was no significant effect of treatment with the synbiotic on antibody titres to H3N2 (Fig. 2b).

Total antibody response to the Brisbane strain

Vaccination increased mean antibody titres to the Brisbane strain (Fig. 2c). There was a significant effect of age ($p < 0.01$), with mean antibody titres to the Brisbane subunit being significantly higher in young subjects after vaccination (Fig. 2c), and there was a significant age*time interaction, reflecting the greater response to vaccination in the young subjects (Fig. 2c).

There was no overall effect of treatment when the young and older cohorts were combined, but when they were considered separately, the synbiotic was associated with a borderline effect (reduction) on the antibody response to vaccine in the young subjects (Fig. 2c).

Effect of B. longum + Gl-OS on seroprotection to seasonal influenza vaccination

Baseline seroprotection to H1N1 was significantly different in the young and older subjects (Table 2). The young subjects already had a significant level of protection at baseline (GMT > 32) compared to older subjects, and this

was apparent in both the placebo and the synbiotic groups (Table 2). After vaccination, seroprotection to the H1N1 strain tended to remain higher amongst the young subjects compared with the older subjects (Table 2), but there was no clear effect of treatment. There were no differences in seroprotection to H3N2 between cohorts and no effect of the synbiotic on seroprotection to H1N1 or H3N2 in either cohort (Table 2).

For the Brisbane strain, seroprotection was significantly greater in the young subjects following vaccination (Table 2), but there was no clear effect of treatment with the synbiotic.

Effect of B. longum + Gl-OS on seroconversion to seasonal influenza vaccination

Seroconversion to H1N1 and H3N2 was not significantly different between the young and older subjects, although there was a trend for better seroconversion to H3N2 in the young subjects (Table 3). Young subjects demonstrated significantly greater seroconversion to the Brisbane strain than older subjects (Table 3). There was no significant effect of supplementation with the synbiotic on seroconversion to Brisbane, although it tended to reduce seroconversion in the older subjects (Table 3).

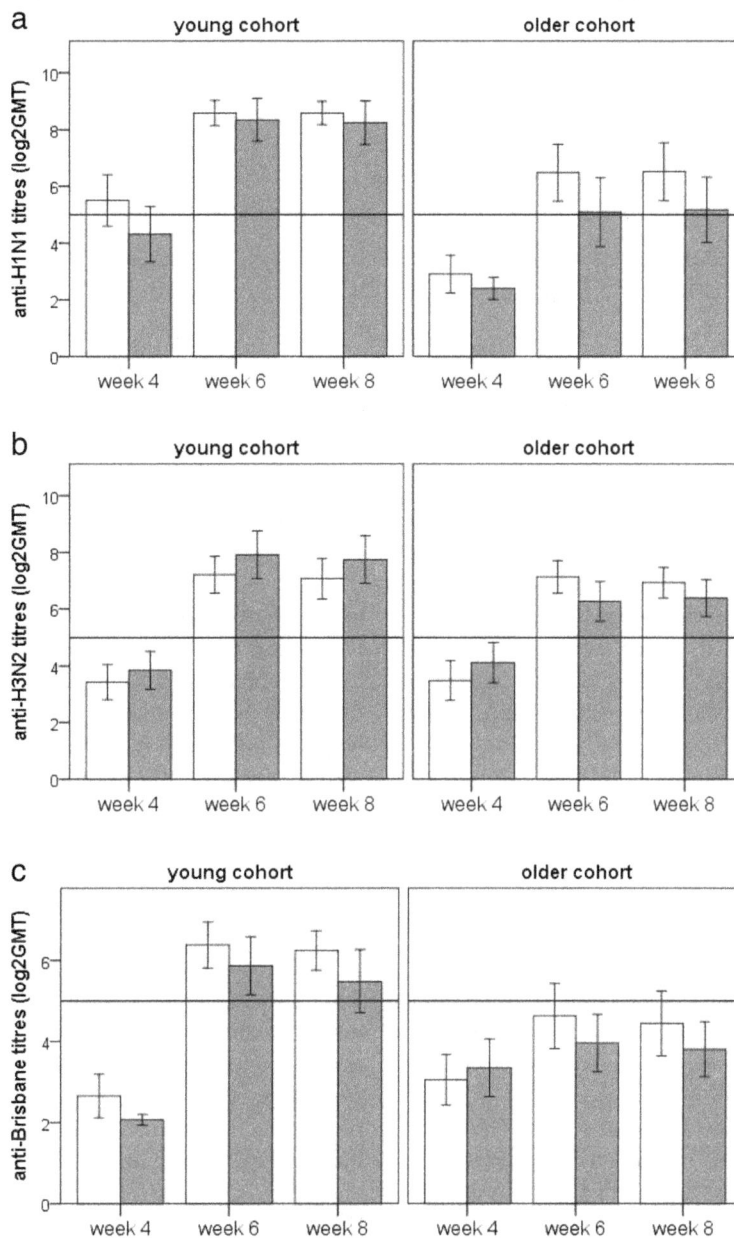

Fig. 2 Effect of *B. longum* + GI-OS on antibody responses to the influenza vaccine in young and older subjects. Data are log$_2$ transformed geometric mean antibody titres (GMT) (±2SEM) at baseline and weeks 6 and 8 for $n = 54$–58 subjects per group. □ Maltodextrin, ▨ *B. longum* + GI-OS. The reference line at the Y axis indicates seroprotection (GMT = 32). Data were analysed using a Linear Mixed Model (LMM) with fixed factors of time, age and treatment. **a** H1N1; For the LMM, there were significant effects of age ($p < 0.001$) and time ($p < 0.001$) and a trend for a treatment effect ($p < 0.02$). For data split by cohorts, there was a significant effect of time in both cohorts ($p < 0.001$), but no significant effect of treatment. **b** H3N2; for the LMM overall, there was a significant effect of time ($p < 0.001$) and an age*time interaction ($p < 0.01$). For data split by cohort there was a significant effect of time ($p < 0.001$) and a time*treatment interaction ($p < 0.01$) in the older cohort, and a significant effect of time ($p < 0.001$) in the young cohort. **c** Brisbane; for the LMM overall, there were significant effects of age ($p < 0.005$), time ($p < 0.001$) and an age*time interaction ($p < 0.001$). For data split by cohort, there was a significant effect of time ($p < 0.001$) and a time*treatment interaction ($p < 0.01$) in the older cohort, and a significant effect of time ($p < 0.001$) in the young cohort. There was a borderline effect of treatment ($p < 0.05$)

Effect of *B. longum* + GI-OS on levels of vaccine-specific IgA, IgG1, IgD and IgM and salivary sIgA following seasonal influenza vaccination

Levels of vaccine-specific IgA, IgG, IgD and IgM were significantly increased following influenza vaccination in both young and older subjects (Additional file 1: Figure S1). In all cases, except for IgM, increases were significantly greater in the young subjects (Additional file 1: Figure S1). There was no effect of the synbiotic on levels of vaccine-specific Ig subclasses, although

Table 2 Effect of *B. longum* + GI-OS on seroprotection status in young and older subjects before and 4 weeks after influenza vaccination

Vaccine strain		Seroprotection status				p
		Young cohort (n = 58)		Older cohort (n = 54)		
		Placebo	B. longum + GI-OS	Placebo	B. longum + GI-OS	
		n/N (%)	n/N (%)	n/N (%)	n/N (%)	
A/California/7/2009 (H1N1)	Before	20/29 (69)[a]	13/29 (45)[a]	5/28 (18)	1/26 (4)	< 0.001
	After	29/29 (100)	27/29 (93)[a]	22/27 (81)	16/26 (62)	< 0.001
A/Perth/16/2009 (H3N2)	Before	10/29 (34)	13/29 (45)	8/28 (29)	12/26 (46)	NS
	After	26/29 (90)	27/29 (93)	25/27 (93)	22/26 (85)	NS
B/Brisbane/60/2008	Before	4/29 (14)	0/29 (0)	4/24 (17)	5/26 (19)	NS
	After	28/29 (97)	20/29 (76)	14/27 (52)	11/26 (42)	< 0.001

Data are numbers of seroprotected (n)/total (N) and % seroprotected subjects in parentheses. 'Before' refers to week 4 samples and 'After' refers to week 8 samples (ie 4 weeks after vaccination). P refers to results of Fisher's exact test for differences between the cohorts with treatment groups combined;
[a]young cohort significantly different from the older cohort within same treatment group ($p < 0.01$, Fisher's Exact test)

there was a tendency for a smaller IgG response in the older subjects on the synbiotic relative to the placebo group ($p = 0.03$; Additional file 1: Figure S1) and an improved induction of vaccine-specific IgM and, to some degree, IgG (only at week 6) in young subjects (Additional file 1: Figure S1). There was no effect of either age or of the synbiotic on concentrations of salivary sIgA at any timepoint (data not shown).

Effect of *B. longum* + GI-OS on copy number of *B. longum* in faecal samples and influence of numbers of bifidobacteria on seroconversion

There was a significant increase in copy numbers of *B. longum* in faecal samples from subjects taking the synbiotic when the young and older cohorts were combined ($p < 0.01$), but although trends remained when the cohorts were analysed separately, they were not statistically significant (Additional file 2: Figure S2). Overall, no significant genus-level changes in the faecal gut microbiota, as assessed by FISH, were observed (data not shown), but seroconverters to all three subunits of the influenza vaccine tended to demonstrate a greater bifidogenic effect of the pre- and probiotic treatment compared with non-seroconverters ($p = 0.057$), suggesting that successful seroconversion may be associated

with increased numbers of bifidobacteria (Additional file 3: Figure S3).

Influence of baseline markers of immunosenescence and CMV status on intervention outcome

Older subjects randomized to the synbiotic had a significantly higher number of senescent (CD28$^-$CD57$^+$) helper T cells at baseline compared with those randomized to the placebo (Fig. 3). They also had significantly higher plasma levels of anti-CMV IgG (Fig. 4) and a greater tendency for CMV seropositivity (66.7 % vs 38.1 %). CD28$^-$CD57$^+$ helper T cells and cytotoxic T cells were significantly higher in CMV$^+$ subjects compared with age-matched CMV$^-$ subjects and were positively correlated with the plasma level of anti-CMV IgG and with telomere length (data not shown). Higher numbers of these CD28$^-$CD57$^+$ helper T cells were associated with failure to seroconvert to Brisbane (Fig. 5), suggesting that differences in immunosenescence between the randomized groups at baseline may have influenced the outcome of the intervention.

Discussion

This paper demonstrates marked impairment of the antibody response to influenza vaccination in older subjects. Intervention with a novel synbiotic, *B. longum* + GI-OS

Table 3 Effect of *B. longum* + GI-OS on seroconversion in young and older subjects 4 weeks after influenza vaccination (week 8)

Vaccine strain	Seroconversion status (≥ fourfold increase in Ab titres)				p
	Young cohort (n = 58)		Older cohort (n = 54)		
	Placebo	B. longum + GI-OS	Placebo	B. longum + GI-OS	
	n/N (%)	n/N (%)	n/N (%)	n/N (%)	
A/California/7/2009 (H1N1)	15/29 (52)	18/29 (62)	21/27 (78)	15/26 (58)	NS
A/Perth/16/2009 (H3N2)	20/29 (69)	22/29 (76)[a]	17/27 (63)	10/26 (38)	0.031
B/Brisbane/60/2008	23/29 (79)[a]	20/29 (69)[a]	7/27 (26)	1/26 (4)	< 0.001

Data are numbers of seroconverted (n)/total (N) and % seroconverted subjects in parentheses. P refers to results of Fisher's exact test for differences between the cohorts with treatment groups combined; [a]young cohort significantly different from the older cohort within same treatment group ($p < 0.01$, Fisher's Exact test)

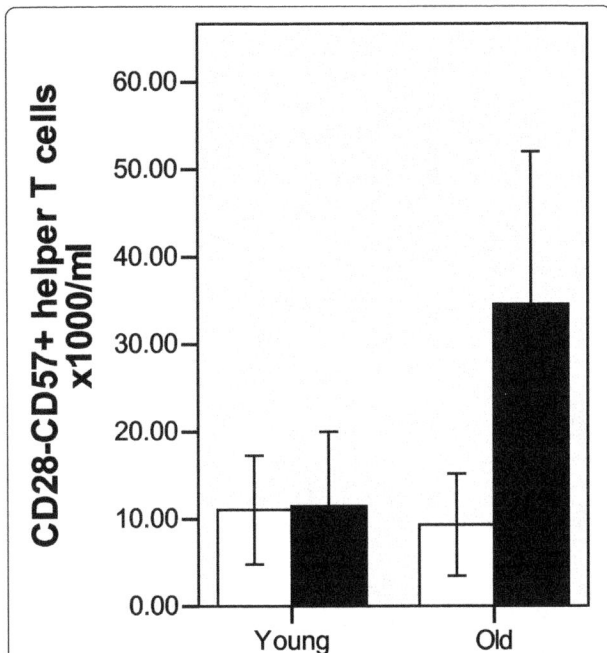

Fig. 3 Numbers of CD28$^-$CD57$^+$ helper T cells at baseline differ in older subjects randomized to *B. longum* + GI-OS and placebo. Data are absolute numbers of T-cell subsets × 1000/ml ± 2SEM for *n* = 58 young and *n* = 54 older subjects randomized to *B. longum* + GI-OS ■ or placebo □. Data were analysed using Student's independent *t*-tests for differences between young and older subjects. ** Denotes significant difference between treatment groups within age cohort (*p* < 0.01)

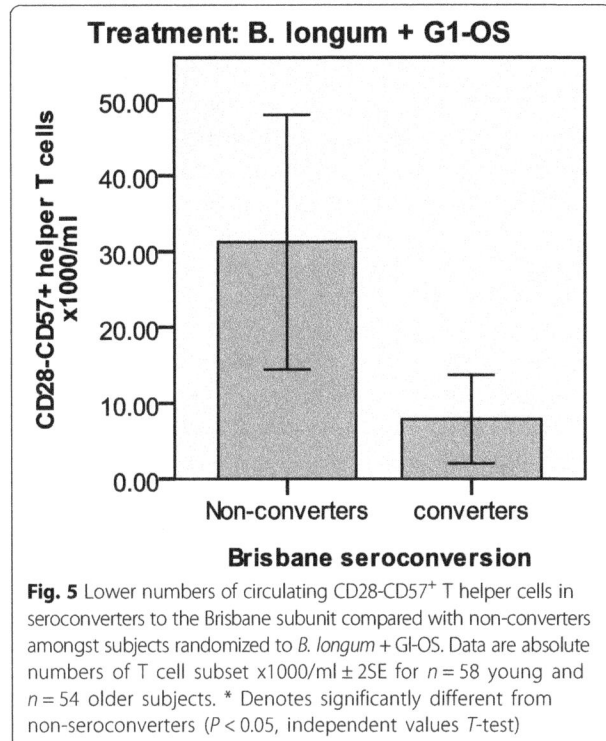

Fig. 5 Lower numbers of circulating CD28-CD57$^+$ T helper cells in seroconverters to the Brisbane subunit compared with non-converters amongst subjects randomized to *B. longum* + GI-OS. Data are absolute numbers of T cell subset x1000/ml ± 2SE for *n* = 58 young and *n* = 54 older subjects. * Denotes significantly different from non-seroconverters (*P* < 0.05, independent values *T*-test)

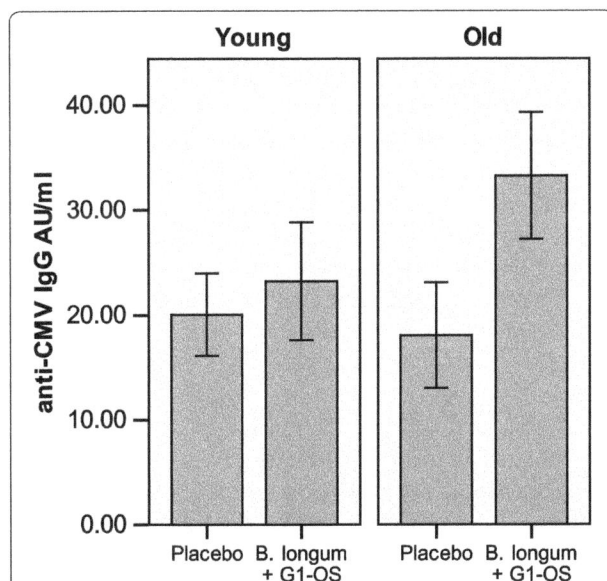

Fig. 4 Baseline levels of anti-CMV IgG differ in older subjects randomized to *B. longum* + GI-OS and placebo. Data are anti-CMV IgG (AU/ml) ± 2SEM for *n* = 45 young and *n* = 45 older subjects randomized to *B. longum* + GI-OS or placebo. Data were analysed using Student's independent t-tests for differences between young and older subjects. * Denotes significant difference between treatment groups within age cohort (*p* < 0.05)

failed to reverse this impairment in older subjects, and in fact there were trends for reduced seroconversion to the Brisbane subunit and a reduced IgG response. However, further immunological characterization revealed a greater degree of immunosenescence at baseline in older subjects randomized to the synbiotic, which could explain the particularly poor response of these subjects to the vaccination. This demonstrates, for the first time, that the interpretation of interventions examining the response to vaccination in older people may be highly dependent on their baseline immunological phenotype.

While there is general consensus that ageing impairs the response to influenza vaccination [13], there are very few robust studies specifically comparing responses of young and older subjects, and the most comprehensive information available is from a meta-analysis published in 2006, which concluded that clinical vaccine efficacy in older subjects was only 17–53 % compared with 70–90 % in young subjects [14]. In the current study, antibody responses to all three subunits of the influenza vaccine were impaired in the older subjects and there was significantly greater seroprotection to the H1N1 and Brisbane subunits and seroconversion to the H3N2 and Brisbane subunits in the young subjects after vaccination. Accounting for differences in baseline seroprotection between individuals and groups was a particular challenge in the current study since the B/Brisbane/60/ 2008 strain had previously been used in the trivalent vaccine in the 2009/2010 season and the H1N1 strain had previously been used in the monovalent swine flu vaccination during the pandemic of 2009/2010 (although only three subjects had previously been vaccinated with this). In the current study, individuals who were seroprotected at baseline were not excluded because it was considered valuable to employ a 'real life' scenario. Notably, the older subjects had high pre-vaccination antibody titres to the Brisbane strain and a poor seroconversion rate compared with the young subjects. On the other hand, baseline seroprotection for the H1N1 strain was greater in the young cohort, yet rates of seroconversion were similar in the two cohorts.

To date, studies which have examined the potential adjuvant properties of probiotics given in conjunction with influenza vaccines in healthy adults have shown promise in their ability to beneficially modulate the humoral response to influenza, but robust data is still lacking [6, 15]. The effects of probiotics on the response to influenza vaccination in older adults is of particular importance, given the consequences of respiratory infections in older people [16]. Among free-living Chilean subjects over 70 years old, a complete nutritional formula containing a range of nutrients and vitamins plus the probiotic *Lactobacillus paracasei* (NCC 2461) and the prebiotic fructo-oligosaccharide was associated with a significantly lower incidence of respiratory infection, but had no effect on antibody responses to vaccination [17]. Provision of a probiotic drink containing *Lactobacillus paracasei* ssp. *paracasei* (Actimel®) to healthy elderly volunteers (> 70 years) resulted in higher influenza virus-specific antibody titres post-vaccination, although these differences were only statistically significant within the confirmatory phase of this study [18]. A small study of 27 elderly (mean age > 85) subjects provided with *Bifidobacterium longum* BB536, reported significantly lower incidence of influenza and fever in the probiotic group [19]. However, the largest study to date investigated the effect of *Lactobacillus casei* Shirota (*Lc*S) on the susceptibility to respiratory symptoms and influenza vaccination responses among 737 nursing home residents (mean age > 80 year) and reported no significant differences in antibody titres, seroconversion or seroprotection 4 and 22 weeks after vaccination, and no effect on reported respiratory symptoms [20]. Thus the evidence is not clear cut and it is possible that there are differences in the immunomodulatory potential of different strains.

In the current study, the response of the young and older subjects to the intervention differed to some degree. In older subjects consuming the synbiotic, there was a trend for reduced seroconversion to the Brisbane subunit, whereas in the young subjects, there were trends for enhanced production of vaccine-specific IgM

and, to some extent, IgG. Increased production of vaccine-specific IgM and IgG following intervention with probiotics has been reported in several other studies [21–25]. The possibility that there is a differential immune response to probiotics in young vs older subjects has also been explored to some extent. You et al. [12] demonstrated that peripheral blood mononuclear cells (PBMC) from older subjects (60–85y) were more responsive to the immunoregulatory effects (IL-10 induction) of two strains of bifidobacteria than young subjects (18–30y), whereas PBMC from young subjects were more responsive to the immunostimulatory effects (IL-12 induction) of two strains of lactobacilli. Further studies demonstrated that probiotics (including the strain employed in the current study) increased the responsiveness of DCs in older subjects to a greater degree than young subjects, but this was not sufficient to overcome the impact of immunosenescence in a mixed leukocyte reaction [26]. The choice of probiotic, particularly for older individuals, is a matter of debate and it has been suggested that 'successfully aged' donors of probiotic strains might survive better in an older host and achieve a more suitable equilibrium with the resident microbiota [9]. *Bifidobacterium longum bv. infantis* CCUG 52,486 is an example of a strain present in particularly healthy subjects aged > 90y, which has subsequently been demonstrated to have particular ecological fitness and anti-pathogenic effects in vitro [27] and immunomodulatory effects which are strongly influenced by the age of the host [12, 26]. The effects of prebiotics on immune function are less well characterized than those of probiotics, but are suggested to be mainly indirect via modulation of the gut microbiota. In the current study, the prebiotic Gl-OS was used chiefly to support the colonization of the probiotic, and although an independent effect of the prebiotic on the gut microbiota cannot be excluded, the fact that the intervention increased copy numbers of *B. longum* while having no significant effect on the fecal microbiota at genus level suggests that the prebiotic was selectively supporting the growth of the probiotic strain *in vivo*.

The results of the intervention must take into account the potential influence of baseline differences in immunosenescence, which in the current study were revealed after the study was completed and occurred entirely by chance. T cells are particularly susceptible to senescence, resulting in loss of CD28; repeated antigenic exposure, for example to cytomegalovirus (CMV), is suggested to play a major role in this [28, 29]. Latent infection with CMV has been demonstrated to result in a poor response to infection and vaccination [29]. In the current study, not only did older subjects randomized to the synbiotic have a significantly higher number of senescent

(CD28⁻CD57⁺) helper T cells at baseline compared with those randomized to the placebo, they also had significantly higher plasma levels of anti-CMV IgG and a greater tendency for CMV seropositivity. Moreover, higher numbers of $CD28^-CD57^+$ helper T cells were associated with failure to seroconvert to Brisbane, strongly suggesting that the subjects randomized to the synbiotic were already at a significant disadvantage in terms of likely ability to respond to the vaccine compared with those randomized to the placebo and that differences in immunosenescence between the randomized groups at baseline may have influenced the outcome of the intervention. Future work therefore needs to consider prospective randomization of subjects based on robust immunological markers; this is challenging given the wide range of potential markers and uncertainty regarding their predictive value.

In this paper, we report the effects of the synbiotic on the humoral arm of the immune response only. However, recognizing the importance of the T cell response following vaccination, and the potential effects of the synbiotic on adaptive immunity [30], we conducted extensive analysis of antigen-specific T cell activation following in vitro vaccine recall challenge. We observed that while the synbiotic increased the responsiveness of cytotoxic T cells to re-stimulation with the vaccine in young subjects, it decreased responsiveness in the older subjects (unpublished data). Thus, the impact of greater immunosenescence in the older subjects randomized to the synbiotic group appears to be significant, extending beyond the humoral arm of the immune response and influencing the T cell response to the vaccine.

Conclusion

In conclusion, we demonstrate marked impairment of the antibody response to influenza vaccination in older subjects and failure of the synbiotic to reverse this impairment. However, the older subjects randomized to the synbiotic were revealed to be at a significant disadvantage due to significantly higher numbers of senescent (CD28⁻CD57⁺) helper T cells at baseline compared with those randomized to the placebo, as well as significantly higher plasma levels of anti-CMV IgG and a greater tendency for CMV seropositivity. Thus, baseline differences in immunosenescence between the randomized groups are likely to have influenced the outcome of the intervention, highlighting the need for detailed immunological characterization of subjects prior to interventions.

Methods
Ethics and trial registration
The study protocol was reviewed and approved by the University of Reading Research Ethics Committee (project number: 10/09) the National Health Service

(NHS) Research Ethics Committee for Wales (10/MRE09/5). The trial was registered with clinicaltrials.gov (Identifier: NCT01066377) and conducted according to the guidelines laid down in the Declaration of Helsinki.

Participants
Prior to the influenza season of 2010–2011, young (18–35 y) and older (60–85 y) healthy adults were recruited from the population in and around Reading (UK) through newspaper and poster advertisements, email and radio. Inclusion criteria were: a signed consent form, age 18–35 y or 60–85 y, body mass index (BMI) 18.5–30 kg/m², good general health, as determined by medical questionnaires and laboratory data from screening blood and urine sample (fasting glucose, erythrocyte sedimentation rate, full blood count, liver function tests, renal profile, dipstick urinalysis), not pregnant, lactating or planning a pregnancy. Exclusion criteria included: allergy to the influenza vaccine, HIV infection, diabetes requiring any medication, asplenia and other acquired or congenital immunodeficiences, any autoimmune disease, including connective tissue diseases, malignancy, cirrhosis, connective tissue diseases, current use of immunomodulating medication (including oral and inhaled steroids), self–reported symptoms of acute or recent infection (including use of antibiotics within last 3 months), taking lactulose or any other treatment for constipation, alcoholism and drug misuse. Additional exclusion criteria for older volunteers included: laboratory data which were outside the normal range for this age group AND outside the ranges specified in the SENIEUR protocol [31], Barthel Index score of < 16/100, cumulative illness rating scale (CIRS) score of > 15 [32]. Additional exclusion criteria for the young subjects included laboratory data which were outside the normal range and influenza vaccination in the previous 12 months.

Sample size
The primary outcome of the trial was the antibody response to vaccination, incorporating mean antibody titres, vaccine-specific Ig subclasses and seroprotection and seroconversion. Power calculations were based on mean antibody titres. Since the influenza vaccine is trivalent, it is unlikely that an intervention will alter the response to all three subunits in the same way. For example, in the study of Davidson et al. [33], there was no effect of probiotic on mean antibody titres in response to the H1N1 subunit, whereas the responses to both H3N2 and the B subunit were improved (72 vs 51 [SD 16.5] for H3N2 and 31 vs 25 [SD 7.1] for B subunit). Based on the smaller effect size for the B subunit, a sample size of 26 subjects per group within each cohort was determined to be sufficient for a two-tailed significance level of 5 % and a power of 80 %; this was adjusted to 30

subjects per group to allow for dropouts. Data on the co-primary endpoints, immunoglobulin subclasses, seroprotection and seroconversion, is very sparse, but a sample size of 26 subjects per group within each cohort was determined to be sufficient for a 376 mg/dL difference in circulating IgG levels in response to influenza vaccination, with an SD of 438 mg/dL, a two-tailed significance level of 5 % and a power of 80 % [23]. A total of 62 young subjects and 63 older subjects entered the study and 58 young and 54 older subjects completed the study (Fig. 1). Two subjects experienced adverse effects (gastrointestinal bloating) during the study, one on the placebo group and one in the *B. longum* + Gl-OS group; both withdrew from the study.

Study design

Subjects consumed *Bifidobacterium longum bv. infantis* CCUG 52,486 (*B. longum*, 10^9 CFU in 1 g skim milk powder/day) combined with gluco-oligosaccharide (Gl-OS (BioEcolians, Solabia); 8 g/day) in a double-blind, placebo controlled randomised parallel study design for 8 weeks. The synbiotic approach was selected because in vitro data examining the growth and survival of this strain indicated that it was very vulnerable compared with other strains, but survived much better in the presence of an oligosaccharide substrate (data not shown). When comparing a number of possible substrates, the low water activity of Gl-OS, combined with its ability to support the growth of the probiotic strain, made it a clear choice for a powdered product. This prebiotic also has bifidogenic effects in batch culture models [34]. The placebo used was maltodextrin (9 g/day); both the placebo and the pre- and probiotic were sourced, packaged and blinded by BioAgro S.A. (Italy). The powders were consumed sprinkled into water or milk or with breakfast cereal. Microbiological safety of the product was independently verified by Leatherhead Food Research associates (UK) prior to commencement of the study and viability of the probiotic strain was confirmed on

random samples on a weekly basis during the study. During the 3 weeks prior to the study and during the intervention itself, subjects were requested not to consume fermented products such as yogurts, kefir etc. or pre- or probiotic products. Dietary records were used to confirm avoidance of such foods. Subjects were randomized by a research nurse not involved in the analysis according to gender, age and BMI to receive the probiotic or placebo by covariate adaptive randomization [35]. All investigators were blinded to the treatments. After 4 weeks, subjects were administered with a single dose of the influenza vaccine (Influvac®sub-unit 2010/2011 season, Abbott Biologicals B.V., lot number 1070166) containing A/California/7/2009 (H1N1), A/Perth/16/2009 (H3N2) and the B/Brisbane/60/2008- like strain by intramuscular injection in the deltoid. Vaccination was carried out by a research nurse in the presence of a qualified clinician (MG). Details of the study schedule and samples collected are detailed in Fig. 6. Compliance was assessed by counting returned sachets and by copy numbers of *B. longum*, assessed by qPCR. None of the subjects in the young cohort had previously received seasonal influenza vaccination or swine flu vaccination. Three subjects in the older cohort had received swine flu vaccination, and forty subjects had previously been vaccinated for seasonal influenza, of whom 37 had been vaccinated in the 2009/2010 period.

Blood sample processing

For serum, blood was collected into serum separator tubes and left at room temperature for 30mins to allow coagulation. Samples were centrifuged at $1300 \times g$ for 10 min and aliquots of serum were collected and stored at −80 °C prior to analysis.

Hemagglutination inhibition assay

Serum samples (in duplicate) were sent to the Health Protection Agency (London, UK) for analysis of total antibody responses to each of the 3 viral subunits. This

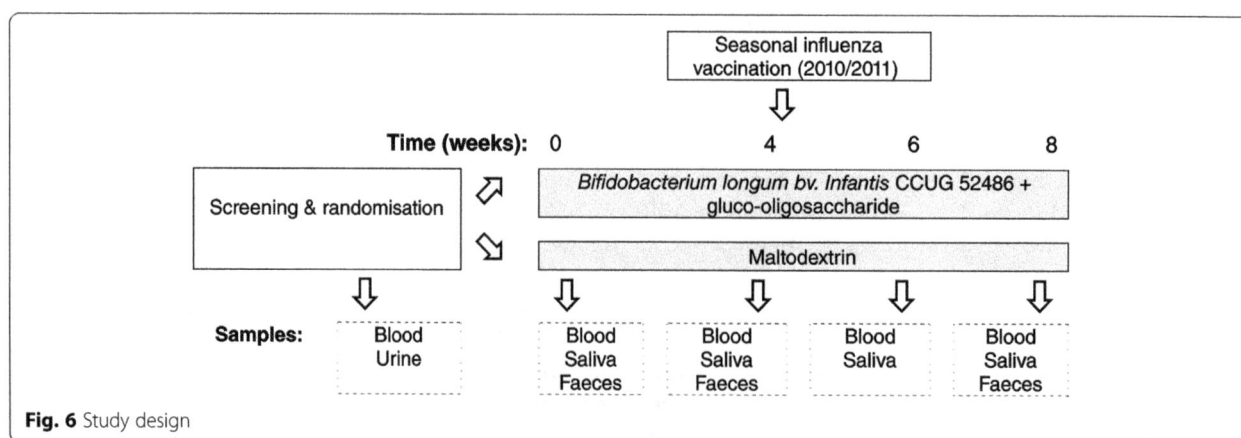

Fig. 6 Study design

technique is based on the ability of specific anti-influenza antibodies to inhibit hemagglutination of red blood cells by influenza virus hemagglutinin protein. Serum antibody titers measured by hemagglutination inhibition (HI) assay was performed using an 8-step dilution protocol (1:8 to 1:1024). Serum samples were titrated in duplicate, and samples showing titres of 1024 were further titrated up to 1:4096. Titres which were < 8 (below the detection limit) were expressed as 4, to represent half of the detection threshold. Post-vaccination antibody titres were not normally distributed, and were therefore log transformed.

Analysis of vaccine-specific Ig subclasses

Vaccine-specific Ig subclasses were analysed using an in-house ELISA method. Briefly, 96-well maxisorb ELISA plates (Serotec) were coated with 500 ng/ml of the vaccine (Influvac sub-unit 2010/2011) in coating buffer (0.5 M Na_2CO_3). After overnight incubation at 4 °C, plates were washed three times with wash solution (50 nM TRIS, 0.14 M NaCl, 1 % BSA, 0.2 % Tween-20 in dH_2O). Blocking buffer (5 % BSA in PBS) was added and plates were incubated for 1 h at 37 °C. After three washes, plasma samples (neat for IgA, IgD, IgM, and diluted 1:100 in PBS for IgG1) were added, and plates were incubated for a further hour at RT. Plates were then washed to remove non-specific binding antibodies and mouse anti-human IgA, IgG, IgM or IgD was added. IgA, IgG1, and IgM were diluted with PBS 1:1000, whereas IgD was diluted 1:500. After a 1 h incubation, diluted horse radish peroxidase conjugated goat anti-mouse IgG (H/L) (AbD Serotec, Oxfordshire, UK) was added and the plate was incubated for a further 1 h at RT. Substrate (3.3', 5.5' tetramethylbenzidine) was added and the reaction was stopped with 0.16 M sulphuric acid. Plates were read at 450 nm in a micro-plate autoreader (Thermo Scientific) and the results were presented as a mean optical density units (OD) ± SEM.

To minimize inter-assay variation, three quality control samples were included in every assay, consisting of post-vaccination plasma samples from two young and one older subject.

Analysis of salivary sIgA

Saliva samples were collected by passive drooling into a sterile screw-cap tube, centrifuged at 13,000 × g for 10 min at 4 °C to remove cells and debris and stored at −80 °C until analysis, which was completed within 6 months. The concentration of sIgA in saliva was analysed by sandwich ELISA using a commercially available kit (Immunodiagnostik AG, Bensheim, Germany) in accordance with the manufacturer's instructions.

Analysis of anti-CMV IgG antibodies

Concentrations of anti-CMV IgG antibodies were analysed by ELISA according to the manufacturer's instructions (ab108724 Anti-Cytomegalovirus (CMV) IgG Human Elisa Kit, Abcam, UK) and read in a microplate reader (GENios) at 450 nm, with 620 nm as a reference wavelength.

T cell phenotyping

Peripheral blood mononuclear cells (PBMC: 1×10^6) were stained with the following fluorochrome-conjugated monoclonal antibodies: (PerCP) labelled anti-CD3, (AmCyan) labelled anti-CD4, (APC-Cy7) labelled anti-CD8, (PE-Cy7) labelled anti-CD25, (Pacifice Blue) labelled anti-CD28, (APC) labelled anti-CD57, (FITC) labelled anti-CD26, (PE) labelled anti-CD127 in TruCOUNT tubes (BD Biosciences), washed and fixed before analysis by multiparamter flow cytometry (FACS Canto II, BD Biosciences) using BD *FACSDiva*™ software.

Relative telomere length

Telomere length of PBMC was measured by using the DAKO Telomere PNA Kit/FITC for Flow Cytometry (DAKO, UK), according to the manufacturer's instructions. Relative telomere length (RTL) was determined by comparing isolated PBMC with a control cell line (1301; subline of the Epstein–Barr virus (EBV) genome negative T-cell leukaemia line CCRF-CEM; Sigma-Aldrich Company Ltd, UK). Quantification of RTL was carried out using an Accuri™ C6 flow cytometer (BD Biosciences, Oxford, UK).

Quantification of faecal *Bifidobacterium longum*

Freshly voided faecal samples were collected in sterile plastic pots and stored at −20 °C.

DNA was extracted from faecal samples using a commercial kit (Fast DNA Spin kit, MP Biomedicals, Cambridge, UK) according to the manufacturers' instructions. Quantity and purity of the DNA was assessed using NanoDrop (Thermo Fisher Scientific Inc., Loughborough, UK). Real-time quantitative PCR was performed in triplicate for enumeration of *Bifidobacterium longum* with the Rotor-Gene 6000 (Corbett, Mortlake, Australia) using 5 μL of extracted faecal DNA in 20 μL PCR master-mix according to Haarman and Knol (2005). The reaction was carried out after 1 cycle at 95 °C for 10 min, followed by 45 cycles at 95 °C × 10, 62 C° per 60 s, 72 °C per 40 s. Standard quantification was carried out using serially diluted DNA extract of *Bifidobacterium longum bv. infantis* CCUG 52,486 strain enumerated by plate count.

Fluorescence in situ hybridisation

Freshly voided faecal samples were collected in sterile plastic pots, diluted 1 in 10 (wt:wt) in PBS and homogenised in a Stomacher 400 (Seward, Norfolk, United Kingdom) for 2 min. A 15 ml sample of faecal slurry was vortexed with 2 g of 3 mm diameter glass beads and then centrifuged to remove particulate matter (1500 × g, 2 min). Supernatant was fixed in paraformaldehyde [1:4 v/v in 4 % PFA in 0.1 mol PBS, pH 7.2] for 4 h at 4 °C, centrifuged (13,000 g 5 mins), washed twice with 0.1 M PBS, resuspended in 1:1 PBS:ethanol and stored at −20 °C. Oligonucleotide probes used were Cy-3 labeled and synthesized by Sigma-Aldrich (Poole, UK). Probes used were Bif164, Bac303, Chis150, Lab158, ATO291, Enter1432, Fprau655 and EUB338I/II/III specific for *Bifidobacterium* spp., *Bacteroides/Prevotella* group, *Clostridium* clusters I and II (including *C. perfringens* and *C. histoliticum*), *Lactobacillus/Enterococcus* subgroup, *Atopobium*, *Enterobacterium* group, *Faecalibacterium* cluster and total bacteria respectively. Samples were hybridized as described [36]. Data is expressed as log10 counts per g dry weight faeces.

Self-reported illness

Subjects in the older cohort who received the influenza vaccination during October/November 2010 in accordance with UK NHS vaccination schedules ($n = 43$) were requested to record incidence of any cold or flu like symptoms in the 6 months post-vaccination. However, the numbers were too small to be statistically meaningful and are therefore not included.

Statistical analysis

Data were analysed using SPSS software (version 21). For the primary and continuous secondary endpoints, a Linear Mixed Model (LMM) was implemented. A first order autoregressive covariance structure was selected AR (1), with fixed factors of time (repeated measures), age and treatment and subject as a random effect. The main effects are reported first, followed by all two-way interactions of the variables. Following this initial analysis, the data were split by cohort (young/older) and the analysis was repeated in the same manner to determine time and treatment effects within each cohort. Vaccine-specific immunoglobulin subclass data were analysed as change following vaccination. The distribution of the data was checked using the Kolmogorov-Smirnov test. If data were not normally distributed, they were log transformed. Antibody titre data were transformed with binary log ($\log_2 n$) and were not analysed as change from baseline. Seroprotection, seroconversion and self-reported illness data were analysed by the Fisher's exact test. To account for multiple primary endpoints, two sided P values of 0.01 or less were considered statistically significant. All

missing data were classed as missing at random and only available data were analysed.

Additional files

Additional file 1: Figure S1. Effect of *B. longum* + GI-OS on levels of vaccine-specific IgA, IgG1, IgD and IgM. Data are optical density units (OD_{450nm}) ± 2 SEM, change from baseline (week 4) for $n = 54$–58 subjects per group, 2 (week 6) and 4 (week 8) weeks after vaccination. □ Maltodextrin, (gray square) *B. longum* + GI-OS. Data were analysed using a Linear Mixed Model (LMM) with fixed factors of time, age and treatment. For IgA (plot A), there was a significant effect of age ($p < 0.001$) and time ($p < 0.001$) and a significant age*time interaction ($p < 0.001$). Data split by cohort showed a significant effect of time in both the young ($p < 0.01$) and older ($p < 0.001$) cohorts. For IgG1 (plot B), there were significant effects of time ($p < 0.001$) and age ($p < 0.001$). Data split by cohort showed a significant effect of time ($p < 0.001$) and a trend for a treatment effect ($p = 0.03$) in the older cohort, and a significant effect of time ($p < 0.001$) in the young cohort. For IgD (plot C), there were significant effects of age ($p < 0.001$) and time ($p < 0.001$) for the combined cohorts and a significant effect of time in both the young ($p < 0.001$) and older cohorts ($p < 0.001$) when considered separately. For IgM (plot D), there was a significant effect of time ($p < 0.001$), but no effect of age or treatment.

Additional file 2: Figure S2. Copy numbers of *B. longum* + GI-OS in faecal samples. Data are mean ± 2SEM for $n = 58$ young and $n = 54$ older subjects. □ Maltodextrin, (gray square) *B. longum* + GI-OS. Data were analysed using a Linear Mixed Model (LMM) with fixed factors of time, age and treatment. There were no statistically significant effects, either

Additional file 3: Figure S3. Effect of *B. longum* + GI-OS on numbers of bifidobacteria in seroconverters vs non converters. Data are mean ± 2SEM for $n = 18$ seroconverters (to all three subunits) and $n = 135$ non-converters in the placebo group and $n = 14$ seroconverters and $n = 36$ nonconverters in the *B. longum* + GIOS group. Trend for greater increase in bifidobacteria in seroconverters compared with non-converters in the *B. longum* + GIOS group (p

Abbreviations

BSA: bovine serum albumin; CIRS: cumulative illness rating scale; ELISA: enzyme-linked immunosorbent assay; GI-OS: gluco-oligosaccharide; Ig: immunoglobulin; PBMC: peripheral blood mononuclear cells; PBS: phosphate-buffered saline; RPMI: Roswell Park Memorial Institute; URTI: upper respiratory tract infection..

Competing interests

The study was supported by a grant (BB/H00470X/1) from the Biotechnology and Biological Sciences Research Council Diet and Health Research Industry Club (BBSRC-DRINC). Clinical trial identifier: clinicaltrials.gov NCT01066377 None of the authors has any competing interests to declare. Data will be made available on request.

Authors' contributions

PY, KT, ST and MG designed the research. CEC, APK, CM, HD, and IBD conducted the research. APK, CEC and KT analyzed the data. PY and CEC wrote the first draft of the paper. PY had primary responsibility for the final content. All authors read and approved the final manuscript.

Acknowledgements

We thank Dr Esme Roads (Research Nurse) for help with screening, recruitment and vaccination and Victoria Austen for assisting with the sIgA analysis.

Author details

[1]Department of Food and Nutritional Sciences, University of Reading, PO Box 226Whiteknights, Reading, Berkshire RG6 6AP, UK. [2]Department of Mathematics and Statistics, University of Reading, Reading, RG6 6AP, UK. [3]Department of Food Quality and Nutrition, Research and Innovation Centre, Fondazione Edmund Mach, via E. Mach, 1, San Michele all'Adige, Trento 38010, Italy.

References

1. Haq K, McElhaney JE. Immunosenescence: influenza vaccination and the elderly. Curr Opin Immunol. 2014;29:38–42.

2. Pang IK, Iwasaki A. Inflammasomes as mediators of immunity against influenza virus. Trends Immunol. 2011;32:34–41.

3. Pang IK, Iwasaki A. Control of antiviral immunity by pattern recognition and the microbiome. Immunol Rev. 2012;245:209–26.

4. Hao Q, Lu Z, Dong BR et al. Probiotics for preventing acute upper respiratory tract infections. Cochrane Database Syst Rev. 2011:CD006895. doi: 10.1002/14651858.CD006895.pub2.

5. MacDonald TT, Bell I. Probiotics and the immune response to vaccines. Proc Nutr Soc. 2010;69:442–6.

6. Maidens C, Childs C, Przemska A, et al. Modulation of vaccine response by concomitant probiotic administration. Br J Clin Pharmacol. 2013;75:663–70.

7. Lomax AR, Calder PC. Prebiotics, immune function, infection and inflammation: a review of the evidence. Br J Nutr. 2009;101:633–58.

8. Biagi E, Candela M, Turroni S, et al. Ageing and gut microbes: perspectives for health maintenance and longevity. Pharmacol Res. 2013;69:11–20.

9. Dominguez-Bello MG, Blaser MJ, Ley RE, Knight R. Development of the human gastrointestinal microbiota and insights from high-throughput sequencing. Gastroenterology. 2011;140:1713–9.

10. Silvi S, Verdenelli MC, Orpianesi C, Cresci A. EU project Crownalife: functional foods, gut microflora and healthy ageing - Isolation and identification of Lactobacillus and Bifidobacterium strains from faecal samples of elderly subjects for a possible probiotic use in functional foods. J Food Eng. 2003;56:195–200.

11. Likotrafiti EMKSF, F.; Tuohy, K.M.; Gibson, G.R.; Rastall, R.A. Molecular identification and anti-pathogenic activities of putative probiotic bacteria isolated from faeces of healthy elderly adults. Microbial Ecology in Health and Disease 2004; 16:8.

12. You J, Yaqoob P. Evidence of immunomodulatory effects of a novel probiotic, Bifidobacterium longum bv. infantis CCUG 52486. FEMS Immunol Med Microbiol. 2012;66:353–62.

13. Derhovanessian E, Pawelec G. Vaccination in the elderly. Microb Biotechnol. 2012;5:226–32.

14. Goodwin K, Viboud C, Simonsen L. Antibody response to influenza vaccination in the elderly: A quantitative review. Vaccine. 2006;24:1159–69.

15. Yaqoob P. Ageing, immunity and influenza: a role for probiotics? Proc Nutr Soc. 2014;73:309–17.

16. Kovaiou RD, Herndler-Brandstetter D, Grubeck-Loebenstein B. Age-related changes in immunity: implications for vaccination in the elderly. Expert Rev Mol Med. 2007;9:1–17.

17. Bunout D, Barrera G, Hirsch S, et al. Effects of a nutritional supplement on the immune response and cytokine production in free-living Chilean elderly. JPEN J Parenter Enteral Nutr. 2004;28:348–54.

18. Boge T, Remigy M, Vaudaine S, et al. A probiotic fermented dairy drink improves antibody response to influenza vaccination in the elderly in two randomised controlled trials. Vaccine. 2009;27:5677–84.

19. Namba K, Hatano M, Yaeshima T, et al. Effects of Bifidobacterium longum BB536 administration on influenza infection, influenza vaccine antibody titer, and cell-mediated immunity in the elderly. Biosci Biotechnol Biochem. 2010;74:939–45.

20. Van Puyenbroeck K, Hens N, Coenen S, et al. Efficacy of daily intake of Lactobacillus casei Shirota on respiratory symptoms and influenza vaccination immune response: a randomized, double-blind, placebo-controlled trial in healthy elderly nursing home residents. Am J Clin Nutr. 2012;95:1165–71.

21. Isolauri E, Joensuu J, Suomalainen H, et al. Improved Immunogenicity of Oral Dxrrv Reassortant Rotavirus Vaccine by Lactobacillus-Casei Gg. Vaccine. 1995;13:310–2.

22. de Vrese M, Winkler P, Rautenberg P, et al. Probiotic bacteria reduced duration and severity but not the incidence of common cold episodes in a double blind, randomized, controlled trial. Vaccine. 2006;24:6670–4.

23. Olivares M, Diaz-Ropero MP, Sierra S, et al. Oral intake of Lactobacillus fermentum CECT5716 enhances the effects of influenza vaccination. Nutrition. 2007;23:254–60.

24. Bosch M, Mendez M, Perez M, et al. Lactobacillus plantarum CECT7315 and CECT7316 stimulate immunoglobulin production after influenza vaccination in elderly. Nutricion hospitalaria: organo oficial de la Sociedad Espanola de Nutricion Parenteral y Enteral. 2012;27:504–9.

25. Rizzardini G, Eskesen D, Calder PC, et al. Evaluation of the immune benefits of two probiotic strains Bifidobacterium animalis ssp. lactis, BB-12(R) and Lactobacillus paracasei ssp. paracasei, L. casei 431(R) in an influenza vaccination model: a randomised, double-blind, placebo-controlled study. Br J Nutr. 2012;107:876–84.

26. You J, Dong H, Mann ER, et al. Ageing impairs the T cell response to dendritic cells. Immunobiology. 2013;218:1077–84.

27. Likotrafiti E, Manderson KS, Fava F, Tuohy KM, Gibson GR, Rastall RA. Molecular identification and anti-pathogenic activities of putative probiotic bacteria isolated from faeces of healthy elderly individuals. Microb Ecol Health Dis. 2004;16:105–12.

28. Vallejo AN. Immune remodeling: lessons from repertoire alterations during chronological aging and in immune-mediated disease. Trends Mol Med. 2007;13:94–102.

29. Derhovanessian E, Maier AB, Hahnel K, et al. Latent Infection with Cytomegalovirus Is Associated with Poor Memory CD4 Responses to Influenza A Core Proteins in the Elderly. J Immunol. 2014;193:3624–31.

30. Frei R, Akdis M, O'Mahony L. Prebiotics, probiotics, synbiotics, and the immune system: experimental data and clinical evidence. Curr Opin Gastroen. 2015;31:153–8.

31. Ligthart GJ, Corberand JX, Fournier C, et al. Admission criteria for immunogerontological studies in man: the SENIEUR protocol. Mech Ageing Dev. 1984;28:47–55.

32. Hudon C, Fortin A, Vanasse A. Cumulative Illness Rating Scale was a reliable and valid index in a family practice context. J Clin Epidemiol. 2005;58:603–8.

33. Davidson LE, Fiorino AM, Snydman DR, Hibberd PL. Lactobacillus GG as an immune adjuvant for live-attenuated influenza vaccine in healthy adults: a randomized double-blind placebo-controlled trial. Eur J Clin Nutr. 2011;65:501–7.

34. Sarbini SR, Kolida S, Gibson GR, Rastall RA. In vitro fermentation of commercial alpha-gluco-oligosaccharide by faecal microbiota from lean and obese human subjects. Br J Nutr. 2013;109:1980–9.

35. Kang M, Ragan BG, Park JH. Issues in outcomes research: an overview of randomization techniques for clinical trials. J Athl Train. 2008;43:215–21.

36. Costabile A, Kolida S, Klinder A, et al. A double-blind, placebo-controlled, cross-over study to establish the bifidogenic effect of a very-long-chain inulin extracted from globe artichoke (Cynara scolymus) in healthy human subjects. British J Nutr. 2010;104:1007–17.

pERK-dependent defective TCR-mediated activation of CD4$^+$ T cells in end-stage renal disease patients

Ling Huang[*], Nicolle H. R. Litjens, Nynke M. Kannegieter, Mariska Klepper, Carla C. Baan and Michiel G. H. Betjes

Abstract

Background: Patients with end-stage renal disease (ESRD) have an impaired immune response with a prematurely aged T-cell system. Mitogen-activated protein kinases (MAPKs) including extracellular signal-regulated kinase (ERK) and p38, regulate diverse cellular programs by transferring extracellular signals into an intracellular response. T cell receptor (TCR)-induced phosphorylation of ERK (pERK) may show an age-associated decline, which can be reversed by inhibiting dual specific phosphatase (DUSP) 6, a cytoplasmic phosphatase with substrate specificity to dephosphorylate pERK. The aim of this study was to assess whether ESRD affects TCR-mediated signaling and explore possibilities for intervening in ESRD-associated defective T-cell mediated immunity.

Results: An age-associated decline in TCR-induced pERK-levels was observed in the different CD4$^+$ ($P < 0.05$), but not CD8$^+$, T-cell subsets from healthy individuals (HI). Interestingly, pERK-levels of CD4$^+$ T-cell subsets from young ESRD patients were in between young and elderly HI. A differentiation-associated decline in TCR-induced ERK and p38 phosphorylation was observed in T cells, although TCR-induced p38 phosphorylation was not significantly affected by age and/or ESRD. Frequencies of TCR-induced CD69-expressing CD4$^+$ T cells declined with age and were positively associated with pERK. In addition, an age-associated tendency of increased expression of DUSP6 was observed in CD4$^+$ T cells of HI and DUSP6 expression in young ESRD patients was similar to old HI. Inhibition of DUSP6 significantly increased TCR-induced pERK-levels of CD4$^+$ T cells in young and elderly ESRD patients, and elderly HI.

Conclusions: TCR-mediated phosphorylation of ERK is affected in young ESRD patients consistent with the concept of premature immunological T cell ageing. Inhibition of DUSP6 specific for pERK might be a potential intervention enhancing T-cell mediated immunity in ESRD patients.

Keywords: ESRD, T cells, ERK, p38, DUSP 6, MAPK

Background

ESRD patients have a defective T-cell mediated immune system that is clinically characterized by an increased risk of a variety of infections [1, 2] and impaired response of vaccination [3–7]. Infections are the second leading cause of mortality following cardiovascular disease and a major cause of morbidity in ESRD patients [8].

Uremia-associated T-cell defects closely resemble premature immunological T-cell ageing [9]. ESRD patients have a discrepancy of 15–20 years between the immunological T-cell age and their chronological age [10]. Declined thymic output, more differentiated memory T cells, T cells lacking co-stimulatory molecules like CD28, skewed T cell receptor (TCR) Vβ repertoire diversity and shorter telomere length are observed in ESRD patients compared to age-matched healthy individuals (HI) [11].

TCR-induced signaling mediates clonal (positive or negative) selection of thymocytes in the thymus and initiates T cell immune responses in the periphery, consisting of T cell proliferation and differentiation [12]. The mitogen-activated protein kinase (MAPK) pathway is one of the major pathways induced upon

* Correspondence: l.huang.1@erasmusmc.nl
Department of Internal Medicine, Section Nephrology and Transplantation, Erasmus University Medical Center, Rotterdam, the Netherlands

TCR stimulation [13]. Activation of MAPK is mediated by phosphorylation of MAPK and downregulated by MAPK phosphatase resulting in inactive MAPK [14]. In particular, the extracellular signal-regulated kinase (ERK) pathway is one of the important MAPK pathways. Phosphorylation of ERK can reduce sensitivity of cells to apoptosis and promote cell proliferation [15]. ERK activity controls the positive feedback loop in the TCR-induced activation cascade and reduced ERK activity affects signal strength and activation of T cells [16, 17]. Reduced phosphorylation of ERK is associated with decreased interleukin-2 (IL-2) production [18] and vice versa [19]. Dual specific phosphatases (DUSPs) represents a family of phosphatases that dephosphorylate phosphor-threonine and phosphor-tyrosine residues on MAPK and that are pivotal regulators of MAPK activities. DUSP6 is a cytoplasmic phosphatase with substrate specificity to dephosphorylate pERK [20]. Ageing is also associated with defective signaling pathways [21, 22]. Recently it was shown that decreased phosphorylation of ERK in naive CD4$^+$ T cells from elderly HI was associated with more time to build up the required signaling strength following stimulation compared to those from young HI. This decreased phosphorylation of ERK can be overcome by inhibiting DUSP6 [16].

P38 is another pivotal protein in the MAPK pathway [23] and of interest with respect to age-related changes is T cell activation. Most stimuli, including engagement of TCR, costimulatory receptors, inflammation, stress, growth factors, as well as DNA damage induce phosphorylation of p38 by various pathways [24, 25]. Although phosphorylation of ERK and p38 from T cells share some upstream molecules after triggering of TCR, such as phosphorylation of CD3 zeta-chain associated protein kinase of 70 kDa (ZAP70) [26], they each have their unique upstream MAPK kinases (MKKs) [14]. Highly differentiated CD4$^+$ T cells lacking expression of CD28 are accumulated in elderly healthy individuals [27], patients with ESRD [28], following chronic viral infection [29], and also in patients suffering from autoimmune disease [30]. Senescent CD27$^-$CD28$^-$CD4$^+$ T cells employ an MKK-independent mechanism for phosphorylating p38 and depend on 5′ adenosine monophosphate-activated protein kinase (AMPK) and transforming growth factor-β-activated protein kinase 1(TAK1)-binding protein 1(TAB1) ex vivo [31].

Little is known as to how MAPK signaling pathways in ESRD patients. Understanding MAPK signaling in ESRD patients may increase knowledge about mechanisms of uremia-associated impaired T-cell mediated immunity and offer possibilities for intervention. Here, we demonstrate that TCR-induced phosphorylation of ERK, and not p38, in CD4$^+$ T cells decreases with age and T cell

differentiation. This pathway is specifically affected in young ESRD patients and at the level of elderly healthy individuals, compatible with the concept of premature immunological T cell ageing in patients with renal failure. In addition, inhibition of DUSP6 may offer a potential intervention for improving T-cell mediated immunity in ESRD patients.

Methods

Study population

In line with our previous studies, young and elderly patients groups were defined based on their chronological age [32, 33]. Twenty-four stable ESRD patients, defined as having a glomerular filtration rate of ≤15 ml/min with or without renal replacement therapy (RRT; i.e. dialysis) and 24 HI were included (Study population characteristics are described in Table 1) at the outpatient clinic. Patients with any clinical or laboratory evidence of acute bacterial or viral infection, malignancy, immunosuppressive drug treatment within 28 days prior to transplantation (except for glucocorticoids) were excluded. Lithium-heparinized blood was drawn of ESRD patients and healthy kidney donors. All individuals included gave informed consent and the local medical ethical committee approved the study (METC number: 2012–022). It was conducted according to the principles of Declaration of Helsinki and in compliance with International Conference on Harmonization/Good Clinical Practice regulations.

Table 1 Clinical characteristics of the study population

	HI	ESRD patients	P value
Number of individuals	24	24	
Age groups (years; mean ± SD)			
young	29,4 ± 5,6	34,6 ± 8,0	ns
elderly	70,5 ± 5,8	70,8 ± 4,2	ns
Sex (% male)	50	79,2	ns
CMV IgG serostatus (% pos)	62,5	62,5	ns
RRT (number; %)		11; (45,8%)	
Duration of RRT in months (median with range)		22 (1—37)	
Hemodialysis (number)		7	
Peritoneal dialysis (number)		4	
Underlying kidney disease (number; %)			
atherosclerosis/hypertensive nephropathy		8; (33%)	
primary glomerulopathy		4; (17%)	
Diabetic nephropathy		6; (25%)	
congenital disorder		3; (13%)	
others		2; (8%)	
unknown		1; (4%)	

PBMCs preparation

Peripheral blood mononuclear cells (PBMCs) were isolated from peripheral blood from HI and ESRD patients as described previously [34] and then cryopreserved for further analysis.

Phosphorylation-specific flow cytometry

PBMCs were stained with eFluor-450-labeled anti-CD7 (eBioscience, Vienna, Austria), allophycocyanin-Cy7 (APC-Cy7)-labeled anti-CD8 (BD, Erembodegem, Belgium), Brilliant Violet (BV)-510-labeled anti-CD16 (BD) and fluorescein isothiocyanate (FITC)-labeled anti-CCR7 (R&D system, Uithoorn, the Netherlands) for 30 min at room temperature. Then 1 million PBMCs/50 µl were prepared for stimulation by labeling cells with 20 µg/ml mouse anti-human CD3 (BD) and mouse anti-human CD28 (BD) each on ice for 20 min, followed by an incubation with goat-anti mouse IgG (BD) for cross-linking on ice for 20 min. Stimulation was initiated by transferring cells to a 37 °C water bath for 10 min. Cells were fixed using Cytofix (BD) at 37 °C for 10 min and then permeabilized in 70% methanol at -20 °C for 30 min. Subsequently, cells were stained with peridinin chlorophyll (PerCP)-labeled anti-CD4 (BD), phycoerythrin (PE)-Cy7-labeled anti-CD45RO (BioLegend, Uithoorn, Netherlands), PE-labeled anti-phospho-p38MAPK (pT180/pY182) (BD), and Alexa Fluor (AF) 647-labeled anti-phospho-ERK1/2 (pThr202/pTyr204) (BD). Phosphorylation was measured on a BD FACSCanto II flow cytometer (BD) and data were analyzed by Kaluza™ software (Beckman Coulter, Woerden, Netherlands). Median fluorescence intensity (MFI) of phosphorylated ERK or p38, generated by Kaluza™, were multiplied by 256 to make them comparable to the data analyzed by FACS Diva software (linear value instead of log-transformed value) (BD). The MFI obtained for anti-CD3/anti-CD28-stimulation were corrected by subtracting the MFI of the unstimulated condition.

CD69 and IL-2 measurement

PBMCs were either not or stimulated with anti-CD3/anti-CD28 T-cell expander beads (Invitrogen Dynal, Oslo, Norway) at different ratios, i.e. 1 cell / 0.1 bead, 1 cell / 0.5 bead, 1 cell / 1 bead for 6 h in human culture medium (HCM; RPMI-1640 with GlutaMAX, 10% heat-inactivated pooled human serum and 1% penicillin and streptomycin) (Lonza, Breda, Netherlands) with Golgistop (BD). Then cells were stained with AmCyan-labeled anti-CD3 (BD), Pacific Blue-labeled anti-CD4 (BD), APC-Cyanin 7 (APC-Cy7)-labeled anti-CD8 (BD), APC-labeled anti-CD45RO (BD) and PE-Cy7-labeled anti-CCR7 (R&D Systems) antibodies and a live–dead marker ViaProbe (7-aminoactinomycin D; 7AAD; BD). Upon fixation with FACS lysing solution (BD) and permeabilization using FACS permeabilizing solution 2 (BD), cells were

stained intracellular using PE-labeled anti-CD69 (BD) and FITC-labeled anti-IL-2 (BD). Percentages CD69-expressing and IL-2 producing CD4$^+$ T cell subsets were evaluated upon measuring the samples on a BD FACSCanto II flow cytometer (BD). Data were analyzed by Kaluza™ software (Beckman Coulter).

DUSP6/1 inhibition

PBMCs were pre-incubated in HCM including 50 µM (E)-2-benzylidene-3-(cyclohexylamino)-2, 3-dihydro-1 H-inden-1-one (BCI) (Merck – Millipore, Amsterdam, Netherlands) at 37 °C for 1 h. BCI has been shown to be an inhibitor of DUSP6 and DUSP1 activity. PBMCs were subsequently washed 3 times and then stimulated by CD3/CD28 antibodies (as described previously) for 10 mins and then MFI of pERK of BCI-pretreated T cells was measured by Phosphorylation-specific flow cytometry as described previously.

DUSP6/1 measurement

PBMCs were stained with AmCyan-labeled anti-CD3 (BD), Pacific Blue-labeled anti-CD4 (BD), APC-Cy7-labeled anti-CD8 (Biolegend); APC-labeled anti-CD45RO (BD) and PE-Cy7-labeled anti-CCR7 (R&D Systems) antibodies and 7-AAD for 30 min at 4 °C. Upon fixation and permeabilization using Fix/Perm buffer (eBioscience), 1% bovine serum albumin (Zwijndrecht, Netherlands) was used to block Fc receptors. Then cells were further stained with AF647-labeled anti-DUSP6 (Santa Cruz Biotechnology, Heidelberg, Germany) and PE-labeled anti-DUSP1 (Santa Cruz Biotechnology) for 30 min at 4 °C. MFI of DUSP6 and DUSP1 was measured on a BD FACSCanto II flow cytometer (BD) and data were analyzed using FACS Diva software version 6.1.2 (BD).

Statistical analyses

Data were analyzed by Graphpad Prism 6 (GraphPad Software, CA, USA). Comparison between two groups (non-parametric data) were using Mann Whitney test. Comparison in multiple groups were using Friedman test followed by Dunn's Multiple Comparison T test or repeated ANOVA test followed by Bonferroni's multiple comparison test. Comparison between DUSP6-treated and non-treated conditions was done by Paired T- test. All reported P-values are two-sided and were considered statistically significant when $P < 0.05$.

Results

Study population

The demographic and clinical characteristics of the study population are given in Table 1. Twelve patients were within the young group (age 22–44 years) and 12 patients belonged to the elderly group (age 66–78 years). Age- and cytomegalovirus (CMV)-matched HI, i.e. 13

young (age 21–40 years) and 11 elderly (age 65–74 years) HI were included for comparison. Approximately half of the ESRD patients received RRT (dialysis) with a median dialysis time of 22 months.

Decreased ERK phosphorylation in young ESRD patients

A typical flow cytometric example for analysis of ERK phosphorylation is given in Fig. 1. First, we compared phosphorylation of ERK and p38 between young and elderly HI or young and elderly ESRD patients. A significant age-related lower TCR-mediated phosphorylation of ERK was observed within all $CD4^+$ T cell subsets from HI (Fig. 2a–d). For example, the median of MFI value of $CD4^+$ phosphorylated ERK (pERK) was 658 in young HI, which was significantly higher than 535 in elderly HI ($p = 0.015$) (Fig. 2a). This trend consistently existed between young and elderly HI when we compared MFI value of pERK in $CD4^+$ naïve (median 722 vs. 612, $p = 0.022$) (Fig. 2b), CM (median 666 vs. 489, $p = 0.021$) (Fig. 2c) and EM subsets (517 vs. 364, $p = 0.018$) (Fig. 2d). Due to the almost absent

EMRA subset within the $CD4^+$ T cells, phosphorylation of ERK and p38 within this subset was not evaluated.

However, no significant differences in expression levels of pERK in total $CD4^+$ T cells or the subsets were found comparing young and elderly ESRD patients (Fig. 2a–c &d). For example, the median (interquartile range)) MFI value of $CD4^+$ pERK in young patients was 613 (490–664) and 541 (413–801) in elderly patients ($p = 0.51$). The median MFI value for $CD4^+$ pERK in young patients was in between the MFI values of young HI 658 (485–1212)) and elderly HI (535 (305–620)) but did not significantly differ from either group (respectively $p = 0.13$ and $p = 0.06$). This age-associated decline in pERK was not found for $CD8^+$ T cell subsets (Fig. 2e–h & i). In addition, an age-related decline in TCR-mediated phosphorylation of p38, was absent in $CD4^+$ T cells (Fig. 3a–c & d) as well as $CD8^+$ T cells (Fig. 3e–h & i) of both HI and ESRD patients. In conclusion, ESRD patients have a defective ERK, but not p38, phosphorylation in $CD4^+$ T cells, that is independent of age and at a level similar to aged HI.

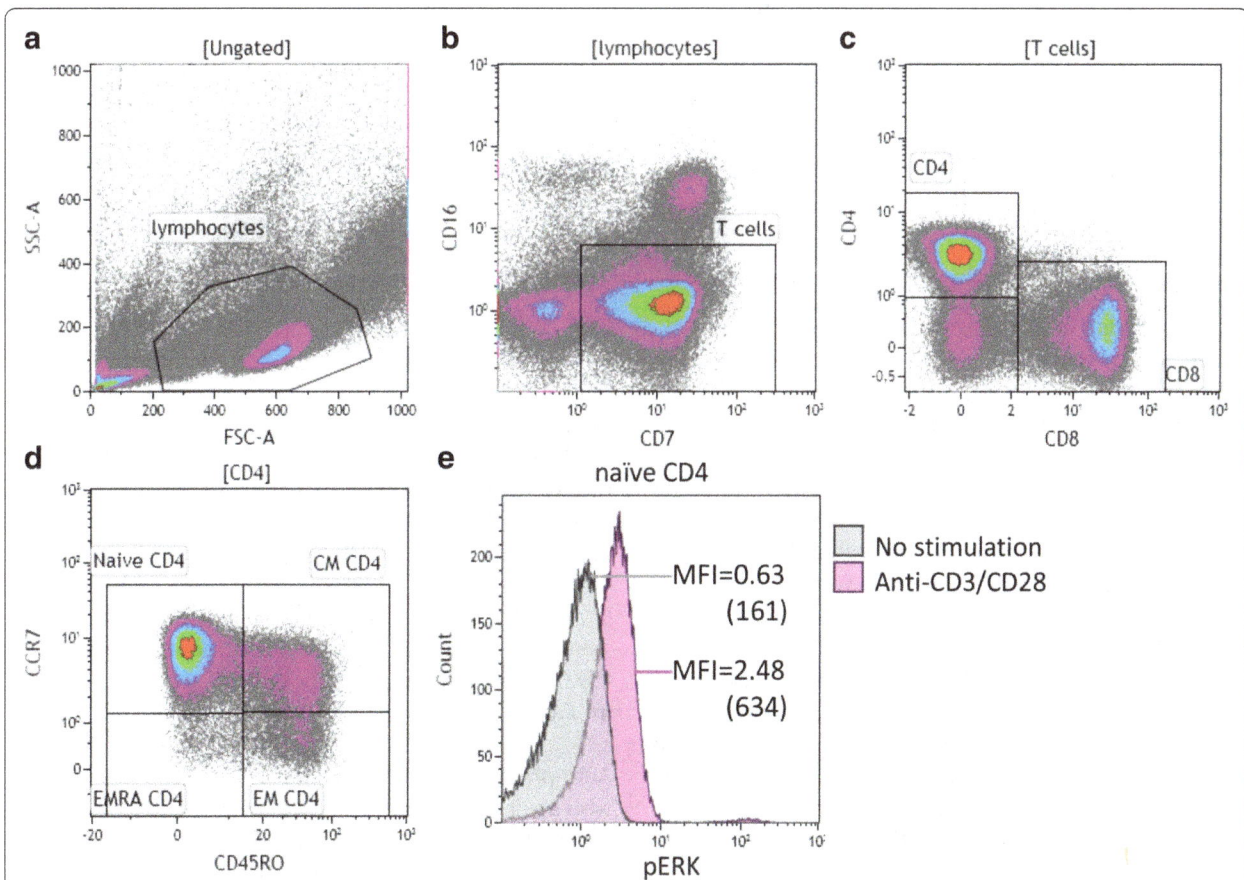

Fig. 1 Typical example of the gating strategy for analysis of phosphorylation of ERK (pERK) in naïve $CD4^+$ T cell subsets. Briefly, (**a**) lymphocytes were identified based on the forward/sideward characteristics followed by (**b**) the selection of $CD7^+$ $CD16^-$ T cells. **c** These T cells were then dissected into $CD4^+$ and $CD8^+$ T cells. **d** CCR7 and CD45RO were used to identify naïve and different memory subsets within $CD4^+$ T cells. Furthermore, (**e**) pERK was measured in naïve $CD4^+$ T cells without and with CD3/CD28 stimulation, and median fluorescence intensities (MFI) were shown (values multiplied by 256 in *brackets*). A similar gating strategy was employed for phosphorylation of ERK and p38 in all T cells subsets

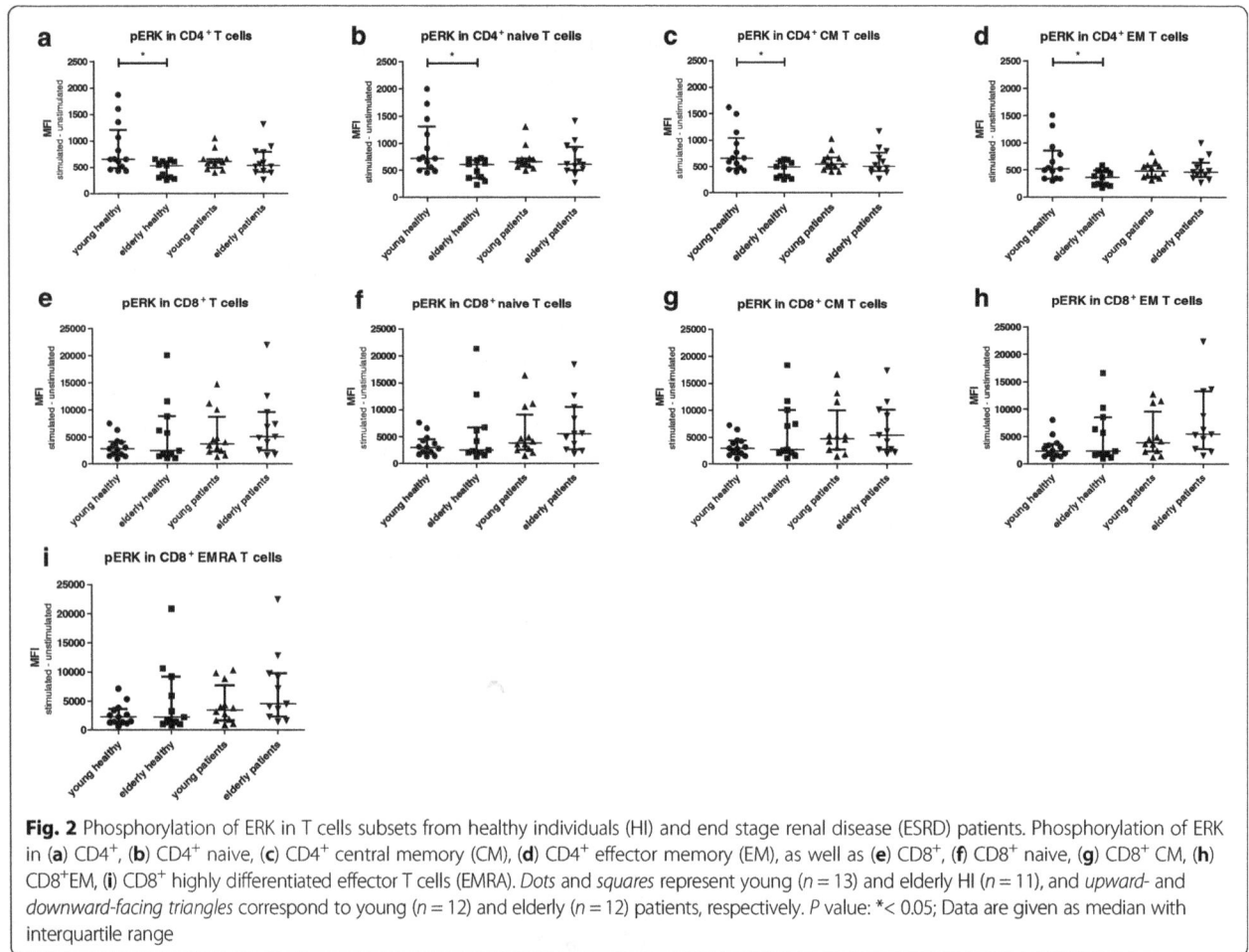

Fig. 2 Phosphorylation of ERK in T cells subsets from healthy individuals (HI) and end stage renal disease (ESRD) patients. Phosphorylation of ERK in (**a**) CD4+, (**b**) CD4+ naive, (**c**) CD4+ central memory (CM), (**d**) CD4+ effector memory (EM), as well as (**e**) CD8+, (**f**) CD8+ naive, (**g**) CD8+ CM, (**h**) CD8+EM, (**i**) CD8+ highly differentiated effector T cells (EMRA). *Dots* and *squares* represent young (*n* = 13) and elderly HI (*n* = 11), and *upward-* and *downward-facing triangles* correspond to young (*n* = 12) and elderly (*n* = 12) patients, respectively. *P* value: *< 0.05; Data are given as median with interquartile range

Phosphorylation of ERK is associated with T-cell differentiation status

Next, we compared phosphorylation of ERK and p38 within different T cell subsets to assess whether differentiation-associated effects exist in the study groups. In all groups, a gradual decrease in TCR-induced phosphorylation capacity was seen with increasing CD4+ T cell differentiation. Phosphorylation of ERK was highest in naive CD4+ T cells of young HI, followed by that in the CM and EM subsets of the memory compartment (Fig. 4a). Median MFI dropped from 722 to 666 and 517 in the naive, CM and EM T cell subset, respectively. Interestingly, in elderly HI as well as both groups of ESRD patients (Fig. 4b, c & d), pERK levels were still highest within naive CD4+ T cells compared to the more differentiated EM T cell subset, but the difference with that observed within CM T cells disappeared. ERK phosphorylation within CM is higher than that within the EM compartment in young and elderly HI (Fig. 4a & b), as well as in young patients (Fig. 4c), but not in elderly patients (Fig. 4d). Differences for the various CD8+ T-cell subsets with respect to TCR-mediated phosphorylation of ERK between naive and CM compartment, or between EM and EMRA were less outspoken and not significantly different in HI (Fig. 4e & f) and patients (Fig. 4g & h). Similar to ERK, phosphorylation of p38 showed a similar trend to decrease with increasing differentiation status but no significant decline in phosphorylation of p38 from naive to CM in CD4+ in HI and patients (Fig. 5a–c & d). In CD8+ T cells, p38 phosphorylation was decreased in highly differentiated EMRA compared to CM in HI and patients (Fig. 5e–g & h). In conclusion, a differentiation-associated decrease in anti-CD3/CD28-induced phosphorylation of ERK and p38 in T cells was present in HI and patients.

Auto-phosphorylation (baseline) of ERK was associated with ageing in HI and increased according to differentiation status in CD4+ T cells

Baseline phosphorylation of ERK (i.e. auto-phosphorylation) was significantly lower for total and naive CD4+T cells in young HI compared with elderly HI, however, this trend was not observed in patients (Fig. 6a & b). Baseline levels of pERK were significantly lower in the CD8+ memory compartment (CM, EM and

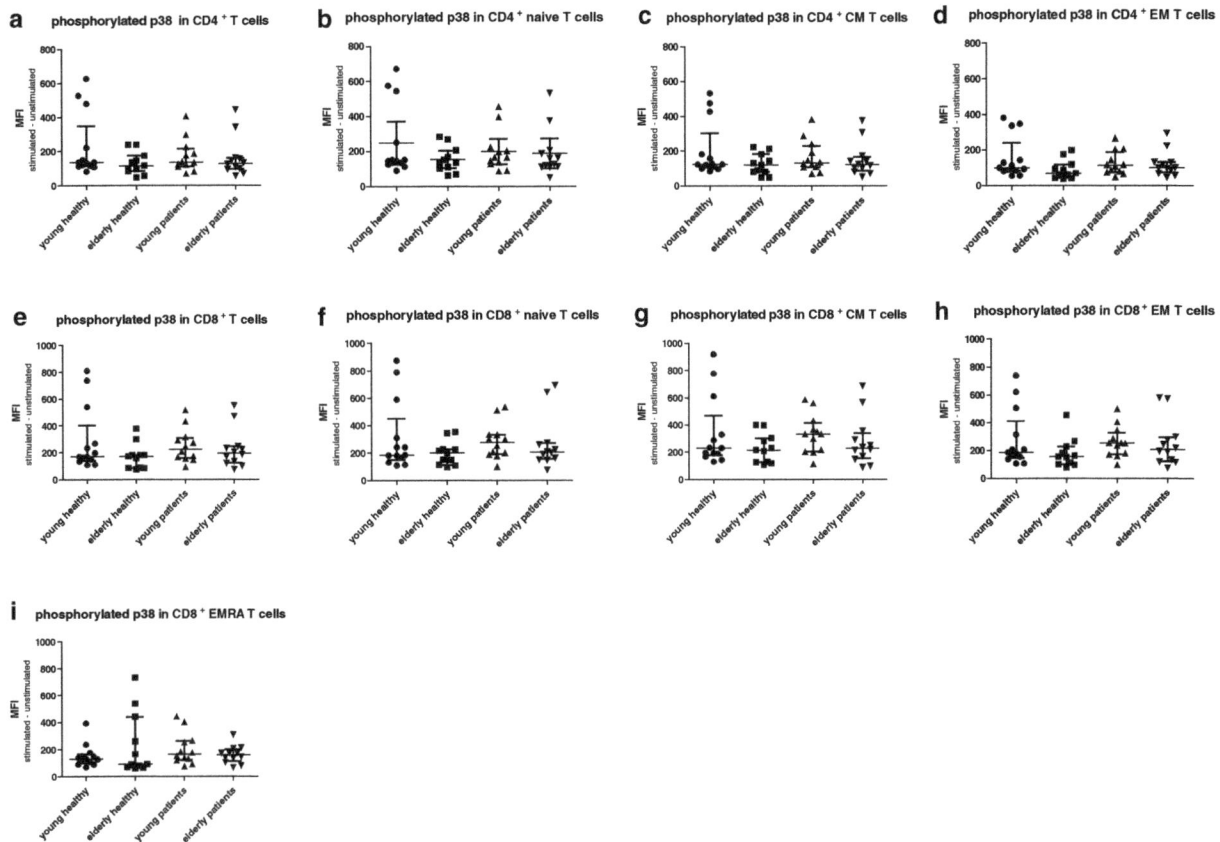

Fig. 3 Phosphorylation of p38 in T cells subsets from healthy individuals (HI) and end stage renal disease (ESRD) patients. Phosphorylation of p38 in (**a**) CD4[+], (**b**) CD4[+] naive, (**c**) CD4[+] central memory (CM), (**d**) CD4[+] effector memory (EM), as well as (**e**) CD8[+], (**f**) CD8[+] naive, (**g**) CD8[+] CM, (**h**) CD8[+]EM, (**i**) CD8[+] highly differentiated effector T cells (EMRA). *Dots* and *squares* represent young ($n = 13$) and elderly HI ($n = 11$), and *upward-* and *downward-facing triangles* correspond to young ($n = 12$) and elderly ($n = 12$) patients, respectively. *P* value: *< 0.05; Data are given as median with interquartile range

EMRA) when comparing young to elderly HI, but no age-related differences were observed for patients (Fig. 6g, h & i). Baseline phosphorylation of ERK was lower in the naive CD4[+] T cells when compared to CM and/or EM in HI (Fig. 7 a & b) and patients (Fig. 7c & d). Naive CD8[+] T cells also had lower baseline pERK when compared to EMRA in elderly HI (Fig. 7f), CM and EM in young patients (Fig. 7g), and EM in elderly patients (Fig. 7h). Naive CD4[+] T cells had lower baseline phosphorylated p38 compared to CM or EM in elderly HI (Additional file 1: Fig. S1b), and lower p38 phosphorylation compared to EM in young patients (Additional file 1: Figure S1c). In CD8[+] T cells, p38 auto-phosphorylation in naive compartment was significantly lower than that of EMRA in young and elderly HI (Additional file 1: Figure S1e & f), but this trend was not observed in the patient population (Additional file 1: Figure S1 g & h). To summarize, an age- as well as differentiation-related increase in baseline levels of pERK was observed for CD4[+] T cells.

Neither CMV-serostatus nor RRT significantly influenced ERK or p38 phosphorylation

CMV-seropositivity may promote immunological T-cell ageing and was therefore analyzed for its association with MAPK pathway activation. However, ERK or p38 phosphorylation within T cells showed no significant difference comparing CMV-seropositive individuals to their CMV- seronegative counterparts in healthy individuals and ESRD patients respectively (Additional file 1: Figure S2 & S3). Moreover, in ESRD patients, ERK or p38 phosphorylation was not significantly different between the patients receiving RRT (i.e. dialysis) and those without RRT (Additional file 1: Fig. S4 & S5). In conclusion, neither CMV-serostatus nor RRT significantly influenced TCR-stimulation induced phosphorylation of ERK or p38.

Age-related decline in anti-CD3/CD28-induced CD69-expressing CD4[+] T cells positively associated with phosphorylation of ERK

A typical flow cytometric example for analysis of frequencies of CD69-expressing and IL-2 producing CD4[+]

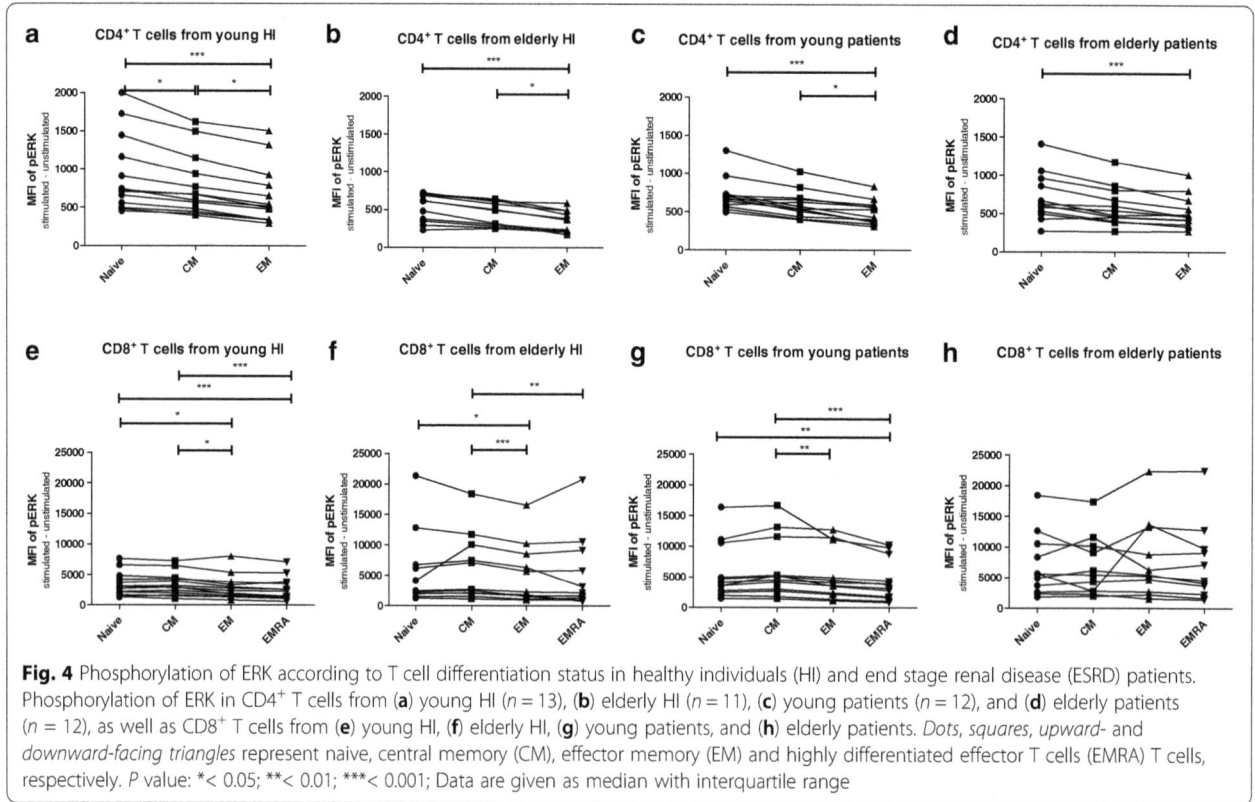

Fig. 4 Phosphorylation of ERK according to T cell differentiation status in healthy individuals (HI) and end stage renal disease (ESRD) patients. Phosphorylation of ERK in CD4⁺ T cells from (**a**) young HI ($n = 13$), (**b**) elderly HI ($n = 11$), (**c**) young patients ($n = 12$), and (**d**) elderly patients ($n = 12$), as well as CD8⁺ T cells from (**e**) young HI, (**f**) elderly HI, (**g**) young patients, and (**h**) elderly patients. *Dots, squares, upward-* and *downward-facing triangles* represent naive, central memory (CM), effector memory (EM) and highly differentiated effector T cells (EMRA) T cells, respectively. *P* value: *< 0.05; **< 0.01; ***< 0.001; Data are given as median with interquartile range

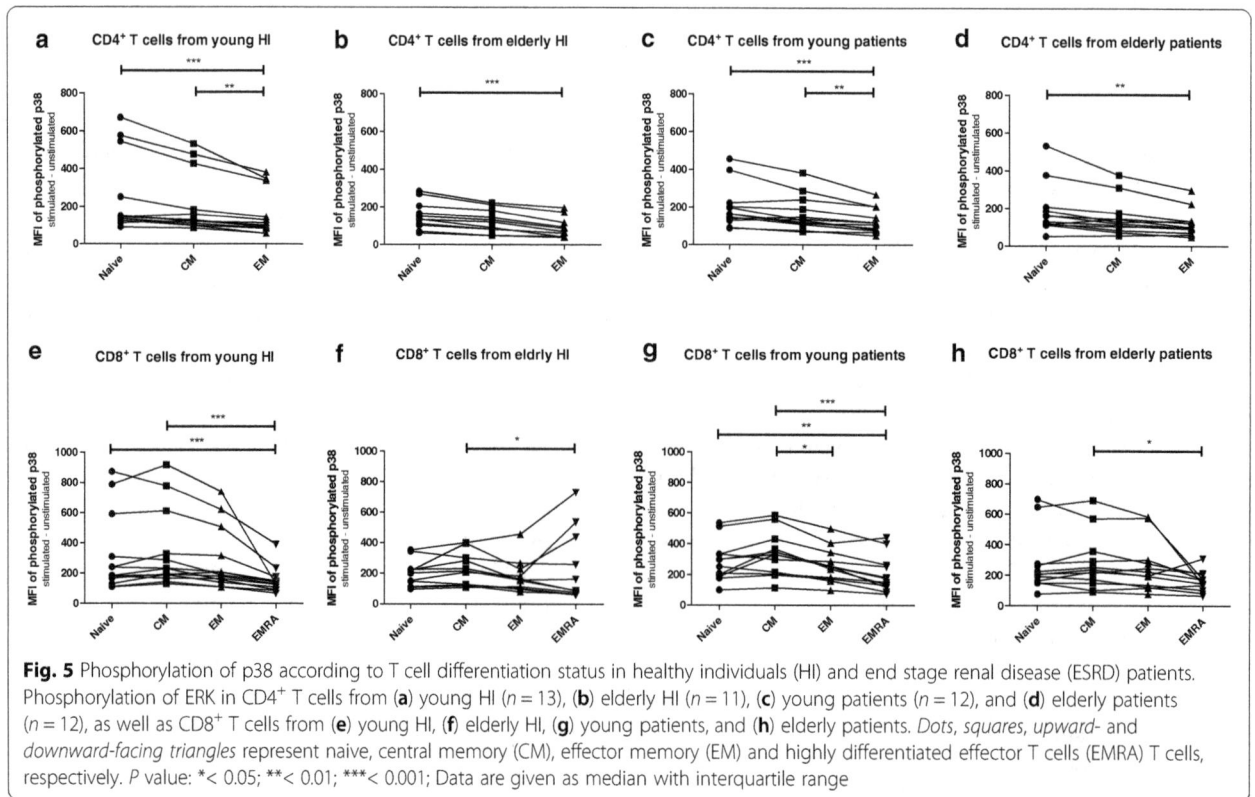

Fig. 5 Phosphorylation of p38 according to T cell differentiation status in healthy individuals (HI) and end stage renal disease (ESRD) patients. Phosphorylation of ERK in CD4⁺ T cells from (**a**) young HI ($n = 13$), (**b**) elderly HI ($n = 11$), (**c**) young patients ($n = 12$), and (**d**) elderly patients ($n = 12$), as well as CD8⁺ T cells from (**e**) young HI, (**f**) elderly HI, (**g**) young patients, and (**h**) elderly patients. *Dots, squares, upward-* and *downward-facing triangles* represent naive, central memory (CM), effector memory (EM) and highly differentiated effector T cells (EMRA) T cells, respectively. *P* value: *< 0.05; **< 0.01; ***< 0.001; Data are given as median with interquartile range

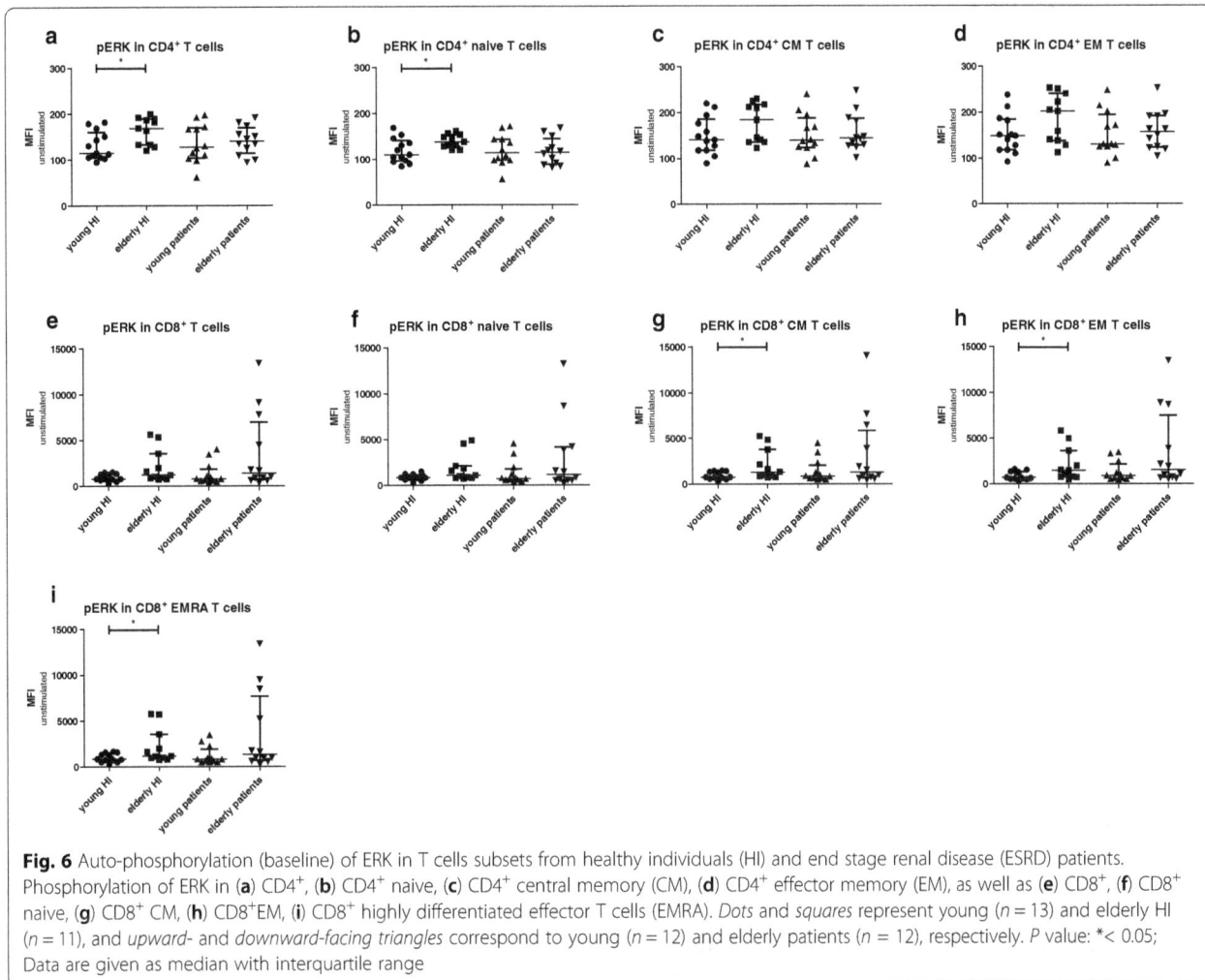

Fig. 6 Auto-phosphorylation (baseline) of ERK in T cells subsets from healthy individuals (HI) and end stage renal disease (ESRD) patients. Phosphorylation of ERK in (**a**) CD4$^+$, (**b**) CD4$^+$ naive, (**c**) CD4$^+$ central memory (CM), (**d**) CD4$^+$ effector memory (EM), as well as (**e**) CD8$^+$, (**f**) CD8$^+$ naive, (**g**) CD8$^+$ CM, (**h**) CD8$^+$EM, (**i**) CD8$^+$ highly differentiated effector T cells (EMRA). *Dots* and *squares* represent young ($n = 13$) and elderly HI ($n = 11$), and *upward-* and *downward-facing triangles* correspond to young ($n = 12$) and elderly patients ($n = 12$), respectively. *P* value: *< 0.05; Data are given as median with interquartile range

T cells after CD3/CD28 stimulation was given in Additional file 1: Figure S6. Higher frequencies of CD69-expressing CD4$^+$ T cells were observed in young HI compared to that in elderly HI when stimulated with different ratios of anti-CD3/CD28 beads to cells (Fig. 8a). This age-related decline in CD69-expressing cells was observed for naive CD4$^+$ T cells in the healthy population at a ratio of 1:0.1 (Fig. 8b) and at 1:0.1 and 1:1 ratios for memory CD4$^+$ T cells (Fig. 8c). Percentages of IL-2 producing CD4$^+$ T cells did not reveal an age-associated decline in our study population (Fig. 8d, e & f). Percentages of CD69-expressing CD4$^+$ T cells following stimulation with anti-CD3/CD28 beads (at ratios 1:0.5 and 1:1) were associated with ERK phosphorylation, presented as the fold increase in MFI dividing the MFI from stimulated samples by that of unstimulated samples (Fig. 8g). Percentages of IL-2 producing CD4$^+$ T cells were not associated with pERK (Fig. 8h). In addition, frequencies of CD69-expressing CD4$^+$ T cells were significantly higher in the naive subset compared to

CM or EM (Fig. 8i). In short, an age-related decline in anti-CD3/CD28-induced percentages of CD69-expressing CD4$^+$ T cells was observed and percentages of CD69-expressing CD4$^+$ T cells were positively associated with phosphorylation of ERK.

BCI promoted TCR-mediated phosphorylation of ERK

BCI is known to inhibit DUSP6 but also decrease levels of DUSP1 (product document, Merck – Millipore). BCI did not significantly enhance phosphorylation of ERK in young HI; in contrast, in elderly HI and both young and elderly ESRD patients, the pERK level was significantly upregulated in all CD4$^+$ T cell subsets pretreated with BCI compared to that without (Fig. 9a–c & d). The average fold increase in pERK levels in naive CD4$^+$ T cell subsets were 3.8, 2.5, and 2.1 in elderly HI, young and elderly ESRD patients, respectively. This was not observed for CD8$^+$ T cells (Additional file 1: Figure S7). In short, BCI promoted TCR-mediated phosphorylation of ERK in CD4$^+$ T

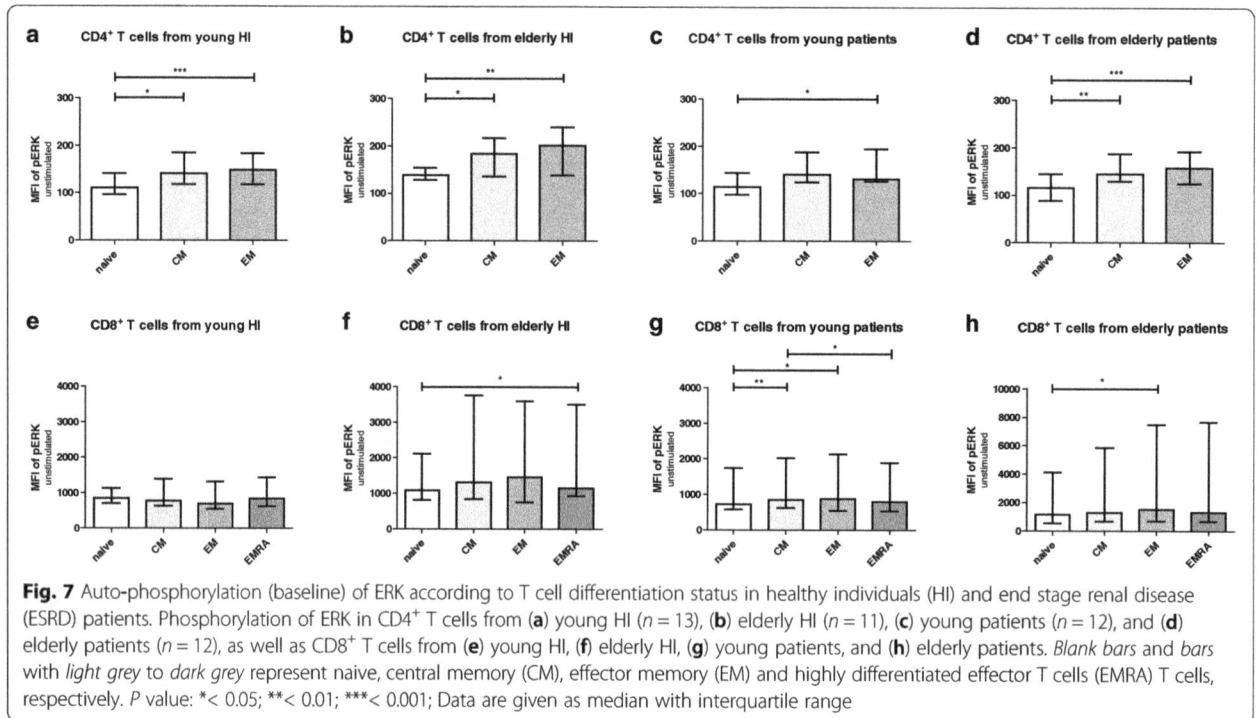

Fig. 7 Auto-phosphorylation (baseline) of ERK according to T cell differentiation status in healthy individuals (HI) and end stage renal disease (ESRD) patients. Phosphorylation of ERK in CD4+ T cells from (**a**) young HI ($n = 13$), (**b**) elderly HI ($n = 11$), (**c**) young patients ($n = 12$), and (**d**) elderly patients ($n = 12$), as well as CD8+ T cells from (**e**) young HI, (**f**) elderly HI, (**g**) young patients, and (**h**) elderly patients. *Blank bars* and *bars* with *light grey* to *dark grey* represent naive, central memory (CM), effector memory (EM) and highly differentiated effector T cells (EMRA) T cells, respectively. *P* value: *< 0.05; **< 0.01; ***< 0.001; Data are given as median with interquartile range

cells of both elderly HI as well as young and old ESRD patients.

DUSP6 and DUSP1 expression in CD4+ T cells

In an attempt to unravel whether effects of BCI on pERK levels were mediated by interfering with DUSP6 and/or DUSP1, we measured DUSP6 and DUSP1 levels within CD4+ T cells in a small fraction of our study cohort. Due to limited availability of materials only 10 HI (4 young and 6 elderly) and 9 ESRD patients (4 young and 5 elderly) could be included. A typical flow cytometric example for analysis of DUSP6 and DUSP1 is given in Additional file 1: Figure S8. An age-associated trend of increased levels of DUSP6 was noted for total and naive CD4+ T cells in HI (Fig. 10a & b). The opposite was present comparing young to old ESRD patients (Fig. 10a, b & c). Levels of DUSP6 in young ESRD patients were similar to old HI. Like observed for pERK, a significant differentiation-associated increase in DUSP6 levels was observed (Fig. 10 d). Interestingly, DUSP1 expression in CD4+ T cells was quite comparable between both young and elderly HI and patients (Fig. 10e, f, & g). To conclude, an age-related tendency of increased levels of DUSP6, but not DUSP1, was observed for HI. Moreover, DUSP6 expression was significantly associated with T-cell differentiation status in CD4+ T cells.

Discussion

The main observation of this study was that TCR-mediated phosphorylation of ERK in CD4+ T cells of young patients was in between young and old HI. Phosphorylation of ERK decreased in highly differentiated T-cell subsets compared to naive T cells. This defective TCR-mediated phosphorylation was specific as it could be restored by addition of a DUSP6 inhibitor. TCR-induced p38 phosphorylation was comparable between ESRD patients and HI.

Beyond midlife, the immune system shows age-related features and its defensive capabilities becomes impaired [35]. The uremia-associated inflammatory environment present in ESRD patients accelerates this age-related immune senescence process. In addition to declined thymic output, accumulation of highly differentiated T cells, short telomere length [10, 33, 36] and narrowed TCR-Vβ repertoire diversity [32], this study indicates that young ESRD patients also have a defective CD4+ TCR activation judging from the reduced capacity to phosphorylate ERK upon TCR-triggering. ERK activity is critical for TCR threshold calibration, as it controls positive feedback loops in TCR-induced activation [17]. Reduced ERK activity impairs TCR signal strength and activation, and favors T cells with higher affinity to antigen to be activated, leading to a contracted immune response to a given antigen [16]. The ERK phosphorylation upregulation of early activation marker CD69 on T cells ensures a proper inducing activation of T cells in the lymph node

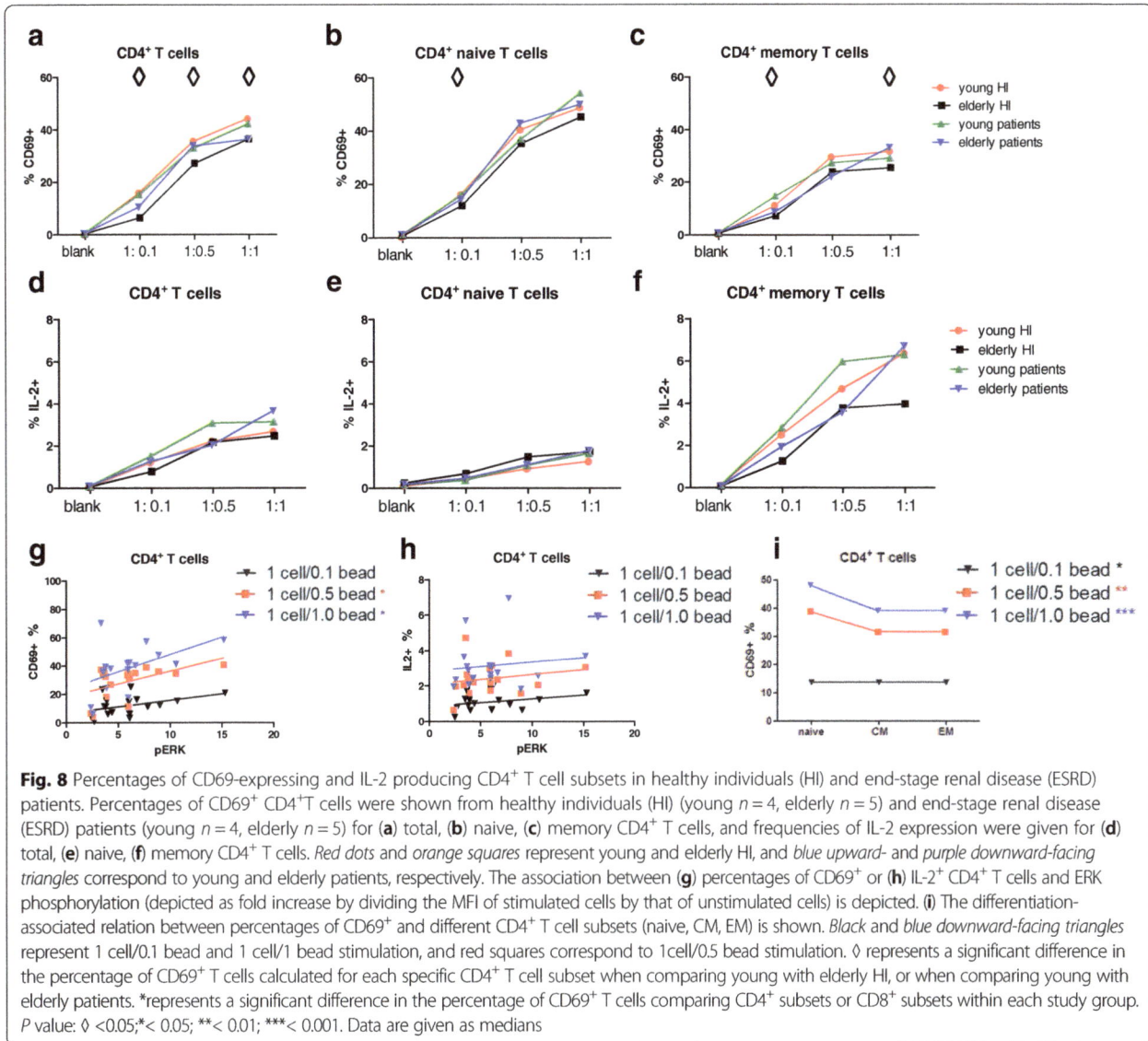

Fig. 8 Percentages of CD69-expressing and IL-2 producing CD4[+] T cell subsets in healthy individuals (HI) and end-stage renal disease (ESRD) patients. Percentages of CD69[+] CD4[+]T cells were shown from healthy individuals (HI) (young $n = 4$, elderly $n = 5$) and end-stage renal disease (ESRD) patients (young $n = 4$, elderly $n = 5$) for (**a**) total, (**b**) naive, (**c**) memory CD4[+] T cells, and frequencies of IL-2 expression were given for (**d**) total, (**e**) naive, (**f**) memory CD4[+] T cells. *Red dots* and *orange squares* represent young and elderly HI, and *blue upward-* and *purple downward-facing triangles* correspond to young and elderly patients, respectively. The association between (**g**) percentages of CD69[+] or (**h**) IL-2[+] CD4[+] T cells and ERK phosphorylation (depicted as fold increase by dividing the MFI of stimulated cells by that of unstimulated cells) is depicted. (**i**) The differentiation-associated relation between percentages of CD69[+] and different CD4[+] T cell subsets (naive, CM, EM) is shown. *Black* and *blue downward-facing triangles* represent 1 cell/0.1 bead and 1 cell/1 bead stimulation, and red squares correspond to 1cell/0.5 bead stimulation. ◊ represents a significant difference in the percentage of CD69[+] T cells calculated for each specific CD4[+] T cell subset when comparing young with elderly HI, or when comparing young with elderly patients. *represents a significant difference in the percentage of CD69[+] T cells comparing CD4[+] subsets or CD8[+] subsets within each study group. *P* value: ◊ <0.05;*< 0.05; **< 0.01; ***< 0.001. Data are given as medians

[37], and also play an important role in T cell proliferation [38] and IL-2 production [39, 40]. In addition, ERK activation impacts cellular apoptosis as it inhibits Fas-mediated apoptosis in T cells [41]. Evaluating ERK phosphorylation is a valuable tool to study more upstream molecules in the defective T-cell mediated immune system from ESRD patients. T cells from rheumatoid arthritis (RA) patients exhibit several defects which can also be viewed as premature immunological ageing [42]. However, ERK phosphorylation in CD4[+] T cells of RA patients selectively increased [43]. This increased ERK activation lowers the TCR threshold in T cells of RA patients to respond to self-antigens, which may partly explain the adaptive immune system of RA patients to exhibit abnormalities that go beyond the local inflammatory response in the synovium [44].

DUSP6 is a cytoplasmic phosphatase with substrate specificity for phosphorylated ERK. In elderly individuals, silencing of DUSP6 increased the expression of T cell activation markers, such as CD69 and CD25, IL-2 production as well as proliferative response [16]. Inhibition of DUSP6 could be a potential intervention to increase CD4[+] TCR-sensitivity by enhancing ERK phosphorylation in ESRD patients. BCI (an inhibitor of DUSP6 and 1) enhanced TCR-induced pERK in CD4[+] T cells from elderly HI, young and elderly ESRD patients, but not young HI, implying a role for DUSP6 and/or DUSP1 in regulation of ERK phosphorylation. Based on the age- as well as differentiation-related expression of DUSP6, but not DUSP1, in our HI, a potential role for DUSP6 may be present in defective TCR-induced ERK phosphorylation, especially in elderly HI and young patients. This needs to

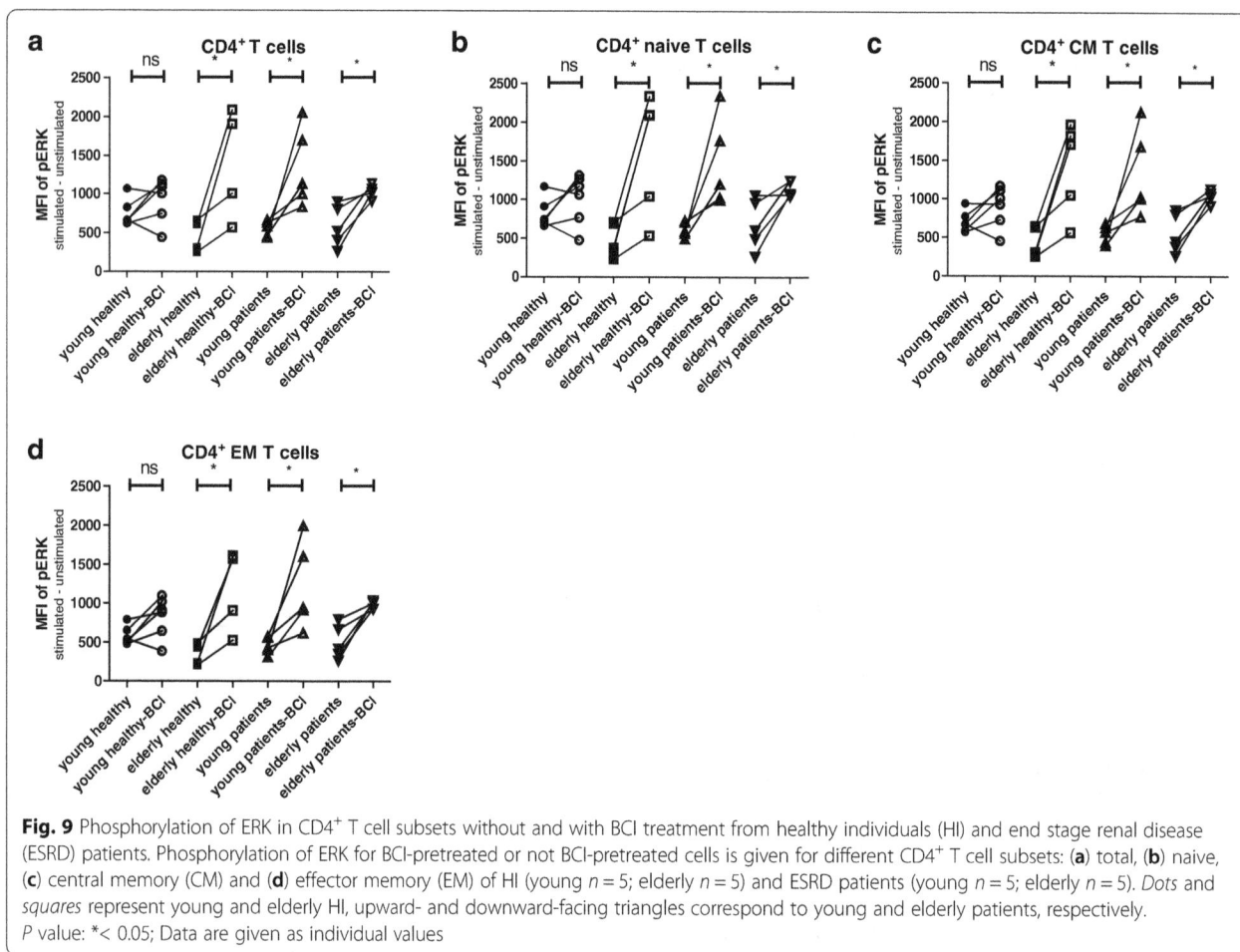

Fig. 9 Phosphorylation of ERK in CD4$^+$ T cell subsets without and with BCI treatment from healthy individuals (HI) and end stage renal disease (ESRD) patients. Phosphorylation of ERK for BCI-pretreated or not BCI-pretreated cells is given for different CD4$^+$ T cell subsets: (**a**) total, (**b**) naive, (**c**) central memory (CM) and (**d**) effector memory (EM) of HI (young $n = 5$; elderly $n = 5$) and ESRD patients (young $n = 5$; elderly $n = 5$). *Dots* and *squares* represent young and elderly HI, upward- and downward-facing triangles correspond to young and elderly patients, respectively. *P* value: *< 0.05; Data are given as individual values

be confirmed in a larger cohort. Furthermore, use of siRNA specific for DUSP6 is required to draw a more definite conclusion with respect to the role of DUSP6 in defective TCR-induced phosphorylation of ERK in ESRD patients. The lack of age-related effects on pERK in CD8$^+$ T cells of ESRD patients and HI, the latter confirming observations done by another study [16], as well as absence of effects of BCI on pERK levels in CD8$^+$ T cells, indicates a different role for DUSP6 in CD8$^+$ T cells compared to CD4$^+$ T cells. We did not observe an association between DUSP6 expression and ERK phosphorylation in CD4$^+$ T cells in ESRD patients. This could be due to the small cohort size or imply other DUSPs (e.g. 2, 4 or 5) [45–49] or upstream signaling molecules to contribute to this defective TCR-induced ERK phosphorylation in ESRD patients.

ERK over-phosphorylation might be as bad as defective ERK phosphorylation. ERK over-activation from kidney cells occurs in the physiologic setting in some chronic kidney diseases, such as compensatory kidney hypertrophy and in pathologic conditions for example glomerular disease [50]. Increased ERK phosphorylation in T cells predisposes for autoimmunity for example rheumatoid arthritis [43]. Over-expression of DUSP6 is also reported to impair

T-cell function in chronic viral infections such as hepatitis C virus infection [51]. Therefore, more research is warranted evaluating inhibition of DUSP in the setting of defective T-cell mediated immunity in ESRD patients.

We analyzed the effect of latency for CMV as it represents chronic antigenic stimulation of T cells, but ERK- or p38-activation of CD4$^+$ or CD8$^+$ T cells was not different between the CMV-IgG seropositive population and CMV-IgG seronegative population following CD3/CD28 stimulation. Highly differentiated memory CD4$^+$ and CD8$^+$ T cells may accumulate in CMV seropositive individuals and are functional CMV-specific T cells [29, 52, 53]. The results of our study show that non-specific TCR stimulation does not identify a defect p38 and ERK signaling associated with CMV seropositivity. In accordance with the results of a previous study, uremia is the major determinant affecting MAPK pathway parameters in ESRD patients and not RRT [9, 11, 33].

In the present study, we induced phosphorylation of p38 in T cells via triggering CD3 [54] and CD28 [26]. Lack of CD28 may only partly explain the decreased p38 activation in more differentiated CD4$^+$ T cells. In addition to that, senescent human CD27$^-$CD28$^-$ CD4$^+$

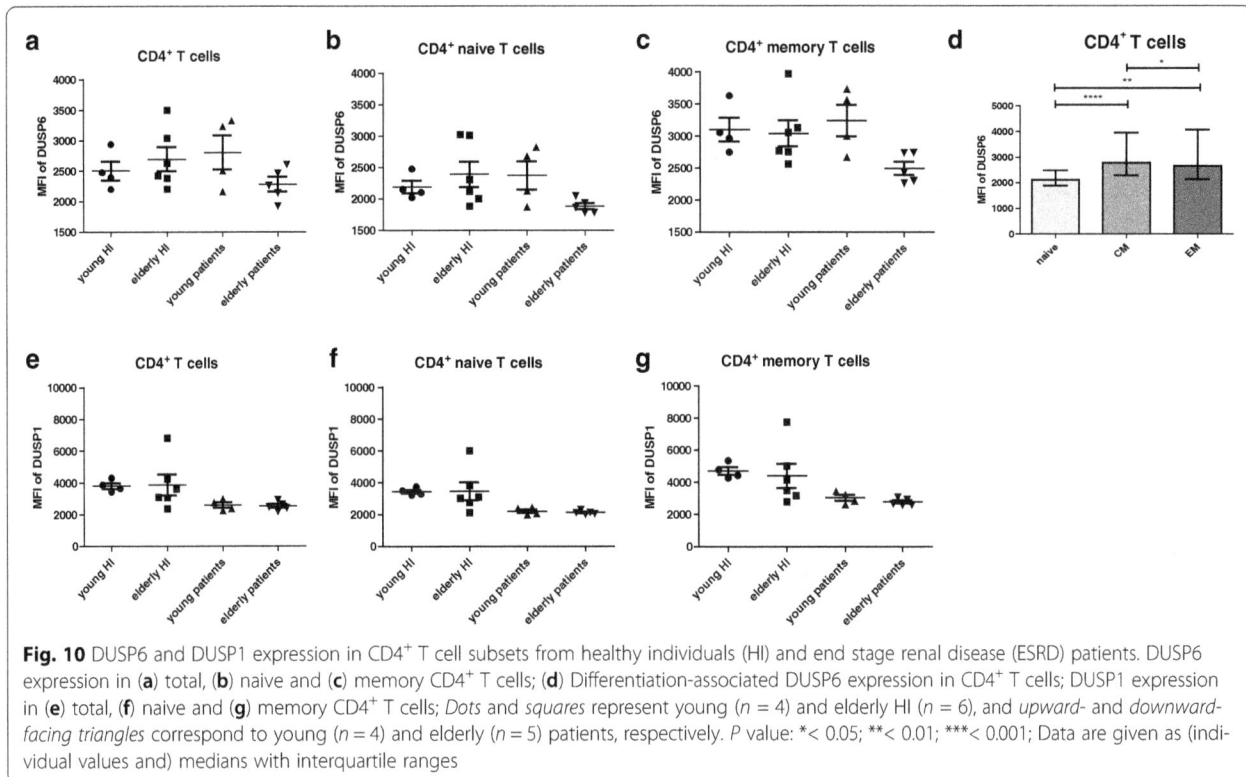

Fig. 10 DUSP6 and DUSP1 expression in CD4$^+$ T cell subsets from healthy individuals (HI) and end stage renal disease (ESRD) patients. DUSP6 expression in (**a**) total, (**b**) naive and (**c**) memory CD4$^+$ T cells; (**d**) Differentiation-associated DUSP6 expression in CD4$^+$ T cells; DUSP1 expression in (**e**) total, (**f**) naive and (**g**) memory CD4$^+$ T cells; *Dots* and *squares* represent young (*n* = 4) and elderly HI (*n* = 6), and *upward-* and *downward-facing triangles* correspond to young (*n* = 4) and elderly (*n* = 5) patients, respectively. *P* value: *< 0.05; **< 0.01; ***< 0.001; Data are given as (individual values and) medians with interquartile ranges

T cells lack several essential upstream components including ZAP70 and the loss of TCR signaling machinery in those cells was associated with a defective calcium influx [31], which may indicate the decreased response of TCR-mediated activation in the more differentiated T cells. Interestingly, in contrast to the p38 activation following CD3/CD28 stimulation, baseline levels (spontaneous phosphorylation) of p38 increased during T cells differentiation [55]. This might be caused by DNA damage in these more differentiated T cells and mediated by TAB1 (MKK-independent molecule), a key molecule involved in this auto-phosphorylation [31].

Conclusion

We have described for the first time a uremia-mediated defect in TCR-induced phosphorylation of ERK which may contribute to the impaired T-cell mediated immune response in ESRD patients. Inhibition of DUSP6 specific for pERK can restore defective p-ERK-mediated activation of CD4$^+$ T cells in ESRD patients.

Additional files

Additional file 1: Figure S1. Auto-phosphorylation (baseline) of p38 according to T cell differentiation status in healthy individuals (HI) and end stage renal disease (ESRD) patients. **Figure S2**. CMV-effects on phosphorylation of ERK in T cells subsets of healthy individuals (HI) and end stage renal disease (ESRD) patients. **Figure S3**. CMV-effects on

phosphorylation of p38 in T cells subsets of healthy individuals (HI) and end stage renal disease (ESRD) patients. **Figure S4**. Effects of renal replacement therapy (RRT) on phosphorylation of ERK in T cells subsets of end stage renal disease (ESRD) patients with and without dialysis. **Figure S5**. Effects of renal replacement therapy (RRT) on phosphorylation of p38 in T cells subsets of end stage renal disease (ESRD) patients with and without dialysis. **Figure S6**. Typical example of the gating strategy for analysis of percentages of CD69$^+$ CD4$^+$ T cell subsets. **Figure S7**. Phosphorylation of ERK in CD8+ T cell subsets without and with BCI treatment from healthy individuals (HI) and end stage renal disease (ESRD) patients. **Figure S8**. Typical example of the gating strategy for analysis of DUSP6 and DUSP1 expression in CD4$^+$

Abbreviations

AF: Alexa Fluor; AMPK: 5' adenosine monophosphate-activated protein kinase; APC: Allophycocyanin; BCI: (E)-2-benzylidene-3-(cyclohexylamino)-2, 3-dihydro-1 H-inden-1-one; BV: Brilliant Violet; CM: Central memory; CMV: Cytomegalovirus; DUSP: Dual specific phosphatase; EM: Effector memory; EMRA: Highly differentiated effector T cells; ERK: Extracellular signal-regulated kinase; ESRD: End-stage renal disease; FITC: Fluorescein isothiocyanate; HCM: Human culture medium; HI: Healthy individuals; IL-2: Interleukin-2; MAPKs: mitogen-activated protein kinases; MFI: Median fluorescence intensity; MKKs: MAPK kinases; PBMCs: Peripheral blood mononuclear cells; PE: Phycoerythrin; PerCP: Peridinin chlorophyll; pERK: Phosphorylation of ERK; RA: Rheumatoid arthritis; RRT: Renal replacement therapy; TAB1: TAK1-binding protein 1; TAK1: Transforming growth factor-β-activated protein kinase 1; TCR: T cell receptor; ZAP70: CD3 zeta-chain associated protein kinase of 70 kDa

Acknowledgements
Not applicable.

Funding
The research was supported by the China Scholarship Council for funding PhD fellowship to Ling Huang (File No. 201307720043).

Authors' contributions

LH participated in design the study, performed the experiments, analyzed the data and wrote the manuscript. NK participated in establishing the experiment protocol and revised the manuscript. MK conducted some experiments and interpreted part of the data. CB participated in design of the study and revised the manuscript. NL and MB designed the study, interpreted the data and revised the manuscript. All authors read and approved the final manuscript.

Competing interests

The authors declare that they have no competing interests.

References

1. Dalrymple LS, Go AS. Epidemiology of acute infections among patients with chronic kidney disease. Clin J Am Soc Nephrol. 2008;3(5):1487–93.
2. Betjes MG. Immune cell dysfunction and inflammation in end-stage renal disease. Nat Rev Nephrol. 2013;9(5):255–65.
3. Eleftheriadis T, Antoniadi G, Liakopoulos V, Kartsios C, Stefanidis I. Disturbances of acquired immunity in hemodialysis patients. Semin Dial. 2007;20(5):440–51.
4. Janus N, Vacher LV, Karie S, Ledneva E, Deray G. Vaccination and chronic kidney disease. Nephrol Dial Transplant. 2008;23(3):800–7.
5. Fabrizi F, Martin P. Hepatitis B vaccine and dialysis: current issues. Int J Artif Organs. 2001;24(10):683–94.
6. Remschmidt C, Wichmann O, Harder T. Influenza vaccination in patients with end-stage renal disease: systematic review and assessment of quality of evidence related to vaccine efficacy, effectiveness, and safety. BMC Med. 2014;12:244.
7. Principi N, Esposito S, Group EVS. Influenza vaccination in patients with end-stage renal disease. Expert Opin Drug Saf. 2015;14(8):1249–58.
8. Sarnak MJ, Jaber BL. Mortality caused by sepsis in patients with end-stage renal disease compared with the general population. Kidney Int. 2000;58(4): 1758–64.
9. Betjes MG, Litjens NH. Chronic kidney disease and premature ageing of the adaptive immune response. Curr Urol Rep. 2015;16(1):471.
10. Betjes MG, Langerak AW, van der Spek A, de Wit EA, Litjens NH. Premature aging of circulating T cells in patients with end-stage renal disease. Kidney Int. 2011;80(2):208–17.
11. Meijers RW, Litjens NH, de Wit EA, Langerak AW, van der Spek A, Baan CC, et al. Uremia causes premature ageing of the T cell compartment in end-stage renal disease patients. Immun Ageing. 2012;9(1):19.
12. Cantrell DA. T-cell antigen receptor signal transduction. Immunology. 2002; 105(4):369–74.
13. Smith-Garvin JE, Koretzky GA, Jordan MS. T cell activation. Annu Rev Immunol. 2009;27:591–619.
14. Johnson GL, Lapadat R. Mitogen-activated protein kinase pathways mediated by ERK, JNK, and p38 protein kinases. Science. 2002;298(5600): 1911–2.
15. Mebratu Y, Tesfaigzi Y. How ERK1/2 activation controls cell proliferation and cell death: is subcellular localization the answer? Cell Cycle. 2009;8(8): 1168–75.
16. Li G, Yu M, Lee WW, Tsang M, Krishnan E, Weyand CM, et al. Decline in miR-181a expression with age impairs T cell receptor sensitivity by increasing DUSP6 activity. Nat Med. 2012;18(10):1518–24.
17. Altan-Bonnet G, Germain RN. Modeling T cell antigen discrimination based on feedback control of digital ERK responses. PLoS Biol. 2005;3(11):e356.
18. Liu B, Carle KW, Whisler RL. Reductions in the activation of ERK and JNK are associated with decreased IL-2 production in T cells from elderly humans stimulated by the TCR/CD3 complex and costimulatory signals. Cell Immunol. 1997;182(2):79–88.
19. Kogkopoulou O, Tzakos E, Mavrothalassitis G, Baldari CT, Paliogianni F, Young HA, et al. Conditional up-regulation of IL-2 production by p38 MAPK inactivation is mediated by increased Erk1/2 activity. J Leukoc Biol. 2006; 79(5):1052–60.
20. Ekerot M, Stavridis MP, Delavaine L, Mitchell MP, Staples C, Owens DM, et al. Negative-feedback regulation of FGF signalling by DUSP6/MKP-3 is driven by ERK1/2 and mediated by Ets factor binding to a conserved site within the DUSP6/MKP-3 gene promoter. Biochem J. 2008;412(2):287–98.

21. Bignon A, Regent A, Klipfel L, Desnoyer A, de la Grange P, Martinez V, et al. DUSP4-mediated accelerated T-cell senescence in idiopathic CD4 lymphopenia. Blood. 2015;125(16):2507–18.
22. Moro-Garcia MA, Alonso-Arias R, Lopez-Larrea C. Molecular mechanisms involved in the aging of the T-cell immune response. Curr Genomics. 2012; 13(8):589–602.
23. Shiryaev A, Moens U. Mitogen-activated protein kinase p38 and MK2, MK3 and MK5: menage a trois or menage a quatre? Cell Signal. 2010;22(8): 1185–92.
24. Ashwell JD. The many paths to p38 mitogen-activated protein kinase activation in the immune system. Nat Rev Immunol. 2006;6(7):532–40.
25. Yan M, Dai T, Deak JC, Kyriakis JM, Zon LI, Woodgett JR, et al. Activation of stress-activated protein kinase by MEKK1 phosphorylation of its activator SEK1. Nature. 1994;372(6508):798–800.
26. Salvador JM, Mittelstadt PR, Guszczynski T, Copeland TD, Yamaguchi H, Appella E, et al. Alternative p38 activation pathway mediated by T cell receptor-proximal tyrosine kinases. Nat Immunol. 2005;6(4):390–5.
27. Weng NP, Akbar AN, Goronzy J. CD28(−) T cells: their role in the age-associated decline of immune function. Trends Immunol. 2009;30(7):306–12.
28. Betjes MG, Huisman M, Weimar W, Litjens NH. Expansion of cytolytic CD4 +CD28- T cells in end-stage renal disease. Kidney Int. 2008;74(6):760–7.
29. Fletcher JM, Vukmanovic-Stejic M, Dunne PJ, Birch KE, Cook JE, Jackson SE, et al. Cytomegalovirus-specific CD4+ T cells in healthy carriers are continuously driven to replicative exhaustion. J Immunol. 2005;175(12): 8218–25.
30. Pawlik A, Ostanek L, Brzosko I, Brzosko M, Masiuk M, Machalinski B, et al. The expansion of CD4+CD28- T cells in patients with rheumatoid arthritis. Arthritis Res Ther. 2003;5(4):R210–3.
31. Lanna A, Henson SM, Escors D, Akbar AN. The kinase p38 activated by the metabolic regulator AMPK and scaffold TAB1 drives the senescence of human T cells. Nat Immunol. 2014;15(10):965–72.
32. Huang L, Langerak AW, Wolvers-Tettero IL, Meijers RW, Baan CC, Litjens NH, et al. End stage renal disease patients have a skewed T cell receptor Vbeta repertoire. Immun Ageing. 2015;12:28.
33. Huang L, Langerak AW, Baan CC, Litjens NH, Betjes MG. Latency for cytomegalovirus impacts T cell ageing significantly in elderly end-stage renal disease patients. Clin Exp Immunol. 2016;186(2):239–48.
34. Litjens NH, Huisman M, Baan CC, van Druningen CJ, Betjes MG. Hepatitis B vaccine-specific CD4(+) T cells can be detected and characterised at the single cell level: limited usefulness of dendritic cells as signal enhancers. J Immunol Methods. 2008;330(1–2):1–11.
35. Moro-Garcia MA, Alonso-Arias R, Lopez-Larrea C. When aging reaches CD4+ T-cells: phenotypic and functional changes. Front Immunol. 2013;4:107.
36. Betjes MG, Meijers RW, Litjens NH. Loss of renal function causes premature aging of the immune system. Blood Purif. 2013;36(3–4):173–8.
37. Shaw AS. How T cells 'find' the right dendritic cell. Nat Immunol. 2008;9(3): 229–30.
38. Sharrocks AD. Cell cycle: sustained ERK signalling represses the inhibitors. Curr Biol. 2006;16(14):R540–2.
39. Koike T, Yamagishi H, Hatanaka Y, Fukushima A, Chang JW, Xia Y, et al. A novel ERK-dependent signaling process that regulates interleukin-2 expression in a late phase of T cell activation. J Biol Chem. 2003;278(18): 15685–92.
40. Tsukamoto H, Irie A, Nishimura Y. B-Raf contributes to sustained extracellular signal-regulated kinase activation associated with interleukin-2 production stimulated through the T cell receptor. J Biol Chem. 2004;279(46):48457–65.
41. Holmstrom TH, Schmitz I, Soderstrom TS, Poukkula M, Johnson VL, Chow SC, et al. MAPK/ERK signaling in activated T cells inhibits CD95/Fas-mediated apoptosis downstream of DISC assembly. EMBO J. 2000;19(20): 5418–28.
42. Goronzy JJ, Weyand CM. Thymic function and peripheral T-cell homeostasis in rheumatoid arthritis. Trends Immunol. 2001;22(5):251–5.
43. Singh K, Deshpande P, Pryshchep S, Colmegna I, Liarski V, Weyand CM, et al. ERK-dependent T cell receptor threshold calibration in rheumatoid arthritis. J Immunol. 2009;183(12):8258–67.
44. Cope AP. T cells in rheumatoid arthritis. Arthritis Res Ther. 2008;10 Suppl 1: S1.
45. Mandl M, Slack DN, Keyse SM. Specific inactivation and nuclear anchoring of extracellular signal-regulated kinase 2 by the inducible dual-specificity protein phosphatase DUSP5. Mol Cell Biol. 2005;25(5):1830–45.

46. Caunt CJ, Armstrong SP, Rivers CA, Norman MR, McArdle CA. Spatiotemporal regulation of ERK2 by dual specificity phosphatases. J Biol Chem. 2008;283(39):26612–23.

47. Cagnol S, Rivard N. Oncogenic KRAS and BRAF activation of the MEK/ERK signaling pathway promotes expression of dual-specificity phosphatase 4 (DUSP4/MKP2) resulting in nuclear ERK1/2 inhibition. Oncogene. 2013;32(5): 564–76.

48. Caunt CJ, Keyse SM. Dual-specificity MAP kinase phosphatases (MKPs): shaping the outcome of MAP kinase signalling. FEBS J. 2013;280(2):489–504.

49. Ferguson BS, Nam H, Stephens JM, Morrison RF. Mitogen-dependent regulation of DUSP1 governs ERK and p38 signaling during early 3T3-L1 Adipocyte differentiation. J Cell Physiol. 2016;231(7):1562–74.

50. Feliers D, Kasinath BS. Erk in kidney diseases. J Signal Transduct. 2011;2011: 768512.

51. Li GY, Zhou Y, Ying RS, Shi L, Cheng YQ, Ren JP, et al. Hepatitis C virus-induced reduction in miR-181a impairs CD4(+) T-cell responses through overexpression of DUSP6. Hepatology. 2015;61(4):1163–73.

52. Labalette M, Salez F, Pruvot FR, Noel C, Dessaint JP. CD8 lymphocytosis in primary cytomegalovirus (CMV) infection of allograft recipients: expansion of an uncommon CD8+ CD57- subset and its progressive replacement by CD8+ CD57+ T cells. Clin Exp Immunol. 1994;95(3):465–71.

53. Lachmann R, Bajwa M, Vita S, Smith H, Cheek E, Akbar A, et al. Polyfunctional T cells accumulate in large human cytomegalovirus-specific T cell responses. J Virol. 2012;86(2):1001–9.

54. Dodeller F, Schulze-Koops H. The p38 mitogen-activated protein kinase signaling cascade in CD4 T cells. Arthritis Res Ther. 2006;8(2):205.

55. Di Mitri D, Azevedo RI, Henson SM, Libri V, Riddell NE, Macaulay R, et al. Reversible senescence in human CD4+CD45RA+CD27- memory T cells. J Immunol. 2011;187(5):2093–100.

Changes in blood lymphocyte numbers with age in vivo and their association with the levels of cytokines/cytokine receptors

Yun Lin[1†], Jiewan Kim[1†], E. Jeffrey Metter[2,3], Huy Nguyen[1], Thai Truong[1], Ana Lustig[1], Luigi Ferrucci[2] and Nan-ping Weng[1*]

Abstract

Background: Alterations in the number and composition of lymphocytes and their subsets in blood are considered a hallmark of immune system aging. However, it is unknown whether the rates of change of lymphocytes are stable or change with age, or whether the inter-individual variations of lymphocyte composition are stable over time or undergo different rates of change at different ages. Here, we report a longitudinal analysis of T- and B-cells and their subsets, and NK cells in the blood of 165 subjects aged from 24 to 90 years, with each subject assessed at baseline and an average of 5.6 years follow-up.

Results: The rates of change of T-(CD4+ and CD8+) and B-cells, and NK cells were relative stable throughout the adult life. A great degree of individual variations in numbers of lymphocytes and their subsets and in the rates of their changes with age was observed. Among them, CD4+ T cells exhibited the highest degree of individual variation followed by NK cells, CD8+ T cells, and B cells. Different types of lymphocytes had distinct trends in their rates of change which did not appear to be influenced by CMV infection. Finally, the rates of CD4+, CD8+ T cells, naïve CD4+ and naïve CD8+ T cells were closely positively correlated.

Conclusion: Our findings provide evidence that the age-associated changes in circulating lymphocytes were at relative stable rates in vivo in a highly individualized manner and the levels of selected cytokines/cytokine receptors in serum might influence these age-associated changes of lymphocytes in circulation.

Keywords: Aging, Human, Peripheral blood, Lymphocytes, CD4 and CD8 T cell, B cell, NK cell, CMV

Background

Decline in immune function with age is viewed as a fundamental problem for the increased risk of age-associated diseases or disabilities [1–3]. One of the hallmark changes in the immune system with age is the alteration of the number and composition of different types of lymphocytes in the circulation. In older individuals, the numbers of CD4+ and CD8+ T cells and B cells are reduced whereas the numbers of NK cells are increased as compared to younger individuals [4, 5]. At the subset level, decreases of naïve T and B cells and increases of memory T and B cells also occurs with aging [6–11]. Such changes may reflect a combination of reduced production of naïve lymphocytes and the accumulation of memory lymphocytes as the results of the reduced overall production of lymphocytes and of the host-environment interaction over time. Despite the overall trend of age-associated changes, striking variations in the numbers of lymphocytes exist between individuals. It is currently unknown whether the observed variations are due to stable characteristics that are maintained over time or whether different subjects have different rates of change with aging.

In the T cell compartment, age associated reduction of CD4+ and CD8+ T cells as a percentage of peripheral blood mononuclear cells (PBMCs) as well as absolute numbers (cell/µl) in blood have been reported [5, 12, 13]. Within the T cell subsets, in addition to reduced

* Correspondence: wengn@mail.nih.gov
†Equal contributors
[1]Laboratory of Molecular Biology & Immunology, National Institute on Aging, 251 Bayview Blvd., Baltimore, MD 21224, USA
Full list of author information is available at the end of the article

naïve and increased memory CD4$^+$ and CD8$^+$ T cells with age, studies have shown that CD4$^+$ regulatory T cells and CD8$^+$CD28$^-$ T cells increase with age [14–16]. Thymic involution is the single most critical contributor of reduction in naïve T cells with age [17] whereas cumulative encounters with antigens over time is the force driving the increase memory T cells [18], CD8$^+$CD28$^-$ T cells [16], as well as Tregs [19]. A similar decrease of naïve and increase of memory B cells also occurs in the B cell compartment but the magnitude of change is not as profound as what is observed in T cells [6, 20]. Interestingly, natural killer cells (NK cells) are the only lymphoid linage cells that increase with aging [4, 21, 22]. However, the cytotoxic activity of NK cells appears to be reduced with age and thus the increase in NK cell number may be interpreted as compensatory. Some of the alterations in lymphocyte composition are considered biomarkers of immunosenenscence (ratio of CD4/CD8, increase of CD28$^-$ T cells, and increase of NK cells) because they are associated with mortality in elderly [23, 24].

Information regarding age-related changes in lymphocyte composition in humans is mostly derived from cross-sectional studies. This approach may be biased by selective mortality or participation attrition and, in addition, lack the time dimension necessary to dissect cross-sectional and longitudinal effects. Data from longitudinal studies should allow for the determination of whether changes in lymphocyte compositions occur at a constant rate or are non-linear over time and whether there are detectable causes of these changes.

Here, we conducted a longitudinal analysis of CD4$^+$ and CD8$^+$ T cells, B cells and their subsets, and NK cells in 165 participants from the Baltimore Longitudinal Study of Aging (BLSA) (https://www.blsa.nih.gov/) assessed at baseline and, on average, after a 5-year follow-up. We analyzed the rates of changes and explored potential causes of variations and correlation among these changes and with CMV infection. Our findings provide detailed longitudinal rates of changes in lymphocytes and their subsets with aging in a relatively healthy population dispersed over a relatively wide age-range.

Methods
Study design and participants
We performed a longitudinal study of T- and B-cells and their subsets, and NK cells in peripheral blood of 165 BLSA participants at first visit and 5-year follow-up under the NIH IRB- approved protocol (GRC98-12-28-01) and performed in accordance with the Declaration of Helsinki. Demographic characterization of these participants was summarized in Additional file 1: Table S1. At each visit, blood cell counts were measured by standard complete blood cell counts by Coulter Counter and PBMCs were isolated from 50 mL blood drawn from

participants under fasting condition and cryopreserved in liquid nitrogen. Two to five cryopreserved PBMCs from each subject with an average of 5.6 years apart were used in the experiments. PBMCs from all time points were thawed and counted on the day of the experiment. The recovery of frozen PBMC was 77 % ± 0.3 % (mean ± SEM). Complete blood cell counts was combined with flow cytometry analysis (see gating strategy in Additional file 1: Figure S1) to obtain the cell count and to estimate rate changes for different cell populations.

Analysis by flow cytometry
Antibodies used for flow cytometry analysis included: CD2-Tri-Color (TC); CD4-Phycoerythrin (PE) and CD4Allophycocyanin (APC); CD28-Fluorescein Isothiocyanate (FITC); CD8-TC; CD19-APC; CD45RA-APC; CD16-FITC from Life Technologies (Grand Island, NY); CD14-PE; CD27-PE; and IgM-FITC from BD Biosciences (San Jose, CA). Freshly thawed PBMCs from each visit were stained with three to five antibodies: T cells (CD2, CD4, CD8, CD45RA, and CD28); B cells (CD19, IgM, and CD27); NK cells (CD16). The data were collected on a BD FACSCalibur or BD FACSCanto II, and analyzed by Cell-Quest (BD Biosciences) and FlowJo. The gating strategies were presented in Additional file 1: Figure S1.

Measurement of selected biomarkers and CMV IgG
Fasting blood was collected at each visit for measurement of complete blood cell count and other routine blood chemistry using the standard method under the BLSA protocol. Sera were isolated from blood and stored in a -80 °C freezer prior to cytokine (IL) measurement using a custom-made multiplex assay (BioRad Luminex Assays) according to the manufacturer's instruction. CMV IgG was measured from sera of 120 subjects (117 of them had two time points and 3 had single time points) using the ELISA kit (Abcam, # ab108639) according to the manufacturer's instruction.

Statistical analysis
Figures were plotted as scatterplots with a linear regression line. The regression lines for rate and percentage rate of change by age were analyzed using linear regression. Regressions of number of cells and percent of cells were tested using mixed effects linear regression on age with a random effect for subject to address the within-subject correlation with the repeated measurements. The inclusion of the time difference between the measurements did not affect the assessment. For the regression models, all tests were performed with a $p < 0.05$. Correlations were calculated between pairs of variables, and after adjusting by FDR [25], p value less or equal to 0.005 is considered as significant. To address the question whether rapid rates of change are present across more

cell types than expected, rates for each cell type were dichotomized and summed to identify subjects in the tertile with the greatest rate of cell loss (except for NK rates which were the highest tertile). The summed score was compared to the expected binomial distribution by chi-squared test. Assuming a binomial distribution, the probability coefficient was estimated from the data using the Bayesian modeling program rstan (http://mc-stan.org/rstan.html). A single sample proportion test was used to test whether the proportion of subject with summed score of 4 or more was greater in the data as compared to the expected summed score of 4 or more from a binomial distribution with probability of 0.33.

All statistical analyses were done using R version 2.12.1 (http://www.r-project.org).

Results

Changes of CD4[+] T cells and their subsets in peripheral blood with age in vivo

In agreement with previous reports, at baseline older age was associated with slightly lower number of CD4[+] T (Additional file 1: Figure S2a) [26, 27]. Rates of change of CD4[+] T cell, reported as cell number per µl blood per year, were quite heterogeneous across study subjects (ranging from -120 to +170 cells/µl/yr and an average of 9.8 cells/µl/yr) and were relatively stable at different ages (Fig. 1a). Next, we examined rates of change in three subsets of CD4[+] T cells, including naïve (CD45RA[+]CD28[+]), Treg (CD25[+]Foxp3[+]), and CD28[-] cells. Similar to previous reports, older age was associated with fewer naïve CD4[+] T cells (Additional file 1: Figure S2b) [28, 29]. Similarly to the total CD4[+] T cells, there were remarkable individual variability in rates of change in naïve CD4[+] T cells (ranging from -80 to +108 cells/µl/yr and average 4.3 cells/µl/yr) but the average trend of change with age was surprisingly flat, suggesting that naïve phenotype CD4[+] T cells were well maintained throughout the adult life span in the absence of apparent new genesis from the thymus (Fig. 1b). In agreement with previous reports [14, 30], Treg (CD4[+]CD25[+]FOXP3[+]) tended to be more numerous in older than in younger individuals (Additional file 1: Figure S2c). However, the degree of individual variations in the rates

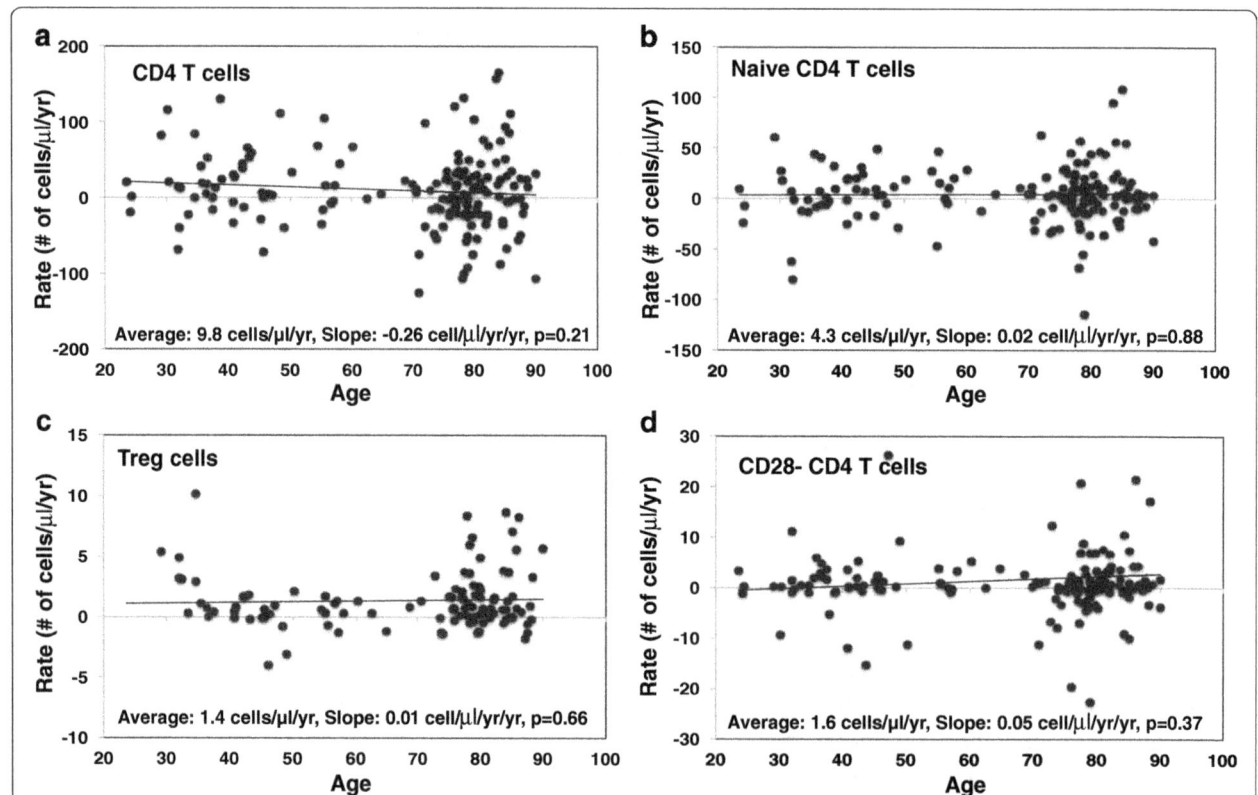

Fig. 1 Rate of CD4[+] T cells and subsets change with age in vivo. **a** Rate of CD4[+] T cells in peripheral blood in number of cells per µl blood. The rate of CD4[+] T cells was calculated based on flow cytometry analysis using the gating strategy described in (Additional file 1: Figure S1) and lymphocyte counts from complete blood counts. The linear regressions rate over time are -0.26 cell/µl/year (N = 165). **b** Rate of naïve CD4[+] T cells in CD4[+] T cells in number of cells per µl blood. The rate of naïve CD4[+] T cell in cell/µl/year was based on flow cytometry analysis and lymphocyte counts from complete blood counts (N = 158). **c** Rate of regulatory CD4 T (Treg) cells in peripheral blood (N = 112). Treg was defined by expression of CD25 and Foxp3. **d** Rate of CD4[+]CD28[-] T cells in peripheral blood (N = 160). P values were calculated by linear regression in this and subsequent figures

of change in Treg (ranging from -4 to +10 cells/μl/yr and average 1.4 cells/μl/yr) was smaller than that of naïve cells but similarly stable in the trend of change with age (Fig. 1c). We observed a similar age-related increase of $CD4^+CD28^-$ T cells from ages 20 to 90 (Additional file 1: Figure S2d). Again, the rate of change in $CD4^+CD28^-$ T cells showed individual variations and the trend of rate of change with age was relatively stable (ranging from -23 to +60 cells/μl/yr and average 1.6 cells/μl/yr) (Fig. 1d). Together, these results showed a great degree of individual variation in the rates of change in $CD4^+$ T cells and their subsets among study subjects. Overall there was a rather stable trend in the rates of changes in $CD4^+$ T cells and their subsets over the adult life time.

Changes in $CD8^+$ T cells and their subsets in peripheral blood with age in vivo

In $CD8^+$ T cells, we observed a similar age related reduction in the number of cells/μl blood in our study cohort of cross-sectional analysis as previously reported [31–33] (Additional file 1: Figure S3a). The rate of change in $CD8^+$

T cells (ranging from -163 to +69 cells/μl/yr and average -1.3 cells/μl/yr) showed a comparable degree of variation as observed in $CD4^+$ T cells and the overall rate of change of $CD8^+$ T cells was remarkably stable throughout the adult lifetime (Fig. 2a). Decrease of naïve $CD8^+$ T cells in blood with age was observed in this study cohort (Additional file 1: Figure S3b) as well as in previous reports [5, 12, 13]. The rates of naïve $CD8^+$ T cells (ranging from -34 to +43 cells/μl/yr and average -1.8 cells/μl/yr) also displayed a high degree of individual variations with no significant change of the average rates at different ages (Fig. 2b). The increase of $CD8^+CD28^-$ T cells with age is considered as a signature of T cell aging and was observed in this study (Additional file 1: Figure S3c). Interestingly, while the rates of change with age of $CD8^+CD28^-$ T cells showed individual variations (ranging from -121 to +53 cells/μl/yr and average 0.9 cells/μl/yr), the average trend was not significantly changed with age, suggesting that the increase of $CD8^+CD28^-$ T cells was accumulated through a relatively constant rate over the adult lifetime (Fig. 2c). Collectively, the individual variations in the rates of changes in $CD8^+$ T cells and

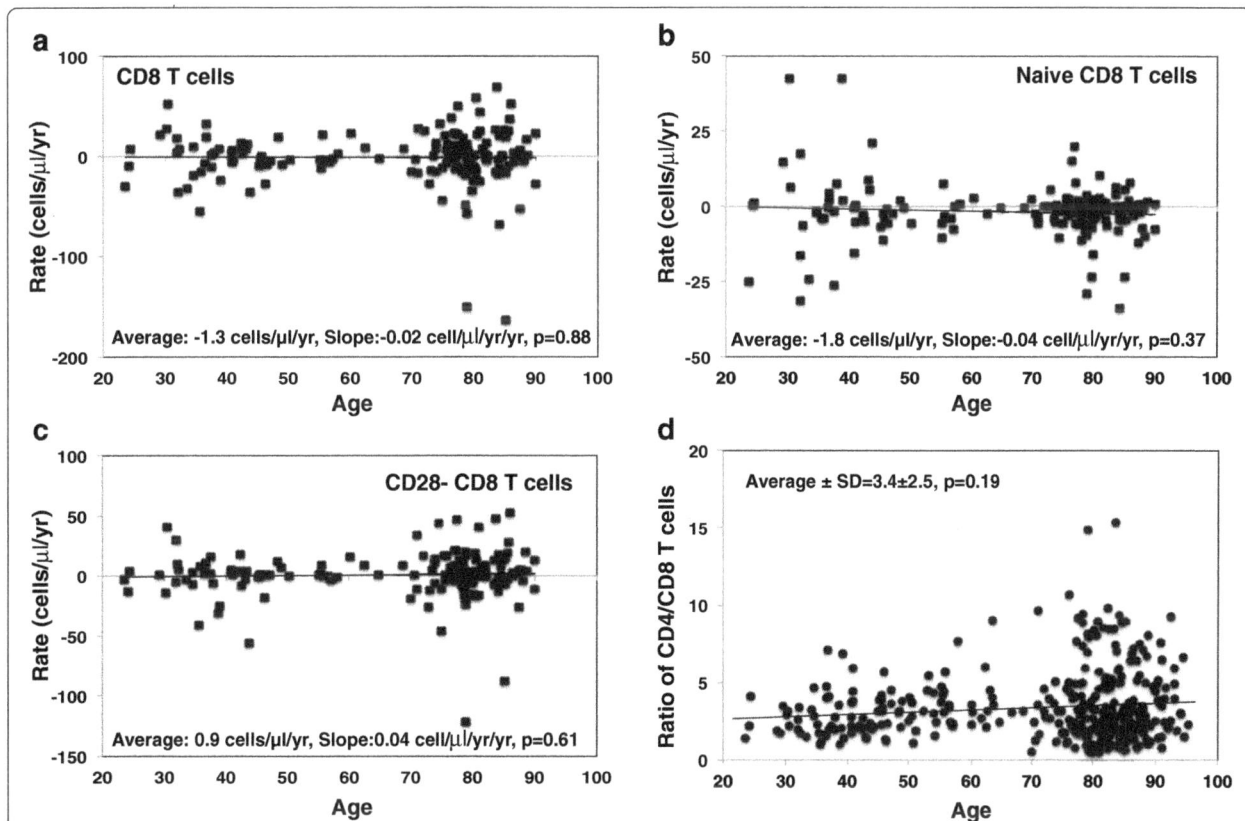

Fig. 2 Rate of $CD8^+$ T cells and subsets change with age in vivo. **a** Rate of $CD8^+$ T cells in peripheral blood in number of cells per μl blood (N = 162). The rate of $CD8^+$ T cells was calculated based on flow cytometry analysis using the gating strategy described in (Additional file 1: Figure S1) and lymphocyte counts from complete blood counts. **b** Rate of naïve $CD8^+$ T cells in $CD8^+$ T cell in cell number per μl blood (N = 159). Naïve $CD8^+$ T cell were defined by $CD45RA^+/CD28^+$. **c** Rate of $CD8^+CD28^-$ T cells in $CD8^+$ T cell in cell number per μl blood (N = 162). **d** Ratio of $CD4^+/CD8^+$ T cells (number of cells/μl) as a function of age (N = 162). P values were calculated by linear regression in this and subsequent figures

their subsets were similar to those of CD4$^+$ T cells; the overall trend of the rates of CD8$^+$ T cells and their subsets were largely stable over the adult life. Previous studies suggest that a reduction of the CD4/CD8 ratio with increasing age is an "Immune Risk Profile (IRP)" [23, 24, 34, 35]. Here, we evaluated whether the CD4$^+$/CD8$^+$ ratio reduced with age along with the number of cells in the blood, and found that the average ratios of CD4/CD8 T cells were relatively stable with age (mean ± SD = 3.4 ± 2.5) (Fig. 2d). Thus, a reduction in CD4$^+$/CD8$^+$ ratio was not observed as a general trend of age in this study cohort.

Changes in B cells and their subsets in peripheral blood with age in vivo

B cells were defined based by the expression of CD19 and naïve and memory B cells were defined based by CD19$^+$IgM$^+$CD27$^-$ and CD19$^+$CD27$^+$, respectively (Additional file 1: Figure S1). We observed a reduction of total B cells as well as naïve B cells with age in our study cohort from the cross-sectional analysis (Additional file 1: Figure S4a-b), and a slight increase in memory B cells with age (Additional file 1: Figure S4c). The average rate of change in B cells was -6.6

cells/µl/yr, and the trend of the rate did not differ across the adult age span (Fig. 3a). Similarly, the average rate of change in naïve B cells was -5.5 cells/µl/yr, and the trend of the rate across the adult age span was flat (Fig. 3b). The average rate of change of memory B cells was -0.1 cells/µl/yr across the age span (Fig. 3c). Overall, these findings showed that the average loss of B cells and naïve B cells with age in vivo did not alter with the subject's age.

Change of NK cell and its subsets in peripheral blood with age in vivo

Increase of NK cells in peripheral blood with aging has been reported [4, 21, 36] and was also observed in this study (Additional file 1: Figure S5). Here, we analyzed the major population of NK cells defined by CD14$^-$CD16$^+$ (Additional file 1: Figure S1), which is composed of around 90 % of NK cells (Le Garff-Tavernier et al., 2011). The rate of change in NK cells displayed wide individual variation among the study subjects (from -180 to 100 cells/µl/yr) (Fig. 4). Among the average rates of T (CD4 and CD8) and B cells, the average rate of NK cells of all subjects was the highest (25.3 cells/µl/yr) with no change in the rate with age (Fig. 4).

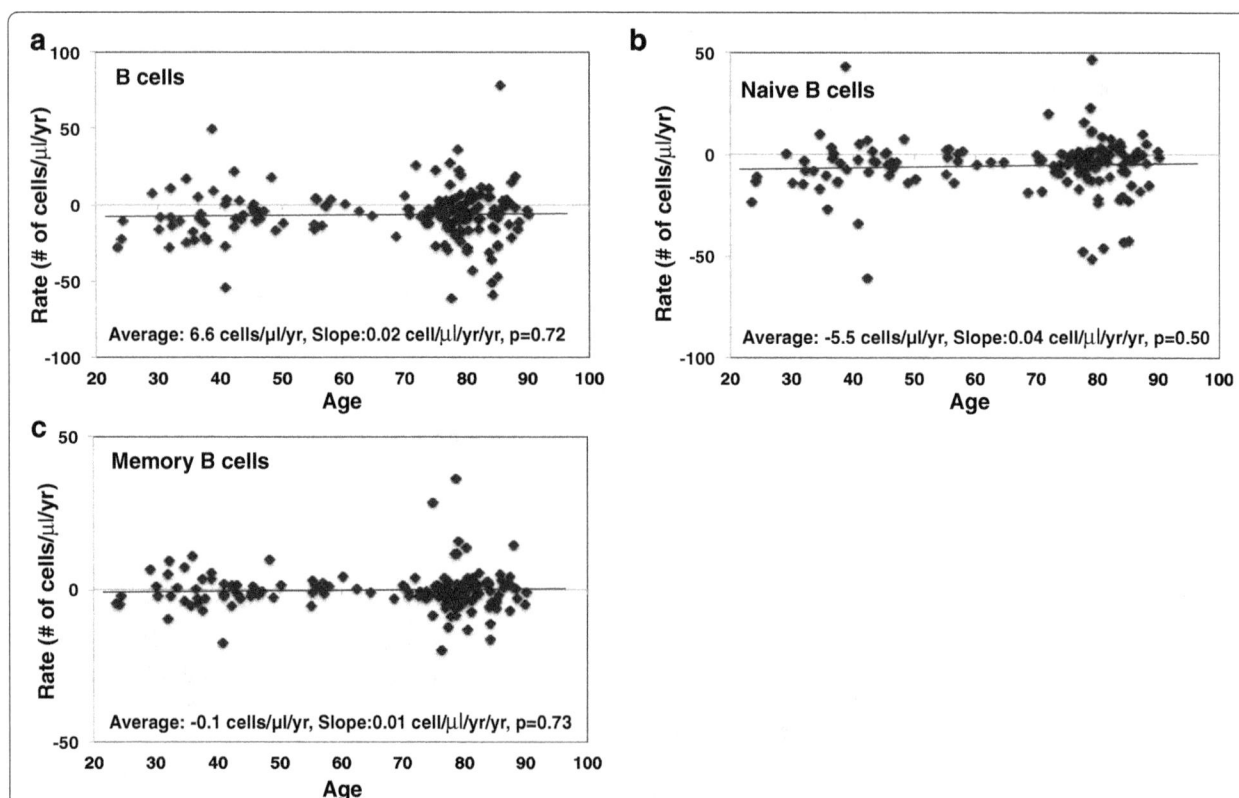

Fig. 3 Rate of B cells and subsets change with age in vivo. **a** Rate of B cells in peripheral blood in cell number per µl blood. The rate of B cell was calculated based on flow cytometry analysis using the gating strategy described in (Additional file 1: Figure S1) and lymphocyte counts from complete blood (N = 162). **b** Rate of naïve B cells in B cell in cell number per µl blood (N = 218). Naïve B cells were defined by CD19$^+$IgM$^+$CD27$^-$. **c** Rate of memory B cells in B cell in cell number per µl blood (N = 162). Memory B cells were defined by CD19$^+$CD27$^+$

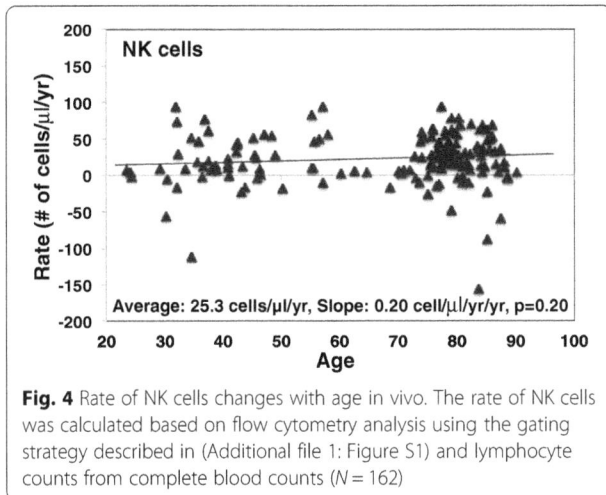

Fig. 4 Rate of NK cells changes with age in vivo. The rate of NK cells was calculated based on flow cytometry analysis using the gating strategy described in (Additional file 1: Figure S1) and lymphocyte counts from complete blood counts ($N = 162$)

Correlation between changes among different types of lymphocytes and selected cytokines and soluble cytokine receptors, and antibodies against cytomegalovirus (CMV) in blood

To determine whether the rates of change in subsets of lymphocytes correlated with each other and with some physiological measurements such as levels of cytokines and soluble cytokine receptors in blood and other physiological parameters, we compared the rate of change of each type of lymphocyte subset with the percents and counts of lymphocytes and a panel of cytokines and physiological parameters (Additional file 1: Table S2) using Pearson's partial correlation coefficient adjusted for age (Fig. 5). Lymphocyte count was positively correlated with body fat and LDL in sera (Fig. 5). The rate of change in $CD4^+$ T cells showed a positive correlation with the rates of change for naïve $CD4^+$ and naïve $CD8^+$ T cells, total $CD8^+$ T cells, $CD4^+CD28^-$ cells and $CD8^+CD28^-$ cells, but a negative correlation with numbers of $CD4^+$ cells and naïve $CD4^+$ cells (Fig. 5).

The rate of naïve $CD4^+$ T cells was positively correlated with the rates of change of $CD4^+$, $CD8^+$ and naïve $CD8^+$ T cells but negatively correlated with numbers of $CD4^+$ and naïve $CD4^+$, and naïve $CD8^+$ T cells (Fig. 5). The rate of Treg cells was positively correlated with numbers of $CD4^+$ and naïve $CD4^+$ T cells, and rate of $CD4^+CD28^-$ cells (Fig. 5). To determine whether there is a tendency for subjects who show rapid rates of change in one cell type to show similar changes in other cell types, we dichotomized the rates for each cell type to identify subjects in the tertile with the greatest rate of cell loss (except for NK rates which were the highest tertile) and the seven dichotomized rates were summed (total score 0 to 7). If the cell rates are independent, the distribution should be binomial with probability 0.33, which was not the case by chi-squared test ($p < 0.0001$). The probability which fits the summed score was 0.38

that is significantly different that the 0.33 used in creating the score ($p < 0.02$). If the cell rates occur together, the expectation would be for an excessive proportion of subjects to have high summed scores. The expected probability of a score of 4 or more is 0.17, while the observed proportion is 0.23 ($p = 0.03$). The high proportion of high counts argues that there is evidence that rapid rates tend to co-occur among cell types far more often than would be expected by chance (i.e. being independent). Finally, the rate of $CD4^+CD28^-$ cells was positively correlated with the rates of $CD4^+$, Treg and $CD8^+CD28^-$ T cells (Fig. 5).

The rate of $CD8^+$ T cells showed a positive correlation with the rates of $CD8^+CD28^-$, naïve $CD8^+$, total $CD4^+$, naïve $CD4^+$ T cells and serum level of IL-15 and a negative correlation with number of $CD8^+$ T cells, $CD8^+CD28^-$ T cells, and rate of naïve B cells (Fig. 5). The rate of change of naïve $CD8^+$ T cells was positively correlated with rates of change of $CD4^+$, $CD8^+$, and naïve $CD4^+$ T cells but negatively correlated with the numbers of naïve $CD8^+$ T cells (Fig. 5). Finally, the rate of change of $CD8^+CD28^-$ T cells was positively correlated with the rates of $CD8^+$, $CD4^+$, $CD4^+CD28^-$ and serum level of IL-15 but negatively corrected with numbers of $CD8^+$ $CD8^+CD28^-$ T cells, and rate of naïve B cells (Fig. 5). The ratio of $CD4^+/CD8^+$ T cell number was positively correlated with numbers of $CD4^+$, Treg, and naïve $CD4^+$ but negatively numbers of $CD8^+$, $CD8^+CD28^-$, and naïve CD8 T cells, and CMV seropositivity defined by the presence of anti-CMV IgG antibodies in sera (Fig. 5). The association CMV seropositivity with the low ratio of $CD4^+/CD8^+$ found here is in agreement with the previous report [37].

The rate of B cells was positively correlated with serum levels of soluble TNFRI and TNFRII, and rates of naïve and memory B cells but was negatively correlated with the numbers of B cells and naïve B cells (Fig. 5). The rate of naïve B cells was positively correlated with rate of B cells but negatively correlated with numbers of naïve B, naïve B cells, rates of $CD8^+CD28^-$ and $CD8^+$ T cells (Fig. 5). The rate of change of memory B cells was positively correlated with serum levels of soluble TNFRI and numbers of NK cells (Fig. 5). Finally, the rate of change of NK cells was negatively correlated with the serum level of triglyceride (Fig. 5).

Discussion

Limited information is available regarding the trajectories of in vivo aging of immune cells in humans. As lymphocyte numbers in peripheral blood exhibit a great degree of individual variation, it is unclear whether inter-individuals differences are due to individual's characteristics that remain stable with aging or result from the different rates of changes in different types of

a

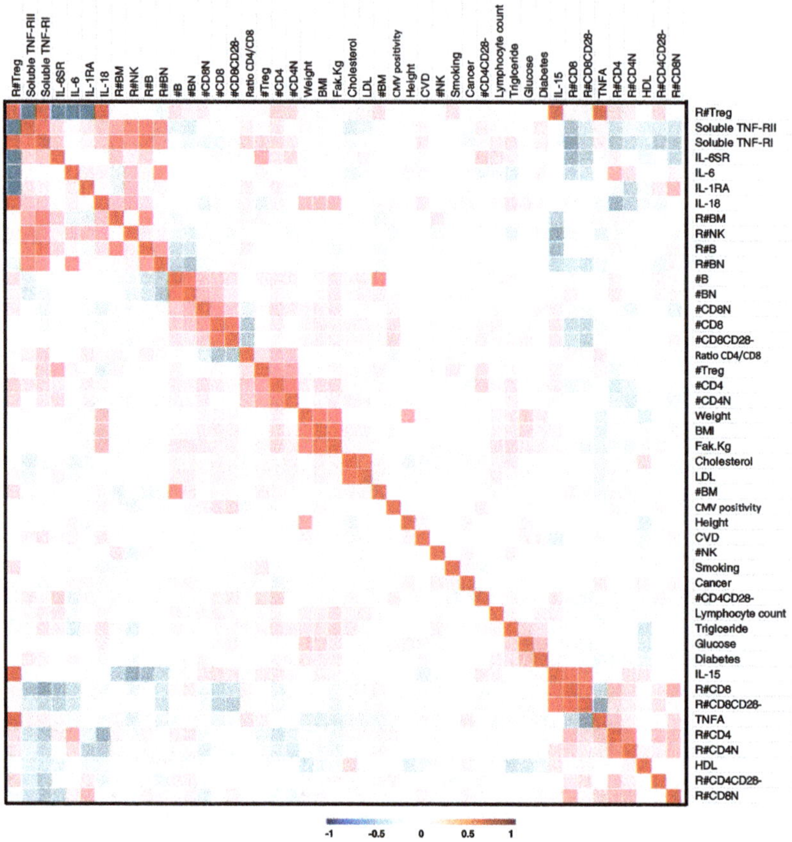

b

Lymphocyte count	R	P
Fat.kg	0.27	0.000
LDL	0.20	0.003

Ratio CD4/CD8	R	P
#CD8	-0.60	0.000
#CD8CD28	-0.55	0.000
#CD8N	-0.29	0.000
CMV positivity	-0.18	0.004
#Treg	0.28	0.000
#CD4N	0.39	0.000
#CD4	0.41	0.000

R-CD4	R	P
#CD4	-0.39	0.000
#CD4N	-0.28	0.002
R-CD8CD28-	0.27	0.003
R-CD4CD28-	0.41	0.000
R-CD8N	0.45	0.000
R-CD8	0.47	0.000
R-CD4N	0.69	0.000

R-CD4N	R	P
#CD4N	-0.35	0.000
#CD4	-0.28	0.003
#CD8N	-0.26	0.005
R-CD8	0.30	0.001
R-CD8N	0.43	0.000
R-CD4	0.69	0.000

R-Treg	R	P
R-CD4CD28-	0.30	0.005
#CD4N	0.31	0.005
#CD4	0.35	0.001

R-CD4CD28-	R	P
R-CD4	0.41	0.000
R-Treg	0.30	0.005
R-CD8CD28-	0.26	0.005

R-CD8	R	P
#CD8	-0.44	0.000
#CD8CD28-	-0.37	0.000
R-BN	-0.35	0.000
R-CD4N	0.30	0.001
R-CD4	0.47	0.000
R-CD8N	0.52	0.000
IL-15	0.86	0.000
R-CD8CD28-	0.88	0.000

R-CD8N	R	P
#CD8N	-0.26	0.005
R-CD4N	0.43	0.000
R-CD4	0.45	0.000
R-CD8	0.52	0.000

R-CD8CD28-	R	P
#CD8CD28-	-0.50	0.000
#CD8	-0.48	0.000
R-BN	-0.42	0.000
R-CD4CD28-	0.26	0.005
R-CD4	0.27	0.003
IL-15	0.83	0.000
R-CD8	0.88	0.000

R-B	R	P
#B	-0.40	0.000
#BN	-0.36	0.000
R-BN	0.61	0.000
R-BM	0.71	0.000
STNF_RII	0.77	0.003
STNF_RI	0.87	0.000

R-BN	R	P
#BN	-0.59	0.000
#B	-0.47	0.000
R-CD8CD28-	-0.42	0.000
R-CD8	-0.35	0.000
R-B	0.61	0.000

R-BM	R	P
#NK	0.75	0.005
STNF_RI	0.25	0.005

R-NK	R	P
Triglyceride	-0.27	0.003

Fig. 5 Correlation of rate changes and cytokines/soluble receptor levels in sera. **a** Correlation coefficient among the rate changes of lymphocytes and selected cytokines/their receptors. The correlation coefficients between pair comparison were analyzed with adjustment for age, and presented as a clustered heat map. # refers to the cell counts (x10^3/μl) and R# refers to the rate of changes used cell counts (cell counts/year). **b** Significant correlations were presented with correlation coefficient (R) and p values. After adjusting by FDR, p value is significant less or equal to 0.005

lymphocytes in across individuals. Our longitudinal analysis showed that the rates of changes of all four major types of lymphocytes (CD4+, CD8+, B, and NK cells) were also highly individualized. The average rates of change of all four major types of lymphocytes were quite stable in the study subjects across 70 years of adult life. It will be necessary to further examine these changes in a longer time follow-up such as 10 or 20 years to understand the contributing genetic and environmental factors that determine the individual variation. Such a study will require long-term commitment and resources but the yield will have the details and resolution needed to better understand these age-associated changes within the immune system.

One of the most prominent signs of an immune system aging is a significant reduction of naïve lymphocytes in blood. The reduction of naïve lymphocytes occurs continuously with advancing age, which has been mainly attributed to a reduction of thymic output after puberty and imperfect peripheral maintenance. However, it is unknown whether the loss of naïve lymphocytes occurs at a constant or increasing rate with age. Our longitudinal analysis showed that the trends of rates of change of naïve CD4+ and CD8+ T cell and naïve B cells over 70 years of adult life were remarkably flat, indicating that the continuous reduction of naïve T and B cells in blood is due to a cumulative effect during aging. This conclusion is further supported by study using ^2H_2O labeling showed similar dynamics of lymphocytes between young and elderly subjects [38]. In contrast to naïve lymphocytes, CD28- T cells (both CD4+ and CD8+) and NK cells increase in blood with age. Interestingly, we observed that the trends of the rates of change of CD4+CD28- T cells and NK cells (Figs. 1c and 4a) but not CD8+CD28- T cells (Fig. 2c) also slightly increase with age. This suggests that age-associated increase of CD4+CD28- T cells and NK cells with age is not only accumulated over time but also increased in pace with age.

A reduced CD4+/CD8+ ratio is considered as one of the immune risk phenotypes (IRP) related to increased morbidity and mortality in elderly [23, 24, 34, 35]. In agreement with previous finding [37], we also found that the ratio of CD4/CD8 T cells is negatively correlated with CMV seropositivity and the trend of the CD4+/CD8+ ratio was not substantially changed with age (Fig. 2e). Collectively, these findings suggest that a reduction in the CD4+/CD8+ ratio is not a general change with age in this study cohort but is more obvious to the CMV infected old subjects.

Correlational analysis of the rates of change of lymphocytes and their subsets with some selected cytokines and soluble cytokine receptors revealed some unexpected findings. We found that the rates of CD8+ and CD8+ CD28-T cells were positively correlated with levels of serum IL-15. In contrast to T cells, rates of B cells and memory B cells were positively correlated with soluble TNF-RI. IL-15 is a critical growth factor for CD8+ T cells [39] and TNF alpha can induce B cell proliferation [40], their positive correlations suggest that cytokine mediated peripheral expansion is an influencing factor of the rate of changes.

We have applied 11 cell lineage/differentiation makers in analyzing 4 major lymphocyte populations in blood. Although using frozen PBMCs in this study prevents selection of those temperature sensitive markers such as CD62L and CCR7, there are more differentiation markers that can be used to improve the resolution and precision of age-associated changes in these lymphocyte subsets. In particular, applying IgD and IgG staining could further separate naïve and memory B cell subpopulations as some of those subpopulations display more obvious age-related changes [41–43]. Therefore, further study is warranted to precisely assess the age-associated change of lymphocyte composition and function in vivo.

Conclusion

In conclusion, our findings showed that the rates of changes in T (CD4+ and CD8+), B, NK cells and their subsets are highly individualized, exhibiting a wide range regardless of the subject's age and the average trends of the rates of changes were relatively flat over 70 years of adult life. Unexpectedly, we observed significant associations of the serum levels of certain cytokines and cytokine receptors with the rates of change in selected lymphocytes and their subjects. Collectively, our findings provide much needed information of the in vivo changes of lymphocyte compositions and numbers in blood with age, the interrelationship among different type of lymphocytes and their subsets, and potential contributions of serum cytokines/cytokine receptors in these age-associated changes. Future study with a longer time span, samples with multiple time points and assessment with more differentiation markers will further enhance our understanding of how and when the alterations of lymphocyte type, composition, and number occur, and will be essential to better guide clinical interventions such as vaccination with improved precision and efficacy in the elderly.

Acknowledgements
We thank the NIA clinical core lab for collecting blood samples; all BLSA participants in this study, and Annette Ko for making the cluster graph.

Funding
This research work was supported entirely by the Intramural Research Program of the National Institute on Aging, National Institutes of Health (NIH).

Authors' contributions

YL, JK, HY, TT, and AL contributed to this manuscript in designing, conducting experiments, and data analysis. JM performed statistical analysis of the data. NPW and LF supervised the project. NPW and JK wrote the manuscript with approval from all authors. All authors discussed and reviewed the results of the project.

Competing interests

The authors declare that they have no competing interests.

Author details

[1]Laboratory of Molecular Biology & Immunology, National Institute on Aging, 251 Bayview Blvd., Baltimore, MD 21224, USA. [2]Translational Gerontology Branch, National Institute on Aging, National Institutes of Health, Baltimore, MD 21224, USA. [3]Department of Neurology, University of Tennessee Health Science Center, Memphis, TN 38111, USA.

References

1. Frasca D, Riley RL, Blomberg BB. Humoral immune response and B-cell functions including immunoglobulin class switch are downregulated in aged mice and humans. Semin Immunol. 2005;17:378–84.
2. Goronzy JJ, Weyand CM. Understanding immunosenescence to improve responses to vaccines. Nat Immunol. 2013;14:428–36.
3. Weng NP. Aging of the immune system: how much can the adaptive immune system adapt? Immunity. 2006;24:495–9.
4. Le Garff-Tavernier M, Beziat V, Decocq J, Siguret V, Gandjbakhch F, Pautas E, et al. Human NK cells display major phenotypic and functional changes over the life span. Aging Cell. 2010;9:527–35.
5. Sansoni P, Cossarizza A, Brianti V, Fagnoni F, Snelli G, Monti D, et al. Lymphocyte subsets and natural killer cell activity in healthy old people and centenarians. Blood. 1993;82:2767–73.
6. Chong Y, Ikematsu H, Yamaji K, Nishimura M, Nabeshima S, Kashiwagi S, et al. CD27+ (memory) B cell decrease and apoptosis-resistant CD27− (naive) B cell increase in aged humans: implications for age-related peripheral B cell developmental disturbances. Int Immunol. 2005;17:383–90.
7. Colonna-Romano G, Bulati M, Aquino A, Scialabba G, Candore G, Lio D, et al. B cells in the aged: CD27, CD5, and CD40 expression. Mech Ageing Dev. 2003;124:389–93.
8. Fagnoni FF, Vescovini R, Passeri G, Bologna G, Pedrazzoni M, Lavagetto G, et al. Shortage of circulating naive CD8+ T cells provides new insights on immunodeficiency in aging. Blood. 2000;95:2860–8.
9. Kang I, Hong MS, Nolasco H, Park SH, Dan JM, Choi JY, et al. Age-associated change in the frequency of memory CD4+ T cells impairs long term CD4+ T cell responses to influenza vaccine. J Immunol. 2004;173:673–81.
10. Kilpatrick RD, Rickabaugh T, Hultin LE, Hultin P, Hausner MA, Detels R, et al. Homeostasis of the Naive CD4+ T cell compartment during aging. J Immunol. 2008;180:1499–507.
11. Stervbo U, Bozzetti C, Baron U, Jurchott K, Meier S, Malzer JN, et al. Effects of aging on human leukocytes (part II): immunophenotyping of adaptive immune B and T cell subsets. Age (Dordr). 2015;37:93.
12. Lin Y, Damjanovic A, Metter EJ, Nguyen H, Truong T, Najarro K, et al. Age-associated telomere attrition of lymphocytes in vivo is co-ordinated with changes in telomerase activity, composition of lymphocyte subsets and health conditions. Clin Sci (Lond). 2015;128:367–77.
13. Simone R, Zicca A, Saverino D. The frequency of regulatory CD3+CD8+. J Leukoc Biol. 2008;84:1454–61.
14. Trzonkowski P, Szmit E, Mysliwska J, Mysliwski A. CD4+CD25+ T regulatory cells inhibit cytotoxic activity of CTL and NK cells in humans-impact of immunosenescence. Clin Immunol. 2006;119:307–16.
15. Czesnikiewicz-Guzik M, Lee WW, Cui D, Hiruma Y, Lamar DL, Yang ZZ, et al. T cell subset-specific susceptibility to aging. Clin Immunol. 2008;127:107–18.
16. Weng NP, Akbar AN, Goronzy J, CD28(−) T cells: their role in the age-associated decline of immune function. Trends Immunol. 2009;30:306–12.
17. Palmer DB. The effect of age on thymic function. Front Immunol. 2013;4:316.
18. Nikolich-Zugich J. Aging of the T cell compartment in mice and humans: from no naive expectations to foggy memories. J Immunol. 2014;193:2622–9.
19. Jagger A, Shimojima Y, Goronzy JJ, Weyand CM. Regulatory T cells and the immune aging process: a mini-review. Gerontology. 2014;60:130–7.
20. Morbach H, Eichhorn EM, Liese JG, Girschick HJ. Reference values for B cell subpopulations from infancy to adulthood. Clin Exp Immunol. 2010;162: 271–9.
21. Chidrawar SM, Khan N, Chan YL, Nayak L, Moss PA. Ageing is associated with a decline in peripheral blood CD56bright NK cells. Immun Ageing. 2006;3:10.
22. Gayoso I, Sanchez-Correa B, Campos C, Alonso C, Pera A, Casado JG, et al. Immunosenescence of human natural killer cells. J Innate Immun. 2011;3: 337–43.
23. Huppert FA, Pinto EM, Morgan K, Brayne C. Survival in a population sample is predicted by proportions of lymphocyte subsets. Mech Ageing Dev. 2003; 124:449–51.
24. Wikby A, Ferguson F, Forsey R, Thompson J, Strindhall J, Lofgren S, et al. An immune risk phenotype, cognitive impairment, and survival in very late life: impact of allostatic load in Swedish octogenarian and nonagenarian humans. J Gerontol A Biol Sci Med Sci. 2005;60:556–65.
25. Benjamini Y, Hochberg Y. Controlling the false discovery rate: a practical and powerful approach to multiple testing. J R Stat Soc Ser B. 1995;57:289–300.
26. Fahey JL, Schnelle JF, Boscardin J, Thomas JK, Gorre ME, Aziz N, et al. Distinct categories of immunologic changes in frail elderly. Mech Ageing Dev. 2000;115:1–20.
27. Utsuyama M, Hirokawa K, Kurashima C, Fukayama M, Inamatsu T, Suzuki K, et al. Differential age-change in the numbers of CD4+CD45RA+ and CD4+CD29+ T cell subsets in human peripheral blood. Mech Ageing Dev. 1992;63:57–68.
28. den Braber I, Mugwagwa T, Vrisekoop N, Westera L, Mogling R, de Boer AB, et al. Maintenance of peripheral naive T cells is sustained by thymus output in mice but not humans. Immunity. 2012;36:288–97.
29. Wertheimer AM, Bennett MS, Park B, Uhrlaub JL, Martinez C, Pulko V, et al. Aging and cytomegalovirus infection differentially and jointly affect distinct circulating T cell subsets in humans. J Immunol. 2014;192:2143–55.
30. Gregg R, Smith CM, Clark FJ, Dunnion D, Khan N, Chakraverty R, et al. The number of human peripheral blood CD4+ CD25high regulatory T cells increases with age. Clin Exp Immunol. 2005;140:540–6.
31. Cossarizza A, Ortolani C, Paganelli R, Barbieri D, Monti D, Sansoni P, et al. CD45 isoforms expression on CD4+ and CD8+ T cells throughout life, from newborns to centenarians: implications for T cell memory. Mech Ageing Dev. 1996;86:173–95.
32. Rea IM, Stewart M, Campbell P, Alexander HD, Crockard AD, Morris TC. Changes in lymphocyte subsets, interleukin 2, and soluble interleukin 2 receptor in old and very old age. Gerontology. 1996;42:69–78.
33. Provinciali M, Moresi R, Donnini A, Lisa RM. Reference values for CD4+ and CD8+ T lymphocytes with naive or memory phenotype and their association with mortality in the elderly. Gerontology. 2009;55:314–21.
34. Ferguson FG, Wikby A, Maxson P, Olsson J, Johansson B. Immune parameters in a longitudinal study of a very old population of Swedish people: a comparison between survivors and nonsurvivors. J Gerontol A Biol Sci Med Sci. 1995;50:B378–82.
35. Pawelec G, Ouyang Q, Colonna-Romano G, Candore G, Lio D, Caruso C. Is human immunosenescence clinically relevant? Looking for 'immunological risk phenotypes'. Trends Immunol. 2002;23:330–2.
36. Borrego F, Alonso MC, Galiani MD, Carracedo J, Ramirez R, Ostos B, et al. NK phenotypic markers and IL2 response in NK cells from elderly people. Exp Gerontol. 1999;34:253–65.
37. Wikby A, Johansson B, Olsson J, Lofgren S, Nilsson BO, Ferguson F. Expansions of peripheral blood CD8 T-lymphocyte subpopulations and an association with cytomegalovirus seropositivity in the elderly: the Swedish NONA immune study. Exp Gerontol. 2002;37:445–53.
38. Westera L, van Hoeven V, Drylewicz J, Spierenburg G, van Velzen JF, De Boer RJ, et al. Lymphocyte maintenance during healthy aging requires no substantial alterations in cellular turnover. Aging Cell. 2015;14:219–27.
39. Weng NP, Liu K, Catalfamo M, Li Y, Henkart PA. IL-15 is a growth factor and an activator of CD8 memory T cells. Ann N Y Acad Sci. 2002;975:46–56.
40. Patke CL, Shearer WT. gp120- and TNF-alpha-induced modulation of human B cell function: proliferation, cyclic AMP generation, Ig production, and B-cell receptor expression. J Allergy Clin Immunol. 2000;105:975–82.
41. Buffa S, Bulati M, Pellicano M, Dunn-Walters DK, Wu YC, Candore G, et al. B cell immunosenescence: different features of naive and memory B cells in elderly. Biogerontology. 2011;12:473–83.
42. Colonna-Romano G, Bulati M, Aquino A, Pellicano M, Vitello S, Lio D, et al. A double-negative (IgD−CD27−) B cell population is increased in the peripheral blood of elderly people. Mech Ageing Dev. 2009;130:681–90.

14

Human longevity: Genetics or Lifestyle? It takes two to tango

Giuseppe Passarino[*], Francesco De Rango and Alberto Montesanto

Abstract

Healthy aging and longevity in humans are modulated by a lucky combination of genetic and non-genetic factors. Family studies demonstrated that about 25 % of the variation in human longevity is due to genetic factors. The search for genetic and molecular basis of aging has led to the identification of genes correlated with the maintenance of the cell and of its basic metabolism as the main genetic factors affecting the individual variation of the aging phenotype. In addition, studies on calorie restriction and on the variability of genes associated with nutrient-sensing signaling, have shown that ipocaloric diet and/or a genetically efficient metabolism of nutrients, can modulate lifespan by promoting an efficient maintenance of the cell and of the organism. Recently, epigenetic studies have shown that epigenetic modifications, modulated by both genetic background and lifestyle, are very sensitive to the aging process and can either be a biomarker of the quality of aging or influence the rate and the quality of aging.

On the whole, current studies are showing that interventions modulating the interaction between genetic background and environment is essential to determine the individual chance to attain longevity.

Keywords: Human longevity, Genetics of aging, Calorie restriction

Background

The research on aging, and in particular the search for the determinants of successful aging and longevity, has been continuously growing in the last decades also due to the social and medical burden correlated to the continuous increase of lifespan in western countries and the consequent grow of the elderly population. One of the main questions in this field is the correlation between the genetic background and lifestyle in determining the individual chance of a delayed aging (possibly without age-related diseases and disabilities) and longevity. The results obtained by biogerontologists in these years, which highlighted most of the biological and biochemical mechanisms involved in the aging process, allowed to better understand such correlation. This has brought to elaborate important strategies focused on possible interventions to improve lifestyle in order to increase the chance to attain longevity by modulating the basic molecular mechanisms of aging.

The genetics of aging

Before the 1990ies it was largely spread the idea that aging is ineluctable and that genetics does not control it. It was important, in this view, the idea that aging occurs after reproduction, and then there is no need, but also no opportunity, for selection to act on genes that are expressed during this late period of life [1].

The researcher who pioneered the genetics of aging and longevity was Tom Johnson, who studied groups of *C. elegans* where he was able to separate long living individuals from short living subjects. The analysis of hybrids obtained from different strains of *C. elegans,* allowed to estimate that the heritability of life-span was between 20 and 50 % [2, 3]. Subsequently, he started the analysis of different mutants and, with M. Klass, found a number of mutants with longer lifespan. Subsequently, Tom Johnson found out that most of the mutants with long lifespan had mutations in the *age1* gene [4]. This gene turned out to be the catalytic subunit of class-I phosphatidylinositol 3-kinase (PI3K).

The studies of Johnson clearly demonstrated that genetic variability could indeed affect lifespan. This triggered many studies in model organisms in order to disentangle the different biochemical pathways which

* Correspondence: g.passarino@unical.it

Department of Biology, Ecology and Earth Science, University of Calabria, 87036 Rende, Italy

could affect lifespan, and to highlight the genes coding for the proteins involved in such pathways. In particular, yeast, C. elegans, drosophila and mice were analyzed and this highlighted numerous genes which could affect lifespan if mutated (for an updated list of these genes see http://genomics.senescence.info/genes/models.html).

Most of these genes are related to the maintenance of the integrity of the cell (especially the integrity of DNA). In C. elegans, however, some of the main genes which have been found to modulate lifespan (daf2, daf16) are related to the ability to enter the dauer status [5, 6], that is a quiescent status (usually entered in case of nutrient deprivation) with a minimum energy expense, which causes an arrest of the reproduction process and allows the organism to live longer "expecting" for the availability of nutrients. This suggested that longevity can be attained by means of an efficient maintenance of the cell but also by diverting resources from reproduction to self maintenance, in line with previous findings that dietary restriction can extend lifespan. After the characterization of these genes in C. elegans, it was found that in mice the ortholog of daf16 (FOXO) could affect lifespan. In mammals, FOXO is correlated to the Insulin/IGF1 axis which is stimulated by nutrient availability and, through FOXO, promotes protein synthesis [7–11].

It is of note that some Authors suggested these molecular mechanisms modulating lifespan could be due to a pleiotropic effect of genes which have evolved for different purposes (such as the genes in the IGF-1 pathway which have evolved to face presence/absence of nutrients) but can, ultimately affect lifespan; others proposed that some genes may have evolved to program aging and avoid "immortality", as this would hamper the continuous substitution of old subjects with new, younger, ones [12, 13].

It was obviously inevitable that the research of the genetic basis of longevity turned to human beings and investigated whether the common genetic variability of human populations could affect inter individual differences in lifespan but also whether the genes found to prolong lifespan in model organisms, on turn, were correlated to human lifespan.

As to the first question (does common genetic variability affect lifespan, and in particular does it affect longevity?), this has been studied by two approaches. The first one was the reconstruction of the sibships of long-lived subjects [14, 15] and the comparison of their survival curves with those of the birth cohorts born in the same geographical area. This approach demonstrated that brothers and sisters of the long-lived subjects had a clear survival advantage (at any age) with respect to the general population. The second approach, with intrafamily controls, was started in order to distinguish the genetic from the "familiar" effect. Montesanto et al. [15] compared the survival function of brothers of centenarians with those

estimated for their brothers in law, that is with the men who married their sisters; these men were supposed to share with the brothers of the long lived subjects the familiar environment. By using this second approach, it has been found that the survival advantage of siblings of long-lived subjects was not completely shared by their brothers in law, despite they shared the same environment for most of their life. This suggested that beyond the family environment, there are genetic factors influencing survival and, consequently, lifespan. Interestingly, in this study, the survival curve of the sisters of long-lived subjects did not differ from the one of sisters in law, suggesting that the genetic component does explain lifespan in men more than in women. The genetic component of lifespan in humans has also been analyzed by comparing the age of death of monozygotic and dizygotic twins. This has allowed to estimate that about 25 % of the variation in human longevity can be due to genetic factors and indicated that this component is higher at older ages and is more important in males than in females [16–18].

In parallel to these studies, many researches have been carried out to search the genetic variants responsible of modulating human longevity. Most of them were carried out by a case/control approach, by comparing the frequency of specific polymorphisms in long-lived subjects and in younger geographically matched controls. The rationale of this study design is that as the population ages, alleles favorable for survival will be present at higher frequency among long-living people, while unfavorable alleles will be eliminated [19–21]. The candidate genes analyzed by this approach were either genes involved in age-related diseases (such as APOE, which had been observed to be involved in the predisposition to Alzheimer Disease and other age-related cognitive impairments), or genes implicated in pathways related to longevity in studies with model organisms (IGF-1, FOXO, Sirtuins) [22–25]. This study design has indeed led to find numerous polymorphic genes the variability of which affects longevity. However, each of these polymorphisms turned out to explain only a very small fraction of the longevity variability. Indeed high-throughput Genome-wide analyses, which have recently been carried out have identified many genes positively associated with longevity but only a very few ones could hold multiple test significance and successfully replicated in different studies and across different populations [26–29]. Population stratification and inadequate sample sizes are among the main plausible explanations [30]. The adoption of innovative study design and the development of new statistical and computational tools for effective processing of genetic data arising from high-throughput DNA technologies will help to better understand the complex genetic architecture underlying human longevity [31, 32].

A new way of looking at the genetic data has been proposed by Raule et al. [33] who analyzed the complete sequences of mitochondrial DNA from long-lived subjects coming from different areas of Europe. The availability of complete sequences allowed to evaluate for the first time the cumulative effects of specific, concomitant mitochondrial DNA (mtDNA) mutations, including those that *per se* have a low, or very low, impact. The analysis indicated that the presence of single mutations on mtDNA complex I may be beneficial for longevity, while the co-occurrence of mutations on both complexes I and III or on both I and V might lower the individual's chances for longevity. Previous analyses on single mutations falling on complex I (either specific mutations or mutations defining groups of haplotypes) had given contrasting results, showing association with longevity in some cases but not in others. It is likely that positive results were obtained in populations were mutations on complex I were not associated with mutations on complex III or V, while negative results were obtained in populations with high prevalence of mtDNA haplotypes carrying mutations on complex I in association with mutations in complex III and V. This approach confirmed that most of the genetic variants have a very limited effect on longevity, and that only their cumulative effect can give a consistent appreciable effect and suggests that a limit of previous analyses has been to search for single mutations instead of cumulative effects. On the other hand, it is very difficult to think of using such approach, which has been successful for mitochondrial DNA, on genomic DNA unless small fractions (or specific regions harboring genes involved in relevant pathways) are analyzed.

On the whole, the genetic association studies suggested that, also in humans, mutations in genes correlated with the maintenance of the cell and of its basic metabolism are essential in modulating lifespan. Indeed, genes involved in DNA repair [34], telomere conservation [35–37], heat shock response [38, 39], and the management of free radicals' levels [33, 40] were found to contribute to longevity or, in case of reduced functionality, to accelerated senescence (cellular aging) and the consequent organism aging. In addition, as suggested by the studies in mice, the pathways involved in nutrient-sensing signaling and in regulating transcription, such as IGF-1/insulin axis [41] and TOR (target of rapamycin) [42] showed to be involved in modulating human longevity. Besides these genes involved in cellular maintenance/metabolism and senescence, concurrent efforts, especially from clinical studies, also showed that genes implicated in important organismal process may have a strong impact on aging and longevity. For instance genes involved in lipoprotein metabolism (especially APOE), cardiovascular homeostasis, immunity, and inflammation

have been found to play an important role in aging, age-related disorders, and organism longevity [43–46].

Human longevity and life style

Life expectancy at birth has been increasing for most of the last century in western societies, thanks to the continuous amelioration of medical assistance, to the improvement of the environment (in particular clean, safe water and food), and to the improvement of nutrients. For instance, in Italy life expectancy went from 29 years in 1861 to 82 in 2011 (Table 1 reports the evolution of this data in women and men). Similarly, the extreme longevity has been growing in these years. Indeed, the number of centenarians (still in Italy) remarkably increased from 165 in 1951 to more than 15000 in 2011. These results have been attained first by a dramatic reduction of infectious diseases, which, on turn, has dramatically reduced infantile mortality, but also mortality in adult age. In fact, in 2011 less than 10 % of deaths occurred in subjects under 60 years of age, while the corresponding figures were 74 % in 1872, 56 % in 1901 and 25 % in 1951. However, in the last decades, the continuous extension of lifespan was mainly due to the improvement of medical assistance with respect to age-related diseases, especially Cardiovascular Diseases and Cancer, which allowed to increase lifespan of 5 years in the last 2 decades and of 2 years in the last 10 years (data from www.mortality.org and www.istat.it).

These data clearly show that environmental factors have a very strong impact on lifespan and on longevity in humans. However, the extension of lifespan that there has been in the last decades have not been accompanied

Table 1 Evolution of lifespan expectancy in Italy from 1861

Year	Male	Female	Total
1861	28	29	29
1871	30	31	30
1881	35	35	35
1891	38	39	38
1901	43	43	43
1911	46	46	46
1921	48	50	49
1931	53	56	55
1941	55	58	56
1951	63	67	65
1961	67	72	69
1971	69	75	72
1981	71	78	75
1991	74	80	77
2001	77	83	80
2011	79	84	82

by a similar extension of healthy lifespan. Indeed, in most cases this lifespan extension is due to the chronicit of the age-related diseases. This has brought the community of biogerontologists to study interventions, possibly modulated on the knowledge emerged from the studies on the genetic and biomolecular basis of longevity, to extend not only lifespan but also healthy lifespan, or, with a new word, "healthspan". In fact, model organisms with mutations that extend lifespan have a healthy life also when they are old. This suggested that health span extension could be attained by targeting (stimulating or silencing) the genes, which had been highlighted to be involved in life extension in both model organisms and humans [47]. In support of this hypothesis, it has been reported that dietary restricted mice, which live much longer and show a very delayed aging phenotype than mice fed *at libitum*, at old age have an expression pattern very different from mice of the same age for a number of genes correlated with life extension, such as those related to DNA repair, stress response, immune response and others [48, 49]. Thus, dietary restriction can trigger a molecular-genetic response which postpones aging and age-related phenotypes. This has brought to search for drugs or interventions which may act on these mechanisms without the side effects of calorie restriction. Among the most important interventions which have been considered in this context, we may name the protein restriction, the use of drugs targeting different genes of IGF-1 axis or of the FOXO/TOR pathway [47]. In addition, these studies have allowed to reconsider previous data on some areas characterized by exceptional longevity (such as Okinawa, Sardinia and Calabria) which are characterized by traditional ipoproteic diets, such as the "Mediterranean diet" [50–53]. In these cases, then, the environment, that is the traditional diet, has allowed to stimulate the molecular mechanisms which can increase life span.

Among the several changes that occur with the aging process, in the last decade Epigenomics has attracted the interest of many researchers. This was mainly due to the fact that epigenetic modifications summarizing, at least in part, the interaction between the individual genetic background and lifestyle characteristics, should be potentially able to capture part of the unexplained susceptibility observed today for complex diseases (the so-called missing heritability problem).

Starting from the pioneeristic observations that epigenetic modifications affect not only the aging process but also its quality (successful aging) [54], EpiGenome-Wide Association Studies identified hundreds of sites spread along the entire genome in which methylation levels change between oldest old and younger subjects. In particular, Horwat and co-workers, on the basis of the methylation levels of 353 CpG units, formulated a mathematical model, the so-called epigenetic clock, that showed some important properties [55]. First, it was able to predict the chronological age of a subject starting from the methylation level of several cells and tissues of his body. Second, it represents one of the most accurate biomarker of age (also superior to the estimates obtained from the telomere length). Third, using methylation levels of blood and brain tissues from subjects affected by Down syndrome, it showed that an accelerated aging occur in such a syndrome [56]. Fourth, it was able to predict all-cause mortality also after adjusting for traditional risk factors [57]. Finally, when it was used to estimate the biological age of several tissues from supercentenarians, it has been demonstrated that brain and muscle represent the youngest tissues of these exceptional individuals [58].

However, even if the cause-effect relationship between methylation process and aging is still not clear, the potential applications of this discovery are very wide, ranging from detailed monitoring of changes occurring with age within individual systems or organs (muscle, brain, etc.) to forensic purposes. For this and several other reasons, future advances in this field could help the understanding of the complex physiology of aging, lifespan and age-associated diseases.

Conclusions

On the whole, although the common variability accounts for only 25 % of human lifespan variability, the knowledge of the genetic basis modulating longevity may give significant hints on modulating lifestyle in order to attain longevity and extend healthspan. That is, a few subjects can attain longevity because a lucky combination of polymorphisms which allow them to have an efficient metabolism or an efficient response to different stress. Most of the others can attain a similar result by targeting the same pathways with appropriate life style or interventions. In this context, the importance of epigenetic factors, both as biomarkers of aging and target of interventions will certainly grow in the forthcoming future.

Abbreviations

APOE: apolipoprotein E; FOXO: forkhead box O; IGF-1: insulin-like growth factor 1; mtDNA: mitochondrial DNA; PI3K: phosphatidylinositol-3-kinase; TOR: target of rapamycin.

Competing interests

The authors declare that they have no competing interests.

Authors' contributions

The authors equally contributed to the drafting and finalization of the manuscript. All authors read and approved the final manuscript.

Acknowledgements

This work was partially supported by the European Union's Seventh Framework Programme (FP7/2007–2011) [grant number 259679] and by funds from Programma Operativo Nazionale [01_00937] - MIUR"Modelli sperimentali biotecnologici integrati per lo sviluppo e la selezione di molecole di interesse per la salute dell'uomo".

References

1. Johnson TE. A personal retrospective on the genetics of aging. Biogerontology. 2002;3(1–2):7–12.

2. Johnson TE, Wood WB. Genetic analysis of life-span in Caenorhabditis elegans. Proc Natl Acad Sci USA. 1982;79(21):6603–7.

3. Johnson TE. Aging can be genetically dissected into component processes using long-lived lines of Caenorhabditis elegans. Proc Natl Acad Sci USA. 1987;84(11):3777–81.

4. Friedman DB, Johnson TE. Three mutants that extend both mean and maximum life span of the nematode, Caenorhabditis elegans, define the age-1 gene. J Gerontol. 1988;43(4):B102–9.

5. Kenyon C, Chang J, Gensch E, Rudner A, Tabtiang R. A C. elegans mutant that lives twice as long as wild type. Nature. 1993;366(6454):461–4. doi:10.1038/366461a0.

6. Gottlieb S, Ruvkun G. daf-2, daf-16 and daf-23: genetically interacting genes controlling Dauer formation in Caenorhabditis elegans. Genetics. 1994; 137(1):107–20.

7. Taguchi A, Wartschow LM, White MF. Brain IRS2 signaling coordinates life span and nutrient homeostasis. Science. 2007;317(5836):369–72. doi:10.1126/science.1142179.

8. Lin K, Dorman JB, Rodan A, Kenyon C. daf-16: An HNF-3/forkhead family member that can function to double the life-span of Caenorhabditis elegans. Science. 1997;278(5341):1319–22.

9. Ogg S, Paradis S, Gottlieb S, Patterson GI, Lee L, Tissenbaum HA, et al. The Fork head transcription factor DAF-16 transduces insulin-like metabolic and longevity signals in C. elegans. Nature. 1997;389(6654):994–9. doi:10.1038/40194.

10. Kenyon C. The plasticity of aging: insights from long-lived mutants. Cell. 2005;120(4):449–60. doi:10.1016/j.cell.2005.02.002.

11. Kenyon CJ. The genetics of ageing. Nature. 2010;464(7288):504–12. doi:10.1038/nature08980.

12. Rose G, Passarino G, Franceschi C, De Benedictis G. The variability of the mitochondrial genome in human aging: a key for life and death? Int J Biochem Cell Biol. 2002;34(11):1449–60.

13. Skulachev VP. The programmed death phenomena, aging, and the Samurai law of biology. Exp Gerontol. 2001;36(7):995–1024.

14. Schoenmaker M, de Craen AJ, de Meijer PH, Beekman M, Blauw GJ, Slagboom PE, et al. Evidence of genetic enrichment for exceptional survival using a family approach: the Leiden Longevity Study. Eur J Human Genet EJHG. 2006;14(1):79–84. doi:10.1038/sj.ejhg.5201508.

15. Montesanto A, Latorre V, Giordano M, Martino C, Domma F, Passarino G. The genetic component of human longevity: analysis of the survival advantage of parents and siblings of Italian nonagenarians. Eur J Human Genet EJHG. 2011;19(8):882–6. doi:10.1038/ejhg.2011.40.

16. vB Hjelmborg J, Iachine I, Skytthe A, Vaupel JW, McGue M, Koskenvuo M, Kaprio J, Pedersen NL, Christensen K. Genetic influence on human lifespan and longevity. Hum Genet. 2006;119(3):312–21.

17. Herskind AM, McGue M, Holm NV, Sorensen TI, Harvald B, Vaupel JW. The heritability of human longevity: a population-based study of 2872 Danish twin pairs born 1870–1900. Hum Genet. 1996;97(3):319–23.

18. Skytthe A, Pedersen NL, Kaprio J, Stazi MA, Hjelmborg JV, Iachine I, et al. Longevity studies in GenomEUtwin. Twin Res Off J Int Soc Twin Studies. 2003;6(5):448–54. doi:10.1375/136905203770326457.

19. Capri M, Salvioli S, Sevini F, Valensin S, Celani L, Monti D, et al. The genetics of human longevity. Ann N Y Acad Sci. 2006;1067:252–63. doi:10.1196/annals.1354.033.

20. Passarino G, Montesanto A, Dato S, Giordano S, Domma F, Mari V, et al. Sex and age specificity of susceptibility genes modulating survival at old age. Hum Hered. 2006;62(4):213–20. doi:10.1159/000097305.

21. Perls TT, Wilmoth J, Levenson R, Drinkwater M, Cohen M, Bogan H, et al. Life-long sustained mortality advantage of siblings of centenarians. Proc Natl Acad Sci U S A. 2002;99(12):8442–7. doi:10.1073/pnas.122587599.

22. Pawlikowska L, Hu D, Huntsman S, Sung A, Chu C, Chen J, et al. Association of common genetic variation in the insulin/IGF1 signaling pathway with human longevity. Aging Cell. 2009;8(4):460–72. doi:10.1111/j.1474-9726. 2009.00493.x.

23. Ziv E, Hu D. Genetic variation in insulin/IGF-1 signaling pathways and longevity. Ageing Res Rev. 2011;10(2):201–4. doi:10.1016/j.arr.2010.09.002.

24. Morris BJ, Willcox DC, Donlon TA, Willcox BJ. FOXO3: A Major Gene for Human Longevity - A Mini-Review. Gerontology. 2015. doi:10.1159/000375235.

25. Bellizzi D, Rose G, Cavalcante P, Covello G, Dato S, De Rango F, et al. A novel VNTR enhancer within the SIRT3 gene, a human homologue of SIR2, is associated with survival at oldest ages. Genomics. 2005;85(2):258–63. doi:10.1016/j.ygeno.2004.11.003.

26. Sebastiani P, Solovieff N, Dewan AT, Walsh KM, Puca A, Hartley SW, et al. Genetic signatures of exceptional longevity in humans. PLoS One. 2012;7(1): e29848. doi:10.1371/journal.pone.0029848.

27. Beekman M, Blanche H, Perola M, Hervonen A, Bezrukov V, Sikora E, et al. Genome-wide linkage analysis for human longevity: Genetics of Healthy Aging Study. Aging Cell. 2013;12(2):184–93. doi:10.1111/acel.12039.

28. Hindorff LA, Sethupathy P, Junkins HA, Ramos EM, Mehta JP, Collins FS, et al. Potential etiologic and functional implications of genome-wide association loci for human diseases and traits. Proc Natl Acad Sci USA. 2009; 106(23):9362–7. doi:10.1073/pnas.0903103106.

29. Deelen J, Beekman M, Uh HW, Broer L, Ayers KL, Tan Q, et al. Genome-wide association meta-analysis of human longevity identifies a novel locus conferring survival beyond 90 years of age. Hum Mol Genet. 2014;23(16): 4420–32. doi:10.1093/hmg/ddu139.

30. Novelli V, Viviani Anselmi C, Roncarati R, Guffanti G, Malovini A, Piluso G, et al. Lack of replication of genetic associations with human longevity. Biogerontology. 2008;9(2):85–92. doi:10.1007/s10522-007-9116-4.

31. Ferrario A, Villa F, Malovini A, Araniti F, Puca AA. The application of genetics approaches to the study of exceptional longevity in humans: potential and limitations. Immun Ageing. 2012;9(1):7. doi:10.1186/1742-4933-9-7.

32. Villa F, Carrizzo A, Spinelli CC, Ferrario A, Malovini A, Maciąg A, et al. Genetic Analysis Reveals a Longevity-Associated Protein Modulating Endothelial Function and Angiogenesis. Circ Res. 2015;117(4):333–45. doi:10.1161/CIRCRESAHA.117.305875.

33. Raule N, Sevini F, Li S, Barbieri A, Tallaro F, Lomartire L, et al. The co-occurrence of mtDNA mutations on different oxidative phosphorylation subunits, not detected by haplogroup analysis, affects human longevity and is population specific. Aging Cell. 2014;13(3):401–7. doi:10.1111/acel.12186.

34. Debrabant B, Soerensen M, Flachsbart F, Dato S, Mengel-From J, Stevnsner T, et al. Human longevity and variation in DNA damage response and repair: study of the contribution of sub-processes using competitive gene-set analysis. Eur J Human Genet EJHG. 2014;22(9):1131–6. doi:10.1038/ejhg.2013.299.

35. Soerensen M, Thinggaard M, Nygaard M, Dato S, Tan Q, Hjelmborg J, et al. Genetic variation in TERT and TERC and human leukocyte telomere length and longevity: a cross-sectional and longitudinal analysis. Aging Cell. 2012; 11(2):223–7. doi:10.1111/j.1474-9726.2011.00775.x.

36. Crocco P, Barale R, Rose G, Rizzato C, Santoro A, De Rango F, et al. Population-specific association of genes for telomere-associated proteins with longevity in an Italian population. Biogerontology. 2015;16(3):353–64. doi:10.1007/s10522-015-9551-6.

37. Atzmon G, Cho M, Cawthon RM, Budagov T, Katz M, Yang X, et al. Evolution in health and medicine Sackler colloquium: Genetic variation in human telomerase is associated with telomere length in Ashkenazi centenarians. Proc Natl Acad Sci U S A. 2010;107 Suppl 1:1710–7. doi:10.1073/pnas.0906191106.

38. Altomare K, Greco V, Bellizzi D, Berardelli M, Dato S, DeRango F, et al. The allele (A)(−110) in the promoter region of the HSP70-1 gene is unfavorable to longevity in women. Biogerontology. 2003;4(4):215–20.

39. Ross OA, Curran MD, Crum KA, Rea IM, Barnett YA, Middleton D. Increased frequency of the 2437 T allele of the heat shock protein 70-Hom gene in an aged Irish population. Exp Gerontol. 2003;38(5):561–5.

40. Rose G, Crocco P, De Rango F, Montesanto A, Passarino G. Further support to the uncoupling-to-survive theory: the genetic variation of human UCP genes is associated with longevity. PLoS One. 2011;6(12):e29650. doi:10.1371/journal.pone.0029650.

41. Junnila RK, List EO, Berryman DE, Murrey JW, Kopchick JJ. The GH/IGF-1 axis in ageing and longevity. Nat Rev Endocrinol. 2013;9(6):366–76. doi:10.1038/nrendo.2013.67.

42. Johnson SC, Rabinovitch PS, Kaeberlein M. mTOR is a key modulator of ageing and age-related disease. Nature. 2013;493(7432):338–45. doi:10.1038/nature11861.

43. Schachter F, Faure-Delanef L, Guenot F, Rouger H, Froguel P, Lesueur-Ginot L, et al. Genetic associations with human longevity at the APOE and ACE loci. Nat Genet. 1994;6(1):29–32. doi:10.1038/ng0194-29.

44. Garasto S, Berardelli M, DeRango F, Mari V, Feraco E, De Benedictis G. A study of the average effect of the 3′APOB-VNTR polymorphism on lipidemic

parameters could explain why the short alleles (<35 repeats) are rare in centenarians. BMC Med Genet. 2004;5:3. doi:10.1186/1471-2350-5-3.

45. Cardelli M, Cavallone L, Marchegiani F, Oliveri F, Dato S, Montesanto A, et al. A genetic-demographic approach reveals male-specific association between survival and tumor necrosis factor (A/G)-308 polymorphism. J Gerontol A Biol Sci Med Sci. 2008;63(5):454–60.

46. Di Bona D, Vasto S, Capurso C, Christiansen L, Deiana L, Franceschi C, et al. Effect of interleukin-6 polymorphisms on human longevity: a systematic review and meta-analysis. Ageing Res Rev. 2009;8(1):36–42. doi:10.1016/j.arr.2008.09.001.

47. Longo VD, Antebi A, Bartke A, Barzilai N, Brown-Borg HM, Caruso C, et al. Interventions to Slow Aging in Humans: Are We Ready? Aging Cell. 2015; 14(4):497–510. doi:10.1111/acel.12338.

48. Prolla TA, Mattson MP. Molecular mechanisms of brain aging and neurodegenerative disorders: lessons from dietary restriction. Trends Neurosci. 2001;24(11 Suppl):S21–31.

49. Ghosh S, Wanders D, Stone KP, Van NT, Cortez CC, Gettys TW. A systems biology analysis of the unique and overlapping transcriptional responses to caloric restriction and dietary methionine restriction in rats. FASEB J Off Publication Federation Am Soc Exp Biol. 2014;28(6):2577–90. doi:10.1096/fj.14-249458.

50. Willcox DC, Willcox BJ, Todoriki H, Suzuki M. The Okinawan diet: health implications of a low-calorie, nutrient-dense, antioxidant-rich dietary pattern low in glycemic load. J Am Coll Nutr. 2009;28(Suppl):500S–16S.

51. Poulain M, Pes GM, Grasland C, Carru C, Ferrucci L, Baggio G, et al. Identification of a geographic area characterized by extreme longevity in the Sardinia island: the AKEA study. Exp Gerontol. 2004;39(9):1423–9. doi:10.1016/j.exger.2004.06.016.

52. Pes GM, Tolu F, Dore MP, Sechi GP, Errigo A, Canelada A, et al. Male longevity in Sardinia, a review of historical sources supporting a causal link with dietary factors. Eur J Clin Nutr. 2015;69(4):411–8. doi:10.1038/ejcn.2014.230.

53. Montesanto A, Passarino G, Senatore A, Carotenuto L, De Benedictis G. Spatial analysis and surname analysis: complementary tools for shedding light on human longevity patterns. Ann Hum Genet. 2008;72(Pt 2):253–60. doi:10.1111/j.1469-1809.2007.00405.x.

54. Bellizzi D, D'Aquila P, Montesanto A, Corsonello A, Mari V, Mazzei B, et al. Global DNA methylation in old subjects is correlated with frailty. Age. 2012; 34(1):169–79. doi:10.1007/s11357-011-9216-6.

55. Horvath S. DNA methylation age of human tissues and cell types. Genome Biol. 2013;14(10):R115. doi:10.1186/gb-2013-14-10-r115.

56. Horvath S, Garagnani P, Bacalini MG, Pirazzini C, Salvioli S, Gentilini D, et al. Accelerated epigenetic aging in Down syndrome. Aging Cell. 2015;14(3): 491–5. doi:10.1111/acel.12325.

57. Marioni RE, Shah S, McRae AF, Chen BH, Colicino E, Harris SE, et al. DNA methylation age of blood predicts all-cause mortality in later life. Genome Biol. 2015;16:25. doi:10.1186/s13059-015-0584-6.

58. Horvath S, Mah V, Lu AT, Woo JS, Choi OW, Jasinska AJ, et al. The cerebellum ages slowly according to the epigenetic clock. Aging. 2015;7(5): 294–306.

15

Transcriptomic evidence of a para-inflammatory state in the middle aged lumbar spinal cord

William Galbavy, Yong Lu, Martin Kaczocha, Michelino Puopolo, Lixin Liu and Mario J. Rebecchi[*]

Abstract

Background: We have previously reported elevated expression of multiple pro-inflammatory markers in the lumbar spinal cord (LSC) of middle-aged male rats compared to young adults suggesting a para-inflammatory state develops in the LSC by middle age, a time that in humans is associated with the greatest pain prevalence and persistence. The goal of the current study was to examine the transcriptome-wide gene expression differences between young and middle aged LSC.

Methods: Young (3 month) and middle-aged (17 month) naïve Fisher 344 rats ($n = 5$ per group) were euthanized, perfused with heparinized saline, and the LSC were removed.

Results: ~70% of 31,000 coding sequences were detected. After normalization, ~ 1100 showed statistically significant differential expression. Of these genes, 353 middle-aged annotated genes differed by > 1.5 fold compared to the young group. Nearly 10% of these genes belonged to the microglial sensome. Analysis of this subset revealed that the principal age-related differential pathways populated are complement, pattern recognition receptors, OX40, and various T cell regulatory pathways consistent with microglial priming and T cell invasion and modulation. Many of these pathways substantially overlap those previously identified in studies of LSC of young animals with chronic inflammatory or neuropathic pain.

Conclusions: Up-modulation of complement pathway, microglial priming and activation, and T cell/antigen-presenting cell communication in healthy middle-aged LSC was found. Taken together with our previous work, the results support our conclusion that an incipient or para-inflammatory state develops in the LSC in healthy middle-aged adults.

Keywords: Transcriptome, Aging, Spinal cord, Microglia, Neuropathic, Complement, T-cell, Inflammation

Background

Numerous studies have documented age-related inflammatory marker expression in the central nervous system (CNS), particularly of pro-inflammatory cytokines interleukin 1β (IL1β), tumor necrosis factor α (TNFα) and IL6, as well as microglial activation markers Cd11b (C3A receptor) and MHCII and the astrogliosis marker glial fibrillary acidic protein (GFAP) in various brain regions of healthy animals, including rats, mice, primates and in post-mortem human samples [1–4]. Challenging the senescent CNS with stimuli that mimic infection or stress, such as LPS, induce exaggerated neuroinflammatory

responses [4, 5]. These results suggested a pre-existing incipient or para-inflammatory state that predisposes the CNS to deleterious neurotoxic response in older animals and humans, and have led to the idea that the CNS undergoes a process of "inflammaging", with important implications for neurodegenerative disorders, such as Alzheimer's dementia and Parkinson's disease [2, 6, 7].

While the effects of aging on inflammatory marker expression in various brain regions are well established, few studies have examined the spinal cord, particularly of animals corresponding to middle-age, a time when chronic pain incidence and persistence reach a maximum in the human populations [8–13]. We have recently demonstrated that changes in expression patterns of inflammatory markers indicate that a para-inflammatory state in the

* Correspondence: mario.rebecchi@stonybrookmedicine.edu
Department of Anesthesiology, School of Medicine, Health Sciences Center L4, Stony Brook University, Stony Brook, New York 11794-8480, USA

lumbar spinal cords (LSC) arises by middle age in healthy rats [14]. This is accompanied by remarkable changes in dorsal horn microglial morphology rarely seen in young adult LSC, that indicated activated M1 and M2 morphologies (shortened, thickened processes, decreased arborization, and hypertrophic cell bodies). In the present study we compared the transcriptomic expression of whole lumbar spinal cords of healthy middle-aged male rats to those of young adults. The results provide further support for a para-inflammatory status in the LSC by middle age and point to development of microglial states previously associated with establishment of neuropathic or inflammatory pain.

Methods

Perfusion, tissue harvesting, RNA extraction and purification

All work conformed to the National Institutes of Health Guidelines for the Care and Use of Laboratory Animals and were approved by the Stony Brook University Institutional Animal Care and Use Committee and conducted under protocol #203692-23. Three-month and 17-month old Fisher 344 rats were were euthanized and transcardially perfused with heparinized saline-buffered with 5 mM H_2NaPO_4 to pH 7. LSC were rapidly removed and immediately frozen on dry ice and stored at -80 °C. Total RNAs were extracted from LSC using Qiazol extraction, and further purified with RNeasy spin columns following the manufacturer's directions and as described previously [14]. Briefly, frozen tissues were placed on ice, Qiazol lysis reagent (Qiagen) was added immediately along with three or six 2.3 mm silica/zirconia beads (DRG and LSC, respectively), and homogenized in a BioSpec mini bead beater for 1.5 min and allowed to stand on ice for 5 min. Chloroform was added to comprise 1/5 of the total volume, and samples were mixed vigorously for 2 min and allowed to settle for 2 min before being centrifuged at 12,000 X g for 15 min at 4 °C. The upper aqueous phase was saved, mixed 1:1 with 70% ethanol, and subjected to RNeasy spin column purification (Qiagen). Final concentrations and 230/260/280 ratios were determined by nanodrop absorbancy using an Eppendorf BioSpectrometer.

Transcriptomic analysis

The RNA's were reversed transcribed, and then, using an in vitro transcription reaction, biotinylated nucleotides were incorporated, converting the cDNA to labeled cRNA. The cRNA pool was purified, fragmented and then hybridized to Rat Genome 230 2.0 arrays (Affymetrix) displaying over 31,000 probe sets, representing 30,000 transcripts and variants from over 28,000 well-substantiated rat genes. Hybridized chips were washed, incubated with fluorescently labeled streptavidin probe,

laser scanned and probe fluorescence intensities were measured. Quality control analysis was performed using the affyQCReport package in Bioconductor. CEL files were quantified and normalized using GenePattern ExpressionFileCreator function at the setting of RMA method and quantile normalization. The relation of samples was displayed in dendrogram that was generated by hclust package in Bioconductor. Comparison of samples was conducted using R statistical project. The FDR values were calculated using the samr package in Bioconductor. The normalized data were then subjected to t-testing with FDR = 10%. Annotation of probe sets was based on Affymetrix Rat230_2.na34 release.

qPCR Analysis

Primers were designed with Primer3 and synthesized by Eurofins MWG Operon LLC (Louisville, KY, USA). The primer pairs used in the qPCR reactions are listed in Additional file 1. cDNA was synthesized with Quanti-Tect Reverse Transcription Kit (Qiagen, Germantown, MD, USA) using the same mRNA that were used in the microarray measurements. qPCR analysis was performed on an Step-One Plus qPCR equipment (Applied BioSystems), using the Quantitect SYBR Green Kit (Qiagen). PCR reactions were followed by melt curve analysis. For data analysis, ΔC_t were acquired by subtracting the C_t values of the genes of interest from the C_t of a reference gene (GAPDH) of the corresponding samples. The ΔC_t's for the young and middle-aged groups were subjected to t-testing (one-tailed). Adjusted p value for multiple comparisons was carried out with R using the method of Benjamini and Hochberg [15].

Pathway analysis

The differential expression gene set was subjected to Pathway analysis using IPA software suite. Three hundred fifty three differentially expressed, annotated genes that were increased or decreased significantly were imported and analyzed using Canonical pathways. Adjusted p values were obtained from a modified Fisher test [15] that compared the ratio of differential gene set to number of pathway members obtained to the probability that such a ratio would be found by chance, after correcting for multiple hypothesis testing.

Results

Transcriptomic expression patterns were determined in LSC from young (3 month) and middle-aged (17 month) male Fisher 344 rats. Of the 28,000 genes probed, over 1,100 showed significant differential expression (Fig. 1). Five hundred twenty eight genes increased or decreased at least 1.5 fold in middle age (Additional file 2). Of these, 353 unique well-annotated genes were subjected to further analyses (Additional file 3). Table 1 lists

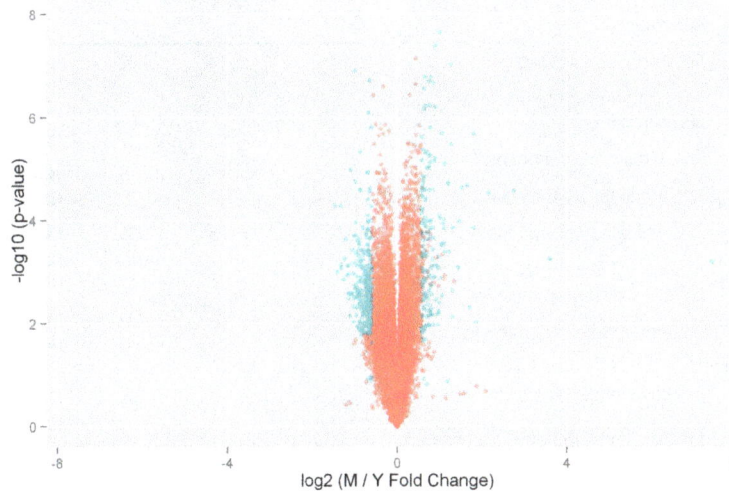

Fig. 1 Transcript expression ratio's in middle-aged compared to young LSC. The mRNA transcript expression in the LSC of 3 month and 17-month-old Fisher 344 male rats were assessed and 21,700 probe sets were measureable. The *horizontal axis* indicates the $\log_2$ ratios of middle aged over young expression and the *vertical axis* is the $-\log_{10}$ of the FDR corrected *p* values. ~ 1100 transcripts were differentially expressed. *Blue dots* represent genes that increased or decreased by at least 1.5 fold (528)

annotated genes with the greatest differential expression. The largest change associated with middle age was expression of Dnajb12 (6.70 fold increase). Dnajb12 and related genes regulate proteasomal degradation of polytopic membrane proteins, particularly ion channels [16]. Gipr transcript, which encodes the receptor for gastric inhibitory polypeptide (GIP), also substantially increased. Agonist analogs of GIP reduce central oxidative stress, and are neuroprotective in Alzheimer's disease [17, 18], and stroke models [19]. Gpnmb transcript levels were elevated over three fold. This mRNA encodes a regulator of immune responses expressed in microglia that appears to have anti-inflammatory properties [20]. Among transcripts reduced in middle age, Herc1 participates in membrane trafficking; its loss increases autophagy and decreases mTOR activity associated with Purkinje cell degeneration [21]. Kif1a expression, which is required for BDNF-induced synaptogenesis in the hippocampus [22], was also significantly diminished in middle age.

To confirm the reproducibility and accuracy of the microarray measurements, we performed qPCR analyses on the same sets of samples measuring the relative change in expression (normalized to GAPDH mRNA). Our results (Table 2) show a close correspondence between qPCR and microarray results for 8 differentially expressed genes: Lgals, Fcr2b, GPNMB, C3, Atf3, Ptprc, Cd163 and Nrg1, as well as induction of the microglial activation marker Cd11b.

The annotated differential gene set consisting of the 353 transcripts, was subjected to pathway analysis (IPA) using its curated pathway database. Of 13 canonical pathways,

complement cascade had the highest proportion of differentially expressed genes and lowest adjusted *p* value (Table 3). In the complement system, 9 differentially expressed aged-related genes were up modulated out of 37 Complement system members (0.243; $p = 1.11 \times 10^{-6}$). Members of the Classical pathway, initiated by C1q activation and the Alternative pathway, initiated by C3 activation were well populated. The positive Z-score = 1.414, indicated significant complement pathway activation. On the other hand, expression of several inhibitory components, Serping1, a C1 esterase inhibitor, and Cfh, which accelerates C3b inactivation, were increased in middle age (1.55 and 1.79 fold, respectively), and could possible suppress these complement activation [23].

Among the remaining 12 pathways, four involved cholesterol metabolism, while nearly all remaining pathways were related to the T-helper cell/antigen presenting cell (APC) or T cell signaling (Table 3). These other pathways overlapped with common immune cell markers including Cd3g, Ptprc, Fcer1g, and MHC-I and MHC-II related genes. This is well illustrated in the Ox 40-signaling pathway, in which APC, such as microglia, present antigen in the context of MHC and Ox 40 receptor ligand to effector T cells, leading to activation of Nfkb, cJun and PI3K/PKB pathways [24].

A number of mechanistic regulatory networks were also populated by the differentially expressed gene set (Table 4), including pro-inflammatory mechanistic networks, IFNG, LPS and TNF. Additionally the inosine network, an immunomodulatory adenosine metabolite, and vancomycin, a neurotoxic antibiotic, were also significantly represented. IFNG, the most well populated

Table 1 Differential gene expression: largest effect sizes

Gene	M/Y	Y Mean	M Mean	Annotation
Abp10	0.46	677	311	Annexin V-binding protein
Aff4	0.45	458	204	Transcription factor and central SEC component
Ago2	0.43	330	141	RISC Catalytic Component 2
Aqp4	0.50	2664	1329	Aquaporin family member
Arl11	2.07	94	195	ADP-ribosylation factor-like 11
Asap1	0.40	524	212	ADP-ribosylation factor (ARF) GTPase-activating protein
Bmpr2	0.46	970	449	Bone morphogenetic protein receptor type II
C3	2.40	830	1996	Central complement component
Chrdl1	2.48	60	148	Ventroptin, antagonizes BMP actions
Clec12a	2.18	99	215	CTL/CTLD member, widely expressed in innate immune system
Cspp1	0.49	207	101	Important for normal neural specific cilia function
Dnajb12	6.70	52	350	DNAJ/HSP40 family member, regulates molecular chaperone activity, protein folding and degradation
Enc1	0.47	135	64	Kelch-related family of actin-binding proteins, role in oxidative stress response, regulates Nrf2
Falz	0.50	482	239	Transcription/epigenetic regulator, up-modulated in neurodegenerative diseases
Fcgr2b	2.89	303	878	Low affinity Fc receptor expressed in microglia
Fcrls	2.78	218	607	Fc receptor; part of TGFb1 microglial signature response
Fmo2	2.35	87	204	Flavin-containing monooxygenase
Fstl3	2.13	66	142	Secreted form binds/antagonizes members of TGF-b family, e.g., BMP2
Gipr	3.49	179	623	Receptor for neuroprotective polypeptide GIP
Golga4	0.42	211	89	Role in Rab6-regulated membrane-tethering events in the Golgi
Gpnmb	3.14	420	1317	Expressed in microglia, inflammatory response gene
Herc1	0.36	294	107	Regulator of membrane trafficking
Kif1a	0.38	3058	1160	Kinesin family protein involved in syaptogenesis
Lgals3	2.44	927	2264	Member galectin family of carbohydrate binding proteins; microglial marker and alt priming gene
Msi2	0.49	304	148	RNA binding protein; role in CNS stem cell proliferation
Nrg1	0.46	553	253	Neuregulin-1, signals through erb2/3 receptors, functions in neural development and plasticity
Pitpnm1	3.50	499	1749	Transfers PtdIns from ER to plasma membrane

Table 1 Differential gene expression: largest effect sizes (Continued)

Gene	M/Y	Y Mean	M Mean	Annotation
Postn	2.73	147	402	Aka periostin; enhances TGF-β signaling, facilitates BMP1, expressed in reactive microglia and astrocytes, neuroprotective
Pou3f1	2.16	266	574	Transcription factor, promotes stem cell commitment to neural fate
RT1-EC2	2.50	75	189	Class I MHC, up-modulated in spinal cord injury and neurodegeneration
S100a8	2.30	85	194	Induced in macrophages and dendritic cells by TLR agonists, oxidative stress and corticosterone
Slc9a3	2.15	195	421	Sodium/proton exchanger; Cation Proton Antiporter 3
Tnc	2.32	75	173	Extracellular matrix protein, up regulated following CNS trauma
Unc5b	0.47	995	469	Netrin receptor family; required for axon guidance; maintains blood–brain barrier
Usp7	0.46	121	56	Uiquitin-specific-processing protease 7, deubiquitinates range Deubiquitinates target proteins

The annotated differential gene set (353) was filtered for largest effect sizes. Mean probe set expression levels (arbitrary units) for Y (young) and M (middle age) genes are shown

network contained the highest density of predicted interactions that correlated to actual changes in target gene expression. This 132-member network, featuring 19 regulatory nodes, was populated by 59 of the differentially expressed age-related genes (50% of the total, $p = 1.24 \times 10^{-16}$). The entire network was activated in middle age with an overall activation Z-score = 2.711. Differentially expressed genes showed large numbers of regulatory inputs including Atf3, Anxa1, Postn, Cp, Cebpd, Fcgr2b, S100a8, C3, Col2a1, Map3k8 And Ppargc1b. Major regulatory nodes include Ctnnb1, Nfkbia, Nfkb, Smad3, Sp1 and Il4.

The transcriptional mechanistic regulatory networks were also well represented. Ctnnb1, part of the canonical WNT pathway, is a co-activator of TCF/LEF family transcription factors, which up-modulates expression of WNT-responsive genes [25]. Out of 124 members, this network contained 36 of the differentially expressed, age-related genes ($p = 3.96 \times 10^{-12}$). Major regulatory nodes included Ctnnb1, Pge2, Smad3, Sp1, and Jun. Differentially expressed genes having multiple regulatory inputs included Igfbp5, Bmp2, Sox2, Ccnd2, Gja1, Ctgf, Mmp14 and Cxcl9. Overall this transcriptional network was significantly inhibited in middle age (Z-score = -2.377) which could explain the down-modulation WNT-responsive genes: Ccnd2, Gja1, Igf1, Ppap2b, Sox2, and Tcf7l2. On the other hand, two Ctnnb1 genes, that are also STAT regulated, were up modulated in older LSC, as are Stat6 and a synergistic co-activator Cepbd.

Table 2 Confirmation of microarray results by qPCR

Results	Lgals	Fcgr2b	Gpnmb	C3	Atf3	Ptprc	Cd163	Nrg1	Cd11b
$\Delta\Delta C_t$ M v Y	1.62	1.68	1.76	1.42	0.94	0.99	0.78	−0.79	0.87
qPCR Fold M/Y	3.08	3.20	3.40	2.68	1.92	1.99	1.72	0.58	1.83
Microarray M/Y	2.44	2.89	3.14	2.40	1.73	1.84	1.59	0.46	N/A
Adjusted p-value	0.004	0.003	0.006	0.010	0.004	0.001	0.001	0.056	1.0E-07

cDNA was synthesized from the same RNA samples analyzed in the microarrays. $\Delta\Delta C_t$ values are expressed as described in Methods

Bio-functional networks were also explored. The top functional populated networks were systemic auto-immune syndrome and activated immune cell adhesion and migration (Network 01). This network had the highest consistency score (10.104) with a total of 21 nodes and 5 regulators and 12 differentially expressed LSC target genes that formed the core of the immune cell regulatory network, under the control of Tmg2, Ifnɑr, Gata4, and/or Hbb-b1. Strong relationships included activation of immune cell adhesion and leukocyte chemotaxis involving S100a8, C3 and Cd74 expression, and migration of antigen presenting cells associated with expression of Tyrobp, Il16, S100a4 and C3. All functional network members are listed in Additional files 4, 5, 6 and 7.

Multiple other functional networks overlapped Bio-functional Network 01. All were related to immune cell function, adhesion and migration. Network 02 had a consistency score of 6.640, with 19 nodes, 5 regulators and 12 targets. Interactions stemming from up-modulation by Nfkb complex of C3, Plau, Tnsf4, Map3k8, and Ctgf expression were associated with activation of macrophage migration; whereas, increased expression of C1qa, S100a8, Cd74, Lgals3, C3 and Plau, under Hrg, Tgm2, Nfκbia, or Nfκb complex control, was associated with immune cell adhesion. Functional networks 03 and 04 (consistency scores of 5.078 and 3.618, respectively) overlapped. Network 03, which had 21 nodes, 6 regulators, and 14 target genes, featured Ifng and/or Ifnɑr driving expression of Cxcl9, Cd74, C3, S100a8, Stat6 and Aif1 expression associated with leukocyte chemotaxis; whereas Network 04, which had 16 nodes, 3 regulators and 11 targets, featured Tlr9, Tlr3, or transcriptional regulator, Ehf, modulating expression of C3, Map3k8, S100a8, Timp1 and, Abca1 that was associated with activation of myeloid lineage cell migration.

Table 3 Canonical pathways populated by the age-related gene set

Pathway	Target Genes	Pathway Genes	Ratio	z-score	B-H p value	Target Gene ID's
Complement	9	37	0.243	1.414	1.11E-06	C3, C1QA, C1QB, C1QC, C1S, CFD, CFH, ITGB2, SERPING1
Cholesterol Biosynthesis	7	28	0.250		2.63E-05	CYP51A1, HMGCR, HMGCS1, HSD17B7, IDI1, LSS, SC5D
iCOS-iCOSL signaling T helper cell	10	108	0.093		6.64E-04	CAMK2B, CD3G, FCER1G, HLA-DQA1, HLA-DQB1, HLA-DRA, HLA-DRB5, PDPK1, PLEKHA4, PTPRC
Cholesterol Biosynthesis I	4	13	0.308		1.84E-03	CYP51A1, HSD17B7, LSS, SC5D
Cholesterol Biosynthesis II (via 24,25-dihydrolanosterol)	4	13	0.308		1.84E-03	CYP51A1, HSD17B7, LSS, SC5D
Cholesterol Biosynthesis II (via desmosterol)	4	13	0.308		1.84E-03	CYP51A1, HSD17B7, LSS, SC5D
Ca-induced T cell Apoptosis	7	64	0.109		2.40E-03	CD3G, FCER1G, HLA-DQA1, HLA-DQB1, HLA-DRA, HLA-DRB5, PRKCE
OX40-signaling	8	89	0.090		2.40E-03	CD3G, FCER1G, HLA-DQA1, HLA-DQB1, HLA-DRA, HLA-DRB5, RT1-EC2, TNFSF4
NFAT regulation of immune response	11	171	0.064	1.89	2.40E-03	BLNK, CD3G, FCER1G, FCGR2B, FCGR3A/FCGR3B, GNAS, GSK3B, HLA-DQA1, HLA-DQB1, HLA-DRA, HLA-DRB5
B Cell development	5	33	0.152		4.35E-03	HLA-DQA1, HLA-DQB1, HLA-DRA, HLA-DRB5, PTPRC
Nur77 signaling in T cells	6	57	0.105		6.70E-03	CD3G, FCER1G, HLA-DQA1, HLA-DQB1, HLA-DRA, HLA-DRB5
Cd28 signaling in T Helper Cells	8	118	0.068		1.15E-02	CD3G, FCER1G, HLA-DQA1, HLA-DQB1, HLA-DRA, HLA-DRB5, PDPK1, PTPRC
PKC-τ signaling in T cells	8	118	0.068	1.414	1.15E-02	CAMK2B, CD3G, FCER1G, HLA-DQA1, HLA-DQB1, HLA-DRA, HLA-DRB5, MAP3K8

The differentially expressed annotated genes (target gene set) were placed in the contexts of canonical biological pathways using the IPA software and its curated database. Ratio = target genes/pathway genes. P values were calculated using a modified Fisher test that corrects for multiple hypothesis testing. Significant Z-score indicate overall pathway modulation (+) for up (-) for down

Table 4 Populated upstream regulatory networks

Upstream Regulator	Molecule Type	p-value of overlap	Target molecules in dataset	Mechanistic Network
IFNG	Pro-inflammatory cytokine produced mainly by activated T cells	1.33E-16	ABCA1,AIF1,ASS1,AVPR1A,BLNK,C1QA,C1QB,C1QC, C3,C4A/C4B,CCND2,CD163,CD74,CDH22,Cebpd,CP, CTGF,FAM107A,FCER1G,FCGR2B,FCGR3A,HLA-DQA1, HLADRA,HMGCR,HMGCS1,IDI1,IFITM1,IGF1,ITGB2, LGALS3,MAP3K8,MERTK,MT1E,PHACTR1,PLEK, PPARGC1B,RT1EC2,SERPING1,SLC6A6,SLC9A3,STAT6, TIMP1,TLR7,TREM2,TYROBP	CEBPA,FOXO3,Hdac,IFNG,IL1B,IL4,LDL, NFkBcomplex,PPARG,RUNX2,SP1,SP3, STAT1,STAT3,STAT5a/b,STAT6,TNF
Inosine	Metabolite with immunomodulatory effects	4.15E-16	AIF1,ANXA1,C1QA,C1QB,C1QC,C1S,C3,C4A/B, CFD,MS4a6b,MT1E,SERPING1,TIMP1	
LPS	Major component of outer membrane of Gram-negative bacteria	2.92E-14	ABCA1,ANXA1,ANXA3,ASAP1,ASS1,AVPR1A, BMP2,C3,CCND2,CD163,CD37,CD53,CD74,CFD, CP,CSF3R,CTGF,DDX6,DIO2,EMR1,FCER1G, FCGR2B,Gp49a/Lilrb4,HLADQA1,IFITM1,IGF1, ITGB2,LGALS3,MAFF,MAP3K8,MERTK,MMP14, MT1E,MT1H,PDE4B,PLD4,PLEK,PPARGC1B, PYCARD,SLC9A3,SLFN13,STAT6,TIMP1, TLR7,TNFSF4,TREM2,TYROBP,VEZF1	CEBPA,FOXO3,HDAC,IFNG,IL1B, IL4,IL6,NCOA1,NFkB (complex), PPARG,RUNX2,SP1,SP3,STAT1, STAT3,STAT4,STAT5a/b,STAT6,TNF, lipopolysaccharide
DYSF	Ca2+ sensor protein involved in synaptic vesicle fusion	4.36E-12	ABCA1,ANXA1,C1QB,CD53,CD74,CFD,FCGR2B, GP49a/Lilrb4,HLA-DQA1,LGALS3,LYZ1/LYZ2,TIMP1	
Vancomycin	Antibiotic that exhibits significant neurotoxicity	8.00E-12	ANXA1,C3,C4A/C4B,CP,FMO2,GPNMB, LGALS3,MS4a6b,S100A11,SCD,TIMP1,TMEM173	
TNF	Pro-inflammatory cytokine; In the CNS, derived mainly from activated microglia	2.31E-11	ABCA1,ANXA1,ASS1,AVPR1A,BIRC7,BMP2,C3, CCND2,CD163,Cebpd,CFD,CP,CTGF, FCER1G,FCGR2B,HERC1,HLADRA,HMGCR, HSD17B7,IFITM1,IGF1,ITGB2,LGALS3,LRG1,LSS, MAFF,MAP3K8,MMP14,MT1E,MT1H,PDE4B, PER2,POSTN,PPARGC1B,PYCARD, RGS4,SCD,SLC9A3,TIMP1,TLR7,TNR,TREM2	CEBPA,CTNNB1,FOXO3,IFNG,IL1B,IL4, NFkB complex),PI3K complex,SP1,SP3, STAT1,STAT3,STAT5a/b,STAT6,TNF, estrogen receptor

Members of the annotated differential gene set (353) were fit to regulatory networks in the IPA data base. P values are the probability that the observed overlap occurred by chance alone

The consistency of each network and the overlaps indicate a strong association of these members of the age-related gene expression set with immune cell adhesion and migration.

We had previously reported that most microglia of healthy middle-aged rat LSC exhibited a activated morphology compared to young adults [14]. Here we find that nearly 10% of the differential gene set was associated entirely or primarily with changing patterns of microglial gene expression (Table 5). Approximately 75% of these transcripts were related to microglial activation [26, 27], and substantially overlapped with neuropathic pain-modulated spinal cord genes that were described in previous transcriptomic studies [28, 29]. In addition to microglial associated genes, other neuropathic pain-related transcripts were differentially expressed, yielding a total of 43 such genes or ~12% of the entire age-related LSC transcriptome (annotated).

Discussion

We have previously published cytokine and immune marker gene expression and immunohistochemical evidence that a para-inflammatory state develops in the LSC by middle age [14]. We reported that microglia of

healthy middle-aged rat LSC showed a predominately activated phenotype, whereas astrocyte morphology and GFAP protein levels indicated quiescence [14]. Results also showed that Cd2, Cd3e, Cd68, Cd45, Tnf-α, Il6, Ccl2, Atf3 and Tgfβ1 mRNA levels were substantially elevated. Here we extend that study and report that the transcriptomic changes associated with middle age are dominated by up-modulation of the innate immune system, including complement, TLR signaling, T-cell/APC interface, microglial priming, and M1 and M2 activation states. A number of other immune regulatory pathways were significantly up modulated including NFAT transcriptional pathways, important for neuronal excitation-transcription coupling and neurotrophin signaling [30], and the T-cell/PKC-Tau pathway. Components of other pathways involved in the regulatory interface between APC's and T-cells were similarly affected with increased expression of components in the OX40, icos-icosL, Nur77, and Cd28 signaling. Many immune regulatory networks were affected by age. Three of the top six networks control or activate central inflammatory responses involving glia and T-cells, which fit well the view that the innate immune system in the healthy LSC in middle age is in a state of incipient activation.

Table 5 Microglial and neuropathic pain-related gene expression

Gene	M/Y	Microglial	Pain	Function
ABCA1	1.62	Y	Y	Transporter of cholesterol and other lipids
AIF1	1.53	Y	Y	Forms complexes with L-fimbrin in membrane ruffles and phagocytic cups; may modulate actin reorganization, facilitates cell migration and phagocytosis
ANXA3	1.55	Y	Y	Annexin family member; up-regulated following tissue injury
ATF3	1.73	Y	Y	Complexes with other transcriptional regulators; up-regulated in response to injury; negative regulator of TLR signaling; suppresses innate immune response
BLNK	1.68	Y		Cytoplasmic linker protein important in B cell development
C1QA	1.61	Y	Y	Part of C1q complex; initial component of classic pathway
C1QB	1.59	Y	Y	Part of C1q complex
C1QC	1.52	Y	Y	Part of C1q complex
C4A	1.98	Y	Y	Cleaved by C1S; combines with C2 cleavage product forms C4b2b complex
CAMK2B	0.64	Y	Y	Ca2+/calmodulin-dependent protein kinase
CD163	1.59	Y		M2 state microglial marker (aka, ED2); Alt priming gene
CD37	1.54	Y	Y	Interacts with dectin; regulates PAMP induced IL6 production; microglial sensome
CD53	1.71	Y	Y	Contributes to transduction of CD2-generated signals in T cells
CD74	1.85	Y	Y	Invariant MHCII component; processes receptor bound PAMP'S and DAMP's for presentation to T cells
CSF3R	1.59	Y	Y	Binds GCSF, which increases M2 state marker expression, and inhibits pro-inflammatory cytokine expression, while promoting neurotrophic factor expression.
CXCL9	1.68	Y	Y	Ligand for Cxcr3 receptor, activated by TLR ligands and pro-inflammatory cytokines; appears to regulate T cell migration
Egr2	1.96	Y		Transcription factor; Alt priming gene
EMR1	1.81	Y	Y	Member of adhesion GPCR receptors; required to activate CD8+ regulatory T cells
FAM105A	2.08	Y	Y	
FCER1G	1.74	Y	Y	High affinity Fc epsilon receptor; binds TREM2; involved in response to apoptotic debris, immune complexes through C1q complex
FCGR2B	2.89	Y	Y	Fc receptor, IgG, low affinity; binds Cxcl7 (CD32B); inhibitory
FCGR3A	1.52	Y	Y	Aka CD16a; similar to FCGR2B
FCRLS	2.78	Y		Fc immunoglobulin receptor; part of TGFb1 microglial signature response
GOLM1	1.53	Y		Assists transport of cargo through Golgi apparatus; AD risk gene
IGF1	0.65	Y		Neurotrophic factor; increased by IL4/MCSF; M2 phenotype and Alt priming gene
IGFBP6	1.53	Y	Y	Binds IGF's and modulates their growth factor effects
ITGB2	1.73	Y	Y	CD18; integrin beta chain beta 2; involved in leukocyte adhesion
LGALS3	2.44	Y		Galectin family; inflammatory factor (MAC2); microglial marker; Alt priming gene
PTPRC	1.84	Y	Y	Protein tyrosine phosphatase; aka CD45; enriched in microglia; opposes microglial activation
PYCARD	1.50	Y	Y	Mediator of apoptosis and inflammation; adapter for inflammasome assembly
TLR7	1.84	Y	Y	TLR (nucleotide sensing); signals via MyD88 pathway; can modulate other TLR's
TMEM173	1.52	Y	Y	Facilitates innate immune signaling; promotes expression of IFN-alpha and IFN-beta;
TREM2	1.74	Y		Forms signaling complex with TYROBP; M2 state and sensome gene; promotes microglial expansion; up-regulated by IL4; critical for normal phagocytosis
TYROBP	1.82	Y	Y	Forms signaling complex with TREM2; activates microglia; required for synaptic pruning

The annotated differentially expressed gene set (353) was compared to previously published consensus genes specific for microglia. Those relevant to establishment of neuropathic pain are indicated

In a detailed study of the mouse life span, 127 genes were identified as aging-related in brain [31]. Eighteen genes associated with middle age in the spinal cord were similarly modulated in in the mouse brain data set, with 8 of these expressed in microglia. A recent combined transcriptomic and proteomic study of aging brain and liver also reported up-modulation of genes associated with antigen processing and presentation and immune system responses in senescent rat brains compared to those of young adults (two of the top three functional classifications) [32]. Thirty of the same genes reported here for middle-aged LSC were identified in the 609 differentially expressed genes in senescent rat brain [32], and 12 of these common genes were related to microglial function and/or establishment of neuropathic pain, including a number of complement components.

While our results are consistent with those previously reported for the senescent brain and other aging tissues, few of the genes we report are represented in the differential gene set previously reported for middle-aged and young adult mouse spinal cord [33]. Only 7, Acbd3, Elovl6, Jam2, Matn2, Nedd4, Pank3, Phactr1, and Ryr2 were found in both differential gene sets. Of these, the directions of modulations in 5 (Elovl6, Jam2, Nedd4, Phactr1, Ryr2) were not in agreement. The reasons underlying the lack of consistency with our study is unclear, though species differences may have contributed, as well as the many variables explored in the previous work (age, gender, tissue), that could have reduced the power to reliably identify differentially expressed genes in middle-aged mouse spinal cord. In two previous transcriptomic studies of middle-aged brain reported by Loerch and co-workers [34] and by Wood and others [35], only 3 (Csnk2a1, Hmgcr, Sgtb) and 4 (RT1-Ba, RT1-Bb, RT1-Da, Sema3b), respectively, were in common with the differential set reported here, suggesting the changes in middle-aged spinal cord we report here may be unique to the spinal cord. It is also possible that dissimilar platforms could have contributed the lack of overlap.

Up-modulation of the complement pathway activation is one of the most common age [36] or neuropathic pain related changes reported for the CNS [37]. A detailed study of complement component expression in aging mouse forebrain also reported significant increases in C1q and C3 transcript levels [38], similar to those reported here. Unlike the LSC, C4 transcript levels were not significantly elevated until 24 months in the mouse forebrain. We also measured significant increases (by qPCR) in transcripts encoding Cd11b or Cr3 (Table 2), a common microglial activation marker and the receptor for C3 complement, which has been reported to increase in a variety of different CNS pathologies [39–41]. While many activating components were up modulated in the middle-aged LSC, so were the transcripts of several counter regulatory components encoding proteins that block formation of C1q protein or increase the degradation of C3a, suggesting that complement activation in middle age could be suppressed.

A substantial fraction of the age-associated LSC transcriptome (Table 5) belongs to the microglial sensome [26, 27]. Most identified here are related to M1 or M2 activation states. Cd74 (MHCII invariant chain) encodes a marker of microglial M1 activation [42–44] and is increased in the brains of aging rodents [27] and nonhuman primates [45]. MHCII complex, identified in the canonical pathways up modulated in LSC, is key on APC/T-cell interface [24]. Consistent with M1 state activation were the increases in transcripts encoding proinflammatory chemokine Cxcl9, Cd16 (Fcgr2a, Fcgr3b), Cd32 (Fcgr2b) and Cd45 (Ptprc) [42–44]. On the other hand, many M2 sub-state activation markers and associated microglial transcripts were also up modulated including Cd163, Trem2, Tyrobp, Lgals3, and Csfr3 [42–44]. Some transcripts identified in the differential gene set are also implicated in activating microglial phagocytosis; these include Trem2, Tyrobp, Fcer1g, Cd32, and Aif1 [44, 46]. Enhanced phagocytosis is associated with M2 activation and with beneficial anti-inflammatory effects and augmented recovery/resolution or lower risk of neurodegenerative changes [42, 46]. Overall the evidence supports the evolution of multiple different microglia activation states during aging in the spinal cord, any one of which could alter the innate immune response to injury or infection, and the trajectory of recovery or resolution.

We also report here a general down modulation of transcripts encoding enzymes involved in cholesterol metabolism including Hmgrc, Hmgcs1, Cyp51, Lss, Sc5d and Scd1; whereas the cholesterol transporter, Abca1, was up-modulated. Implications for spinal cord cholesterol, however, are unclear. Comparable changes have been previously reported, in a study of aging cervical spinal cord, that were associated with perturbation of cholesterol homeostasis (increased white matter cholesterol ester concentrations) and inflammatory activation in the cervical spinal cord [47]. Age-related changes in CNS cholesterol metabolism are believed to play a key role in the development of some forms of Alzheimer's disease and other degenerative disorders [48].

Overall, these results provide further support for "inflammaging" of the LSC by middle age in rat, which has been amply demonstrated in other senescent tissues of many species, including humans [6]. Such emerging inflammatory changes in the LSC may be most relevant to human spinal cord neuropathies, particularly the increased risk of chronic pain, which is strongly associated with middle age, rather than senescence [8, 10–13, 49, 50]. The spinal cord is the primary site of first order nociceptive signal processing; the first relay in transmission to higher centers; and is the origin of hyperalgesia and spontaneous pain, all driven by activated microglia, astrocytes and the innate immune system [51–53]. Nonetheless, our study did not investigate changes in the aging rat proteome, nor did we explore here any alterations in the responses to injury or to degeneration of the somatosensory system; therefore these potential implications remain speculative. Furthermore, to test whether our results are relevant to the risks of chronic pain or the failures of current treatments in middle-aged humans will require investigations of post-mortem spinal cords.

Conclusions

Transcriptomic analysis of healthy middle-aged LSC demonstrated up-modulation of complement pathway, microglial priming and activation, and T cell/antigen-presenting cell communication. Taken together with previous work, the results support our conclusion that an incipient or para-inflammatory state develops in the LSC in healthy middle-aged adults.

Additional files

Additional file 1: Primer sequences used in the qPCR measurements.

Additional file 2: Up and down modulated genes. Description: all genes significantly up or down modulated in LSC comparing young to

Additional file 3: Differentially expressed gene set. Description: all annotated genes included in the differentially expressed gene set that

Additional file 4: Bio-functional Network 01. Description: differentially expressed gene set: pink to red (intensity indicates degree of up-modulation), while green denotes down-modulation). Colors of upstream regulators and downstream biological processes are related to predicted activation states with orange indicating activation and blue denoting inhibition. Lines connecting nodes are orange when leading to activation, blue when inhibition is predicted, and yellow if relationships are not consistent with the downstream node state shown. Gray lines denote lack of evidence to form a prediction. Solid lines show direct relations and dashed indirect. Blunted ends indicate expected inhibition if

Additional file 5: Bio-functional Network 02. Description: as for

Additional file 6: Bio-functional Network 03. Description: as for

Additional file 7: Bio-functional Network 04. Description: as for

Abbreviations

APC: Antigen presenting cell; CNS: Central nervous system; LSC: Lumbar spinal cord; qPCR: Quantitative polymerase chain reaction

Acknowledgements
Not applicable.

Funding
This research did not receive any specific grant from funding agencies in the public, commercial, or not-for-profit sectors.

Authors' contributions
WG extracted RNA, conducted quality controls, performed qPCR assays, assisted in analyzing the results and helped to write the manuscript; YL performed qPCR assays, assisted in analyzing the results and helped to write the manuscript, MK helped design the study, analyzed data and assisted in editing the manuscript; MP assisted in analyzing the data, and editing the manuscript; LL helped design the study and edit the manuscript; and MR designed and supervised the study, analyzed data, and edited the manuscript. All authors read and approved the final manuscript.

Competing interests
The authors declare that they have no competing interests.

References

1. Jurgens HA, Johnson RW. Dysregulated neuronal-microglial cross-talk during aging, stress and inflammation. Exp Neurol. 2012;233(1):40–8. doi:10.1016/j.expneurol.2010.11.014. PubMed PMID: 21110971, PubMed Central PMCID: PMC3071456, Epub 2010/11/30S0014-4886(10)00415-2 [pii].
2. Mosher KI, Wyss-Coray T. Microglial dysfunction in brain aging and Alzheimer's disease. Biochem Pharmacol. 2014;88(4):594–604. doi:10.1016/j.bcp.2014.01.008. PubMed PMID: 24445162, PubMed Central PMCID: PMC3972294, Epub 2014/01/22.
3. Norden DM, Godbout JP. Review: microglia of the aged brain: primed to be activated and resistant to regulation. Neuropathol Appl Neurobiol. 2013; 39(1):19–34. doi:10.1111/j.1365-2990.2012.01306.x. PubMed PMID: 23039106, PubMed Central PMCID: PMC3553257, Epub 2012/10/09.
4. Norden DM, Muccigrosso MM, Godbout JP. Microglial priming and enhanced reactivity to secondary insult in aging, and traumatic CNS injury, and neurodegenerative disease. Neuropharmacology. 2015;96(Pt A):29–41. doi:10.1016/j.neuropharm.2014.10.028. PubMed PMID: 25445485; PubMed Central PMCID: PMC4430467.
5. Sparkman NL, Johnson RW. Neuroinflammation associated with aging sensitizes the brain to the effects of infection or stress. Neuroimmunomodulation. 2008;15(4–6):323–30. doi:10.1159/000156474. PubMed PMID: 19047808, PubMed Central PMCID: PMC2704383, Epub 2008/12/03000156474 [pii].
6. Franceschi C, Capri M, Monti D, Giunta S, Olivieri F, Sevini F, et al. Inflammaging and anti-inflammaging: a systemic perspective on aging and longevity emerged from studies in humans. Mech Ageing Dev. 2007;128(1): 92–105. doi:10.1016/j.mad.2006.11.016. Epub 2006/11/23.
7. von Bernhardi R, Tichauer JE, Eugenin J. Aging-dependent changes of microglial cells and their relevance for neurodegenerative disorders. J Neurochem. 2010;112(5):1099–114. doi:10.1111/j.1471-4159.2009.06537.x. Epub 2009/12/17JNC6537 [pii].
8. Blyth FM, March LM, Brnabic AJ, Jorm LR, Williamson M, Cousins MJ. Chronic pain in Australia: a prevalence study. Pain. 2001;89(2–3):127–34. Epub 2001/02/13.
9. Blyth FM, Van Der Windt DA, Croft PR. Chronic Disabling Pain: A Significant Public Health Problem. Am J Prev Med. 2015;49(1):98–101. doi:10.1016/j.amepre.2015.01.008. Epub 2015/06/22.
10. Fernandez-de-las-Penas C, Hernandez-Barrera V, Alonso-Blanco C, Palacios-Cena D, Carrasco-Garrido P, Jimenez-Sanchez S, et al. Prevalence of neck and low back pain in community-dwelling adults in Spain: a population-based national study. Spine. 2011;36(3):E213–9. doi:10.1097/BRS.0b013e3181d952c2. Epub 2010/11/17.
11. Hoy D, Bain C, Williams G, March L, Brooks P, Blyth F, et al. A systematic review of the global prevalence of low back pain. Arthritis Rheum. 2012; 64(6):2028–37. doi:10.1002/art.34347. Epub 2012/01/11.
12. Leboeuf-Yde C, Nielsen J, Kyvik KO, Fejer R, Hartvigsen J. Pain in the lumbar, thoracic or cervical regions: do age and gender matter? A population-based study of 34,902 Danish twins 20–71 years of age. BMC Musculoskelet Disord. 2009;10:39. doi:10.1186/1471-2474-10-39. PubMed PMID: 19379477, PubMed Central PMCID: PMC2678974, Epub 2009/04/22.
13. Rustoen T, Wahl AK, Hanestad BR, Lerdal A, Paul S, Miaskowski C. Age and the experience of chronic pain: differences in health and quality of life among younger, middle-aged, and older adults. Clin J Pain. 2005; 21(6):513–23. Epub 2005/10/11.
14. Galbavy W, Kaczocha M, Puopolo M, Liu L, Rebecchi MJ. Neuroimmune and Neuropathic Responses of Spinal Cord and Dorsal Root Ganglia in Middle Age. PLoS One. 2015;10(8):e0134394. doi:10.1371/journal.pone.0134394. PubMed PMID: 26241743, PubMed Central PMCID: PMC4524632, Epub 2015/08/05.
15. Hochberg Y, Benjamini Y. More powerful procedures for multiple significance testing. Stat Med. 1990;9(7):811–8. Epub 1990/07/01.
16. Grove DE, Fan CY, Ren HY, Cyr DM. The endoplasmic reticulum-associated Hsp40 DNAJB12 and Hsc70 cooperate to facilitate RMA1 E3-dependent degradation of nascent CFTRDeltaF508. Mol Biol Cell. 2011;22(3):301–14. doi:10.1091/mbc.E10-09-0760. PubMed PMID: 21148293, PubMed Central PMCID: PMC3031462, Epub 2010/12/15.

17. Duffy AM, Holscher C. The incretin analogue D-Ala2GIP reduces plaque load, astrogliosis and oxidative stress in an APP/PS1 mouse model of Alzheimer's disease. Neuroscience. 2013;228:294–300. doi:10.1016/j.neuroscience.2012.10.045. Epub 2012/10/30.

18. Ji C, Xue GF, Li G, Li D, Holscher C. Neuroprotective effects of glucose-dependent insulinotropic polypeptide in Alzheimer's disease. Rev Neurosci. 2016;27(1):61–70. doi:10.1515/revneuro-2015-0021. Epub 2015/09/10.

19. Han L, Holscher C, Xue GF, Li G, Li D. A novel dual-glucagon-like peptide-1 and glucose-dependent insulinotropic polypeptide receptor agonist is neuroprotective in transient focal cerebral ischemia in the rat. Neuroreport. 2016;27(1):23–32. doi:10.1097/WNR.0000000000000490. Epub 2015/11/12.

20. Huang JJ, Ma WJ, Yokoyama S. Expression and immunolocalization of Gpnmb, a glioma-associated glycoprotein, in normal and inflamed central nervous systems of adult rats. Brain Behav. 2012;2(2):85–96. doi:10.1002/brb3.39. PubMed PMID: 22574278, PubMed Central PMCID: PMC3345354, Epub 2012/05/11.

21. Sanchez-Tena S, Cubillos-Rojas M, Schneider T, Rosa JL. Functional and pathological relevance of HERC family proteins: a decade later. Cell Mol Life Sci. 2016;73(10):1955–68. doi:10.1007/s00018-016-2139-8. Epub 2016/01/24.

22. Kondo M, Takei Y, Hirokawa N. Motor protein KIF1A is essential for hippocampal synaptogenesis and learning enhancement in an enriched environment. Neuron. 2012;73(4):743–57. doi:10.1016/j.neuron.2011.12.020. Epub 2012/03/01.

23. Morgan BP, Harris CL. Complement, a target for therapy in inflammatory and degenerative diseases. Nat Rev Drug Discov. 2015;14(12):857–77. doi:10.1038/nrd4657. Epub 2015/10/24.

24. Croft M, So T, Duan W, Soroosh P. The significance of OX40 and OX40L to T-cell biology and immune disease. Immunol Rev. 2009;229(1):173–91. doi:10.1111/j.1600-065X.2009.00766.x. PubMed PMID: 19426222, PubMed Central PMCID: PMC2729757, Epub 2009/05/12.

25. Clevers H, Nusse R. Wnt/beta-catenin signaling and disease. Cell. 2012;149(6):1192–205. doi:10.1016/j.cell.2012.05.012. Epub 2012/06/12.

26. Butovsky O, Jedrychowski MP, Moore CS, Cialic R, Lanser AJ, Gabriely G, et al. Identification of a unique TGF-beta-dependent molecular and functional signature in microglia. Nat Neurosci. 2014;17(1):131–43. doi:10.1038/nn.3599. PubMed PMID: 24316888, PubMed Central PMCID: PMC4066672, Epub 2013/12/10.

27. Hickman SE, Kingery ND, Ohsumi TK, Borowsky ML, Wang LC, Means TK, et al. The microglial sensome revealed by direct RNA sequencing. Nat Neurosci. 2013;16(12):1896–905. doi:10.1038/nn.3554. PubMed PMID: 24162652, PubMed Central PMCID: PMC3840123, Epub 2013/10/29.

28. Costigan M, Moss A, Latremoliere A, Johnston C, Verma-Gandhu M, Herbert TA, et al. T-cell infiltration and signaling in the adult dorsal spinal cord is a major contributor to neuropathic pain-like hypersensitivity. J Neurosci. 2009;29(46):14415–22. Epub 2009/11/20. doi: 29/46/14415 [pii] 10.1523/JNEUROSCI.4569-09.2009. PubMed PMID: 19923276; PubMed Central PMCID: PMC2813708.

29. Griffin RS, Costigan M, Brenner GJ, Ma CH, Scholz J, Moss A, et al. Complement induction in spinal cord microglia results in anaphylatoxin C5a-mediated pain hypersensitivity. J Neurosci Nurs. 2007;27(32):8699–708. doi:10.1523/JNEUROSCI.2018-07.2007. Epub 2007/08/10.

30. Kim MS, Shutov LP, Gnanasekaran A, Lin Z, Rysted JE, Ulrich JD, et al. Nerve growth factor (NGF) regulates activity of nuclear factor of activated T-cells (NFAT) in neurons via the phosphatidylinositol 3-kinase (PI3K)-Akt-glycogen synthase kinase 3beta (GSK3beta) pathway. J Biol Chem. 2014;289(45):31349–60. doi:10.1074/jbc.M114.587188. PubMed PMID: 25231981, PubMed Central PMCID: PMC4223335, Epub 2014/09/19.

31. Jonker MJ, Melis JP, Kuiper RV, van der Hoeven TV, Wackers PF, Robinson J, et al. Life spanning murine gene expression profiles in relation to chronological and pathological aging in multiple organs. Aging Cell. 2013;12(5):901–9. doi:10.1111/acel.12118. PubMed PMID: 23795901, PubMed Central PMCID: PMC3772962, Epub 2013/06/26.

32. Orre M, Kamphuis W, Osborn LM, Melief J, Kooijman L, Huitinga I, et al. Acute isolation and transcriptome characterization of cortical astrocytes and microglia from young and aged mice. Neurobiol Aging. 2014;35(1):1–14. doi:10.1016/j.neurobiolaging.2013.07.008. Epub 2013/08/21.

33. Xu X, Zhan M, Duan W, Prabhu V, Brenneman R, Wood W, et al. Gene expression atlas of the mouse central nervous system: impact and interactions of age, energy intake and gender. Genome Biol. 2007;8(11):R234. doi:10.1186/gb-2007-8-11-r234. PubMed PMID: 17988385, PubMed Central PMCID: PMC2258177, Epub 2007/11/09.

34. Loerch PM, Lu T, Dakin KA, Vann JM, Isaacs A, Geula C, et al. Evolution of the aging brain transcriptome and synaptic regulation. PLoS One. 2008;3(10):e3329. doi:10.1371/journal.pone.0003329. PubMed PMID: 18830410, PubMed Central PMCID: PMC2553198, Epub 2008/10/03.

35. Wood SH, Craig T, Li Y, Merry B, de Magalhaes JP. Whole transcriptome sequencing of the aging rat brain reveals dynamic RNA changes in the dark matter of the genome. Age. 2013;35(3):763–76. doi:10.1007/s11357-012-9410-1. PubMed PMID: 22555619, PubMed Central PMCID: PMC3636386, Epub 2012/05/05.

36. de Magalhaes JP, Curado J, Church GM. Meta-analysis of age-related gene expression profiles identifies common signatures of aging. Bioinformatics. 2009;25(7):875–81. doi:10.1093/bioinformatics/btp073. PubMed PMID: 19189975, PubMed Central PMCID: PMC2732303, Epub 2009/02/05.

37. LaCroix-Fralish ML, Austin JS, Zheng FY, Levitin DJ, Mogil JS. Patterns of pain: meta-analysis of microarray studies of pain. Pain. 2011;152(8):1888–98. doi:10.1016/j.pain.2011.04.014. Epub 2011/05/13.

38. Reichwald J, Danner S, Wiederhold KH, Staufenbiel M. Expression of complement system components during aging and amyloid deposition in APP transgenic mice. J Neuroinflammation. 2009;6:35. doi:10.1186/1742-2094-6-35. PubMed PMID: 19917141, PubMed Central PMCID: PMC2784442, Epub 2009/11/18.

39. Brennan FH, Anderson AJ, Taylor SM, Woodruff TM, Ruitenberg MJ. Complement activation in the injured central nervous system: another dual-edged sword? J Neuroinflammation. 2012;9:137. doi:10.1186/1742-2094-9-137. PubMed PMID: 22721265; PubMed Central PMCID: PMCPMC3464784.

40. Cribbs DH, Berchtold NC, Perreau V, Coleman PD, Rogers J, Tenner AJ, et al. Extensive innate immune gene activation accompanies brain aging, increasing vulnerability to cognitive decline and neurodegeneration: a microarray study. J Neuroinflammation. 2012;9:179. doi:10.1186/1742-2094-9-179. PubMed PMID: 22824372, PubMed Central PMCID: PMC3419089, Epub 2012/07/25.

41. Mastellos DC. Complement emerges as a masterful regulator of CNS homeostasis, neural synaptic plasticity and cognitive function. Exp Neurol. 2014;261:469–74. doi:10.1016/j.expneurol.2014.06.019. Epub 2014/07/01.

42. Cherry JD, Olschowka JA, O'Banion MK. Neuroinflammation and M2 microglia: the good, the bad, and the inflamed. J Neuroinflammation. 2014;11:98. doi:10.1186/1742-2094-11-98. PubMed PMID: 24889886, PubMed Central PMCID: PMC4060849, Epub 2014/06/04.

43. David S, Kroner A. Repertoire of microglial and macrophage responses after spinal cord injury. Nat Rev Neurosci. 2011;12(7):388–99. doi:10.1038/nrn3053. Epub 2011/06/16.

44. Walker DG, Lue LF. Immune phenotypes of microglia in human neurodegenerative disease: challenges to detecting microglial polarization in human brains. Alzheimers Res Ther. 2015;7(1):56. doi:10.1186/s13195-015-0139-9. PubMed PMID: 26286145, PubMed Central PMCID: PMC4543480, Epub 2015/08/20.

45. Sheffield LG, Berman NE. Microglial expression of MHC class II increases in normal aging of nonhuman primates. Neurobiol Aging. 1998;19(1):47–55. Epub 1998/04/30.

46. Painter MM, Atagi Y, Liu CC, Rademakers R, Xu H, Fryer JD, et al. TREM2 in CNS homeostasis and neurodegenerative disease. Mol Neurodegener. 2015;10:43. doi:10.1186/s13024-015-0040-9. PubMed PMID: 26337043, PubMed Central PMCID: PMC4560063, Epub 2015/09/05.

47. Parkinson GM, Dayas CV, Smith DW. Perturbed cholesterol homeostasis in aging spinal cord. Neurobiol Aging. 2016;45:123–35. doi:10.1016/j.neurobiolaging.2016.05.017. Epub 2016/5/24.

48. El Gaamouch F, Jing P, Xia J, Cai D. Alzheimer's disease risk genes and lipid regulators. J Alzheimers Dis. 2016;53(1):15–29. doi:10.3233/JAD-160169.

49. Blyth FM, Cumming RG, Nicholas MK, Creasey H, Handelsman DJ, Le Couteur DG, et al. Intrusive pain and worry about health in older men: the CHAMP study. Pain. 2011;152(2):447–52. doi:10.1016/j.pain.2010.11.022. Epub 2010/12/21.

50. Johannes CB, Le TK, Zhou X, Johnston JA, Dworkin RH. The prevalence of chronic pain in United States adults: results of an Internet-based survey. J Pain. 2010;11(11):1230–9. doi:10.1016/j.jpain.2010.07.002. Epub 2010/08/28.

51. Costigan M, Scholz J, Woolf CJ. Neuropathic pain: a maladaptive response of the nervous system to damage. Annu Rev Neurosci. 2009;32:1–32. doi:10.1146/annurev.neuro.051508.135531. PubMed PMID: 19400724, PubMed Central PMCID: PMC2768555, Epub 2009/04/30.

52. Grace PM, Hutchinson MR, Maier SF, Watkins LR. Pathological pain and the neuroimmune interface. Nat Rev Immunol. 2014;14(4):217–31. doi:10.1038/nri3621. Epub 2014/03/01.

β-glucans: ex vivo inflammatory and oxidative stress results after pasta intake

Annalisa Barera[1], Silvio Buscemi[2], Roberto Monastero[3], Calogero Caruso[1], Rosalia Caldarella[4], Marcello Ciaccio[1,2,3,4] and Sonya Vasto[5,6*]

Abstract

Background: It is well known that Mediterranean Diet can positively influence the health of each individual, in particular it is know that fibers have an important role. However, in Mediterranean cities most people do not have a close adherence to Mediterranean diet. Thus, in our study, we considered fibers like β-glucans that have been added to pasta with a percentage of 6 %. Our study aimed to evaluate the capacity of β-glucans intake on oxidative stress and inflammation in a cohort of middle aged slightly overweight subjects.

Methods: We used a longitudinal study design. The study lasted 30 days during which time, each participant acted with no food restriction. Participants underwent morning fasting blood venous sample for blood chemistry and other biological parameters at the beginning of the study and after 30 days of pasta supplemented with 6 % of β-glucan intake 4 times a week. We performed anthropometric, biochemical, oxidative stress and cytokine analysis at the beginning and the end of study.

Results: After the 30 days of pasta intake we obtained a significant decrease of LDL-cholesterol, IL-6 and AGEs levels.

Conclusion: The results confirmed a capacity of β-glucans intake to lower oxidative stress. Additional longitudinal observation on community-based cohorts are needed to confirm these data and investigate the biological mechanisms through which effects are induced, and to fully explore the therapeutic potential of β-glucans.

Keywords: Mediterranean diet, β-glucans, Diet, Inflammation, Oxidative stress

Background

Mediterranean diet (MD) is a set of eating habits around the Mediterranean basin, actually it is not a specific diet but a set of practices of cultivation, fishing, processing and traditions in the preparation and intake of food among the different Mediterranean countries (Spain, Italy, Greece and Morocco). Since 2010, MD is part of the Intangible Cultural Heritage of UNESCO [1]. This set of eating habits consists mainly in a daily intake of whole grains, legumes, fruit and nuts. In addition, there is a moderate intake of fish (along the sea coast), white meat, dairy products and eggs. Intake of red meat and wine is limited compared to the diets of other areas of the world. To ensure the intake of fat, among the people of the Mediterranean basin, intake of olive oil is widespread. Overall, the MD has the following key features: low content of saturated fatty acids, rich in carbohydrates and fibers, high in monounsaturated fatty acids (derived mainly from olive oil), poor animal proteins [2, 3].

It is quite difficult to define the type of fibers in MD because this term expresses a nutritional and physiological concept rather than a class of chemicals. It was originally used to designate the plant residues that are resistant to digestion by enzymes from the intestinal lumen. This definition is still not complete because it does not take into account the heterogeneity of the chemical composition, the diversity of the plant matrix and the physiological characteristics of the multiple components of the fibers. The fibers are distinguished, by an analytical point of view, in soluble and insoluble: soluble fibers act mainly in the first part of the digestive tract (stomach and small intestine), while the insoluble fibers are more active in the terminal part of the digestive tract (large intestine). The fibers also affect the small intestine transit. In particular, soluble fibers delay while insoluble fibers speed up the luminal content. An additional effect of the fibers is their ability to sequester bile acids in the lumen of the ileum: this effect involves, among other things, the absence of the formation of micelles, which are

---

* Correspondence: sonya.vasto@unipa.it
[5]Department of Biological Chemical and Pharmaceutical Sciences and Technologies (STEBICEF), University of Palermo, Viale delle Scienze, Building 16, Palermo, Italy
[6]Institute of biomedicine and molecular immunology "Alberto Monroy" CNR, Palermo, Italy
Full list of author information is available at the end of the article

necessary for the absorption of cholesterol and fats. Another possible effect of the fibers is to bind the minerals (Ca, Mg, Fe, Cu, Zn, etc.), reducing their absorption and bioavailability [4].

Despite the beneficial effects of the fibers their intake in the Mediterranean world has sharply declined: a possibility is then to add fibers like β-glucans in the typical foods of the MD such as pasta.

The β-glucans are one of the most abundant forms of polysaccharides found in the cell wall of yeasts, fungi, some bacteria, algae and cereals. All the β-glucans are polysaccharides consisting of linear molecules of D-glucose joined together by glycosidic bonds linear β (1-3) and β (1-4) and differ between them for the length and branched structures. The branches derived from the nuclear chain glycoside are highly variable and the two main groups are branching chains glycosidic β (1-4) and β (1-6). These ramifications appear to be specific, for example, the β-glucans of mushrooms have side branches $1 \rightarrow 6$ while those of bacteria have side branches $1 \rightarrow 4$ [5, 6]. The presence of the bond β (1-3) leads to the formation of folds in the linear chain that allow water to enter; for this reason the β-glucans are classified as soluble fibers. Characteristics of β-glucans are their effect on cholesterol that depends on the ability to form a viscous layer on the surface of the small intestine. The higher viscosity reduces the intestinal absorption of cholesterol and the reabsorption of bile acids. The inhibition of the reabsorption of bile acids can increase the synthesis of bile acids from endogenous cholesterol, and reduces the circulation of cholesterol LDL by about 8 % [7]. A minimum dose of 3 g/day of β-glucans has been suggested reducing the levels of cholesterol in the blood and decrease the risk of cardiovascular diseases [6].

Furthermore, the β-glucans have potent immunomodulatory effects on innate and adaptive immunity. In fact, they have been demonstrated to bind directly to specific receptors of immune cells including Dectin-1, complement receptor 3 (CR3), and TLR-2/6 thus triggering a group of cells of the immune system including macrophages, neutrophils, monocytes, NK cells and dendritic cells [5].

Therefore, the nutraceutical use of β-glucans is an interesting perspective. This action has already been investigated using breakfast drinks [8], biscuits and crackers added with less of 3 % of β-glucans [9]. The aim of the present pilot study was to evaluate the effect of 30 days of regular intake of pasta supplemented with 6 % β-glucans on biological parameters of overweight otherwise healthy individuals.

Results and discussion
Hematochemical tests

Physical characteristics and biochemical measurements including cytokines did not change after 30 days of pasta added with β-glucans consumption with the exception of IL-6 blood concentrations as reported in Table 1. The

Table 1 Characteristics of the cohort and blood measurements before and 30 days after regular consumption of pasta added with β-glucans

	Before	After	P*
Gender (Females/Males)	20/20	20/20	
Age (years)	64 ± 9	64 ± 9	
Body weight (kg)	78.8 ± 3.3	78.7 ± 2.4	0.4
BMI (kg/m2)	28.6 ± 2.1	28.5 ± 1.5	0.2
Fasting blood measurements:			
Glucose (mg/dl)	92 ± 10	91 ± 9	0.3
Cholesterol (mg/dl)	212 ± 32	204 ± 33	0.4
HDL-cholesterol (mg/dl)	56 ± 13	56 ± 11	0.8
LDL-cholesterol (mg/dl)	139 ± 39	127 ± 45	0.03
Triglycerides (mg/dl)	116 ± 69	120 ± 65	0.1
Uric acid (mg/dl)	5.1 ± 1.3	5.5 ± 1.0	0.2
hs-CRP (mg/dl)	0.24 ± 0.20	0.23 ± 0.17	0.2
TNF-alpha (pg/ml)	17.2 ± 13.0	18.3 ± 2.8	0.9
IFN-gamma (pg/ml)	0.6 ± 0.6	1.1 ± 0.8	0.3
IL-8 (pg/ml)	41.4 ± 59.3	45.1 ± 103.8	0.81
IL-10 (pg/ml)	2.3 ± 2.4	1.6 ± 1.7	0.6
IL-6 (pg/ml)	6.3 ± 3.0	7.2 ± 1.7	0.02

All values are presented as means ± SD or in absolute values
*Wilcoxon test: $p > 0.01 p < 0.5$
BMI: body mass index; HDL: high-density lipoproteins; LDL: low density lipoproteins; hs-CRP: high-sensitivity-C-reactive protein; TNF-: tumor necrosis factor; IFN-: Interferon; IL-: Interleukin

analysis considers weight, BMI, the blood level of glucose, total cholesterol, HDL-cholesterol, LDL-cholesterol, triglycerides, uric acid, creatinine, AST, ALT, γ-GT, total proteins, hematocrit and hs-CRP. In agreement with data reported by a recent meta-analysis [10] the treatment induced a reduction (although not significant) of serum LDL-cholesterol concentrations whereas no significant effect was observed on HDL-cholesterol and triglycerides concentrations or the other parameters considered in this study. In addition, glucose blood concentrations slightly decreased following treatment confirming what reported in previous studies [4]. AST and ALT concentrations were in the range of normality and did not show any significant modification along the study. As stated in the Background section, it is believed that the cholesterol-lowering effect depends on its viscosity in the small intestine, which, in turn, is affected by the molecular weight (MW) and the amount of β-glucans in solution [4]. Body weight and BMI did not vary along the 30 days since the participant were asked to do not modify their nutritional habits.

Cytokines

Cytokines are small glycoprotein messengers involved in biological function with several immunological effects. They possess a pleiotropic and potent effector function as in acute and in chronic inflammatory processes and are considered reliable markers of inflammation. The Table 1 shows that, 30 days after the regular intake of the studied food uniquely the IL-6 blood concentrations were significantly decreased. IL-6 is a pleiotropic cytokine capable of regulating proliferation, differentiation and activity in a variety of cell types. In particular, it plays a pivotal role in acute phase responses and in the balancing of the pro and anti-inflammatory pathways. IL-6 is involved in impaired lipid metabolism and in the production of triglycerides. Moreover, it decreases lipoprotein lipase activity and monomeric lipoprotein lipase levels in plasma, which contributes to increased macrophage uptake of lipids [11]. The latter result suggests that a regular intake of the pasta investigated in this study may have an anti-inflammatory effect, probably linked to the immunomodulatory effects of β-glucans [12].

Oxidative stress analyses

Only few studies described an antioxidant effect of β-glucans [13, 14]. Thus, we have analysed the effects of pasta supplemented with β-glucans intake on oxidized LDL-cholesterol (Ox-LDL), 8-hydroxy-2' –deoxyguanosine (8-OHdG) and 3-nitrotyrosine (3NT) concentrations.

The Ox-LDL represents a modified form of circulating LDL-cholesterol which, accumulates in macrophage by LDL scavenger receptors and play a key-role in the pathophysiology of atherosclerotic plaques. Among the different types of oxidative DNA damage, the formation of 8-OHdG is a marker of oxidative stress [15–17].

While all tyrosine residues in proteins might be targets for nitration, the amount and efficacy of tyrosine nitration might vary according to different biological conditions that may vary from the local production and concentration of reactive oxygen species (ROS), antioxidants and scavengers availability to the presence of inflammatory mediators. Fasting blood levels of oxidized LDL were unchanged 30 days after pasta added with β-glucans intake (17.7 ± 16 vs 10.4 ± 6; $P = 0.9$), also unchanged were the fasting blood concentrations of 8OHdG (110.3 ± 133 vs 37.2 ± 32; $P = 0.07$). Furthermore, 30 days after the intake of pasta supplemented with β-glucans blood concentrations of 3NT significantly increased (6.1 ± 3.1 vs 6.8 ± 3.2; $P = 0.02$; Fig. 1) while those of AGEs decreased (3.4 ± 2.5 vs 2.2 ± 1.5; $P = 0.01$. Fig. 2). We cannot exclude that this lack of effect is probably due to the need of longer time of food exposure.

The mechanism that leads to the formation of AGEs starts with a non-enzymatic covalent bond of an aldehyde or ketone group of a reducing sugar with the free amino groups of the proteins and other molecules; subsequently, a series of events consisting in rearrangements and reactions lead to the production of AGEs takes irreversibly place inducing the production of ROS. It has been proposed that the binding and activation of specific receptors, with changing in the extracellular matrix and circulating lipoproteins, which leads to atherosclerosis, realize the vascular toxicity of AGEs.

The present data, although indirectly, are indicative of an antioxidant effect of pasta supplemented with β-glucans.

Conclusions

It is well known that MD can positively influence the health of each individual, in particular it is know that fibers have an important role. However, in Mediterranean cities most people do not have a close adherence to MD [2]. Thus, in our study, we considered fibers like β-glucans that have been added to pasta with a percentage of 6 %, far higher concentration of commercially available products on the market.

After the 30 days of pasta intake we obtained encouraging results with a significant decrease of LDL-cholesterol, IL-6 and AGEs levels.

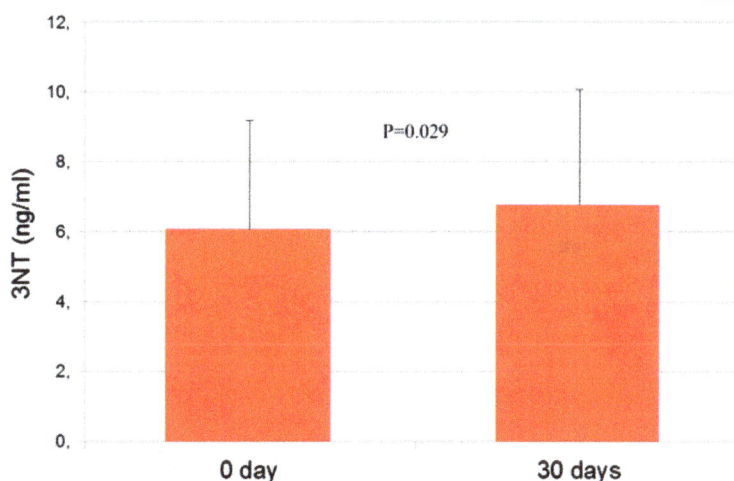

Fig. 1 The figure shows 3NT blood levels at time 0 and after 30 days of pasta intake

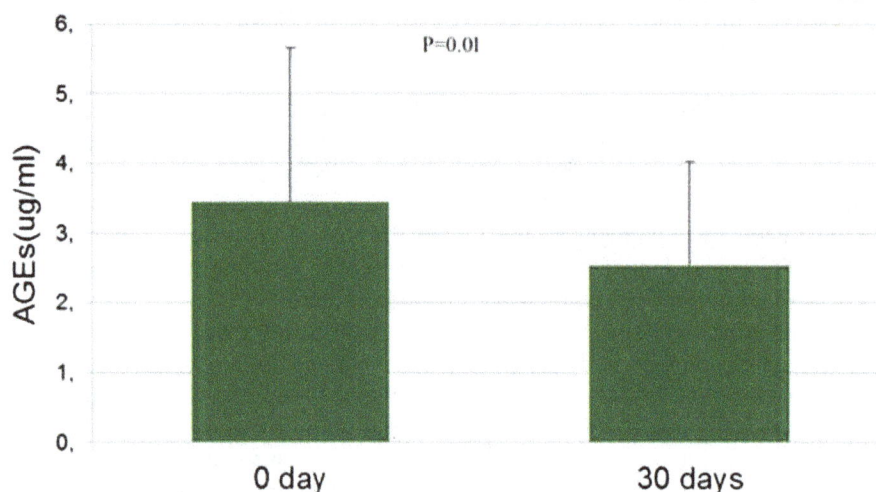

Fig. 2 The figure shows AGEs blood levels at time 0 and after 30 days of pasta intake

According to the results of this pilot trial, we might speculate that a system of well-balanced diet of carbohydrates and fats, as appears to be the MD, may be suitable for helping to correct metabolic abnormalities thus contributing to the clinical management of metabolic syndrome.

Additional longitudinal observation on community-based cohorts are needed to confirm these data and investigate the biological mechanisms through which effects are induced, and to fully explore the therapeutic potential of β-glucans.

Subjects and methods

Study design and participants

We used a longitudinal study design. The study lasted 30 days during which time, each participant acted with no food restriction (see flowchart, Fig. 3). Inclusion criteria were: range of age 40–60 years, overweight (body mass index [BMI] 25–29.9 kg/m^2), normal glucose tolerance (fasting plasma glucose < 100 mg/dL), slight dyslipidemia (total cholesterol ≤ 240 mg/dL, HDL-cholesterol 40–59 mg/dL, LDL 130–160 mg/dL, triglyceride level ≤ 170 mg/dL) any treatment for specific disease, including psychotropic drugs and drugs to treat metabolic disorders. Exclusion criteria were: a diagnosis of a severe systemic disorder (including heart disease and hypertension, obesity, diabetes mellitus, dyslipidemia, rheumatological disease, liver, kidney and gastroenterological disorders); psychosis; a history of significant head injury or substance abuse; severe neurological diseases (including stroke, dementia, Parkinson's disease and other neurodegenerative disorders),eating behaviour disease based on the VAS Questionnaire [18] or under any restrictive dietary

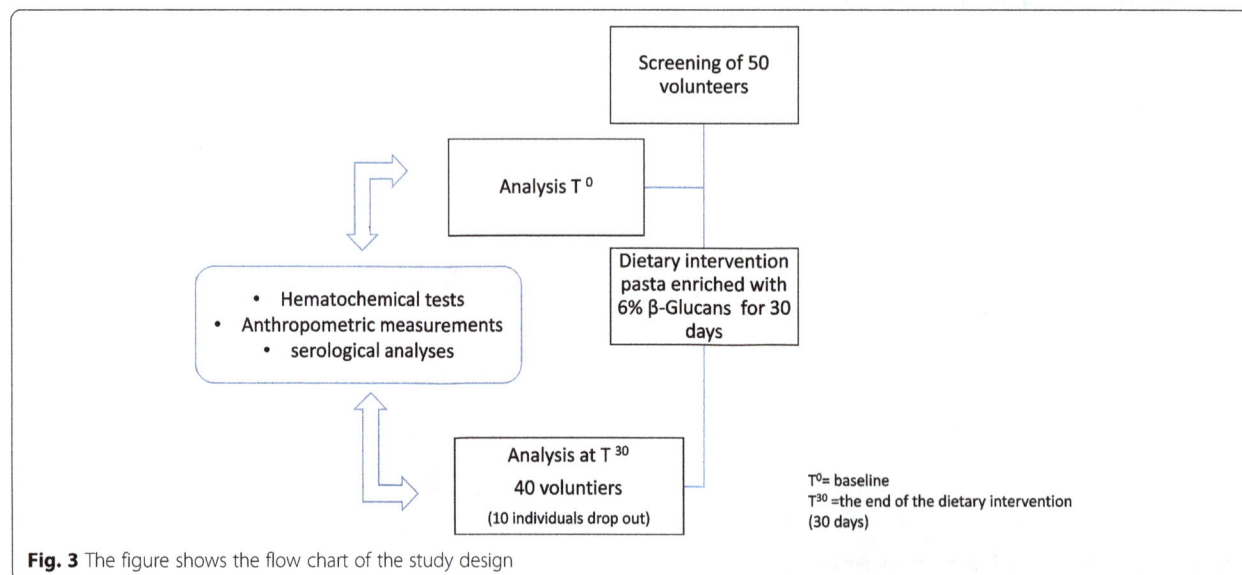

Fig. 3 The figure shows the flow chart of the study design

treatment. Enrolled subjects underwent a complete internal medicine and neurological examination with trained physicians (SB and RM).

After a complete description of the study, written informed consent was obtained from all participants. Before entering the study, participants were asked not to vary their food and\or physical activity during the period of the study. Accordingly, 40 subjects ended the pilot study (80 % of trial completion) while ten participants abandoned the study before completion for personal reasons.

Participants underwent morning fasting blood venous sample for blood chemistry and other biological parameters at the beginning of the study and after 30 days of pasta supplemented with 6 % of β-glucan intake 4 times a week. Body weight, height and blood pressure of all participants were measured and blood samples were collected at the beginning of the study and after 30 ± 2 days.

β-glucans preparation
β-glucans extraction, characterization and pasta have been prepared according to Montalbano et al. 2016 [19].

Blood analyses
Plasma and serum samples were used for hematocrit and chemistry analysis (total cholesterol, LDL-cholesterol, HDL-cholesterol, alanine aminotransferase (ALT), aspartate aminotransferase (AST), glucose, triglycerides, creatinine, gamma-glutamyl transferase (GGT), total protein, uric acid, high sensitivity c-reactive protein (hs-CRP).

Elisa test
Human Oxidized LDL (MDA-LDL Quantitation) (Oxiselect, cod. STA-369, Cell Biolabs, Inc), Human 3-nitrotyrosine (3-NT) ELISA kit (cod. CSB-E14324H, Cusabio Biotech Co), Human 8-OHdG ELISA Kit (cod. CSB-E10140H, Cusabio Biotech Co), Human advanced glycation end-products (AGE) kit (cod. CSB-E14324H, Cusabio Biotech Co) were used according to manual or data sheet.

Cytokines assay
Citokines analysis of High Sensitivity IL-6; High Sensitivity TNF-alfa; High Sensitivity INT-gamma; High Sensitivity –IL-8; High Sensitivity IL-10, were measured by -LHSCM000 Human Mag Luminex Performance Assay Base Kit.

Statistical analysis
The results were analysed by the Biostat 2009 software. Descriptive statistic and non-parametric statistic were used (Wilcoxon test).

Abbreviations
MD: Mediterranean Diet; BMI: body mass index; MW: molecular weight; HDL: high-density lipoproteins; LDL: low density lipoproteins; hs-CRP: high-sensitivity-C-reactive protein; TNF: tumor necrosis factor; IFN: Interferon; IL: Interleukin; ALT: alanine aminotransferase; AST: aspartate aminotransferase; GGT: gamma-glutamyl transferase; Ox-LDL: LDL-cholesterol; 8-OHdG: 8-hydroxy-2′–deoxyguanosine; 3NT: 3-nitrotyrosine; AGE: advanced glycation end-products; ROS: reactive oxygen species.

Competing interests
The authors declare that they have no competing interest.

Authors' contributions
SV, SB and CC conceived and designed the study; AB and LC performed experiments. All authors analyzed and interpreted data; SV drafted the paper and CC made critical revisions to the draft. All authors read and approved the final manuscript.

Acknowledgments
This work was supported by PON DIMESA (Programma Operativo Nazionale Ricerca e Competitività 2007/2013 - Progetto "DI.ME.Sa." PON02_00451_3361785. Valorisation of typical products of the Mediterranean diet and their nutraceutical use to improve health) to CC.

Author details
[1]Pathobiology Department and Biomedical Technologies (DIBIMED), University of Palermo, Palermo, Italy. [2]Biomedic Department of Internal and Specialistic Medicine (DIBIMIS), University of Palermo, Palermo, Italy. [3]Department of Experimental Biomedicine and Clinical Neuroscience (BioNeC), University of Palermo, Palermo, Italy. [4]CORELAB, Policlinico Paolo Giaccone, University of Palermo, Palermo, Italy. [5]Department of Biological Chemical and Pharmaceutical Sciences and Technologies (STEBICEF), University of Palermo, Viale delle Scienze, Building 16, Palermo, Italy. [6]Institute of biomedicine and molecular immunology "Alberto Monroy" CNR, Palermo, Italy.

References
1. Unesco web site; www.unesco.it; accessed on 26th December 2015
2. Vasto S, Buscemi S, Barera A, Di Carlo M, Accardi G, Caruso C. Mediterranean diet and healthy ageing: a Sicilian perspective. Gerontology. 2014;60:508–18.
3. Vasto S, Barera A, Rizzo C, Di Carlo M, Caruso C, Panotopoulos G. Mediterranean diet and longevity: an example of nutraceuticals? Curr Vasc Pharmacol. 2014;12:735–8.
4. Otles S, Ozgoz S. Health effects of dietary fiber. Acta Sci Pol Technol Aliment. 2014;13:191–202.
5. Rieder A, Samuelsen AB. Do cereal mixed-linked β-glucans possess immune-modulating activities? Mol Nutr Food Res. 2012;56:536–47.
6. Lazaridou A, Biliaderis CG. Molecular aspects of cereal β-glucan functionality: physical properties, technological applications and physiologycal effects. J Cereal Sci. 2007;46:101–18.
7. Othman RA, Moghadasian MH, Jones PJ. Cholesterol-lowering effects of oat β-glucan. Nutr Rev. 2011;69:299–309.
8. Barone Lumaga R, Azzali D, Fogliano V, Scalfi L, Vitaglione P. Sugar and dietary fibre composition influence, by different hormonal response, the satiating capacity of a fruit-based and a β-glucan-enriched beverage. Food Funct. 2012;3:67–75.
9. Dhingra D, Michael M, Rajput H, Patil RT. Dietary fibre in foods: a review. J Food Sci Technol. 2012;49:255–66.
10. Whitehead A, Beck EJ, Tosh S, Wolever TM. Cholesterol-lowering effects of oat β-glucan: a meta-analysis of randomized controlled trials. Am J Clin Nutr. 2014;100:1413–219.
11. Ershler WB, Keller ET. Age-associated increased interleukin-6 gene expression, late-life diseases, and frailty. Annu Rev Med. 2000;51:245–70.
12. Wang S, Zhou H, Feng T, Wu R, Sun X, Guan N, et al. β-Glucan attenuates inflammatory responses in oxidized LDL-induced THP-1 cells via the p38 MAPK pathway. NMCD. 2014;24:248–55.
13. Saluk-Juszczak J, Krolewska K, Wachowicz B. Beta-glucan from Saccharomyces cerevisiae as a blood platelet antioxidant. Platelets. 2010;21:451–9.
14. Kofuji K, Aoki A, Tsubaki K, Konishi M, Isobe T, Murata Y. Antioxidant Activity of β-Glucan. ISRN Pharmaceutics. 2012;2012:125864.

15. Basu SK, Brown MS, Ho YK, Goldstein JL. Degradation of low density lipoprotein.dextran sulfate complexes associated with deposition of cholesteryl esters in mouse macrophages. J Biol Chem. 1979;254:7141–46.

16. Patel PR, Bevan RJ, Mistry N, Lunec J. Evidence of oligonucleotides containing 8-hydroxy-2'-deoxyguanosine in human urine. Free Radic Biol Med. 2007;42: 552–8.

17. Toth P, Tarantini S, Springo Z, Tucsek Z, Gautam T, Giles CB, et al. Aging exacerbates hypertension-induced cerebral microhemorrhages in mice: role of resveratrol treatment in vasoprotection. Aging Cell. 2015;14:400–8.

18. Rogers PJ, Blundell JE. Effect of anorexic drugs on food intake and the micro-structure of eating in human subjects. Psychopharmacology (Berl). 1979;66:159–65.

19. Montalbano A, Tesoriere L, Diana P, Barraja P, Carbone A, Spanò V, at al. Quality characteristics and in vitro digestibility study of barley flour enriched ditalini pasta. LWT - Food Science and Technology. In press

17

Prescription database analyses indicates that the asthma medicine montelukast might protect against dementia: a hypothesis to be verified

Bjørn Grinde[*] and Bo Engdahl

Abstract

Background: It has recently been shown that the leukotriene receptor antagonist montelukast rejuvenates aged brains in rats. The question is whether this commonly used, systemic, anti-asthmatic medicine has a similar effect in humans?

Results: We approached this issue by doing statistical analyses based on the Norwegian Prescription Database. The Database lists all prescription-based medications in Norway, but not drugs given to people who are in hospitals or nursing homes. The question asked was whether users of montelukast, compared to users of inhalation asthma medicine, live longer, and are less likely to develop dementia. A small, non-significant protective effect on the use of dementia medicine became significant when adjusting for other prescriptions (based on the notion that montelukast users on average are less healthy). A possible protective effect was substantiated by looking at the lack of prescriptions as a proxy for dementia-related residency in nursing homes, and the risk of death.

Conclusions: The present results suggest that montelukast may alleviate the cognitive decline associated with human aging. However, further data, preferably based on controlled clinical trials, are required.

Keywords: Montelukast, Prescription database, Dementia, Cognitive decline, Leukotriene

Background

According to Marschallinger et al. [1], six weeks of treatment with the asthma medicine montelukast rejuvenates the brain of aging, but otherwise healthy, rats (20 months old, considered equivalent to 60 years in humans). The observation offers hope for finding a remedy that can reduce human, age-related cognitive decline. Montelukast inhibits inflammatory processes by acting as a leukotriene receptor antagonist. There are considerable data suggesting that inflammation plays a role in age-associated disorders of both body and brain [1–4].

The question of whether montelukast has a positive effect on humans is difficult to resolve, as it is ethically questionable to set up clinical trials that involve the use of prescription medicine on healthy individuals. To circumvent this problem, we analysed data from the Norwegian Prescription Database (NorPD) http://www.norpd.no/. A clinical trial should be more acceptable if there is sufficient data suggesting a protective effect. NorPD registers all prescriptions in Norway, but does not cover medication given to people in hospitals or nursing homes. The database allows for asking questions such as whether subjects given montelukast are later less likely to receive medication related to dementia, when compared with individuals using inhalation asthma medicine.

In Norway, with a population of about 5 million, there were 37,445 registered users of montelukast in 2014, of which approximately half were 50 years or older. The use dates back to the nineties. The primary indication (in adults) is the additional treatment of asthma in cases where inhalation medications are insufficient to control the condition. Previous data suggest that asthma patients

* Correspondence: bjorn.grinde@fhi.no
Department of Aging, Norwegian Institute of Public Health, Box 4404 Nydalen, 0403 Oslo, PO, Norway

have an increased risk of both dementia [5, 6] and death [7], which is why we used subjects receiving inhalation medication as a control group. It is, however, expected that users of montelukast have a more severe form of asthma; a conjecture that was supported by the present data. In separate analyses, it was therefore corrected for the use of additional medication as a proxy for general health.

One problem when looking at the use of dementia medicine in Norway is that these drugs are in principle prescribed to people with Alzheimer's disease (AD). It is, however, likely that some of the patients offered medication have other forms of dementia. With this in mind, we considered it useful to compare with patients taking medication associated with Parkinson's disease (PD). Approximately half of those diagnosed with PD will develop dementia [8, 9], but this diagnosis is less likely to be confused with other forms of dementia. Both AD and PD are likely to reflect aetiologies somewhat different from the normal cognitive decline associated with aging [10], aetiologies that may or may not involve the leukotriene signalling pathway. Based on the above discussion, one might expect a limited protective effect of montelukast on the use of dementia medicine, but perhaps not on Parkinson's medication.

NorPD offers two alternative options for probing the effect of montelukast. Individuals who stop receiving prescriptions for an extended period, while still being alive, are likely to be admitted to an institution. Long-term stay in institutions for elderly people generally means nursing homes, and dementia is the most common reason why people are committed to nursing homes in Norway (the prevalence of dementia in nursing homes residents has been estimated to be approximately 80% [11]). We consequently used the lack of prescriptions for a period of at least one year as a proxy for cognitive decline. This group would include all forms of dementia, of which perhaps half suffers from other forms than those related to AD or PD [8, 12]. A final option was to consider whether montelukast protects against death.

Results

The subset of NorPD data used in the present analyses included all prescriptions given to people offered asthma-related medicine who were 60 years or older in 2014. The current version of the database includes the period from 2004 to 2015. Drugs are defined according to the Anatomical Therapeutic Chemical (ATC) classification system, and can be listed as the number of Defined Daily Doses (DDDs) dispensed. The study cohort was further limited to individuals (203,473) who had at least two prescriptions of montelukast (ATC code R03DC03) or inhalation type asthma medication (codes R03AK or R03BA – that is, primarily corticosteroids) during the period covered in the

database (Table 1). The mean age of the study cohort was 75.2 years in 2014.

The follow-up groups included: 1) users of *montelukast* (11.6%); 2) users of *dementia medicine* (code N06D; 3.2%); 3) those who presumably had been admitted to a *nursing home* (2.9%); 4) those who *died* (30.2%); 5) users of *Parkinson's medicine* (code N04; 3.5%); and 6) users of type 2 *diabetes medicine* (codes A10BA, A10BB, and A10BH; 11.7%). Based on total drug consumption, subjects belonging to most follow-up groups had more health problems compared to the overall average (Table 1). Similar results were found when looking at prescription of cardiovascular medicine (codes B01A, C07, and C09; data not shown). In separate analyses, it was consequently adjusted for a combination of total DDDs, cardiovascular medications, and sex (as women tended to be overrepresented).

The prevalence of montelukast use was lower in the following three groups: dementia, nursing home, and death – compared to the complete study group – while slightly higher in the PD and diabetes groups (Tables 1 and 2). Although these figures are indicative, further analyses are required in order to propose a protective effect.

The calculation of hazard ratios (HRs), based on Cox regression analysis, suggested a slight, but not significant, tendency toward a protective effect of montelukast on the later use of dementia medication (Table 2, unadjusted). The effect did reach significance when adjusting for the above mentioned factors. However, as pointed out in the Introduction, the use of dementia medicine is not a good indicator of general, age-related cognitive decline. We therefore analysed a lack of prescriptions for at least a year as a proxy for subjects being committed to nursing homes. Nursing home residency implies a high risk for any form of dementia [11]. In this case, the data had to be split between those below and above 75 years for analytical reasons. There was a highly significant protective effect on subjects 60–75 years (HR 0.65 and 0.67 for unadjusted and adjusted), while no effect on those above 75. A protective effect was further corroborated by analysing for risk of death during the study period. Again, the data had to be split in two age groups, but in this case, both groups displayed a significant effect of montelukast. Subjects for whom the first prescription of montelukast or inhaling corticosteroids happened after the follow-up events (e.g., the use of dementia or PD medicine), were removed from the regression analyses (truncated).

As these analyses only provide correlates, and may be biased by unknown confounders, we decided to see how two other types of medication would perform in similar analyses. PD and type 2 diabetes presumably have aetiologies where leukotrienes have limited impact. We found a slightly increased prevalence of montelukast use in both groups (Tables 1 and 2). Based on Cox regression

Table 1 Characteristics of the study cohort (elderly on asthma medicine)

Study group	Total	Mean age (SD)[a]	Males (%)	Montelukast[b] (%)	Total drugs in DDDs (SD)[c]
All subjects	203,473	75.2 (9.7)	89,755 (44.1)	23,636 (11.6)	5.1 (4.6)
Montelukast	23,636	73.1 (9.0)	8964 (37.9)	-	6.3 (4.3)
Dementia medicine	6453	83.6 (7.7)	2502 (38.8)	602 (9.3)	5.6 (3.2)
Nursing home[d]	5970	77.8 (10.4)	2463 (41.3)	507 (8.5)	4.2 (3.5)
Death	61,434	82.7 (9.5)	31,152 (50.7)	5514 (9.0)	7.1 (6.3)
Parkinson's medicine	7140	76.1 (9.3)	2849 (39.9)	955 (13.4)	6.3 (3.9)
Diabetes medicine	23,747	74.8 (9.1)	11,920 (50.2)	2887 (12.2)	7.8 (4.3)

[a]Age in 2014
[b]At least two prescriptions
[c]Mean Defined Daily Doses (DDDs) prescribed of any drug
[d]It was assumed that a majority of those who did not receive any prescription for more than a year were admitted to a nursing home. Living in a nursing home can be used as a proxy for cognitive decline in that some 80% of Norwegian nursing home residents have dementia [11]

analyses, montelukast users had an increased risk of PD, which became not significant in the adjusted model (Table 2). In the case of diabetes, there was no effect in the unadjusted analysis, but an apparent protective effect in the adjusted model.

Discussion

The present data indicate that the use of montelukast might protect against dementia and extend lives in humans. The study cohort included users of asthma medicine who were 60 years or older in 2014. Based on Cox regression analyses, subjects who received montelukast were less likely later to use dementia drugs (Table 2); although the HR was only significant when adjusting for the consumption of other drugs. The protective effect on the use of dementia medicine was relatively small, but further evidence, discussed below, support the conjecture.

Cognitive impairment, which may lead to dementia, is presumably a natural consequence of normal aging; but dementia may also have more specific causes, such as infections, plaque formation, and stroke. The leukotriene-signalling pathway, which is inhibited by montelukast, is primarily expected to contribute to the general, age-related deterioration; although it has been suggested that leukotrienes may also play a role in more specific forms of dementia such as AD [1, 13, 14]. Dementia medicine is, in principle, given to patients with AD (or, more rarely, PD dementia). There are no drugs intended for other forms of dementia, but the NorPD allows for examining a proxy. The study group used on average more than 5 DDDs, which means that each individual was expected to receive several prescription over the course of a year. Those who did not, while still being alive, were likely to live in an institution. Nursing homes are the main type of institution offering long-term stay

Table 2 Association between montelukast use and risk of different out-comes (significantly protective hazard ratios in bold)[a]

Study group	Cases/Total (%)		Hazard ratios (95% CI)		
	Montelukast pos	Montelukast neg	Age[b]	Unadjusted	Adjusted
Dementia medicine[c]	489/23,521 (2.1)	4967/178,884 (2.9)	>60	0.94 (0.85–1.03)	**0.89** (0.81–0.98)
Nursing home[d]	507/23,634 (2.2)	5459/179,768 (3.1)	60–75	**0.65** (0.57–0.74)	**0.67** (0.59–0.77)
			>75	1.00 (0.88–1.13)	0.99 (0.87–1.13)
Death[d]	5512/23,634 (30.4)	55,857/179,768 (45.1)	60–75	**0.86** (0.82–0.89)	**0.64** (0.61–0.67)
			>75	**0.95** (0.92–0.98)	**0.81** (0.78–0.84)
Parkinson's medicine[e]	691/23,371 (3.0)	4550/178,134 (2.6)	>60	1.21 (1.12–1.32)	1.06 (0.98–1.15)
Diabetes medicine[e]	1523/22,270 (7.3)	11,247/170,157 (7.1)	>60	1.01 (0.96–1.07)	**0.85** (0.80–0.90)

[a]The hazard ratios are based on comparing subjects using montelukast with those using only inhaling corticosteroids. The adjusted ratios are adjusted for sex, receiving drugs for heart conditions, and having a high consumption of drugs during the follow up period. The discrepancies between the sum of users in each analysis, and the grand total of 203,473 in Table 1, are due to truncations. The total number of person-years follow-up was between 1,346,308 and 1,480,476 (average 7.0–7.3 years per subject)
[b]As of 2014
[c]The adjusted analysis was stratified on having a high consumption of drugs dispensed per day, because this covariate did not meet the proportional hazards assumption
[d]As the effect of montelukast did not meet the proportional hazards assumption, the model was fitted by splitting into two age-periods, 60–75 years and >75 years
[e]The adjusted analysis was stratified on having a high consumption of drugs dispensed per day, and prescription of cardiovascular medicine, because these covariates did not meet the proportional hazards assumption

for elderly. The prevalence of dementia in Norwegian nursing homes has been estimated to be approximately 80% [11]. The use of montelukast reduced the HR for ending up in the nursing home group (Table 2); that is, for the younger fraction of the study group. In order to satisfy the proportional hazards assumption for the Cox regression, we needed to split the study group in two age fractions. A similar age-effect was observed with the dementia group (data not shown).

The above data are compatible with the following account: Montelukast has none, or limited, protective effect against AD, but may help prevent other forms of dementia, and a minor fraction of these is given dementia drugs. A larger fraction of nursing home residents has a form of dementia that can be prevented or alleviated by montelukast; however, the medicine needs to be taken while the person is still relatively young.

Drugs associated with two other diseases were included as controls. PD, and thus Parkinson's dementia, is likely to have an aetiology different from that of the previously mentioned conditions. According to the present analyses, montelukast users appeared to have an elevated risk of using PD medicine, but the HR was not significant in the adjusted model. These data suggests that the leukotriene-signalling pathway is not involved as a causal agent. The increased risk may reflect either a protective effect of this pathway, or that montelukast users are less healthy and thus more at risk.

A range of data support the idea that the immune system can impact on the aetiology of perhaps most forms of neurodegenerative disorders (for a broader discussion, see [1–4]), yet the overall effect could be either protective or causal [15, 16]. Inflammation helps remove cellular debris (including plaque-forming proteins). It is conceivable that in the early stages of neurodegeneration, inflammation is destructive – as it also cause tissue damage – while in later stages, with a greater burden of debris, the balance tips in favour of inflammation. Additional information comes from the use of non-steroidal anti-inflammatory drugs (NSAIDs). NSAIDs have not been successful in the treatment of AD [17]; on the other hand, previous use has been associated with a reduced risk of AD and general dementia [18, 19], but not PD [20]. Moreover, a study of genetic polymorphisms for key genes associated with inflammation (cyclooxygenase-2 and 5-lipoxygenase) found that alleles expected to cause increased expression, and thus an increase in inflammatory factors, are overrepresented in AD patients [21]. 5-Lipoxygenase is involved in the generation of leukotrienes. A short-term, randomized controlled trial with NSAIDs did not find any significant protective effect on AD [22]. These observations support the view that early use of drugs designed to reduce inflammatory processes may have a beneficial role, at least in the case

of certain forms of dementia. The balance, as to positive or negative effect of inflammation, may depend on stage of neurodegeneration, aetiology, dose/duration of treatment, and the branch of the inflammatory machinery being inhibited. NSAIDs affect the cox/prostaglandine pathway, while montelukast is a leukotriene antagonist.

We also analysed the effect of montelukast on dying. Again, the data had to be split in two age groups. In this case, montelukast had a protective effect on both groups, but a more pronounced effect on the younger fraction. As suggested above, this observation may reflect that the drug is less useful for those at advanced stages of aging; but other factors may also be involved. For example, in the very old, both dying and admission to a nursing home could be due to a larger variety of causes, of which the leukotriene signalling pathway is only involved in some.

A protective effect on dying is in line with the idea that pro-inflammatory processes are associated with a range of age-related disorders, including cardiovascular conditions, and as such act as predictors of mortality [23–26]. In fact, Swedish register data indicate that montelukast reduces the risk of recurrent stroke and myocardial infarction [27]. As to the present data, most follow-up groups had a higher level of DDDs (Table 1), and cardiovascular medication (data not shown), compared to the overall average. One interesting exception was that the montelukast users received slightly less than average heart medication.

Medicine prescribed to people with type 2 diabetes was used as another control. In this case, there was no effect in the unadjusted data, while the adjusted model appeared to indicate a protective effect. Pointing in the opposite direction, there were actually more montelukast users in the diabetes group compared to the total study group. Although inflammation has been proposed as part of the aetiology of type 2 diabetes [23], the observed reduction in HR reflects, perhaps, that these subjects use a particularly high level of other medications (Table 1). The adjusted data may consequently be biased. The diabetes data emphasize the caution required when interpreting correlates obtained from NorPD. The adjustments performed may be more or less pertinent, and there may be confounders that are not adjusted for.

The use of psychotropic drugs may affect brain aging. We consequently investigated whether there was a bias as to the use of the following drugs: N02 – Analgesics, N05 – Psycholeptics, N06A – Antidepressants, N06B – Psychostimulants, and N07 – Other nervous system drugs. The use was slightly more prevalent among the montelukast group, reflecting their elevated, total DDDs (data not shown). If psychotropic drugs increase the likelihood of dementia, the difference would imply that the present results underestimate the positive effect of montelukast.

Limitations

Besides the obvious problem that the hazard ratios are based on correlations and not causation, we see two main caveats regarding the present study. For one, it employs prescription data as proxies for various conditions, as there is no direct information as to diagnostics in NorPD; and two, the database offers limited options for testing confounders. The main issues regarding these two caveats are discussed below.

The primary indication for prescribing dementia medicine is AD, although one of them (rivastigmine, which stands for some 30% of the prescriptions), can also be used for PD-related dementia. We do not know how often these drugs are prescribed for non-AD dementia. The primary use of PD medication is to alleviate symptoms associated with this disease, but one of the drugs, pramipeksol (code N04 BC05), can also be dispensed for restless legs syndrome. This is a relatively common syndrome; prevalence estimates for our age set range from 5 to 15%, [28], compared to 0.1–1% for PD [29], both increasing with age. However, most likely only a small fraction of restless legs sufferers takes pramipeksol. In 2014, 42% of the subjects on PD medication, received pramipeksol, suggesting that the majority of the PD group has this condition. As to asthma medicine, the code R03 stands for *Drugs for obstructive airway diseases*. The majority presumably has an asthmatic ailment, but the inhalation drugs (not montelukast) may also be prescribed for related conditions such as chronic obstructive pulmonary disease. Montelukast, on the other hand, may be prescribed to treat allergic rhinitis. On a similar note, although lack of prescriptions are likely to be a reasonable proxy for admission to nursing homes, some individuals may end in this group if they have permanently moved abroad, or stop using prescriptions for other reasons. Norway has approximately 40,000 nursing home residents in a population where 700,000 are 65 years or older [30]. Our nursing home group comprised 2.9% of those 60 years or older (Table 1), the numbers are at least compatible with the conjecture that a majority of those included actually are nursing home residents.

The above limitations seem more likely to point in the direction of underestimating, rather than overestimating, a possible effect of montelukast on cognitive decline. The second caveat is perhaps the more problematic. A bias in prescription practises can easily confound the data. For example, the educated and rich may be more likely to seek medical help and obtain medications. Although Norway has a National Insurance Scheme that includes everyone, we would still have preferred to evaluate the effect of socioeconomic factors, but relevant data is not available in NorPD. Moreover, we see no obvious reasons why such a bias should bend the data in any particular direction. Another example is confounding by contraindication. If the prescription of montelukast is contraindicated for some conditions related to the outcomes, the effects may have been inflated. Again, we are not aware of any particular problem pointing in this direction.

Conclusion

Dementia is arguably the biggest challenge for the future of health-care systems worldwide [31], any measure that can alleviate this burden is highly desirable. The present results do not prove that montelukast will help, placebo-based trials are required to obtain more conclusive evidence. We hope the present data is sufficient to make this option ethically acceptable.

Methods

Study cohort

The analyses were based on data from the Norwegian Prescription Database (NorPD; www.norpd.no). The present version of NorPD contains information about all prescribed drugs dispensed at pharmacies to individual patients by any prescriber (within Norway) between January 1, 2004 and December 31, 2015. Medication given patients in nursing homes or hospitals are not recorded in the NorPD, nor are over-the-counter drugs. Available information includes sex, age, the dates on which drugs were dispensed, drug information, and number of Defined Daily Doses (DDDs) [32].

The present study cohort included all who had received two or more prescriptions of either montelukast (ATC code R03DC03) or inhaling corticosteroids (code R03AK or R03BA), and who were 60 years or older in 2014. Two prescriptions, rather than just one, were chosen in order to avoid including subjects who did not actually use the medication. Information on all other prescriptions, and year of death, were also retrieved. Individuals included in the *montelukast group* may have dispensed inhaling corticosteroids, whereas individuals in the *inhaling corticosteroids group* did not have any recorded prescription of montelukast. Drug prescriptions were also used as a proxy for other diseases: Individuals who had received at least one prescription of dementia drugs (code N06D; i.e., memantine, donepezil, rivastigmine, or galantamine) were included in the *dementia group*; Parkinson's drugs (code N04) in *Parkinson's group*; and type 2 diabetes drugs (codes A10BA, A10BB, and A10BH) in the *diabetes group*.

Assessment of potential covariates

The mean number of DDDs dispensed was used as a proxy for drug consumption. The number of DDDs used by an individual was calculated by the following equation:

$$DDDs = \frac{\text{number of tablets dispensed} \times \text{amount of drug per tablet (mg)}}{\text{DDD of the drug (mg)}}$$

As a gross measure of health, we calculated the mean DDD of all drugs dispensed per day by dividing the sum of DDDs during the study period for each individual by the number of days between the first date of inclusion and the end of the follow-up or when censored. The total drug consumption was categories into four categories: <=5 DDDs/day, 5–10 DDDs/day, 10–15 DDDs/day, and >15 DDDs/day. Drug exposure, assessed as at least one prescription of the following drugs, was used to construct proxies for cardiovascular problems: Antithrombotic agents (code B01A), beta blocking agents (code C07), and agents acting on the renin-angiotensin system (code C09). These proxies were dichotomized into exposed or not and used as covariates in the analyses to adjust for medical conditions that involve higher risk of the different outcomes.

Statistical analyses

All descriptive analyses and survival analyses were conducted using Stata version 14.0.

We computed the age for each participant at the date exiting the study as either the date of failure (for example the first prescription of an anti-dementia drug), the year of death, or the end of follow-up (2015), whichever came first. The relative risk of the outcomes associated with dispensing montelukast, compared to the reference group who only dispensed inhaling corticosteroids (the hazard ratio), was calculated using Cox regression. Age was treated as survival-time in the analyses. These analyses were performed unadjusted as well as by adjusting for sex, cardiovascular medication, and the mean number of DDDs dispensed of any drugs.

The effect parameters are possible to estimate in Cox regression without any consideration of the underlying hazard function, if the proportional hazards assumption holds. Testing the assumption of proportional hazards was performed by the stphtest in Stata. Analyses were stratified on covariates for which the effect did not meet the proportional hazards assumption. In models in which the assumption did not hold for the exposure variable montelukast, we estimated separate effects for two different age periods, 60–75 years and above 75 years.

All statistical tests were two-tailed and calculated at a 95% confidence interval ($p < 0.05$).

Censoring and truncation

Subjects were censored at the date of their last prescription. Drugs received by patients in nursing homes or other institutions are not reported to the NorPD. Hence, people in the present data set, for whom the NorPD registrations stopped and who still remained alive for one year or more, were included in the *"nursing home"* group (other institutions, such as hospitals, are unlikely to retain patients for extended periods). Individuals who died before their last prescription were censored at the year of death.

Subjects who dispensed a dementia drug, a Parkinson drug, or a type 2 diabetes drug before the second prescription of montelukast or inhaling corticosteroids were truncated.

Abbreviations

AD: Alzheimer's disease; ATC: Anatomical Therapeutic Chemical; DDD: Defined Daily Dose; HR: Hazard ratio; NorPD: Norwegian Prescription Database; NSAID: Non-steroidal anti-inflammatory drugs; PD: Parkinson's disease

Acknowledgements

We would like to thank Professor Ludwig Aigner for critical reading of the manuscript and helpful advice.

Funding

Not applicable.

Authors' contributions

BG conceptualized the study and obtained the data. BE performed the statistical analyses. Both authors were involved in the design, writing, and reviewing of the manuscript. Both authors read and approved the final manuscript.

Competing interests

The authors declare that they have no competing interests.

References

1. Marschallinger J, et al. Structural and functional rejuvenation of the aged brain by an approved anti-asthmatic drug. Nat Commun. 2015;6:1–16.
2. Zhang G, et al. Hypothalamic programming of systemic ageing involving IKK-beta, NF-kappaB and GnRH. Nature. 2013;497:211–6.
3. Wyss-Coray T. Ageing, neurodegeneration and brain rejuvenation. Nature. 2016;539:180–6.
4. Franceschi C, Campisi J. Chronic inflammation (inflammaging) and its potential contribution to age-associated diseases. J Gerontol A Biol Sci Med Sci. 2014;69:S4–9.
5. Chen MH, et al. Risk of dementia among patients with asthma: a Nationwide longitudinal study. J Am Med Dir Assoc. 2014;15:763–7.
6. Peng YH, et al. Adult asthma increases dementia risk: a nationwide cohort study. J Epidemiol Commun H. 2015;69:123–8.
7. Ali Z, Dirks CG, Ulrik CS. Long-term mortality among adults with ASTHMA ASTHMA a 25-year follow-up of 1,075 outpatients with asthma. Chest. 2013; 143:1649–55.
8. Hoegh M, Ibrahim AK, Chibnall J, Zaidi B, Grossberg GT. Prevalence of Parkinson disease and Parkinson disease dementia in community nursing homes. Am J Geriatr Psychiatry. 2013;21:529–35.
9. Aarsland D, Zaccai J, Brayne CA. Systematic review of prevalence studies of dementia in Parkinson's disease. Mov Disord. 2005;20:1255–63.
10. Makin S. Pathology: the prion principle. Nature. 2016;538:S13–6.
11. Selbaek G, Kirkevold O, Engedal K. The prevalence of psychiatric symptoms and behavioural disturbances and the use of psychotropic drugs in Norwegian nursing homes. Int J Geriatr Psychiatry. 2007;22:843–9.
12. Prince M, et al. The global prevalence of dementia: a systematic review and metaanalysis. Alzheimers Dement. 2013;9:63–75.

13. Firuzi O, Zhuo J, Chinnici CM, Wisniewski T, Pratico D. 5-Lipoxygenase gene disruption reduces amyloid-beta pathology in a mouse model of Alzheimer's disease. FASEB J. 2008;22:1169–78.
14. Tang SS, et al. Leukotriene D4 induces cognitive impairment through enhancement of CysLT(1) R-mediated amyloid-beta generation in mice. Neuropharmacology. 2013;65:182–92.
15. Abeliovich A, Gitler AD. Defects in trafficking bridge Parkinson's disease pathology and genetics. Nature. 2016;539:207–16.
16. Lucin KM, Wyss-Coray T. Immune activation in brain aging and neurodegeneration: too much or too little? Neuron. 2009;64:110–22.
17. Miguel-Alvarez M, et al. Non-steroidal anti-inflammatory drugs as a treatment for Alzheimer's disease: a systematic review and meta-analysis of treatment effect. Drugs Aging. 2015;32:139–47.
18. Cote S, et al. Nonsteroidal anti-inflammatory drug use and the risk of cognitive impairment and Alzheimer's disease. Alzheimers Dement. 2012;8: 219–26.
19. Vlad SC, Miller DR, Kowall NW, Felson DT. Protective effects of NSAIDs on the development of Alzheimer disease. Neurology. 2008;70:1672–7.
20. Manthripragada AD, et al. Non-steroidal anti-inflammatory drug use and the risk of Parkinson's disease. Neuroepidemiology. 2011;36:155–61.
21. Listi F, et al. Role of cyclooxygenase-2 and 5-Lipoxygenase polymorphisms in Alzheimer's disease in a population from northern Italy: implication for pharmacogenomics. J Alzheimer Dis. 2010;19:551–7.
22. Alzheimer's Disease Anti-inflammatory Prevention Trial Research, G. Results of a follow-up study to the randomized Alzheimer's Disease Anti-inflammatory Prevention Trial (ADAPT). Alzheimers Dement 2013;9:714–23.
23. Esser N, Legrand-Poels S, Piette J, Scheen AJ, Paquot N. Inflammation as a link between obesity, metabolic syndrome and type 2 diabetes. Diabetes Res Clin Pract. 2014;105:141–50.
24. Woods JA, Wilund KR, Martin SA, Kistler BM. Exercise, inflammation and aging. Aging Dis. 2012;3:130–40.
25. Rosano C, Marsland AL, Gianaros PJ. Maintaining brain health by monitoring inflammatory processes: a mechanism to promote successful aging. Aging Dis. 2012;3:16–33.
26. Candore G, Caruso C, Jirillo E, Magrone T, Vasto S. Low grade inflammation as a common pathogenetic denominator in age-related diseases: novel drug targets for anti-ageing strategies and successful ageing achievement. Curr Pharm Des. 2010;16:584–96.
27. Ingelsson E, Yin L, Back M. Nationwide cohort study of the leukotriene receptor antagonist montelukast and incident or recurrent cardiovascular disease. J Allergy Clin Immunol. 2012;129:702–7.
28. Ohayon MM, O'Hara R, Vitiello MV. Epidemiology of restless legs syndrome: a synthesis of the litterature. Sleep Med Rev. 2012;16:283–95.
29. Pringsheim T, Jette N, Frolkis A. Steeves TD. The prevalence of Parkinson's disease: a systematic review and meta-analysis. 2014;29:1583–90.
30. Helvik AS, Engedal K, Benth JS, Selbaek G. Prevalence and severity of dementia in nursing home residents. Dement Geriatr Cogn Disord. 2015;40:166–77.
31. Dolgin E. The three things that could help prevent a meltdown in health-care systems worldwide. Nature. 2016;539:156–8.
32. Rønning M, et al. Legemiddelstatistikk 2009:2 Reseptregisteret 2004–2008. (2009).

18

ESRD-associated immune phenotype depends on dialysis modality and iron status: clinical implications

Didier Ducloux[1,2,3,4*], Mathieu Legendre[1,2,3,5], Jamal Bamoulid[1,2,3,4], Jean-Michel Rebibou[1,2,3,5], Philippe Saas[1,2,3,6], Cécile Courivaud[1,2,3,4] and Thomas Crepin[1,2,3,4]

Abstract

Background: End-stage renal disease (ESRD) causes premature ageing of the immune system. However, it is not known whether hemodialysis (HD) and peritoneal dialysis (PD) similarly affect the T cell system.

Methods: The aim of our study was to analyse whether dialysis modality may mitigate ESRD-induced immune senescence. We explored a large population of patients (675 ESRD patients) and both confirmed and refined the results in a second cohort (84 patients).

Results: HD patients exhibited higher inflammatory monocytes counts ($44/mm^3$ (1–520) vs $36/mm^3$ (1–161); $p = 0.005$). Patients on HD also had higher frequency of CD8 T cells (24% (7–61) vs 22% (8–42); $p = 0.003$) and reduced CD4/CD8 ratio. Such results were confirmed in the second cohort. Moreover, both CD4 + CD57 + CD28- (3.25% (0–38.2) vs 1.05% (0–28.5); $p = 0.068$) and CD8 + CD57 + CD28- (38.5% (3.6–76.8) vs 26.1 (2.1–46.9); $p = 0.039$) T cells frequencies were increased in HD patients. Telomere length did not differ according to dialysis modality, but was inversely related to ferritin levels ($r = - 0.33$; $p = 0.003$). There was a trend towards higher telomerase activity in PD patients (11 ± 13 vs 6 ± 11; $p = 0.053$). Thymic function was not different in PD and HD patients. Patients on PD before transplantation had a higher risk of acute rejection after kidney transplantation (HR, 1.61; 95%CI, 1.02 to 2.56; $p = 0.041$).

Conclusions: More pronounced inflammation with hemodialysis may induce premature aging of the immune system. This observation correlates with a lower risk of acute kidney rejection in patients previously on HD. Clinical consequences in patients maintained on dialysis should be determined.

Keywords: Immune senescence, Dialysis, Inflammation, Iron overload, Acute rejection

Background

End-stage renal disease patients are more prone to infection [1], have a greater risk of virus-related cancer [2], and poorly respond to vaccination [3]. These comorbidities are at least in part related to a premature aging of the immune system. Accordingly, concordant studies reported accelerated thymus attrition, accumulation of terminally differentiated activated memory T cells (TEMRA), and reduction in telomere length in ESRD patients [4, 5]. Although the underlying mechanisms are not fully understood, chronic low-grade inflammation, oxidative stress, and epigenetics modifications have been implicated in immune senescence associated with loss of renal function [6, 7]. However, CMV infection also plays a major role in ESRD-induced immunological aging [4].

The uremia-associated immune dysregulation is amplified after the start of renal replacement therapy [8]. However, it is not known whether hemodialysis and peritoneal dialysis similarly affect the T cell system.

---

* Correspondence: dducloux@chu-besancon.fr
[1]INSERM, UMR1098, Federation Hospitalo-Universitaire, INCREASE, Besançon, France
[2]Univ. Bourgogne-Franche-Comté, Faculté de Médecine et de Pharmacie, LabEx LipSTIC, Besançon, France
Full list of author information is available at the end of the article

The aim of our study was to analyze whether dialysis modality may mitigate ESRD-induced immune senescence. We first explored a large population of patients before transplantation. This cohort was initially designed to define pre-transplant immune profile and subsequent post-transplant clinical outcomes. Main lymphocytes subsets (Naïve and memory CD4+ T cells, CD8+ T cells, recent thymic emigrants, B cells, and NK cells) and monocytes were analysed. The results were confirmed and refined in a second cohort designed to explore uremia-related immune senescence. More specifically, thymic function (T cell receptor TREC), replicative senescence (CD4 + CD28-CD57+ and CD8 + CD28-CD57+ T cells (TEMRA)), and telomere length were assessed. Clinical outcomes were analyzed.

Materials and methods
Patients and methods
Exploratory cohort
Research has been conducted in the 833 first consecutive RTR from the ORLY-EST study [9]. Briefly, ORLY-EST is an observational prospective study including incident renal transplant recipients (RTR) in seven French transplant centers (Besançon, Clermont-Ferrand, Dijon, Kremlin-Bicêtre, Nancy, Reims, Strasbourg). The main objective of this study is to describe interactions between immune status and post-transplant atherosclerosis. For each patient, blood samples were collected at time of transplantation and one year after. Sample collection was performed after regulatory approval by the French ministry of health (agreement number # DC-2008-713, June 11th 2009). The ethic committee of Franche-Comté study has approved the study (2008). Patients enrolled in the ORLY-EST study gave their written informed consent. Clinical data were prospectively collected.

Among 833 patients, 747 received a first transplant. Seventy-two patients (9.6%) had never been dialyzed. 675 patients (81%) were included in this cohort. One hundred and thirty eight patients were on PD (20.4%) and 537 on HD.

Calcineurin inhibitors and Mycophenolate Mofetil were widely used as immunosuppressive regimen.

Cytomegalovirus (CMV) prophylaxis was given according to each center practice. Almost all CMV-exposed patients received valganciclovir for 3 months. All CMV-naïve patients having received a CMV positive kidney received valganciclovir for 3 or 6 months. All patients received Pneumocystis antimicrobial prophylaxis with trimethoprim-sulfamethoxazole for at least 6 months.

Cognitive cohort
Research has been conducted in the 84 patients under dialysis from the IRIS study [5]. Briefly, two hundred and twenty-two patients from the Nephrology department of the University Hospital of Besançon have been prospectively included between September 1st 2013 and August 1st 2016. Patients were split in 3 groups according to CKD stage: group 1 with normal renal function (estimated Glomerular Filtration Rate (eGFR) > 60 ml/min/1.73m^2, Modification of Diet in Renal Disease (MDRD) study equation or creatininemia < 120 µmol/l, $n = 85$), group 2 with severe chronic kidney disease stage IV (eGFR 15–30 ml/min/1.73m^2, MDRD, $n = 53$), and group 3 with ESRD on dialysis (hemodialysis [HD]: $n = 47$ and peritoneal dialysis [PD]: $n = 37$, arbitrary eGFR at 10 ml/min/1.73m^2). Exclusion criteria were history of cancer, viral infections (HBV, HCV and HIV viruses), past history of transplantation, immunosuppressive treatments or a recent infectious episode (< 3 months). Clinical parameters including: body mass index, diabetes mellitus (type 1 or 2), chronic heart failure diagnosed by a cardiologist, history of cardiovascular events (myocardial ischemia, stroke, peripheral arterial disease, and carotid endarterectomy), active tobacco defined by consumption of at least 1 cigarette per day, and statin treatment were recorded. Dialysis patients were included at least 6 months after the onset of renal replacement therapy. Dose and duration of dialysis were also recorded. All patients were previously informed and gave their consent.

T and B cell immunophenotypic analysis
Absolute numbers of CD4$^+$ and CD8$^+$ T cells were determined on fresh samples by a single platform flow cytometry approach using TetraCXP® method, Flow-Count® fluorospheres and FC500 cytometer (Beckman Coulter, Villepinte, France) according to manufacturer's recommendations. PBMCs were isolated by density gradient centrifugation (Pancoll, Pan-Biotech GmBH Aidenbach, Germany) and cryopreserved. After thawing, PBMCs were washed twice in RPMI 1640 + GlutaMAX™-I medium (Invitrogen, Cergy-Pontoise, France) containing 10% fetal calf serum (Invitrogen), thereafter referred as complete medium. Cells were stained with the following conjugated antibodies directed against: CD3, CD4, CD8, C25, CD28, CD31, CD45RA, CD45RO, CD57, CD16, CD19, CD56. To detect intracellular FoxP3, surface staining PBMCs were processed using fixation buffer and permeabilization buffer (BD Biosciences, Le Pont de Claix, France) and incubated with the anti-FoxP3 antibody. Cell debris and doublets were excluded on the basis of side versus forward scatter. Cells were analyzed

on a FACS CANTO II cytometer (BD Biosciences) using FACS Diva (BD Biosciences) software.

Recent thymic emigrants (RTE) were defined as $CD45RA^+CD31^+CD4^+$ T cells [10]. Data were analyzed by considering the percentage of RTE among $CD4^+$ T cells (RTE frequency or RTE%) and the absolute numbers of circulating RTE/mm^3. Naive $CD4^+$ and $CD8^+$ T cells was defined as $CD45RA^+CD28^+$, and terminally differentiated $CD4^+$ and $CD8^+$ T cells was defined as $CD57^+CD28^-$.

Pro-inflammatory monocytes were stained on fresh samples with the following conjugated antibodies directed against CD45 (APC, Pharmingen), CD14 (ECD, Immunotech), CD16 (PC-7, Immunotech), HLA-DR (FITC, Pharmingen), CD86 (PE, Immunotech) according to the manufacturer's recommendations.

Regulatory T cells (Treg) were defined as CD4 + CD25 + Foxp3+. This T cell population was analysed in a subset of patients from the exploratory cohort ($n = 60$ with the same proportion of patient on HD and PD).

Relative telomere length (RTL)

DNA was extracted from isolated PBMC according to manufacturer's instructions (QIAMP DNA Blood mini kit reference 51,106, Qiagen, Courtaboeuf, France). A Nanodrop ND-1000 spectrophotometer (Labtech, Palaiseau, France) was used to quantify genomic DNA. Genomic DNA was stored in TE buffer (10 mM Tris-HCl, 0.1 mM EDTA, pH 7.5) at 4 °C at a concentration of 10 ng/μL. DNA samples were diluted into pure water before starting real-time quantitative multiplex PCR runs described in supplementary data Thermocycler was CFX96 Real Time System (Bio-Rad) with Bio-Rad CFX Manager software to generate standard curve and calculate T/S ratio. Two T/S results were obtained for each sample, and the final reported result for one sample in a given run is the average of the 2 T/S values. Average T/S is expected to be proportional to the average telomere length per cell.

Relative telomerase activity (RTA) measurement

Telomerase activity of T cells was examined using the TeloTAGGG Telomerase PCR ELISA PLUS kit (Applied, Roche Diagnostics, France) according to the manufacturer's instructions and as described previously [11].

Outcomes
Exploratory cohort

Acute rejection Acute rejection was considered in the presence of serum creatinine elevation. Only biopsy-proven acute rejections were considered. Acute rejection was defined according to the Banff classification. Only cellular acute rejections were taken into account.

Infections Methods to assess infectious complications have been previously described [11].

Briefly, diagnosis of severe bacterial infections required bacterial infection-related hospitalization. SBI was considered only if infection was the primary diagnosis for hospitalization.

All opportunistic infections (pneumocystis carinii, tuberculosis, toxoplasmosis, aspergillosis, zoster infection, legionella pneumophilia, etc.) were recorded. BK infections were not recorded.

Diagnosis of CMV disease required the presence of viral replication and clinical symptoms.

Diagnosis was blinded from biological evaluation. Most centres performed weekly monitoring until months 2 and at each visit after the second month.

Statistical analysis

Arithmetic mean was calculated and expressed as + SD. For normally distributed variables, t test was used for continuous variables and chi-2 test for dichotomous variables. Abnormally distributed variables were either log-transformed or split in tertiles.

Correlations were calculated through Spearman test. Multiple regressions were used to determine factors associated with insulin sensitivity and secretion.

Outcomes were studied in the exploratory cohort. Using log rank tests on Kaplan Meier nonparametric estimates of the survival without outcome distribution in the first year post-transplant, we selected variables with a p value lower than, or equal to, 0.20. The selected variables were included into a Cox proportional hazards model, and a backward stepwise selection process was performed, this time at a classical $α = 0.05$. Results are expressed as hazard ratio (HR) and 95% confidence interval (CI), with a p value testing the null hypothesis: $HR = 1$. Therefore when p value is less than 0.05, HR is significantly different from 1, either greater than 1 (i.e., risk of acute rejection is increased) or less than 1 (i.e., risk of acute rejection is decreased). Assumptions of Cox models (log-linearity, proportionality of risk in time) were met in this analysis.

Results
Exploratory cohort
Demographic characteristics

Demographic and clinical characteristics of the study population are depicted in Table 1. HD and PD patients did not differ for any parameters.

Importantly, age and CMV exposure were similar in the two groups.

Immune phenotype

Patients on HD exhibited higher frequency of both CD4 + CD45RO+ (62% (15–97) vs 56% (23–95); $p = 0.001$)

Table 1 Demographic and clinical characteristics of the study population (exploratory cohort)

	PD n = 138	HD n = 537	p
Age (years)	51 ± 15	53 ± 13	0.093
Gender (% male)	75%	68%	0.626
Dialysis duration (months)	33 + 20	63 + 123	0.168
Diabetes (%)	19%	20%	0.775
BMI	25.8 ± 4.9	25.8 ± 4.8	0.988
Pre-transplant CMV exposure	55%	54%	0.822
Induction therapy (% of patients having received ATG)	33%	36%	0.567
Tacrolimus (%)	62%	58%	0.348
MMF (%)	97%	97%	0.960
Scheduled stéroids withdrawal (%)	8%	9%	0.720

(Fig. 1a) and CD8+ (24% (7–61) vs 22% (8–42); $p = 0.003$) T cells (Fig. 1b). Other T cell subsets number and frequencies were similar between PD and HD patients.

We separately studied the association between CD8+ T cell frequency and dialysis modality in CMV-exposed and CMV-naïve patients. HD was marginally associated with higher CD8+ T cell frequency in CMV-naïve (OR, 1.71 95%CI [0.92–3.17], $p = 0.084$), but strongly in CMV-exposed (OR, 1.97 95%CI [1.19–3.28], $p = 0.009$) patients.

HD patients had reduced CD4/CD8 ratio as compared with PD patients (2.36 + 1.36 vs 2.81 + 1.45; $p = 0.007$).

CD4 + CD25 + FoxP3+ Treg were similar in the two groups (3.6 + 2.2% vs 3.4 + 3.2%, in HD and DP patients respectively; $p = 0.814$).

NK cell count (139/mm^3 (4–1404) vs 3144/mm^3 (12–999); $p = 0.328$) did not differ between the two groups of patients.

Although B cell frequency was similar in the two groups, total B cell count was higher in PD patients (104/mm^3 (87–116) vs 89/mm^3 (81–96); $p = 0.029$) (Fig. 1c).

Total monocytes count was similar in the two groups of patients. Nevertheless, those on HD had higher inflammatory monocytes counts compared to patients on PD (44/mm^3 (1–520) vs 36/mm^3 (1–161); $p = 0.005$) (Fig. 1d). CRP levels did not differ between the two groups.

Outcomes

Acute rejection 119 patients (17.6%) experienced acute rejection.

In univariate analysis, PD was marginally associated with acute rejection (HR, 1.47; 95%CI, 0.93 to 2.33; $p = 0.109$). The rate of acute rejection was 21.5 and 17.6% in HD and PD patients, respectively (Table 2).

In multivariate Cox model, both delayed graft function (HR, 1.84; 95%CI, 1.19 to 2.84; $p = 0.006$) and PD (HR, 1.61; 95%CI, 1.02 to 2.56; $p = 0.041$) were associated with acute rejection.

Age was not associated with acute rejection.

Infection We did not observe any differences in the incidence of infectious complications between HD and PD patients (Table 2).

Cognitive cohort
Demographic characteristics
Demographic and clinical characteristics of the study population are depicted in Table 3. HD and PD patients did not differ for any parameters.

Importantly, age and CMV exposure were similar in the two groups.

Ferritin levels markedly differ between HD and PD patients (481 ± 396 vs 277 ± 277 ng/ml; $p = 0.007$).

Immune phenotype

Inflammation CRP levels did not significantly differ between PD and HD patients.

CD4 Both CD4 T cell count and frequency were similar in HD and PD patients.

Nevertheless, CD4 + CD57 + CD28- T cell frequency was marginally higher in HD patients (3.25% (0–38.2) vs 1.05% (0–28.5); $p = 0.068$) (Fig. 2a). CMV exposure was the major determinant of CD4 + CD57 + CD28- T cell frequency ($p < 0.001$). Whereas haemodialysis was associated with higher CD4 + CD57 + CD28- T cell frequency in CMV-exposed patients (OR, 3.27 95% CI [1.01–10.62], $p = 0.048$), such a difference between dialysis modalities w as not observed in CMV-naïve patients (OR, 3.00 95%CI [0.28–32.46], $p = 0.366$). There was a trend towards a correlation between dialysis duration

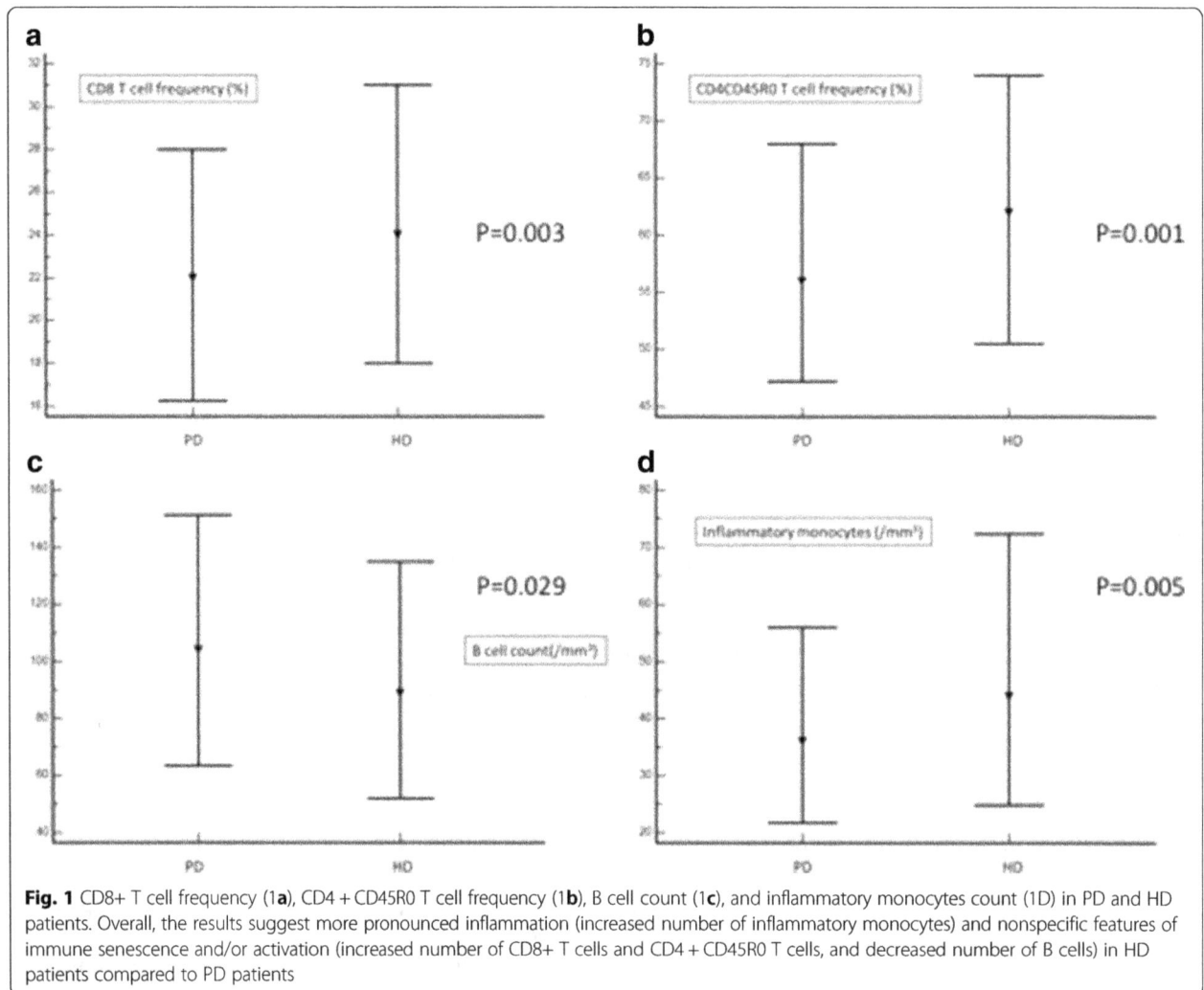

Fig. 1 CD8+ T cell frequency (1**a**), CD4 + CD45R0 T cell frequency (1**b**), B cell count (1**c**), and inflammatory monocytes count (1D) in PD and HD patients. Overall, the results suggest more pronounced inflammation (increased number of inflammatory monocytes) and nonspecific features of immune senescence and/or activation (increased number of CD8+ T cells and CD4 + CD45R0 T cells, and decreased number of B cells) in HD patients compared to PD patients

and CD4 + CD57 + CD28- T cell frequency (r = 0.20; p = 0.066).

Both hemodialysis (OR, 3.06 95%CI [0.95–9.83], p = 0.061) and CMV exposure (OR, 5.05 95%CI [1.31–19.43], p = 0.018) predicted high frequency of CD4 + CD57 + CD28- T cells.

CD8 Patients on HD exhibited higher frequency of CD8 + T cells (33% (11–60) vs 24% (11–55); p = 0.012) (Fig. 2b). Both CD8 + CD57 + CD28- T cell count (110/

mm^3 (52–173) vs 57/mm^3 (29–61); p = 0.034) and frequency (38.5% (3.6–76.8) vs 26.1 (2.1–46.9); p = 0.039) were higher in HD patients. The difference was mainly due to higher TEMRA cells in CMV-exposed patients on

Table 2 Incidence of post-transplant outcomes according to pre-transplant dialysis modality

	PD n = 138	HD n = 537	p
Acute rejection	17,6%	21,5%	0.109
CMV disease	18.2%	17%	0.745
Opportunistic infection	23.1%	27.2%	0.342
Severe bacterial infection	34.1%	35.4%	0.771

Table 3 Demographic and clinical characteristics of the study population (cognitive cohort)

	PD n = 37	HD n = 47	p
Age (years)	67 ± 19	68 ± 14	0.770
Gender (% male)	75%	68%	0.626
Dialysis duration (months)	33 ± 20	63 ± 123	0.168
Diabetes (%)	36	34	0.900
BMI	27.1 ± 4.7	26.7 ± 4.7	0.703
25OH D3 (ng/ml)	24 + 9	30 + 11	0.018
PTH (pg/ml)	393 + 313	401 + 253	0.961
Ferritin (ng/ml)	277 ± 277	481 ± 396	0.007
Albumin (g/l)	32 ± 4	34 ± 3	0.049

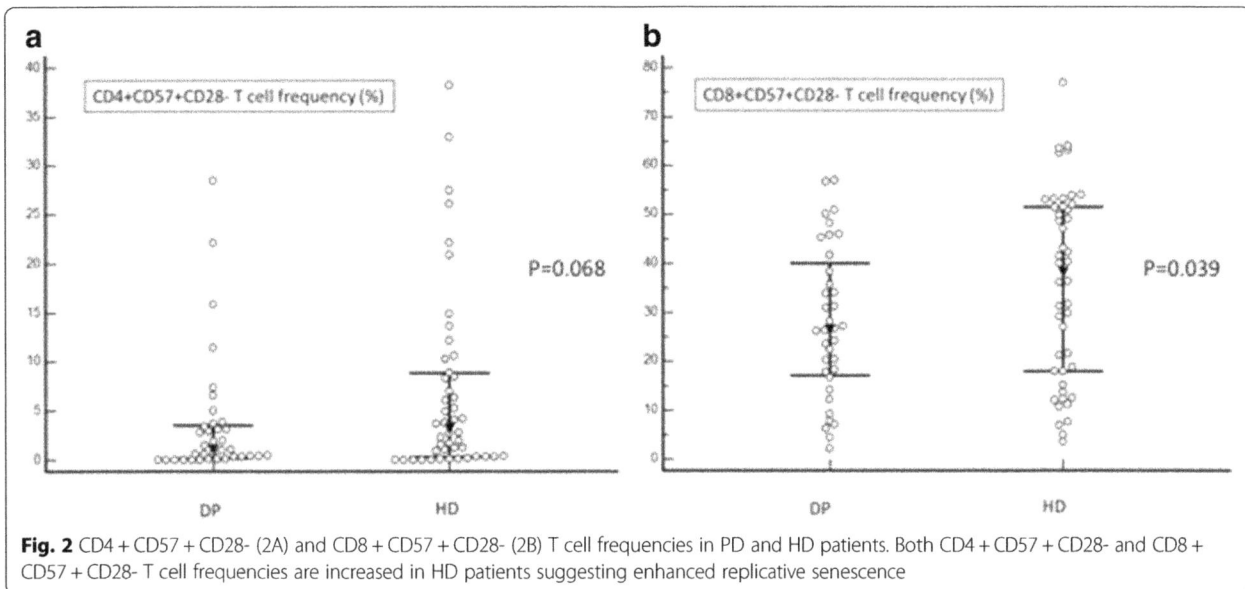

Fig. 2 CD4 + CD57 + CD28- (2A) and CD8 + CD57 + CD28- (2B) T cell frequencies in PD and HD patients. Both CD4 + CD57 + CD28- and CD8 + CD57 + CD28- T cell frequencies are increased in HD patients suggesting enhanced replicative senescence

HD compared to those on PD. Indeed, HD was strongly associated with higher TEMRA frequency in CMV-exposed patients (OR, 3.70 95%CI [1.14–13.18], p = 0.023). This association was not observed in CMV-naïve patients (OR, 0.59 95% CI [0.11–3.20], p = 0.540). The effect was independent of age. The difference was not significant in CMV-naïve patients.

Neither CD8+ T cell frequency (r = 0.05; p = 0.686) nor CD8 + CD57 + CD28- T cell frequency (r = – 0.02; p = 0.914) were related to dialysis duration.

CD4/CD8 ratio was higher in PD patients (3.3 ± 1.7 vs 2.6 ± 1.8; p = 0.015).

TREC TREC numbers did not differ between HD and PD patients.

Telomere length and telomerase activity Telomere length did not differ according to dialysis modality. Nevertheless, we observed a trend towards higher telomerase activity in PD patients (11 ± 13 vs 6 ± 11; p = 0.053).

Iron overload
Because ferritin levels markedly differed between PD and HD patients and because intravenous iron administration, more widely used in HD patients, may induce oxidative stress, a supposed trigger of ESRD-induced immune senescence, we studied whether iron overload may explain at least in part our result.

Iron overload was defined by ferritin levels above 290 ng/ml [12].

TEMRA counts and frequencies were similar in patients with or without iron overload.

By contrast, telomere length was shorter in those with iron overload (0.86 (0.45–1.48) vs 1.01 (0.61–1.56); p = 0.002) (Fig. 3). Ferritin levels and telomere length were closely related (r = – 0.33; p = 0.003) (Fig. 4).

In logistic regression, high ferritin level predicted low telomere length (OR, 5.56 95% CI [1.78–16.67], p = 0.002, for telomere length < 0.87 (median value)). The association persisted after adjustment for age (OR, 4.76 95% CI [1.81–12.50], p = 0.023).

Discussion
Our study reports different immune profile according to dialysis modality. Hemodialysis is associated with more sustained inflammation and lymphocyte activation/exhaustion. The differential immune profile may contribute to an increased incidence of acute rejection in patients on PD before transplantation. By contrast, HD-related accelerated aging may favour infections and ESRD-related cardiovascular disease.

Peritonitis, bio-incompatible solutions, and peritoneal catheter may induce inflammation and T cell activation and aging. Nevertheless, whether PD aggravates systemic ESRD-related inflammation is unclear. Whereas some studies reported higher IL-6 concentrations with longer PD duration [13, 14], others did not observe any burden in IL-6 or CRP levels [15]. Several studies demonstrated inflammation burst with HD procedure [16–18]. Moreover, whereas TLR2 and TLR4 are over-expressed on monocytes from patients on haemodialysis [19], the expression of TLR4 has been reported to be reduced on monocytes in patients with chronic kidney disease (CKD) not receiving dialysis [20]. This suggests

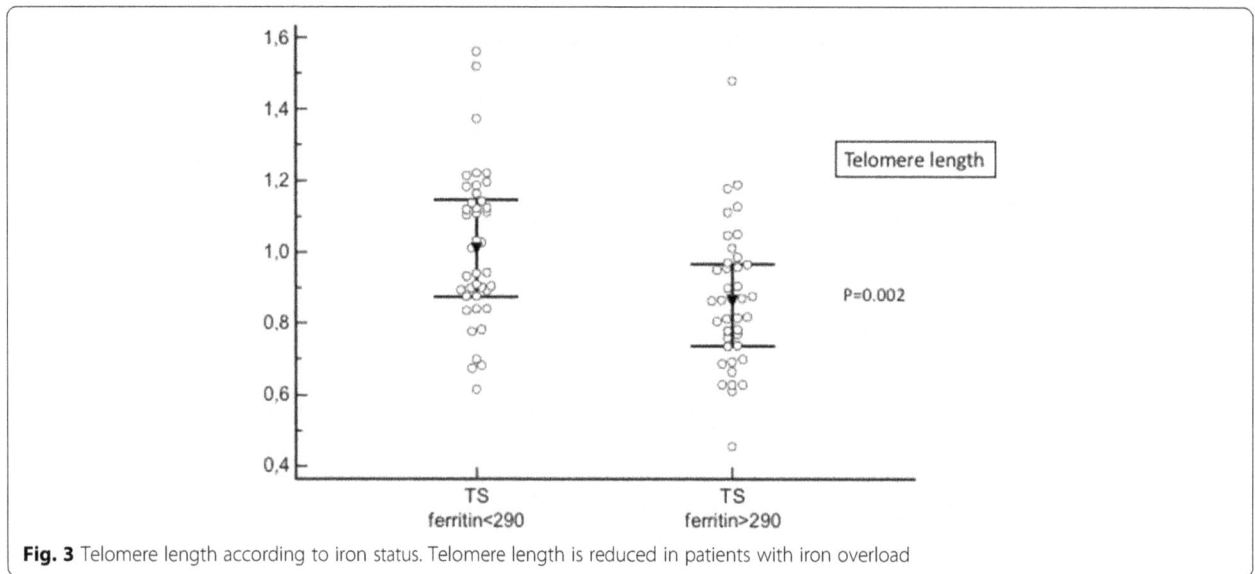

Fig. 3 Telomere length according to iron status. Telomere length is reduced in patients with iron overload

that intermittent activation of monocytes by the dialyzer might result in up-regulation of TLR4. Accordingly, we observed both higher inflammatory monocytes counts in patients on HD as compared to those on PD. We hypothesized that sustained low-grade inflammation may contribute to immune responses to self-antigens and pathological aging by promoting stem cell exhaustion [21]. Alternatively, sustained repeated antigenic stimulation of T cells during hemodialysis procedure may cause more intense proliferation and accelerated aging compared to PD.

It is reported that in cell types with high proliferative capacity, telomerase may be induced in response to

different signal to maintain telomere length and protect chromosomes against damage [22–25]. Nevertheless, we observed higher telomerase activity in patients on PD as compared to those on HD. This result suggests a possible inhibition of telomerase activity. Indeed, certain cytokines secreted during hemodialysis session, such as IFN-α, may inhibit telomerase activity in hematopoietic cells [26, 27].

ESRD-induced T cell exhaustion may play a relevant role in accelerated atherosclerosis observed in dialysis patients. Both CD4 + CD28- and CD8 + CD28- T cells may promote endothelial cell damage, inflammation and destabilization of atherosclerotic plaques, and arterial calcification. Such T cell populations have been

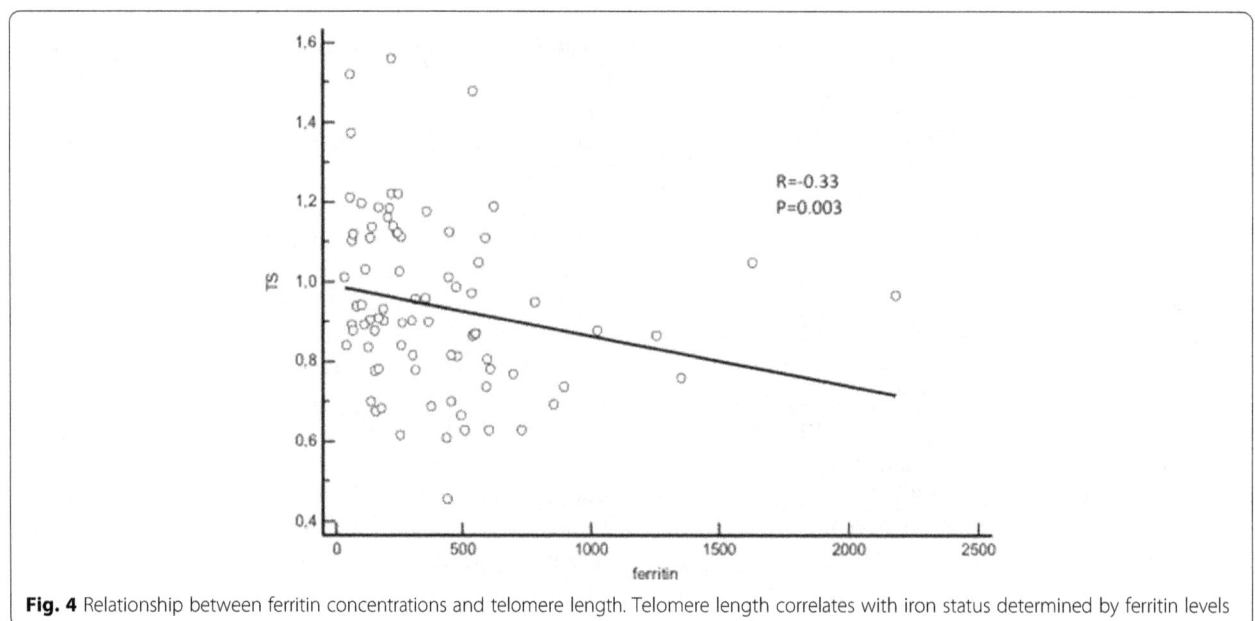

Fig. 4 Relationship between ferritin concentrations and telomere length. Telomere length correlates with iron status determined by ferritin levels

previously associated with cardiovascular outcomes in HIV-infected patients [28]. More recently, we reported that CD8 + CD28-CD57+ T cell number was associated with major cardiovascular outcomes in dialysis patients [5]. CD4 + CD28- T cell expansion was previously reported in ESRD patients and strongly associated with CMV seropositivity [4]. Moreover, CMV-driven expansion of CD28- T lymphocytes may explain the association between CMV seropositivity and atherosclerotic events in both dialysis [29] and kidney transplant patients [30]. We also observed marked TEMRA expansion in CMV-exposed patients. The large majority of CD28- T cells are likely to be CMV-specific and to only proliferate in responses to CMV. This would suggest more frequent CMV reactivation in HD patients compared to PD patients. Otherwise, the differential effect of haemodialysis in CMV-exposed and CMV-naïve patients suggests that haemodialysis procedures may amplify rather than generate the TEMRA pool. Alternatively, some cytokines, such interferon-α, may accelerate the loss of CD28- on T cells as well as inhibit telomerase activity in the absence of CMV antigenic challenge [27, 31].

Previous studies reported that the degree of ESRD-related T cell dysfunction may affect the incidence of acute rejection after kidney transplantation. Betjes et al. showed that patients with higher frequency of terminally differentiated CD8+ TEMRA cells had a decreased risk of acute rejection [32]. Increased CD8+ TEMRA cells number is associated with reduced T cell diversity that may result in reduced diversity of alloreactive T cells [33–35]. Alternatively, these cells may have suppressive effects by reducing the efficacy of antigen-presenting cells to induce T- cell proliferation. Our group reported a tendency for high late stage differentiated CD4 T cell frequency at transplant to be associated with acute rejection in ATG-treated patients [11]. Similar findings have been reported in liver transplantation [36]. By contrast, PD before transplantation has not been previously associated with an increased risk of acute rejection [37]. Delayed graft function is likely to be more frequently reported in HD patients than in PD patients because of better residual renal function in those in PD. This may have masked the association between PD and acute rejection. By contrast, HD was not associated with an increased incidence of post-transplant infections. However, previous studies suggest pre-transplant TEMRA frequency may mitigate the risk of post-transplant infections. Indeed, we previously reported that immune risk profile is associated with post-transplant infectious outcomes [38]. The absence of association may result from confounding parameters (including short duration of follow-up, consideration of different kinds of infections, immunosuppressive drugs, ...) or alternatively from a differential impact of TEMRA on allo-immune and anti-infectious responses.

Ferritin levels were higher in HD patients. Many studies reported better iron supplementation in HD patients compared to PD patients [39]. Intravenous iron administration induces oxidative stress [40]. Nevertheless, we did not observe differences in TEMRA counts or frequencies according to iron status. By contrast, iron overload was associated with shorter telomere length. Other studies reported associations between iron overload and telomere length [41–43]. We previously reported reduced telomere length to be associated with mortality in dialysis patients [5]. Excessive iron load also contributes to ferroptosis [44]. Ferroptosis has an important role in sterile inflammatory conditions such as tissue acute injury, ischemic-reperfusion injury, and neurotoxicity. Further studies should determine whether iron-induced oxidative stress may contribute to morbidity and mortality in dialysis patients.

Association does not preclude causality. As a consequence, we cannot assume a selection bias in the choice of dialysis modality resulting in different immune profiles. Nevertheless, the absence of relevant clinical differences between HD and PD patients make this very unlikely. In fact, this comparison does not suffer usual bias of studies comparing PD and HD patients because we compared a more homogenous subgroup of patients listed on the transplant waiting list. Consequently, major differences between patients are not attempted. Because of the cross-sectional nature of the study, we cannot analyse changes in immunological parameters after and during renal replacement therapy. Nevertheless, we included a very large population in the exploratory cohort and we confirmed primary results in the cognitive cohort.

Conclusions

Our study provides new data concerning ESRD-associated immune senescence. We analysed whether dialysis modality may interfere with immune status. We observed accelerated aging of the immune system in hemodialysis patients as compared with those on peritoneal dialysis. The increase in terminally differentiated CD4[+] and CD8[+] T cells may explain a lower risk of acute kidney rejection in patients previously on HD. Finally, we reported that iron overload correlates with shorter telomere length. Telomere shortening has been associated with excess in mortality in dialysis patients. This result clearly raises the question of the current iron use in dialysis patients.

Abbreviations

CKD: Chronic kidney disease; CMV: Cytomegalovirus; eGFR: Estimated glomerular filtration rate; ESRD: End-stage renal disease; HD: Hemodialysis; MDRD: Modified diet in renal disease; PD: Peritoneal dialysis; RTA: Relative telomerase activity; RTL: Relative telomere length; RTR: Renal transplant recipients; TEMRA: Terminally effector memory

Funding

Supported by grants from the Fondation Transplantation, the PHRC 2005 and 2011 (to DD), the Fondation de France (Appel d'offre "Maladies Cardiovasculaires" 2007 #2007 001859 to PS), the DHOS/INSERM/INCa (Appel d'offre Recherche Translationnelle 2008 to DD and PS) and the APICHU 2010 (to JB), from the Agence Nationale de la Recherche (**Labex LipSTIC**, ANR-11-LABX-0021) and the Région de Franche-Comté (support to **Labex LipSTIC** to PS). JB, CC, TC, and CR received financial support from the Fondation Transplantation (#ET-031211 and #ET-050320, respectively). This work is a part of the RIALTO (**R**esearch in **I**mmunology of **A**therosc**L**erosis after **T**ransplant-ati**O**n) program. This work is supported by the Fédération hospitalo-universitaire INCREASE (**IN**tegrated **C**entre for **R**esearch in Inflammatory Dis**EASE**s).

Authors' contributions

DD, JB, CC, and TC designed the study concept and drafted the manuscript. TC, CC, ML, and JMR participated to acquisition of data and patient follow up. ML, TC, and PS participated in T cell subset analysis in patients. DD did statistical analysis. All authors saw and approved the final version of the manuscript. All the authors approved the final manuscript.

Competing interests

The authors declare that they have no competing interests.

Author details

[1]INSERM, UMR1098, Federation Hospitalo-Universitaire, INCREASE, Besançon, France. [2]Univ. Bourgogne-Franche-Comté, Faculté de Médecine et de Pharmacie, LabEx LipSTIC, Besançon, France. [3]Univ. Bourgogne-Franche-Comté, Faculté de Médecine et de Pharmacie, LabEx LipSTIC, Dijon, France. [4]CHU Besançon, Department of Nephrology, Dialysis, and Renal Transplantation, Besançon, France. [5]CHU Dijon, Department of Nephrology, Dialysis, and Renal Transplantation, Dijon, France. [6]EFS Bourgogne Franche-Comté, Plateforme de Biomonitoring, INSERM CIC 1431/UMR1098, Besançon, France.

References

1. Sakhuja A, Nanchal RS, Gupta S, Amer H, Kumar G, Albright RC, Kashani KB. Trends and outcomes of severe sepsis inpatients on maintenance dialysis. Am J Nephrol. 2016;43:97–103.

2. Stewart JH, Vajdic CM, van Leeuwen MT, Amin J, Webster AC, Chapman JR, McDonald SP, Grulich AE, McCredie MR. The pattern of excess cancer in dialysis and transplantation. Nephrol Dial Transplant. 2009;24:3225–31.

3. Soni R, Horowitz B, Unruh M. Immunization in end-stage renal disease: opportunity to improve outcomes. Semin Dial. 2013;26:416–26.

4. Betjes MGH, Huisman M, Weimar W, Litjens NHR. Expansion of cytolytic CD4+CD28- T cells in end-stage renal disease. Kidney Int. 2008;74:760–7.

5. Crepin T, Legendre M, Courivaud C, Rebibou JM, Ferrand C, Laheurte C, Vauchy C, Gaiffe E, Saas P, Ducloux D, Bamoulid J. Uremia-induced immune senescence and clinical outcomes in chronic disease patients. Nephrol Dial Transplant 2018 (in press).

6. Betjes MG, Meijers RW, Litjens NH. Loss of renal function causes premature aging of the immune system. Blood Purif. 2013;36:173–8.

7. Betjes MG. Immune cell dysfunction and inflammation in end-stage renal disease. Nat Rev Nephrol. 2013;9:255–65.

8. Meijers RWH, Litjens NHR, de Wit EA, Langerak AW, van der Spek A, Baan CC, Weimar W, Betjes MGH. Uremia causes premature ageing of the T-cell compartment in end-stage renal disease patients. Immun Ageing. 2012;9:19.

9. Bamoulid J, Courivaud C, Crepin T, Carron C, Gaiffe E, Roubiou C, Laheurte C, Moulin B, Frimat L, Rieu P, Mousson C, Durrbach A, Heng A-E, Rebibou JM, Saas P, Ducloux D. Pre-transplant thymic function predicts acute rejection in ATG-treated renal transplant recipients. Kidney Int. 2016;89: 1136–43.

10. Ducloux D, Courivaud C, Bamoulid J, Vivet B, Chabroux A, Deschamps M, Rebibou JM, Ferrand C, Chalopin JM, Tiberghien P, Saas P. Prolonged CD4 T cell lymphopenia increases morbidity and mortality after renal transplantation. J Am Soc Nephrol. 2010;21:868–75.

11. Crepin T, Carron C, Roubiou C, Gaugler B, Gaiffe E, Simula-Faivre D, Ferrand C, Tiberghien P, Chalopin J-M, Moulin B, Frimat L, Rieu P, Saas P, Ducloux D, Bamoulid J. ATG-induced accelerated immune senescence: clinical implications in renal transplant recipients. Am J Transplant. 2015;15:1028–38.

12. Rostoker G, Griuncelli M, Loridon C, Magna T, Machado G, Drahi G, Dahan H, Janklewicz P, Cohen Y. Reassessment of iron biomarkers for prediction of dialysis iron overload: an MRI study. PLoS One. 2015:e0132006.

13. Lambie M, Chess J, Donovan L, Kim YL, Do JY, Lee HB, Noh H, Williams PF, Williams AJ, Davison S, Dorval M, Summers A, Williams JD, Bankart J, Davies SJ, Topley N. Independent effects of systemic and peritoneal inflammation on peritoneal dialysis survival. J Am Soc Nephrol. 2013;24:2071–80.

14. Pecoits-Filho R, Carvalho MJ, Stenvinkel P, Lindholm B, Heimbürger O. Systemic and intraperitoneal interleukin-6 system during the first year of peritoneal dialysis. Perit Dial Int. 2006;26:53–63.

15. Cho JH, Hur IK, Kim CD, Park SH, Ryu HM, Yook JM, Choi JY, Choi HJ, Choi HJ, Park JW, Do JY, Kim YL. Impact of systemic and local peritoneal inflammation on peritoneal solute transport rate in new peritoneal dialysis patients: a 1-year prospective study. Nephrol Dial Transplant. 2010;25: 1964–73.

16. Oldani S, Finazzi S, Botazzi B, Garlanda C, Baldassarre E, Valaperta S, Cuccovillo I, Albino M, Child M, Montanelli A, Graziani G, Badalamenti S. Plasma pentraxin-3 as a marker of biocompatibility in hemodialysis patients. J Nephrol. 2012;25:120–6.

17. Yamamoto T, Nascimento MM, Hayashi SY, Qureshi AR, Waniewski J, Brodin LA, Anderstam B, Lind B, Riella MC, Seeberger A, Lindholm B. Changes in circulating biomarkers during a single hemodialysis session. Hemodialysis Int. 2013;17:59–66.

18. Bitla AR, Reddy PE, Manohar SM, Vishnubhotla SV, Pemmaraju Venkata Lakshmi Narasimha SR. Effect of a single hemodialysis session on inflammatory markers. Hemodialysis Int. 2010;14:411–7.

19. Gollapudi P, Yoon JW, Gollapudi S, Pahl MV, Vaziri ND. Leukocyte toll-like receptor expression in end-stage kidney disease. Am J Nephrol. 2010;31: 247–54.

20. Ando M, Shibuya A, Tsuchiya K, Akiba T, Nitta K. Reduced expression of toll-like receptor 4 contributes to impaired cytokine response of monocytes in uremic patients. Kidney Int. 2006;70:358–62.

21. Lopez-Otin C, Blasco MA, Partridge L, Serrano M, Kroemer G. The hallmarks of aging. Cell. 2013;153:1194–217.

22. Chiu CP, Dragowska W, Kim NW, Vaziri H, Yui J, Thomas TE, et al. Differential expression of telomerase activity in hematopoietic progen-itors from adult human bone marrow. Stem Cells. 1996;14:239–48.

23. Engelhardt M, Kumar R, Albanell J, Pettengell R, Han W, Moore MA. Telomerase regulation, cell cycle, and telomere stability in primitive hemato-poietic cells. Blood. 1997;90:182–93.

24. Plunkett FJ, Franzese O, Finney HM, Fletcher JM, Belaramani LL, Salmon M, et al. The loss of telomerase activity in highly differentiated CD8+CD28-CD27- T cells is associated with decreased Akt (Ser473) phos-phorylation. J Immunol. 2007;178:7710–9.

25. Akbar AN, Vukmanovic-Stejic M. Telomerase in T lymphocytes: use it and lose it? J Immunol. 2007;178:6689–94.

26. Xu D, Erickson S, Szeps M, Gruber A, Sangfelt O, Einhorn S, et al. Interferon alpha down-regulates telomerase reverse transcriptase and telomerase activity in human malignant and nonmalignant hematopoietic cells. Blood. 2000;96:4313–8.

27. Reed, J. R., M. Vukmanovic-Stejic, J. M. Fletcher, M. V. Soares, J. E. Cook, C. H. Orteu, S. E. Jackson, K. E. Birch, G. R. Foster, M. Salmon, et al. 2004. Telomere erosion in memory T cells induced by telomerase inhibition at the site of antigenic challenge in vivo. J Exp Med 2004;199; 1433–1443.

28. Kaplan RC, Sinclair E, Landay AL, et al. T cell activation predicts carotid artery stiffness in HIV-infected women. Atherosclerosis. 2011;217:207–13.

29. Betjes MG, Litjens NH, Zietse R. Seropositivity for cytomegalovirus in patients with end-stage renal disease is strongly associated with atherosclerotic disease. Nephrol Dial Transplant. 2007;22:3298–303.

30. Courivaud C, Bamoulid J, Chalopin JM, Gaiffe E, Tiberghien P, Saas P, Ducloux D. Cytomegalovirus exposure and cardiovascular disease in kidney transplant recipients. J Infect Dis. 2013;207:1569–75.

31. Borthwick NJ, Lowdell M, Salmon M, Akbar AN. Loss of CD28 expression on CD8 T cells is induced by IL-2 receptor _ chain signalling cytokines and type I IFN, and increases susceptibility to activation-induced apoptosis. Int Immunol. 2000;12:1005–13.

32. Betjes MGH, Meijers RWJ, de Wit EA, Weimar W, Litjens NHR. Terminally differentiated CD8+ Temra cells are associated with the risk of acute kidney allograft rejection. Transplantation. 2012;94:63–9.

33. Franceschi C, Bonafe M, Valensin S. Human immunosenescence: the prevailing of innate immunity, the failing of clonotypic immunity, and the filling of immunological space. Vaccine. 2000;18:1717–20.

34. Tulunay A, Yavuz S, Direskenell H, Eksioglu-Demiralp E. CD8+CD28-, suppressive T cells in systemic lupus erythematosus. Lupus. 2008;17:630–7.

35. Cortesini R, LeMaoult J, Ciubotariu R, et al. CD8+CD28ʲ T suppressor cells and the induction of antigen-specific, antigen- presenting cellϒmediated suppression of Th reactivity. Immunol Rev. 2001;182:201.

36. Gerlach UA, Vogt K, Schlickeiser S, Meisel C, Streitz M, Kunkel D, Appelt C, Ahrlich S, Lachmann N, Neuhaus P, Pascher A, Sawitzki B. Elevation of CD4+ differentiated memory T cells is associated with acute cellular and antibody-mediated rejection after liver transplantation. Transplantation 2013; 27–1512–1520.

37. Tang M, Li T, Liu H. A comparison of transplant outcomes in peritoneal and hemodialysis patients: a meta-analysis. Blood Purif. 2016;42:170–6.

38. Crepin T, Gaiffe E, Courivaud C, Roubiou C, Laheurte C, Moulin B, Frimat L, Rieu P, Mousson C, Durrbach A, Heng A-E, Saas P, Bamoulid J, Ducloux D. Pre-transplant end-stage renal disease-related immune risk profile in kidney transplant recipients predicts post-transplant infections. Transplant Inf Dis. 2016;18:415–22.

39. Wetmore JB, Peng Y, Monda KL, Kats AM, Kim DH, Bradbury BD, Collins AJ, Gilbertson DT. Trends in anemia management practices in patients receiving hemodialysis and peritoneal dialysis: a retrospective cohort analysis. Am J Nephrol. 2015;41:354–61.

40. Liakopoulos V, Roumeliotis S, Gomy X, Dounousi E, Mertens PR. Oxidative stress in hemodialysis patients : a review of literature. Oxidative Med Cell Longev 2017; 2017: 3081856.

41. Shin C, Baik I. Transferrin saturation concentrations associated with telomeric ageing: a population-based study. Br J Nutr. 2017;117:1693–701.

42. Murillo-Ortiz B, Ramirez Emiliano J, Hernandez Vazquez WI, Martinez-Garza S, Solorio-Meza S, Albarran-Tamayo F, Ramos-Rodriguez E, Benitez-Bribiesca L. Impact of oxidative stress in premature aging and iron overload in hemodialysis patients. Oxidative Med Cell Longev. 2016;2016:1578235.

43. Kepinska M, Szyller J, Milnerowicz H. The influence of oxidative stress induced by iron on telomere length. Environ Toxicol Pharmacol. 2015;40: 931–5.

44. Xie Y, Hou W, Song X, Yu Y, Huang J, Sun X, Kang R, Tang D. Ferroptosis: process and function. Cell death Diff. 2016;23:369–79.

Molecular changes associated with increased TNF-α-induced apoptotis in naïve (T_N) and central memory (T_{CM}) CD8+ T cells in aged humans

Sudhir Gupta[1,2*], Houfen Su[1], Sudhanshu Agrawal[1] and Sastry Gollapudi[1]

Abstract

Background: Progressive T cell decline in aged humans is associated with a deficiency of naïve (T_N) and central memory (T_{CM}) T cells. We have previously reported increased Tumor necrosis factor-α (TNF-α)-induced apoptosis in T_N and T_{CM} T cells in aged humans; however, the molecular basis of increased apoptosis remains to be defined. Since expression of TNF receptors (TNFRs) was reported to be comparable in young and aged, we investigated signaling events downstream of TNFRs to understand the molecular basis of increased TNF-α-induced apoptosis in aged T_N and T_{CM} CD8+ cells.

Results: The expression of TRAF-2 and RIP, phosphorylation of JNK, IKKα/β, and IκBα, and activation of NF-κB activation were significantly decreased in T_N and T_{CM} CD8+ cells from aged subjects as compared to young controls. Furthermore, expression of A20, Bcl-x_L, cIAP1, and FLIP-$_L$ and FLIP-$_S$ was significantly decreased in T_N and T_{CM} CD8+ cells from aged subjects.

Conclusions: These data demonstrate that an impaired expression/function of molecules downstream TNFR signaling pathway that confer survival signals contribute to increased apoptosis of T_N and T_{CM} CD8+ cells in aged humans.

Keywords: TNF-α, A20, TRAF-2, RIP, cFLIP, NF-κb

Background

Aging is associated with a progressive decline in immune responses including impaired proliferative and effector responses, impaired T cell signaling, and increased frequency of infections [1–12]. However, molecular mechanisms for immune dysfunction with age are poorly understood. Following antigenic stimulation naïve CD8+ T cells (T_N) undergo activation and clonal expansion to generate effector CD8+ T cells. After clearance of antigen, majority of effector cells undergo apoptosis, and a subpopulation of effectors cells is retained as long-term memory cells [13]. Based upon their homing properties, and expression of adhesion molecules and chemokine receptors, memory T cells are classified into central memory (T_{CM}) and effector memory (T_{EM}) CD8+ T cells [14–22]. We, and others have reported their characteristics with regard to proliferative response, cytokine production, effector properties, and sensitivity to apoptosis via death receptors, mitochondrial, and endoplasmic reticulum stress signaling pathways [21, 23–25].

TNF-α is a pleiotropic cytokine that activates T cells via both TNF-RI and TNF-RII and mediates both apoptotic and survival signals [26–35]. TNFα-mediates its biological functions predominantly via TNFR-I. Following binding of TNF-α to TNFR-I, the TNFR-associated death domain (TRADD) is recruited to TNFR-I forming a platform for downstream signaling. TNRF-associated factor 2 (TRAF2) and receptor-interacting protein kinase 1 (RIPK1) are recruited to TRADD forming a signaling complex. TRADD also recruits fas-associated death

* Correspondence: sgupta@uci.edu
[1]Program in Primary Immunodeficiency and Aging, Division of Basic and Clinical Immunology, University of California, Irvine, USA
[2]Division of Basic and Clinical Immunology, Medical Sci. I, C-240, University of California at Irvine, Irvine, CA 92697, USA

domain (FADD), which initiates activation of apical caspases resulting in activation of effector caspases, and apoptosis. Both RIPK1 and TRAF2 recruit IKKα and IKKβ to the signaling complex resulting in NF-κB activation [36, 37]. NF-κB translocates to the nucleus, binds to the promoter, and induces a number of anti-apoptotic genes, including FLIP, IAPs, A20, Bcl-x_L [32–34]. TRAF2 also activates MAP kinase/JNK pathway; prolonged JNK activation may result in apoptosis [38].

In human aging, TNF-α production is increased [9–12]. A number of investigators have reported increased sensitivity of T cells, CD4+ and CD8+ T cells and their subsets to death receptors (CD95 and TNF-) mediated apoptosis [25, 39–41]. In aging humans, there is a deficiency in T_N, which in part appears to be associated with increased sensitivity to death-receptor-induced apoptosis [42–47]. In addition, we have reported a deficiency of T_{CM} CD8+ T cells in aging [22]. Furthermore, we have reported that the expression of TNF receptors is comparable between young and aged subjects [23, 48], therefore suggesting that mechanism(s) for increased sensitivity of T_N and T_{CM} CD8+ cells to apoptosis in aging must lie in signaling pathway downstream of TNFRs. In contrast, effector memory CD8+ T cells (T_{EM} and T_{EMRA}) are resistant to apoptosis, and there is no significant different in TNF-α-induced apoptosis in these subsets between young and aged subjects [48].

In this study we present molecular mechanisms of increased sensitivity of purified T_N and T_{CM} CD8+ T in aged humans to TNF-α-induced apoptosis by investigating signaling downstream of TNFRs. Our data show that increased apoptosis in T_N and T_{CM} CD8+ cells from aged subjects is due to decreased expression/function of molecules involved in the signaling pathway involved in cell survival.

Methods

Subjects

Peripheral blood was obtained from 15 healthy young (age 21–35 years with a mean age of 34 years; 9 female and 6 male) and 15 aged (age 65–88 years with a mean age of 72 years, 9 female and 6 male) subjects. Aging subjects belong to middle-class social status and living independently in senior community of Laguna Woods, California. Aging subjects were required to discontinue any and all nutritional supplements at least one week prior to blood draw, to avoid any effect of anti-oxidants, which are commonly used by aging population.

Reagents and monoclonal antibodies

Directly conjugated monoclonal antibodies against CD8 and CD45RA and their isotypes and unconjugated CD8 antibodies were obtained from BD Biosciences (San Diego, CA). Anti-CCR7 and isotypes were purchased from R & D systems, Minneapolis, MN, and anti-CD3/CD28 was Life Technology, Camarillo, CA. TNF-α was obtained from Laguna Scientific, Laguna Niguel, CA. Antibodies to FLIP and IAP were purchased from Transduction Laboratories, San Diego, CA, and antibodies to phospho IKKα/β, phospho IκB, phospho JNK, phosphor TAK1 TAK1, and TAB2 were purchased from Cell Signaling Technologies, Inc. Beverly, MA. Antibodies to A20, TRAF2 and RIPK1 were obtained from Santa Cruz Biotechnology, Dallas, TX. In Situ Cell Death Detection Kit was purchased from Boehringer-Manheim, Indianapolis, IN.

Isolation of T_N and T_{CM} CD8+ T cells and culture conditions

Purified T_N and T_{CM} CD8+ T were separated from healthy young and aged subjects to determine age-related changes rather than simple differences between young and aged subjects. Peripheral blood mononuclear cells (MNCs) were activated with anti-CD3/CD28 monoclonal for 48 h. Cells are washed and used for purification of T_N and T_{CM} CD8+ T cells (cells are activated because freshly isolated human T cells are resistant to all types of death receptor induced apoptosis). First, CD8+ T cells were isolated by negative selection with EasySep CD8+ enrichment cocktail and magnetic nanoparticles (Stem cell Technologies, Vancouver, BC, Canada). Briefly, unwanted cells were specifically-labelled with bispecific tetrameric antibody complexes that recognize unwanted cells and dextran. Dextran-coated magnetic nanoparticles were added and magnetically labeled cells were then separated from unlabeled target cells (CD8+ T cells) using a magnet. Cells obtained are more than 98% CD8 +. T_N (CD8+, CD45RA+ CCR7+) and T_{CM} T-cells (CD8 + CD45RA- CCR7+) were purified to more than 95% by a two-step procedure. First, CD8+ T cells are separated into CD45RA+ and CD45RA- subpopulations by anti-CD45 RA antibody coated Petri dishes. In the second step, CCR7+ T cells are isolated by positive selection using EasySep PE selection kit (Stem cell Technologies). Briefly, CD45RA+ and CD45RA- T cells are labeled with phycoerythrin (PE)-conjugated anti-CCR7 antibody. The labeled cells are then incubated with bispecific tetrameric antibody complexes that recognize PE labeled cells and dextran. After 15 min incubation at room temperature, dextran-coated magnetic nanoparticles are added and magnetically labeled cells are separated from unlabeled cells using a magnet. Positively enriched cells are labeled with APC conjugated anti-CD45 and PerCp-conjugated anti-CD8 and the purity of isolated populations are determined by multicolor analysis using FACSCalibur. Purified T_N and T_{CM} CD8+ T cells were activated with TNF-α to study phosphorylation of signaling molecules by Western blotting.

TNF-α-induced apoptosis was assayed in activated T_N and T_{CM} CD8+ because ex-vivo freshly isolated T cell subsets are resistant to TNF-α-induced apoptosis. Furthermore, phenotypes of T_N cells and T_{CM} were largely maintained following 48 h of anti-CD3/CD28 stimulation of MNCs.

Apoptosis

Purified T_N and T_{CM} CD8+ T cells were stimulated with TNF-α for 48 h to assay for apoptosis. Apoptosis was measured by TUNEL assay (terminal deoxyribonucleotidyl transferase (TDT)-mediated dUTP- nick end labeling). Briefly, TNF-activated purified T_N and T_{CM} CD8+ cells were fixed with 2% formaldehyde for 30 min at room temperature, washed with phosphate buffer saline (PBS), and permeabilized with sodium citrate buffer containing 0.1% Triton X-100 for 2 min on ice. Following washing, cells were incubated with FITC-conjugated dUTP in the presence of TdT enzyme solution containing 1 M potassium cacodylate and 125 mM Tris-Hcl, Ph 6.6 for an hour at 37 °C. Following incubation, cells were washed with PBS, and 10,000 cells were acquired and analyzed by multicolor flow cytometry using FACSCalibur.

Flow cytometry

MNCs activated with anti-CD3/CD28 for 48 h and, then exposed to TNF-α for 10 min. Cell were first surface stained by CCR7 FITC, CD45RA APC, CD8PerCP antibodies and isotype controls. Stained cells were then fixed by 2% paraformaldehyde for 10 min at room temperature, washed and permeabilized by 90% methanol for 15 min on ice. Cells were washed and kept in PBS/2% FBS for 60 min for rehydration and then stained with purified antibodies to cIAP1 and A20 and isotype controls. Cells were washed and stained with secondary PE conjugated goat anti- rabbit antibody.. First cells were gated for CD8+ T cells, and then gated for T_N (CD8+, CD45RA+ CCR7+) and T_{CM} T-cells (CD8 + CD45RA- CCR7+) cells. These gated cells were then analyzed for the expression of cIAP1 and A20. Ten thousand sells were acquired, and were enumerated using FACSCalibur. Data were analyzed by Flow jo software.

Western blotting

Purified T_N and T_{CM} cells activated with TNF-α were lysed with lysis buffer (Cell Signaling). Aliquots of cell lysates containing 50µg of total protein were resolved by SDS-PAGE and transferred onto membranes (Millipore, Bedford, MA) by electro blotting. The membranes were blocked for 1 h at room temperature in TBS-T buffer with 5% nonfat dried milk and incubated with 1µg/ml primary antibodies listed above in reagents and anti-β

actin antibody as loading control used dilution 1:5000 overnight at 4C. The blots were washed three times for 20 min with TBS-T buffer and then incubated with HRP-conjugated secondary antibodies (1:5000–1:10,000 dilution) for 1 h at room temperature. After washing three times for 20 min in TBS-T buffer, blots were developed using enhanced chemiluminescence reagents (ECL, Thermo Scientific Pierce Biotech, Rockford, IL) and exposed to Clear Blue X-Ray Film. Blots were scanned with densitometer.

ELISA for NF-κB activity

DNA-binding activity of NF-κB was measured using an ELISA kit for NF-κB p65 according to manufacturer's protocol (Active Motif, San Diego, CA). The 96-well plates were coated with the oligonucleotide specific for NF-κB binding and the bound NF-κB was measured using anti-NF-κB p65 antibody as described (23). This method provides advantage over traditional EMSA assay in that it is a sensitive assay without using radioactivity, and a large number of samples with smaller number of cells can be analyzed simultaneously.

Statistical analysis was performed by student t test.

Results

Increased sensitivity to TNF-α-induced apoptosis in T_N and T_{CM} CD8 cells in aged subjects

Purified activated T_N and T_{CM} CD8+ cells from young and aged subjects were incubated in the absence or presence of TNF-α for 48 h. Apoptosis was measured by TUNEL assay. Fig. 1 shows data from 10 young and 10 aged subjects. No significant difference was observed in

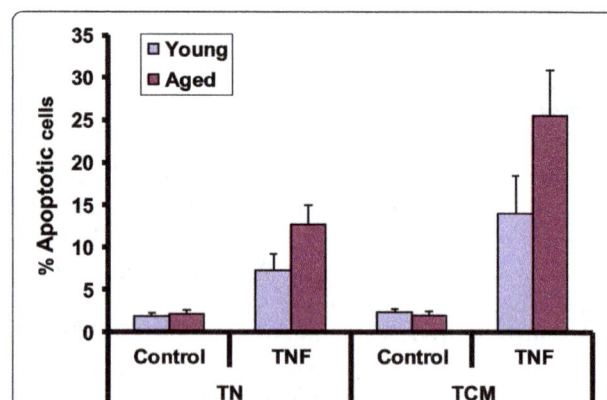

Fig. 1 TNF-α-induced apoptosis in T_N and T_{CM} CD8+ T cells. Activated purified T_N and T_{CM} CD8+ T cells subsets were incubated in the absence or presence of TNF-α for 48 h and apoptosis was measured by TUNEL assay using FACSCalibur. Ten thousand cells were acquired. Data for spontaneous and TNF-α-induced apoptosis from 10 young and 10 aged subjects are presented as percent of TUNEL positive cells. A significantly increased ($P < 0.001$) apoptosis was observed in aged subjects. No significant difference was observed in spontaneous apoptosis between young and aged subjects

spontaneous apoptosis between young and aged group. However, a significantly higher ($P < 0.001$) TNF-α-induced apoptosis was observed in both T_N and T_{CM} CD8+ T cells from aged as compared to young controls. This is in agreement with previous reports [23, 48].

TRAF-2 and RIP expression is decreased in aged T_N and T_{CM}

Since TNFRI and TNFRII expression on aged T_N and T_{CM} CD8+ cells is comparable to young subjects [23, 48] we reasoned that an impaired expression/function of adapter molecule TRAF2 may play an important role in increased sensitivity of T_N and T_{CM} CD8+ T cells in aged humans, via decreased activation of RIP and TAK1 resulting in decreased NF-κB activity and an impaired induction of NF-κB target anti-apoptotic genes. Therefore, first we examined the expression of TRAF-2 and RIPK1 in T_N and T_{CM} CD8+ T cells. Proteins were extracted from purified subsets from young and aged subjects and the expression of these molecules was analyzed by Western blotting with specific antibodies and analyzed by densitometry. Actin was used as a loading internal control. Fig. 2a shows a representative Western blots and Fig. 2b shows data from densitometry of Western blot normalized for actin loading control. Figures 2c shows cumulative densitometry data of Western blot of T_N and T_{CM} CD8+ T cells from five young and five aged subjects normalized for actin

loading control. The expression of TRAF-2 and RIPK1 was significantly decreased ($P < 0.001$) in T_N and T_{CM} CD8+ T cells from aged subjects.

Phosphorylated TAK1 is decreased in aged T_N and T_{CM} CD8 cells

RIPK1 activates TAK-1 via recruitment of TAK-1 complex and interaction of K^{63}ubiquitin chains to TAB2 and subsequent phosphorylation of TAK1 [49]. Since RIPK1 levels are decreased in T_N and T_{CM} CD8+ T cells in aged, we examine the expression of TAB2 and TNF-α-induced phosphorylation of TAK-1 in T_N and T_{CM} CD8 + T cells. Purified T_N and T_{CM} CD8 + T cells were incubated in the presence or absence of TNF-α, and the expression of TAB2 and TAK1, and phosphorylation of TAK-1 was measured with specific antibodies and flow cytometry. Isotype antibodies were used as background control. Figure 3 represents cumulative data of mean fluorescence intensity (density of molecules) from five each young and aged subjects. TAB2 and TAK1 expression was comparable; however, phosphorylated TAK-1 was significantly decreased ($P < 0.004$) in aged cells.

TNF-α-induced phosphorylation of IKKα/β, IκBαand activation of NF-kB is impaired in aged T_N + T_{CM} CD8 cells

TAK1 phosphorylates IKKβ, which in turn phosphorylates IκBα, resulting in the release and activation of NF-κB (p65/p50), providing a survival signal [50]. In

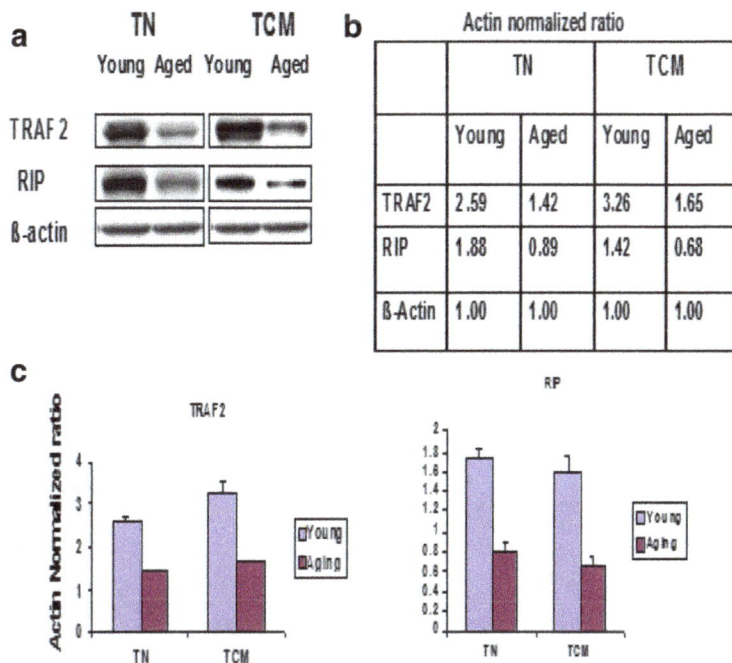

Fig. 2 TRAF-2 and RIP expression in T_N and T_{CM} CD8+ T cells. Protein extracted from purified T_N and T_{CM} CD8+ T cells from aged and young subjects was analyzed by Western blotting using specific antibodies. [**a**] Western blots from a representative experiment, [**b**] densitometry data, and [**c**] cumulative densitometry data from five each young and aged subject. Both TRAF-2 and RPI expression was significantly increased ($P < 0.001$) in aged subjects

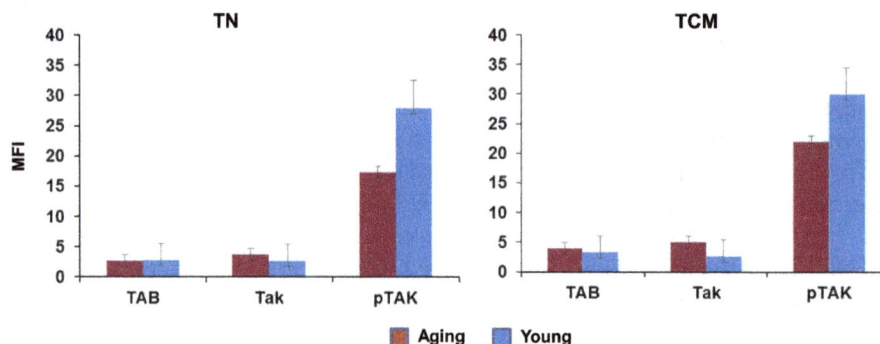

Fig. 3 Expression of TAB2, TAK1 and phospo TAK1. Purified T_N and T_{CM} CD8 + T cells were incubated in the absence or presence of TNF-α for 10 min, and the expression of TAB2 and TAK1, and phosphorylation of TAK-1 were measured with specific antibodies and flow cytometry. Isotype antibodies were used as background control. Data were analyzed for fluorescence intensity (MFI) as an indicator of density of molecules. Cumulative data from 5 young and 5 aged subjects show a significantly decreased ($P < 0.004$) pTAK1 in aged subjects as compared to young subjects

contrast, TAK1 activates JNK that promotes apoptosis [51]. Therefore, we examined TNF-α-induced phosphorylation of JNK, IKKα/β, IκBα, and activation of NF-κB in young and aged subjects.

Purified T_N and T_{CM} CD8+ T cells were activated with TNF-α for 10 min, and the protein was extracted and analyzed by Western blotting, using specific antibodies against phospho IKKα/β, phospho IκBα, and phospho JNK. A representative Western blot is shown in Fig. 4a and the densitometry data from these blots normalized for actin loading control are shown in Fig. 4b. Fig. 4c shows cumulative densitometry data of Western blots from five aged subjects and five young subjects. The levels of phospho JNK, IKKα/β, and IκBα in T_N and

T_{CM} CD8+ T cells from aged subjects were significantly decreased ($P < 0.05-< 0.01$) as compared to young subjects. No difference was observed in the expression of NEMO (data not shown). While JNK signaling can contribute to TNF-induced apoptosis, it is unlikely that decreased JNK activation contributes to increased apoptosis in aged subjects under these experimental conditions.

We also compared NF-κB activity in T_N and T_{CM} CD8 + T cells in young and aged subjects. Purified subsets were activated with TNF-α for 10 min, and NF-κB activity was measured by ELISA-based DNA binding activity. Data from five young and five aged subjects are shown in Fig. 5. Both T_N and T_{CM} CD8+ T cells from aged

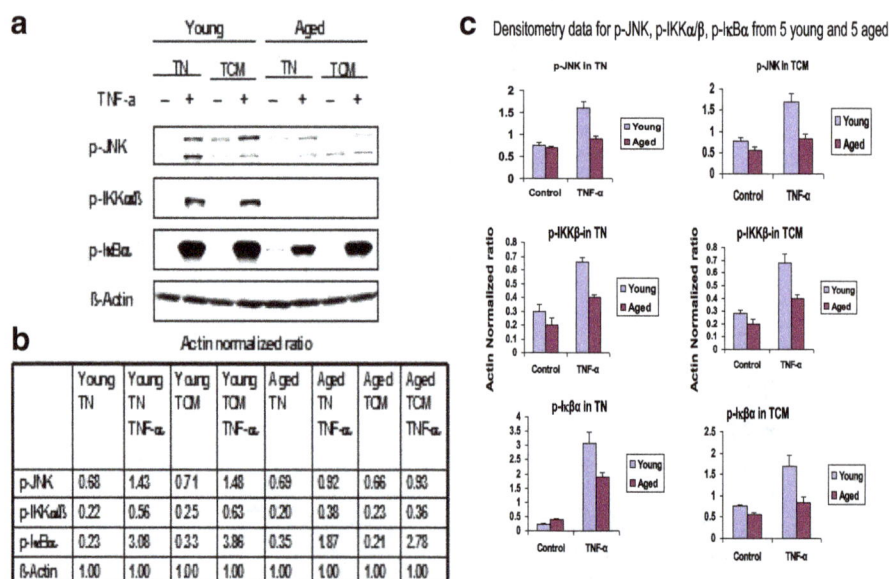

Fig. 4 Effect of TNF-α on the phosphorylation of JNK, IKKβ, IκB in T_N and T_{CM} CD8+ T cells. Purified T_N and T_{CM} CD8+ T cells from young and aged subjects were stimulated with TNF-α for 10 min and then analyzed for expression of phospho JNK, IKKβ, IκB, using specific antibodies. β-actin was used as a loading control. [a] Western blot from one such experiment, [b] densitometry data, and [c] shows densitometry data from 5 each young and aged subjects. A significant decrease in pJNK, pIKKβ, and pIκB ($P < 0.05$, $P < 0.01$) was observed in aged subjects as compared to young subjects

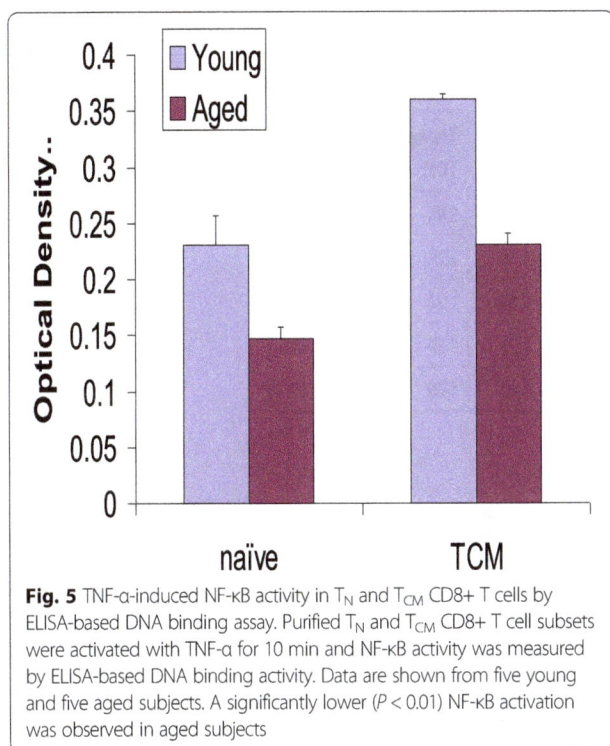

Fig. 5 TNF-α-induced NF-κB activity in T_N and T_{CM} CD8+ T cells by ELISA-based DNA binding assay. Purified T_N and T_{CM} CD8+ T cell subsets were activated with TNF-α for 10 min and NF-κB activity was measured by ELISA-based DNA binding activity. Data are shown from five young and five aged subjects. A significantly lower ($P < 0.01$) NF-κB activation was observed in aged subjects

subjects show significantly lower NF-κB activity following TNF-α activation ($P < 0.01$) as compared to young subjects.

Bcl-X$_L$, FLIP$_L$, FLIP$_S$, A20 and cIAP expression is decreased in T_N + T_{CM} CD8 cells from aged humans

Since NF-κB activates a number of anti-apoptotic genes [52–60], next we examined the expression of cIAP, A20, FLIP and Bcl-x$_L$ in purified T_N and T_{CM} CD8+ T cells in aged and young subjects. Protein extracted from purified T_N and T_{CM} CD8+ T cells from aged and young subjects was analyzed by Western blotting using specific antibodies. A representative Western blot for A20, Bcl-X$_L$, and FLIP$_L$, FLIP$_S$ expression in T_N and T_{CM} CD8+ T cells is shown in Fig. 6a and densitometry data from these blots are shown in Fig. 6b. Fig. 6c shows cumulative densitometry data (mean ± sd) of Western blots from five young and five aged subjects. The expression of A20, FLIP$_L$ and FLIP$_S$, and Bcl-x$_L$ was significantly ($P < 0.05- < 0.001$) decreased in aged subjects.

Since antibodies to A20 and cIAP for flow cytometry became available, and flow cytometry is experimentally less cumbersome and less time consuming than Western blotting, we analyzed the expression of A20 and cIAP in T_N and T_{CM} CD8+ T cells from aged and young subjects by flow cytometry. Data in Fig. 7a is a representative FACS plots, and data in Fig. 7b is cumulative from 4 young and 4 aged subjects (mean ± sd). The expression of A20 (similar to Western blot data in Figure 6) and

cIAP1 is significantly decreased ($P < 0.001$) in T_N and T_{CM} CD8+ T cells from aging as compared to young subjects. These data show that flow cytometry for the analysis of these molecules is a reliable technique, and has advantage over Western blotting in that [a] analysis can be performed on small number of cells, [b] there is no requirement of purification of T_N and T_{CM} CD8+ T cells, and [c] provide better quantitative analysis.

Discussion

Following virus infection or antigen stimulation, naïve T cells undergo a series of proliferative and differentiation steps resulting in the development of effector and memory cells [3]. The differential expression of adhesion molecule (CD62L) and chemokine receptor (CCR7) on memory T cells results in their homing either to lymph nodes (T_{CM}) or to extra nodal sites such as liver and lung (T_{EM}) [14–21]. Both our group, and others have reported decreased in T_N and T_{CM} T cells in aged humans [22, 42–47]. Although a role of thymus in decreased out put of naïve T cells is well-established, we and others have also shown that an increased apoptosis may also contributes to decreased T_N cells in aging [42, 47]. Previously we have reported that T_N and T_{CM} CD8+ T cells are more sensitive to both TNF-α-and CD95-induced apoptosis via activation of caspases as compared to T_{EM} and T_{EMRA} CD8+ T cells [23, 42, 48]; however, expression of TNFRs is comparable to young subjects [23, 48]. Our present data also show increased TNF-α-induced apoptosis in both T_N and T_{CM} CD8+ from aged subjects, which may contribute to their deficiency in aged humans.

TNF-α is a proinflammatory molecule that plays an important role in diverse cellular events including induction of cytokines, cellular proliferation, differentiation, survival and apoptosis [26, 35]. TNF-α-mediates these processes via TNFR-I and/or TNFR-II, apoptosis is predominantly mediated via TNFR-I.

Previously, we have shown that expression of TNFR-I and TNFR-II is comparable in all four subsets of CD8+ T cells (T_N, T_{CM}, T_{EM}, T_{EMRA}); however, T_{EM} and T_{EMRA} CD8+ T cells are resistant to TNF-α-induced apoptosis [48]. Furthermore, in aging, apoptosis and activation of caspase 3 and caspase 8 are increased only in T_N and T_{CM} CD8+ T cells [48]. Therefore, these data suggest that the differences in TNF-α-induced apoptosis in aged T_N and T_{CM} are due to differences in signaling pathway downstream of TNFRs.

The interaction and binding of TNF-α to TNFR-I leads to trimerization of TNFR-I and via death domain and by protein-protein interaction recruits TRADD, which acts as a platform to recruit other proteins including FADD, TRAF2, and RIPK1, forming a signaling complex that activates NF-κB, which induces anti-apoptotic genes. We

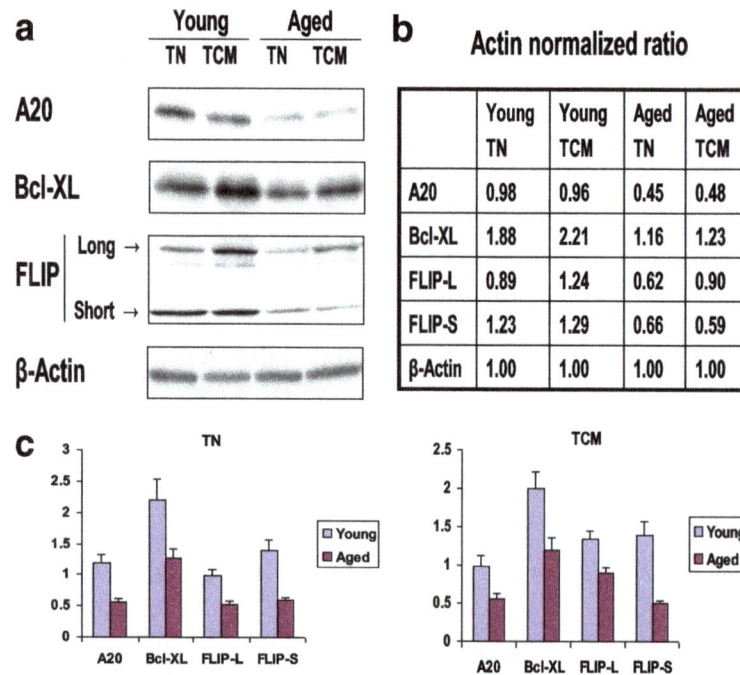

Fig. 6 Expression of A20, Bcl-X$_L$, and FLIP$_L$ and FLIPs in T$_N$ and T$_{CM}$ CD8+ T cells. Protein extracted from purified T$_N$ and T$_{CM}$ CD8+ T cells from aged and young subjects was analyzed by Western blotting using specific antibodies. [**a**] shows a representative Western blot for A20, Bcl-X$_L$, and FLIP expression in T$_N$ and T$_{CM}$ CD8+ T cells [**b**] shows densitometry data from these blots, [**c**] shows cumulative densitometry data (mean ± sd) of Western blots from five young and five aged subjects. T$_N$ and T$_{CM}$ CD8+ T cells subsets from aged subjects display significantly decreased expression of A20 (P < 0.05), Bcl-X$_L$, (P < 0.01), FLIP$_L$ (P < 0.05) and FLIPs (P < 0.05)

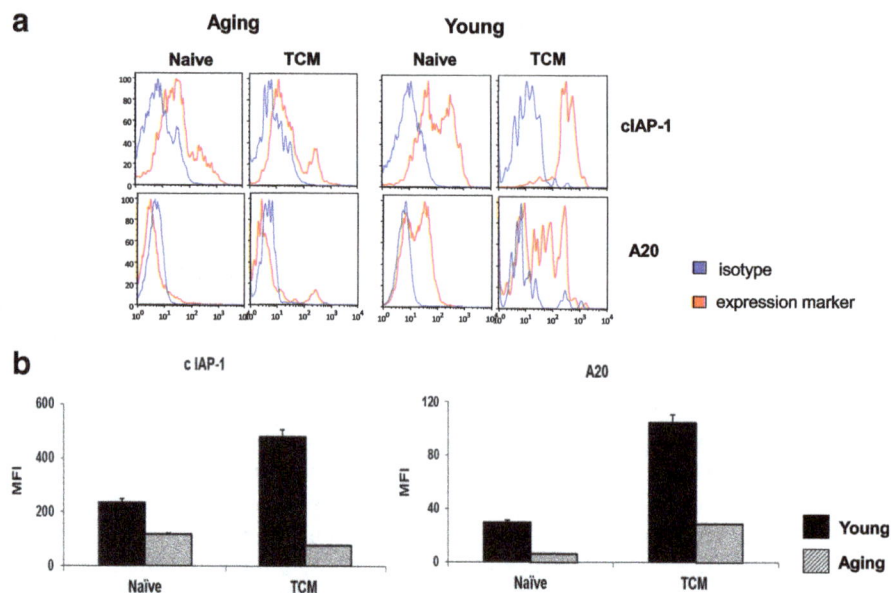

Fig. 7 Expression of A20 and cIAP1 by flow cytometry. MNCs activated with anti-CD3/CD28 for 48 h and, then exposed to TNF-α for 10 min. Cell were first surface stained by CCR7 FITC, CD45RA APC, CD8PerCP antibodies and isotype controls. Stained cells were then fixed and permeabilized, and then stained with purified antibodies to cIAP1and A20 and isotype controls. Cells were washed and incubated with secondary PE conjugated goat anti- rabbit antibody. First cells were gated for CD8+ T cells, and then gated for T$_N$ (CD8+, CD45RA+ CCR7+) and T$_{CM}$ T-cells (CD8 + CD45RA- CCR7+) cells. These gated cells were then analyzed for the expression of cIAP1 and A20. **a** is a representative FACS plot. Blue line represents isotype control, and red line is for A20 and cIAP1. **b** shows cumulative data for MFI from 5 young and 5 aged subjects. T$_N$ and T$_{CM}$ CD8+ T cells from aged subjects show significantly decreased (P < 0.001) expression of both A20 and cIAP

have shown that deficiency of FADD plays an important role in an increased apoptosis of lymphocytes from aged humans [61]. FADD expression is increased in lymphocytes from aged subjects, and transfection of aged lymphocytes with FADD dominant negative plasmid significantly reduced TNF-induced apoptosis in aged lymphocytes comparable to young subjects. Furthermore, we demonstrated that an overexpression of FADD in lymphocytes from young subjects with wild-type FADD resulted in an increased apoptosis of young lymphocytes to a level similar to aged subjects.

RIPK1, a multifunctional protein, and TRAF-2 are required for the activation of NF-κB. It has been demonstrated that in TNF-induced apoptosis caspase-8 cleaves RIPK1 [62]. TRAF2 together with ubiquitin conjugating enzyme complex catalyzes the synthesis of a unique polyubiquitin chain K^{63} of ubiquitin [63–66]. K^{63} polyubiquitination of RIPK1 leads to its activation and recruitment of TAK1 complex and IKK complex [50, 67–70]. This results in the activation of TAK1 kinase complex through interaction between the K^{63} polyubiquitin chain and an ubiquitin-binding domain on TAB2 regulatory units of TAK1 complex [50] and of IKKγ (NEMO) via interaction with K^{63} polyubiquitin chain [69]. TAK1 phosphorylates and activate IKKβ, resulting in phosphorylation and degradation of IκBα, and activation of NF-κB activation [50, 71]. In the current study, we observed decreased expression of both TRAF2 and RIP. TAK1 and not TAB1 or TAB2 plays a role in multiple signaling pathways [72]. In this study we did not see any difference in TAB2 expression in T_N and T_{CM} CD8 cells between young and aged; however, we observed decreased phosphorylation of TAK1, IKKβ, and IκBα, and decreased activation of NF-κB in T_N and T_{CM} CD8 cells. Taken together signaling molecules downstream of TNFR appear to be responsible for increased sensitivity to TNF-α-induced apoptosis in T_N and T_{CM} CD8 cells from aged humans.

The anti-apoptotic genes that are target of NF-κB activation include *cIAP1, cIAP2, Bcl-x_L, A20 and FLIP* show decreased expression in aged naïve and T_{CM} CD8+ T cells [52–60].

A20 (tumor necrosis factor alpha-induced protein 3), a ring finger ubiquitin-modifying enzyme, is essential for the termination of TNF-α-induced activation of NF-kB and inhibition of TNF-induced apoptosis [56–58]. A20 has dual activity in that it inhibits apoptosis as well as activates NF-κB [56, 73]. Interaction of A20 and cIAP with TRAF2 results in the releases of cIAP from the TRAF2-signaling complex, and allows these proteins to exert their anti-apoptotic effects. Our data show decreased expression of A20 and cIAP in aged T_N and T_{CM} CD8+, which are more sensitive to TNF-α-induced apoptosis as compared to young. Therefore, A20

deficiency in aging may be contributing to both increased apoptosis and inflammation. Our data suggest that in primary human CD8+ T cells A20 may function preferentially as an anti-apoptotic molecule.

IAP family proteins have a key role in the inhibition of apoptosis [55, 74, 75]. The cIAP-1 and cIAP2 are structurally homologous proteins. cIAP1 is recruited to DISC of TNFR-I by TRAF-2. Previously we have reported decreased expression of cIAP in CD4+ and CD8+ T cells in aging [76]. In this study we observed decreased expression of cIAP1 in aged T_N and T_{CM} CD8 cells as compared to young subjects, which may contribute to increased sensitivity to TNF-α-induced apoptosis in aged.

cFLIP, an apoptosis inhibiting molecules is a target of NF-κB [52]. FLIP comes in two alternatively spliced forms, the $cFLIP_L$ and cFLIPs. cFLIPs contains two death effector domains (DED) and inhibits procaspase-8 activation, whereas, c-$FLIP_L$ is enzymatically inactive. In addition to its inhibitory effect on procaspase-8 activation, cFLIP by associating with Raf-1activate MEK1, which subsequently activates ERK. cFLIP associates with TRAF2, resulting in NF-κB activation [53, 54, 77, 78]. $cFLIP_L$ inhibits the interaction of caspase 8 prodomain with RIP1 death domain, and regulates caspase 8-dependent NF-κB activation [79]. Our data show a significant decreased expression of both $cFLIP_L$ and $cFLIP_S$ in T_N and T_{CM} CD8+ T cells in aged as compared to young subjects. It remains to determine whether decreased FLIP expression contribute to increased TNF-a-induced activation of caspase-8 and caspase-3 in T_N and T_{CM} CD8+ T cells in aged humans (48).

Conclusions

Our data demonstrate that an impaired expression of adaptor proteins resulting in decreased activation of IKK pathway and decreased NK-κB activation, and decreased expression of anti-apoptotic molecules that are target of NF-κB might play a role in increased sensitivity of T_N and T_{CM} CD8+ T cells, thus contributing to their deficiency and T cell dysfunction in aged humans. However, data presented are correlative, and in vitro overexpression of these molecules may provide the mechanistic explanation for increased sensitivity of T_N and T_{CM} CD8+ T cells in aged humans.

Abbreviations

c-FLIP: FLICE-like inhibitory protein; cIAP1: cellular inhibitor of apoptosis 1; FADD: fas-associated death domain; RIPK1: receptor-interacting protein kinase 1 (RIPK1); T_{CM}: Central memory T cells; T_N: Naïve T cells; TNFR-1 and TNF-R-II: Tumor necrosis factor I and II; TRADD: TNFR-associated death domain; TRAF2: TNRF-associated factor 2

Funding

Was provided by unrestricted research funds of the Division of Basic and Clinical Immunology, University of California, Irvine.

Authors' contributions

SGu conceptualized and designed experiments, interpreted data and wrote the manuscript. HS performed Western blotting, SA was responsible for flow cytometry analysis, and SGo supervised HS, performed apoptosis and NF-κB ELISA assay, compiled all data, and performed statistical analysis. All authors read and approved the final manuscript.

Competing interests

The authors declare that the research was conducted in the absence of any commercial or financial relationships that could be construed as a potential conflict of interest.

References

1. Gruver AL, Hudson LL, Sempowsi GD. Immunosenescence of ageing. J Pathol. 2007;211:144–56.
2. Vallejo AN. Immune aging and challenges for immune protection of the graying population. Aging Disease. 2011;2:339–45.
3. Sansoni P, Vescivini R, Biasini C, Zanni F, Telera A, Lucchini G, Passeri G, Monti G, Frnchesi C, Passeri M. The Imune system in extreme longevity. Exp Gerontol. 2008;43:61–5.
4. Pawlec G, Larbi A, Derhovanessian E. Senescence of the human immune system. J Compl Pathol. 2010;42(suppl 1):S39–44.
5. Pawelec G, Hirokawa K, Fulop T. Altered T cell signaling in ageing. Mech Ageing Dev. 2001;122:1613–37.
6. Ershler WB. Interleukin-6: a cytokine for gerontologists. J Am Geriatric Soc. 1993;41:176–81.
7. Gupta S. Membrane signal transduction in T cells in aging humans. Annals of NY Acad Sciences. 1989;568:277–82.
8. Powlec G, Barnett Y, Effros R, Forsey R, Frasca D, Globerson A, Mariani E, McLeod J, Caruso C, Franceschi C, Fulop T, Gupta S, Mocchegiani E, Solana R. T cells and aging. Front Biosci. 2002;7:d1058–183.
9. Fagiola U, Cossarizza A, Scala E, Fanales-Belasio E, Ortolani C, Cozzi E, Monti D, Franceschi C, Paganelli R. Increased cytokine production in mononuclear cells of healthy elderly people. Eur J Immunol. 1993;23:2375–8.
10. Brunnsgaard H, Andersen-Ranberg K, Hjelmborg JB, Pedersen BK, Jeu B. Elevated tumor necrosis factor alpha and mortality in centenarians. Amer J Med. 2003;115:278–83.
11. Trzonkowski P, Myslizska J, Godlewska B, Szmit E, Lukaszuk K, Wieckiewicz J, Brydak L, Machala M, Landowski J, Mysliwski A. Immune consequences of the spontaneous pro-inflammatory status in depressed elderly patients. Brain Behav Immun. 2004;18:135–48.
12. Penninx BWJH, Kritchevsky SB, Newman AB, Nicklas BJ, Simonsick EM, Rubin S, Nevitt M, Visser M, Harris T, Pahor M. Inflammatory markers and incident mortality limitation in the elderly. J Amer Gerontol Soc. 2004;52:1105–13.
13. Kaech SM, Ahmed R. Memory CD8+ T cell differentiation: initial antigen encounter triggers a developmental program in naïve cells. Nature Immunol. 2001;2:415–22.
14. Sallusto F, Lenig D, Forster R, Lipp M, Lanzavecchia A. Two subsets of memory T lymphocytes with distinct homing potentials and effector functions. Nature. 1999;401:708–12.
15. Masopust D, Vezys V, Marzo AL, Lanzavecchia A. Preferential localization of effector memory cells in nonlymphoid tissue. Science. 2001;291:2413–7.
16. Weninger W, Crowley MA, Manjunath N, von Andriane UH. Migratory properties of naïve, effector, and memory CD8(+) T cells. J Exp Med. 2001; 194:953–66.
17. Tomiyama H, Matsuda T, Takiguchi M. Differentiation of CD8+ T cells from a memory to memory/effector phenotype. J Immunol. 2002;168:5538–50.
18. Geginat J, Lanzvecchia A, Sallusto F. Proliferation and differentiation of human CD8+ memory T-cell subsets in response to antigen or homeostatic cytokines. Blood. 2003;101:4260–6.
19. Van Lier RAW, ten Berge IJM, Gamadia LE. Human CD8+ T cell differentiation in response to viruses. Nat Rev Immunol. 2003;3:931–8.
20. Gupta S, Bi R, Su K, Yel L, Chiplunkar S, Gollapudi S. Characterization of naïve/memory effector subsets of CD8+ T cells: changes in aged humans. Exp Gerontology. 2004;20:545–50.
21. Gupta S, Gollapudi S. Molecular mechanisms of TNF-α-induced apoptosis in naïve and memory T cell subsets. Autoimmun Rev. 2006;5:264–8.

22. Gupta S. Molecular mechanisms of TNF-α-induced apoptosis in naïve and memory T cell subsets: effect of age. Immunol Rev. 2005;205:114–25.
23. Gupta S, Bi R, Gollapudi S. Differential sensitivity of naïve and central and effector memory CD8+ T cells to TNF-α-induced apoptosis. J Clin Immunol. 2006;26:193–203.
24. Gupta S, Gollapudi S. Central and effector memory CD4+ and CD8+ T cells display differential sensitivity to TNF-α-induced apoptosis. N Y Acad Sci. 2005;1050:108–14.
25. Salvioli S, Capri M, Scarcella E, Mangherini S, Faranca I, Volterra V, De Ronchi D, Marini M, Bonafe M, Franceschi C, Monti D. Age-dependent changes in the susceptibility to apoptosis of peripheral blood CD4+ and CD8+ T lymphocytes with virgin or memory phenotype. Mech Ageing Dev. 2003; 124:409–18.
26. Chen G, Goeddel DV. TNF-R1 signaling: a beautiful pathway. Science. 2002; 296:1634–5.
27. Screaton G, Xu X-N. T cell life and death signaling via TNF-receptor family members. Curr Opin Immunol. 2000;12:316–3222.
28. Wajant H, Pfizenmaier K, Scheurich P. Tumor necrosis factor signaling. Cell Death Differ. 2003;10:45–65.
29. Gupta S. Molecular steps of TNF receptor-mediated apoptosis. Curr Mol Med. 2001;1:299–306.
30. Hayden MS, Ghosh S. Shared principles in NF-kappaB signaling. Cell. 2008; 132:344–62.
31. Vallabhapurapu S, Karin M. Regulation and function of NFkappaB transcription factors in the immune system. Annu Rev Immunol. 2009;27: 693–733.
32. Ghosh S, Karin M. Missing pieces in the NF-κB puzzle. Cell. 2002;109:S81–S96.
33. Li Q, Verma IM. NF-κB regulation in the immune system. Nature Rev Immunol. 2002;2:725–34.
34. Li X, Stark GR. NF-κB-dependent signaling pathways. Exp Hematol. 2002; 30:285–96.
35. Varfolomeev EE, Ashkenazi A. Tumor necrosis factor: an apoptosis JunKie. Cell. 2004;116:491–7.
36. Devin A, Cook A, Lin Y, Rodriguez Y, Kelliher M, Z-g L. The distinct role of TRAF2 and RIP in IKK activation by TNFR1: TRAF2 recruits IKK to TNF-R1 while RIP mediates IKK activation. Immunity. 2000;12:419–29.
37. Michaeu O, Tschopp J. Induction of TNF receptor I-mediated apoptosis via two sequential signaling complexes. Cell. 2003;114:181–90.
38. Deng Y, Ren X, Yang L, Lin Y, Wu X. A JNK-dependent pathway is required for TNF-α-induced apoptosis. Cell. 2003;115:61–70.
39. Aggarwal S, Gollapudi S, Gupta S. Increased TNF-α-induced apoptosis in lymphocytes from aged humans: changes in TNF-α receptor expression and activation of caspases. J Immunol. 1999;162:2154–61.
40. Aggarwal S, Gupta S. Increased apoptosis of T cell subsets in aging humans: altered expression of Fas (CD95), Bcl-2 and Bax. J Immunol. 1998;160:1627–37.
41. Gupta S, Gollapudi S. Susceptibility of naïve and subsets of memory T cells to apoptosis via multiple signaling pathways. Autoimmunity Rev. 2007;6: 476–81.
42. Gupta S, Gollapudi S. CD95-mediated apoptosis in naïve, central, and effector memory subsets of CD4+ and CD8+ T cells in aged humans. Exp Gerontol. 2008;43:266–74.
43. Fagnoni FF, Vescovini R, Passeri G, Bologna G, Pedrazzoni M, Lavagetto G, Casti A, Francechi C, Passeri M, Sansoni P. Shortage of circulating naïve CD8+ T cells provides new insights on immunodeficiency in aging. Blood. 2000;95:2860–8.
44. Romanyukha AA, Yashin AI. Age-related changes in population of peripheral T cells: towards a model of immunosenescence. Mech Ageing Dev. 2003; 124:433–43.
45. Effros RB, Boucher N, Porter V, Zhu X, Spaulding C, Walford RL, Kronenberg M, Cohen D, Schachter F. Decline in CD28+ T cells in centenarians and in long-term T cell cultures: a possible cause of both in vivo and in vitro immunosenescence. Exp Gerontol. 1994;29:601–9.
46. Nociari MM, Telford W, Russo C. Postthymic development of CD28-CD8+ T cell subsets: age-associated expansion and shift from naïve to memory phenotype. J Immunol. 1999;162:3327–35.
47. Brzezinska A, Magalska A, Szybinska A, Sikora E. Proliferation and apoptosis of human CD8+CD28+ and CD8+CD28- lymphocytes during aging. Exp Gerontol. 2004;39:539–44.

48. Gupta S, Gollapudi S. TNF-α-induced apoptosis in human naïve and memory CD8+ T cells in aged humans. Exp Gerontol. 2006;41:69–77.

49. Broglie P, Matsumoto K, Akira S, Brautigan DL, Ninomiya-Tsuji J. Transforming growth factor beta-activated kinase 1 (TAK1) kinase adaptor, TAK1-binding protein 2, plays dual roles in TAK1 signaling by recruiting both an activator and an inhibitor of TAK1 kinase in tumor necrosis factor signaling pathway. J Biol Chem. 2010;285:2333–9.

50. Adhikari A, Xu M, Chen ZJ. Ubiquitin-mediated activation of TAK-1 and IKK. Oncogene. 2007;26:3214–26.

51. Huang C-H, Omori E, Akira S, Matsumoto K, Ninomiya-Tsuji J. Osmotic stress activates the TAK1-JNK opathway while blocking TAK1-mediated NF-κB activation: TAO2 regulates TAK1. J Biol Chem. 2006;281:28802–10.

52. Micheau O, Lens S, Gaide O, Alevizopolous K, Tshopp J. NF-κB signals induce the expression of c-FLIP. Mol Cell Biol. 2001;21:5299–305.

53. Irmler M, Thome M, Hahne M, Schnieder P, Hoffmann K, Steiner V, Bodmer J-L, Schroter M, Burns K, Mattmann C, Rimoldi D, French LE, Tschopp J. Inhibition of death receptor signals by cellular FLIP. Nature. 1997;388:190–5.

54. Kataoka T, Budd RC, Holler N, Thome M, Martinon F, Irmler M, Burns K, Hahne M, Kennedy N, Kovacsovics M, Tschopp J. The caspases-8 inhibitor FLIP promotes activation of NF-kappaB and ERK signaling pathways. Curr Biol. 2000;10:640–8.

55. Salvesen GS, Duckett CS. IAP proteins: blocking the road to death's door. Nature Rev Mol Cell Biol. 2004;3:401–10.

56. Heyninck K, Beyaert R. A20 inhibits NF-κB activation by dual ubiquitin-editing functions. Trends Biochem Sci. 2005;30:1–4.

57. Lin S-C, Chung JY, Lamothe B, Rajashanker K, Lu M, Lo Y-C, Lam AY, Darnay BG, Wu H. Molecular basis for the deubiquitinating activity of the NF-κB inhibitor A20. J Mol Biol. 2008;376:526–40.

58. Komander D, Barford DS. Structure of the A20 OUT domain and mechanistic insight into deubiquitination. Biochem J. 2008;408:77–85.

59. Tamatani M, Che YH, Matsuzaki H, Ogawa S, Okado H, Miyake S, Mizuno T, Tohyama M. Tumor necrosis factor-induces Bcl-2 and Bcl-x expression through NF-κB activation in primary hippocampus neurons. J Biol Chem. 1999;274:8531–8.

60. Chen C, Edelstein LC, Gelinas C. The Rel/NF-κB family directly activates expression of the apoptotic inhibitor Bcl-x (L). Mol Cell Biol. 2000;20:2687–95.

61. Gupta S, Kim H, Yel L, Gollapudi S. A role of fas-associated death domain (FADD) in increased apoptosis in aged humans. J Clin Immunol. 2004;24:24–9.

62. Lin Y, Devin A, Rodriguez Y, Liu ZG. Cleavage of the death domain kinase RIP by caspase-8 prompts TNF-induced apoptosis. Genes Dev. 1999;13:2514–26.

63. Xia Z-P, Chen ZJ. TRAF2: a double edge sword? Science Stke. 2005;72:1–4.

64. Chung JY, Park YC, Ye H, Wu H. All TRAFs are not created equal: common distinct molecular mechanisms of TRAF-mediated signal transduction. J Cell Sci. 2002;115:679–88.

65. Sun L, Chen J. The novel functions of ubiquiination in signaling. Curr Opin Cell Biol. 2004;16:119–26.

66. Chen ZJ. Ubiquitination in signaling to and activation of IKK. Immunol Rev. 2012;246:95–106.

67. Wu C-J, Conze DB, Li T, Srinivasula SM, Ashwell JD. Sensing of Lys63-linked polyubiquitination by NEMO is a key event in NF-κB activation. Nature Cell Biol. 2006;8:398–406.

68. Ea CK, Deng L, Xia ZP, Pineda G, Chen ZJ. Activation of IKK by TNFalpha requires site-specific ubiquitination of RIP1 and polyubiquitin binding by NEMO. Mol Cell. 2006;22:245–57.

69. Li H, Kobayashi M, Blonska M, You Y, Lin X. Ubiquitination of RIP is required for tumor necrosis factor-α-induced NF-κB activation. J Biol Chem. 2006;281:13636–43.

70. Israel A. NF-kB activation. Nondegenerative ubiquitination implicates NEMO. Trends Immunol. 2006;27:395–7.

71. Morioka S, Broglie P, Omori E, Ikeda Y, Takaesu G, Matsumoto K, Ninomiya-Tsuji J. TAK1 kinase switches cell fate from apoptosis to necrosis following TNF stimulation. J Cell Biol. 2014;204:607–23.

72. Shim J-H, Xiao C, Paschal AE, Bailey ST, Rao P, Hayden MS, Lee K-Y, Bussey C, Steckel M, Tanaka N, Yamada AS, Matsumoto K, Ghosh S. TAK1, but not TAB1 or TAB2, plays an G essential role in multiple signaling pathways in vivo. Genes Dev. 2005;19:2668–81.

73. Pujari R, Hunte R, Khan WN, Shembade N. A20-mediated negative regulation of canonical NF-kB signaling pathway. Immunol Res. 2013;57:166–71.

74. Deveraux QL, Reed JC. IAP family ptoteins: suppressor of apoptosis. Genes Dev. 1999;13:239–52.

75. Mahoney DJ, Cheung HH, Mrad RL, Plenchette S, Simard C, Enwere E, Arora V, Mak TW, Lacasse EC, Waring J, Korneluk RG. Both cIAP1 and cIAP2 regulate TNF-α-mediated NF-κB activation. Proc Nat Acad Sci (USA). 2008;105:11778–83.

76. Gupta S. A role of inhibitor of apoptosis (IAP) proteins in increased TNF-α-induced apoptosis in lymphocytes from aged humans. Mech Ageing Dev. 2004;125:99–101.

77. Golks A, Brenner D, Krammer PH, Lavrik IN. The c-FLIP-NH2 terminus (p22-FLIP) induces NF-κB activation. J Exp Med. 2006;203:1295–305.

78. Kataoka T, Tschopp J. N-termina fragment of cFLIP (L) processed by caspase 8 specifically interacts with TRAF2 and induces activation of the NF-κB activation. Mol Cell Biol. 2004;24:2627–36.

79. Matsuda I, Matsuo K, Matsushita Y, Haruna Y, Niwa M, Kataoka T. The C-terminal domain of the long form of cellular FLICE-inhibitory protein (c-FLIPL) inhibits the interaction of the caspase 8 prodomain with the receptor-interacting protein 1 (RIP1) death domain and regulates caspase 8-dependent nuclear factor κB (NF-κB) activation. J Biol Chem. 2014;289:3876–87.

Gene and protein expression of *CXCR4* in adult and elderly patients with chronic rhinitis, pharyngitis or sinusitis undergoing thermal water nasal inhalations

Monica Neri[1*] [iD], Luigi Sansone[2,3], Luisa Pietrasanta[4,5], Aliaksei Kisialiou[1], Eloisa Cabano[6], Marina Martini[4,5], Matteo A. Russo[7], Donatella Ugolini[8], Marco Tafani[2,3] and Stefano Bonassi[1,9]

Abstract

Background: Chronic rhinitis, pharyngitis and sinusitis are common health problems with a significant impact on public health, and are suspected to be influenced by ageing factors. Nasal inhalation with thermal water may be used to reduce symptoms, inflammation and drug intake. A pre-post clinical study was conducted in 183 consecutive adult and elderly patients with chronic rhinitis, pharyngitis or sinusitis, to evaluate whether thermal water nasal inhalations could improve their symptoms, clinical signs and rhinomanometry measurements, and influence inflammatory biomarkers levels in nasal epithelial cells.

Results: Participants profile revealed that they were aged on average (mean age and SD 60.6 ± 15.2 years, median 65, range 20–86, 86 aged ≤ 65 years (47%), 96 aged > 65 years (53%)) and extremely concerned about wellbeing. Older age was associated with better compliance to inhalation treatment. Total symptom and clinical evaluation scores were significantly ameliorated after treatment ($p < 0.001$), with no substantial difference according to age, while rhinomanometry results were inconsistent. Persistence of symptom improvement was confirmed at phone follow up 1 year later ($n = 74$). The training set of 48 inflammatory genes (40 patients) revealed a strong increase of *CXCR4* gene expression after nasal inhalations, confirmed both in the validation set (143 patients; 1.2 ± 0.68 vs 3.3 ± 1.2; $p < 0.0001$) and by evaluation of CXCR4 protein expression (40 patients; 1.0 ± 0.39 vs 2.6 ± 0.66; $p < 0.0001$). CXCR4 expression was consistently changed in patients with rhinitis, pharyngitis or sinusitis. The increase was smaller in current smokers compared to non-smokers. Results were substantially unchanged when comparing aged subjects (≥ 65 years) or the eldest quartile (≥ 71 years) to the others. Other genes showed weaker variations (e.g. FLT1 was reduced only in patients with sinusitis).

Conclusions: These results confirm the clinical impact of thermal water nasal inhalations on upper respiratory diseases both in adults and elders, and emphasize the role of genes activating tissue repair and inflammatory pathways. Future studies should evaluate CXCR4 as possible therapeutic target or response predictor in patients with chronic rhinitis, pharyngitis or sinusitis.

Keywords: Clinical trial, CXCR4, Gene expression profiling, Balneology, Inflammation, Respiratory tract infections

---

* Correspondence: monicaneri2008@gmail.com
[1]Unit of Clinical and Molecular Epidemiology, IRCCS San Raffaele Pisana, Via di Val Cannuta, 247, 00166 Rome, Italy
Full list of author information is available at the end of the article

Background

Chronic rhinitis, pharyngitis and sinusitis are common health problems with a significant impact on public health in term of costs and quality of life [1]. Upper airways inflammation is accompanied by a variety of symptoms that can be rather disabling, and ageing factors are suspected to influence both clinical presentation and management of these diseases [2].

Patients are generally treated with antibiotics, steroids, and saline irrigation, but poor compliance when therapy must be pursued for long time has been reported, which in some cases may end up in corticophobia [3, 4]. Six Cochrane reviews have been recently conducted on these treatments for chronic rhinosinusitis, with a common criticism concerning the low quality of several clinical studies [5–10].

Thermal water inhalation therapy for the diseases of the upper respiratory tract has a longstanding tradition and may be used in addition to pharmacological treatment, with the aim of attenuating symptoms and reducing drug intake. This is a major issue particularly in older patients, which often use several drugs to treat chronic diseases or control complex conditions. The effectiveness of thermal treatment in upper airways diseases, of both allergic and non-allergic origin, has been the object of several studies [11]. A bibliometric study conducted by our group showed recently that scientific interest in thermal hydrotherapy applied to nose diseases was quite high in the period between the 1950's and the 1970's, decreased dramatically in the subsequent decade to re-expand again thereafter, with a constant grow of scientific production in number and quality of publications (*personal results*).

A beneficial effect of the treatment in terms of nasal symptoms and functionality has been shown with thermal water of diverse origins. Improvements of several endpoints, including cytology, microbiology, IgE, and some inflammation biomarkers, have been reported in patients of all ages [12–18], but only recently these issues have been investigated specifically in aged patients (> 65 years; [12]). A meta-analysis summarized the results of 13 studies published between 1998 and 2013 on thermal water applications in the treatment of diseases of the upper respiratory tract [11]. Meta-results showed statistically significant improvements in terms of mucociliary clearance time, IgE level, nasal resistance and nasal flow at different time points after treatment with thermal water. The mechanisms are not completely clear. Among the possible effectors, the gasotransmitter H_2S has attracted scientific interest recently, as it is contained in several thermal waters and has anti-inflammatory, antibacterial and antifungal properties [19]. The curative effect of thermal water nasal inhalation could depend on regulation of the expression of different components of the innate immunity system in cells of the nasal epithelia, which can vary with age [2].

Innate immunity is part of the orchestrated homeostatic response to a damaging stimulus. This implies the ability to recognize external noxious agents or molecules (alarmins) released by necrotic cells [20] and to express specific genes in order to repair damaged cells and tissues. Therefore, the families of proteins involved in this process include (a) cell-surface alarmin receptors, such as toll-like receptors [21], the receptor for advanced glycation end products (RAGE) [22] or the purine receptor P2X7R [23], (b) cytokine receptors such as CXCR4, involved mainly in recruiting stem cells into injured organs [24] (c) inducible enzymes, such as cyclooxygenase 2 (COX2), nitric oxide synthase-2(NOS2), 5-lipoxygenase and NAD(P)H-oxidase, (d) growth factors such as epidermal growth factor and fibroblast growth factor along with their receptors, and (e) acute-phase proteins, such as pentraxins (PTX) [25]. Estrogens and their receptors also have well documented immuno-regulatory properties in target tissues and they play an important role in the reparative phase of innate immunity [26]. An age-related reduction in cytokine expression and release, phagocytosis, chemotaxis in the cellular components of the innate immunity has been documented in elderly humans and has been associated with a altered response to pathogens [27].

Among the innate immunity receptors, CXCR4 in particular is the receptor of the cytokine SDF-1 (stromal derived factor 1), physiologically involved in concentrating stem cells into injured organs [24]. Once activated, CXCR4 transduces the molecular signal by activating multiple pathways to control cell migration, proliferation, survival, differentiation [24]. In fact, SDF-1/CXCR4 activation stimulates repair after myocardial infarction [28] as well as wound healing [29].

Aim of the study

We conducted a *pre–post* clinical study to evaluate with a comprehensive approach whether a standard cycle of nasal inhalations with thermal water was able to influence the level of inflammatory biomarkers, ameliorate short-term symptoms, rhinomanometry measurements, and clinical objective evaluation in adult and elderly patients with chronic rhinitis, pharyngitis or sinusitis. The confounding effect of cigarette smoking, age, occupational exposures and diet was taken into account.

Secondary aims of the study were to evaluate the compliance to the treatment, the occurrence of side-effects, and the persistence of beneficial effects of thermal water nasal inhalations on patients' symptoms 1 year later. In addition, the potential interaction of the patients' clinical, demographic, socio-economic and lifestyle profile with the effect of the treatment was investigated.

Methods

Patients recruitment

The study population included adult and elderly consecutive patients with chronic rhinitis, pharyngitis or sinusitis (International Classification of Disease - tenth revision (ICD10): J30 vasomotor and allergic rhinitis, J31 chronic rhinitis, nasopharyngitis and pharyngitis, J32 chronic sinusitis) admitted at Terme di Genova spa (Genoa, Italy) for nasal inhalations with thermal water, male and female.

Approval has been obtained by the competent Ethics Committees of IRCCS San Raffaele Pisana, Rome, and of the Liguria Region.

"Nasal inhalations with thermal water" or "inhalation treatment" mean a cycle of combined warm vapor inhalation and aerosol by nasal adapter for 12 days in 2 weeks with "Cappelletta" source water. The mineral water of this source, which is located in Acquasanta (Genoa, Italy), has an appreciable hydrogen sulfide degree and is a salty earthy alkaline water, due to a prevalence of sodium, calcium and chloride ions, with a pH higher than 11 on average. This water has been used for the treatment of respiratory diseases since ancient times.

Exclusion criteria were systemic or topic treatment within the last 2 week with mucolytics, corticosteroids, anticongestants, antihistamine or NSAIDs, severe chronic diseases, acute disease or surgery in the last month, previous thermal treatment less than 12 months before.

Conditions which determined exclusion from the study were interruption of the treatment before completion, receiving less than 10 sessions, treatment lengthening for more than 4 days, and a new diagnosis of acute or chronic severe disease, hospital admission or surgery during the study period.

All eligible patients admitted to the spa received detailed information about the study by the physician in charge of the treatment, and thereafter were asked to sign an informed consent. All patients who accepted to participate to the study and signed the consent were requested to donate biological samples and were administered a questionnaire.

As is shown in Fig. 1, 233 eligible patients meeting the inclusion/exclusion criteria were asked to participate to the project and 183 (78.5%) entered in the study (T0), while 50 refused, mainly due to time constraints.

Among the patients enrolled, 18 (10%) discontinued the treatment and were considered as dropouts. In sensitivity analysis, they did not show any statistically significant difference from the others neither in terms of diseases of interest nor smoking habits (Pearson χ^2 test), nor as regards total symptom score (TSS) and clinical evaluation score (CES) at enrolment. On the other hand, they were significantly younger on average (49.4 ± 15.3 vs. 61.8 ± 15.3, $p = 0.001$).

Fifteen patients, out of the 165 who completed the treatment and underwent the final evaluations (T1) did not fully respect the protocol, e.g. extension of the end-of-treatment date was longer than 4 days (generally due to personal reasons or to the difficulty to reach the spa, which was located in the countryside). Finally this small group was kept in the analysis, because in sensitivity analysis treatment efficacy was not statistically different when comparing these subjects to the whole study group in terms of TSS, CES and CXCR4 expression, although they were significantly younger (Kruskal-Wallis test).

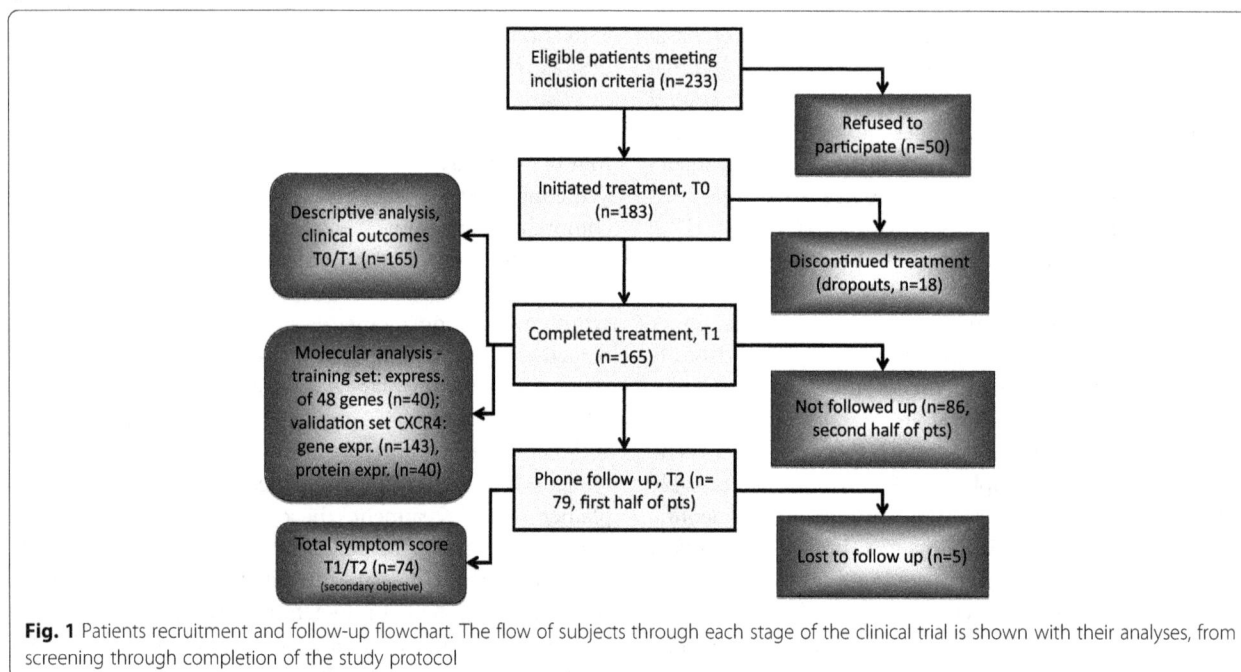

Fig. 1 Patients recruitment and follow-up flowchart. The flow of subjects through each stage of the clinical trial is shown with their analyses, from screening through completion of the study protocol

The first 79 patients enrolled were called on the phone 12 months after the end of the treatment (T2), to administer a questionnaire on their upper respiratory symptoms. Only 74 replied while 5 of them could not be reached (6.3% lost to follow up).

Data and sample collection

A trained physician visited each patient at admission (T0), filling a custom structured questionnaire to collect socio-demographic information and data on job (including exposure to inhalable noxious substances), lifestyle (including smoking habit, exposure to second-hand smoke and diet), clinical history (general and ORL, both remote and specifically referring to the last year), symptom score and clinical evaluation score. The symptom questionnaire was a simplified version of that used in the Naiade survey [30], and was based on 10 items, including cough, nasal obstruction, and nasal discharge with 4 degrees of intensity (0 to 3). TSS were calculated for each subject by summing all the scores assigned to each symptom in the scale. CES were calculated assigning a score 0 to patients without pathologic signs and a score 1 to patients with any pathologic features referring to nasal/pharyngeal mucosa or secretion (e.g.: normal, red, pale or hypertrophic nasal mucosa in left and right nostril; maximum possible CES: 6).

During clinical evaluation, a sample of nasal epithelial cells was collected with a rhinoprobe from the two nostrils for inflammatory biomarkers measurement. An active anterior rhinomanometry was performed in order to measure nasal resistance in a subgroup of patients.

After 2 weeks, at the end of the inhalation therapy (T1), nasal specimen and data on symptoms, clinical evaluation, and rhinomanometry were collected again. The patient was asked about side-effects.

One year after the end of the study (T2), the first 50% of patients enrolled were searched by phone and interviewed using the structured questionnaire for symptom scale, and they were requested to report on any major changes in domicile, job, smoking habit and diet.

Specimen tubes and questionnaires were labeled with unique numerical codes, representing the identity codes for each subject, ensuring blindness of the study and respect of privacy.

A customized database was developed to store patients and specimen information. Access to personal data was restricted.

The samples were stored at − 30 °C no longer than 2 weeks, then transferred at − 80 °C and periodically shipped in dry ice to the laboratory in Rome for analysis.

Additionally, we have included in the study 10 healthy subjects, to ensure a proper comparison of inflammatory biomarker levels with the patients affected by upper respiratory tract diseases. These subjects were enrolled in the

Department of Sense Organs of the Sapienza University of Rome and did not suffer from allergic rhinitis, chronic rhinitis, sinusitis, nasopharyngitis and pharyngitis nor were under anti-inflammatory therapies. They were 7 men and 3 women with a mean age of 50 ± 6 years, non-smokers and without any major inflammatory event in the 3 months preceding sampling of nasal epithelial cells.

Real-Time Quantitative Polymerase Chain Reaction (RT-PCR)

Samples of nasal epithelial cells were lysed to extract total RNA with the Ambion Paris system (Life technologies). After isolation, approximately 1 µg of RNA was reverse transcribed using the High-Capacity cDNA Archive Kit (Applied Biosystems, Milan, Italy) following manufacturer's instructions. Aliquots of cDNA were subjected to real time PCR in 50 µl of 1 x Universal PCR Master Mix, 0.5 µM TaqMan probe and 5 ng of cDNA. Primers and probes for HIF-1α, NF-kB, P2X7R, RAGE, NOS2, COX2, PTX3, CXCR4, VEGF, etc. (see Additional file 1: Table S1) were designed using Assays on-Demand facility (Applied Biosystems). Each sample was loaded in duplicate, and negative and positive controls were included. Amplification of 18S rRNA was used as internal reference gene. PCR amplifications were performed using an ABI PRISM 7900 sequence detector (Applied Biosystems). Amplification data were analyzed using the Sequence Detector version 1.7 software (Applied Biosystems). Statistical analysis of real-time PCR results were done using mean normalized cycle threshold (ΔC_t) values and the pooled standard deviation of the mean ΔC_t.

Western blot assay

Samples were lysed to extract total proteins with the Ambion Paris system (Life technologies). Lysates were clarified by centrifugation (10 min at 4 °C) and the supernatant collected. Protein concentration was determined by the Bradford assay (Bio-Rad). Equivalent amounts of protein were electrophoresed on SDS-polyacrylamide gels. The gels were then electroblotted onto PVDF membranes. After blocking with 5% milk, membranes were incubated with the primary antibody overnight. Finally, the relevant protein was visualized by staining with the appropriate secondary horseradish peroxidase-labeled antibody for 1 h followed by enhanced chemiluminescence.

The following primary antibodies were used: mouse anti-CXCR4, rabbit anti P2X7R, goat anti-AGER, rabbit anti-SOCS1 (Santa Cruz Biotechnology, Santa Cruz, CA), rabbit anti-PTX3 (Alexis Biochemical, San Diego, U.S.A.) and mouse anti-ACTB (Sigma-Aldrich, St Louis, MO). The following secondary antibodies were used: mouse anti-rabbit HRP, goat anti-mouse HRP (Amersham Biosciences, Piscataway, NJ), donkey anti-goat HRP (Santa Cruz).

Statistical analysis

The primary endpoint of the study was the assessment of the safety and efficacy of thermal water nasal inhalations administered to the patients diagnosed with chronic rhinitis, pharyngitis or sinusitis. Measures of effect included changes of symptoms and clinical conditions, rhinomanometry measurements, and inflammatory biomarkers levels from T0 to T1 (primary outcome) and T2 (only for symptoms; secondary outcome). The intent-to-treat (ITT) set included all subjects who were enrolled in the trial. The per protocol (PP) population was the subset of the ITT set that included subjects who completed the study with no major protocol violations.

Descriptive analyses were performed to report on the distribution of clinical and epidemiological variables among the patients, while the variation of the frequency of study endpoints within study intervals was evaluated with the paired samples t-tests (a "repeated measures" t-test). Whenever the distribution of parameters did not allow the use of parametric statistics, non parametric tests such as Mann-Whitney U Test or Wilcoxon signed rank sum test were used instead. In some cases log-transformation was applied. Statistical significance was set at $p < 0.05$ and appropriately adjusted by Bonferroni correction for multiple comparisons when required. Statistical analyses have been conducted using STATA/SE version 12·1 statistical software and MedCalc for Windows, version 15.0 (MedCalc Software, Ostend, Belgium).

Results

Patients profile

Table 1 describes the profile of the 183 enrolled patients: mean age was 61 years, median 65 (range 20–86), and 61% were women. The proportion of subjects aged < 65 years was 47%, while 53% were 65 years or older.

Nine percent had a low education level, while 15% had a university degree. Half of the patients were retired and 12% housewives, while more than one third held an employment.

As regards the pathologies of interest, half of the patients suffered from sinusitis (ICD10 code: J32), 29% from (naso) pharyngitis (J31.1-J31.2), a quarter had chronic, vasomotor or allergic rhinitis (J30, J31.0), with 10 subjects declaring two pathologies at once. The proportions of each disease differed according to age: among the most aged (≥65 years), sinusitis ranked first, followed by rhinitis and pharingitis (42, 35 and 28% respectively), while the youngest were affected mostly by sinusitis (60%), then pharingitis (30%) and rhinitis (14%). The percentages of subjects with two diseases at once were similar (5–6%).

Seventy-one percent of the subjects declared no allergy and 16% a respiratory allergic condition.

Current substantial contact with potentially noxious inhalable substances during work or leisure was reported by a minority of patients ($n = 5$), and for 13% this exposure was considered sporadic or low. Fifty percent of patients never smoked cigarettes, while 14% were current smokers. A low percentage of the subjects declared to be exposed to second-hand smoke at work or at home (7%).

Half of the patients had normal weight, while 38% were overweight and 10% obese. The proportion of subjects eating two portions or less of fruit and vegetables per day was limited to 14%, with 44% of the sample in the intermediate category and 42% declaring to consume at least 6 portions per day. One subject out of four consumed vitamin or antioxidant dietary supplements.

Total symptom score and clinical evaluation score

Symptoms reported by the patients in T0, T1 and T2 are illustrated in Fig. 2. The percentage of patients who declared to suffer with nasal obstruction, nasal discharge, scratchy sore throat, etc. was slightly diminished after treatment among the subjects with low intensity symptoms (panel A) and strongly decreased among those who had symptoms with an intermediate to strong intensity (panel B). The average TSS was 5.7 ± 3.3 at admission, and was reduced by more than 50% after the inhalation treatment (2.7 ± 2.3, statistically significant difference), as is shown in Table 2A. No major changes were found after stratification for age, for pathology or for smoking habit (not shown). Symptoms remained at substantially low levels at T2, that is at the phone follow up 1 year after treatment (mean TSS 2.3 ± 2.6).

At admission, the patients underwent an objective clinical examination: about one quarter of the subjects had deviated septum, 4 out of 10 had pathologic signs in their nasal or pharyngeal mucosa (41 and 38% respectively), 9% had nasal hypersecretion and one patient had pharyngeal hypersecretion. The percentage of patients with any pathological signs in the nasal or pharyngeal mucosa decreased to less than 50% in T1 as compared to T0, while similar but less pronounced patterns were shown for nasal or pharyngeal secretion, which were basically observed only in a minority of the subjects. More in detail, after treatment 17% of the patients had pathologic signs in their nasal mucosa and 14% in their pharyngeal mucosa, while nasal or pharyngeal hypersecretion was found in 4 and 11% of the patients, respectively. Globally, mean CES was 1.4 ± 1.2 at admission and 0.6 ± 0.7 after treatment (statistically significant difference). Results were unchanged when stratifying for age or pathology, while never smokers had lower values with respect to current or former smokers (not shown).

Rhinomanometry

Table 2B shows the main results of active anterior rhinomanometry. Total nasal resistance was globally higher after inhalation treatment (statistically significant in the

Table 1 Sociodemographic, clinical and lifestyle characteristics of the study subjects

Characteristics	N (%)
Total	183 (100%)
Gender	
Men	72 (39.3%)
Women	111 (60.7%)
Age (years)	
mean ± SD (range)	60.6 ± 15.2 (20–86)
1° quartile – median – 3° quartile	51–65-71
≤ 65.	86 (47.0%)
> 65	96 (52.5%)
Education	
Elementary school	17 (9.3%)
Middle school	58 (31.9%)
High school	80 (44.0%)
University	27 (14.8%)
Job or condition (ISCO-08 codes [42])	
Retired	93 (50.8%)
Housewive	22 (12.0%)
Clerical Support Workers (code 4)	15 (8.2%)
Services and Sales Workers (code 5)	15 (8.2%)
Professionals (code 2)	14 (7.7%)
Craft and Related Trades Workers (code 7)	8 (4.4%)
Others[a]	15 (8.2%)
Pathology[b]	
J30-J31.0 rhinitis	46 (25.1%)
J31.1-J31.2 faryngitis	53 (29.0%)
J32 sinusitis	93 (50.8%)
Two pathologies	10 (5.5%)
Allergy	
No	130 (71.0%)
Respiratory	30 (16.4%)
Other allergic condition	23 (12.6%)
Current contact with inhalable substances (work or leisure)[c]	
Never	154 (84.2%)
Sporadic/low	23 (12.6%)
Frequent/heavy	5 (2.7%)
Smoking habit	
Never smokers	87 (47.5%)
Former smokers (1 year or more)	70 (38.2%)
Current smokers	25 (13.7%)
Cigarette pack/years mean ± SD (range)	19.4 ± 20.3 (0.3–102)
Second-hand tobacco smoke (at home, at work)	13 (7.1%)
Body Mass Index kg/m²	
mean ± SD (range)	25.3 ± 3.7 (17.6–40.4)

Table 1 Sociodemographic, clinical and lifestyle characteristics of the study subjects (Continued)

Characteristics	N (%)
Underweight (< 18.5)	5 (2.8%)
Normal weight [18.5;25)	90 (50.0%)
Overweight [25;30)	68 (37.8%)
Obese (≥30)	18 (10.0%)
Vitamin/antioxidants supplementation	
Yes	42 (23.0%)
Fruits+Vegetables consumption	
≤ 2 portions/day	25 (13.7%)
3–5 portions/day	80 (44.0%)
≥ 6 portions/day	77 (42.3%)

Figures may not add up due to missing data
SD standard deviation
[a]Technicians and Associate Professionals (code 3), Elementary Occupations (code. 9), Managers (code 1), Armed Forces Occupations (cod. 0), students and unemployed
[b]Figures do not add up because 10 patients declared two pathologies simultaneously
[c]Solvents and paints, motor-vehicle emissions, cement/plaster/asbestos/silica dust, other dusts, welding fumes, cleaning products

case of exhalation resistance). The differences between T0 and T1 inhalation and exhalation resistances were correlated (Spearman, rho = 0.74, $p < 0.0001$). After stratification by pathology, a statistically significant variation was shown only for exhalation resistance among patients with sinusitis, while the values in T0 and T1 were almost identical among subjects affected with pharyngitis.

No statistically significant difference between measurements in T0 and in T1 remained after stratification of the sample by smoking habit, however never smokers had the lowest values, and current smokers the highest. In addition, increases in T1 tended to be more pronounced among men than women, among elderly patients compared to other adults, and for strong consumers of vegetables and fruits with respect to low or medium consumers (data not shown).

Gene and protein expression

A panel of 48 genes implicated in the innate immunity system and inflammation were analyzed in nasal epithelial cells with High Throughput real-time PCR with a dedicated mini-wells card. This analysis was preliminarily conducted in 40 patients randomly selected among those who reached T1, to identify the candidate gene (s) to be considered for further analyses, among those whose expression was most altered after the inhalation treatment.

Results are shown in Table 3. Mean gene expression of CXCR4 was 3-fold increased at T1 respect to T0 and expression of FLT1 was reduced by one quarter (both highly statistically significant, even after Bonferroni correction), while no other gene showed notable alterations.

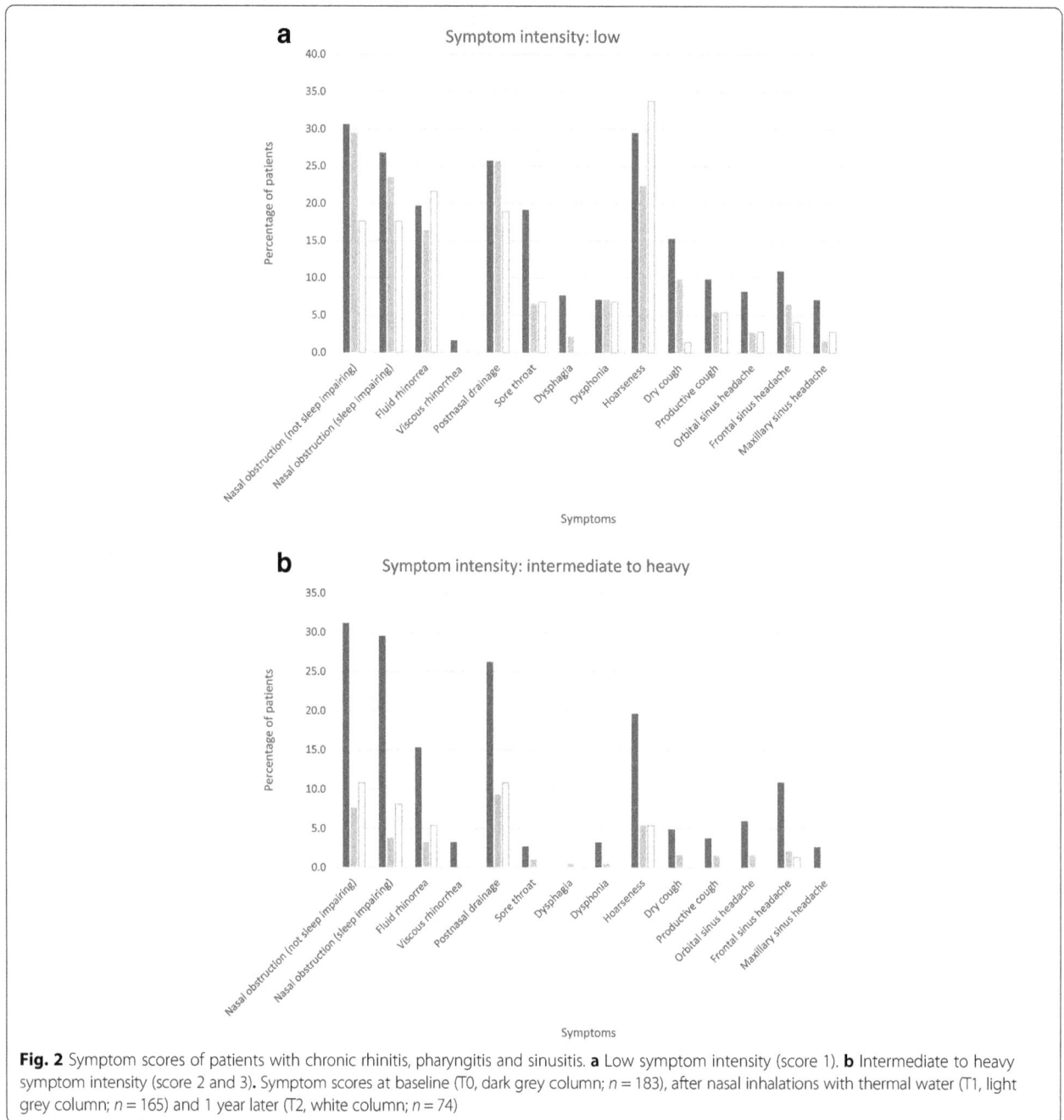

Fig. 2 Symptom scores of patients with chronic rhinitis, pharyngitis and sinusitis. **a** Low symptom intensity (score 1). **b** Intermediate to heavy symptom intensity (score 2 and 3). Symptom scores at baseline (T0, dark grey column; $n = 183$), after nasal inhalations with thermal water (T1, light grey column; $n = 165$) and 1 year later (T2, white column; $n = 74$)

After stratifying for pathology, we found that *CXCR4* expression was consistently changed in patients suffering from all three diseases of interest, while *FLT1* demonstrated a statistically significant post-treatment reduction only in those affected by sinusitis. Other genes showed weaker changes, although in some cases the change reached statistical significance, namely *SOD2* average expression was more than double after treatment among patients with pharyngitis ($p = 0.007$), *TLR4* was one third lower in subjects affected with rhinitis ($p = 0.02$), and *NFKB1* was 20% higher in the subgroup with sinusitis ($p = 0.04$).

When stratifying by smoking habit (data not shown), the increase of *CXCR4* mean expression in T1 was confirmed in all subgroups, while *FLT1* was significantly altered only among non-smokers. The small subgroup of current smokers ($n = 4$) showed a somehow peculiar profile, with highly significant changes in the expression of *ICAM1* and *NFKB1* ($p < 0.0001$ and $p = 0.002$ respectively) and some other minor variations.

Finally, we decided to focus on *CXCR4* in further analyses, considering the notable difference in absolute figures between mean expression in T0 and in T1, the high

Table 2 Total symptom score and clinical evaluation score (panel A), and rhinomanometry measurements (panel B) of patients with chronic rhinitis, pharyngitis or sinusitis at admission (T0), after nasal inhalations with thermal water (T1) and at phone follow up 1 year later (T2)

A) Total symptom scores in T0 - T1 - T2, and clinical examination scores in T0 – T1

	T0 Mean ± SD (range) N = 183	T1 Mean ± SD (range) N = 165	T2 Mean ± SD (range) N = 74	P - value[a] (T0 vs. T1)	P - value[a] (T0 vs. T2)
Total symptom score (TSS)	5.7 ± 3.3 (0–18)	2.7 ± 2.3 (0–12)	2.3 ± 2.6 (0–12)	< 0.00001	< 0.00001
Clinical examination score (CES)	1.4 ± 1.2 (0–5)	0.6 ± 0.7 (0–4)	n.a.	< 0.0001	n.a.

B) Rhinomanometry measurements in T0 - T1

	Inhalation resistance (Pa/ml s)				Exhalation resistance (Pa/ml s)			
	N	T0 Mean ± SD	T1 Mean ± SD	P - value[b]	N	T0 Mean ± SD	T1 Mean ± SD	P - value[b]
All patients	105	0.40 ± 0.35	0.51 ± 0.61	NS	103	0.40 ± 0.35	0.53 ± 0.60	=0.01
Pathology[c]								
J30-J31.0 Rhinitis	28	0.40 ± 0.38	0.63 ± 1.00	NS	28	0.40 ± 0.32	0.67 ± 0.96	NS
J31.1-J31.2 Pharyngitis	24	0.43 ± 0.43	0.44 ± 0.37	NS	24	0.46 ± 0.41	0.45 ± 0.26	NS
J32 Sinusitis	57	0.38 ± 0.28	0.49 ± 0.44	NS	55	0.36 ± 0.31	0.49 ± 0.43	=0.009
Cigarette smoke								
Never smokers	47	0.39 ± 0.32	0.44 ± 0.38	NS	49	0.39 ± 0.34	0.46 ± 0.38	NS
Former smokers	46	0.39 ± 0.34	0.53 ± 0.11	NS	41	0.37 ± 0.33	0.60 ± 0.74	NS
Currentsmokers	12	0.52 ± 0.45	0.69 ± 0.84	NS	13	0.48 ± 0.40	0.62 ± 0.81	NS

n.a. not assessed, SD standard deviation, NS not statistically significant (p > 0.05), SD standard deviation
[a]Wilcoxon signed rank sum test
[b]Wilcoxon signed rank sum test T0 vs. T1
[c]Figures do not add up because 10 patients declared two pathologies simultaneously

statistical significance and the consistency in subgroups, while the other genes were discarded, also taking account of the multiple comparison issue.

CXCR4 protein was visualized by Western blot of the cell lysate with the appropriate antibodies in the same 40 patients plus 10 reference subjects (Fig. 3 and Table 4). The mean value of the patients' CXCR4 expression at baseline was similar to that of the controls and was 2.5-fold increased after inhalation treatment, confirming the results obtained with High Throughput real-time PCR, although no statistical correlation was demonstrated between the two endpoints. The same results were found in the three pathologies of interest or among never smokers and former smokers even after stratifications. On the other hand, the mean value of CXCR4 expression at baseline resulted to be higher in the small subgroup of current smokers than in the non-smokers ($p = 0.05$), and the increase after treatment was smaller and non significant.

Results were substantially unchanged when comparing aged subjects (≥ 65 years) or the eldest quartile (≥ 71 years) to the others. No major changes were shown after stratifying for gender, allergy, exposure to second-hand smoke, exposure to noxious inhalable substances or fruit and vegetables consumption.

Finally, expression levels of the gene CXCR4 were measured through RT-PCR in all the available samples (143 patients and 10 controls; Table 4). The results obtained with the first 40 patients were substantially confirmed in this larger group, with a 2.75-fold increase of the mean values in T1 respect to T0, a highly statistically significant increase. In addition, CXCR4 gene expression at baseline was significantly augmented in patients compared to controls.

The considerable increase after treatment was substantially maintained after stratifying for the three groups of pathologies or according to smoking habit. The increase was smaller in the subgroup of current smokers than in non-smokers (CXCR4 gene expression level in T1: 2.7 ± 0.93 vs. 3.4 ± 1.2, $p = 0.02$).

Results were substantially unchanged after stratifying for age, gender, allergy, exposure tosecond-hand smoke and exposure to noxious inhalable substances.

Associated events
Among the 163 patients who completed the inhalation treatment, 7 (3.8%) suffered from the so-called "thermal crisis" (a temporary exacerbation of their symptoms lasting 1–2 days, which is considered a systemic reaction to the treatment and has no pathologic meaning [31]), and

Table. 3 Expression of inflammatory-reparative genes in patients undergoing thermal water nasal inhalation

Genes	All patients (n = 40)[a]			J30-J31.0 Rhinitis (n = 10)			J31.1-J31.2 Pharyngitis (n = 7)			J32 Sinusitis (n = 24)		
	T0 Mean ± SD	T1 Mean ± SD	P-value[b]	T0 Mean ± SD	T1 Mean ± SD	P-value[b]	T0 Mean ± SD	T1 Mean ± SD	P-value[b]	T0 Mean ± SD	T1 Mean ± SD	P-value[b]
AGER	2.2 ± 2.0	1.9 ± 1.7	NS	2.3 ± 2.4	2.2 ± 2.6	NS	1.5 ± 1.3	1.5 ± 1.0	NS	2.3 ± 2.0	1.9 ± 1.5	NS
CXCR2	1.5 ± 1.3	1.6 ± 1.2	NS	1.2 ± 1.1	1.5 ± 1.2	NS	1.0 ± 1.0	1.1 ± 0.8	NS	1.7 ± 1.4	1.9 ± 1.3	NS
CXCR4	1.4 ± 0.8	4.4 ± 0.7	< 0.0001[c]	1.4 ± 0.5	4.9 ± 0.9	< 0.0001[c]	1.4 ± 0.5	4.8 ± 0.5	< 0.0001[c]	1.4 ± 0.9	4.1 ± 0.6	< 0.0001[c]
FLT1	1.9 ± 1.4	1.4 ± 0.9	0.005	1.9 ± 0.8	1.7 ± 1.0	NS	1.0 ± 1.0	0.7 ± 0.6	NS	2.2 ± 1.5	1.5 ± 0.9	0.004
FUT7	1.1 ± 1.0	1.3 ± 1.6	NS	1.6 ± 1.4	2.1 ± 1.7	NS	1.1 ± 0.7	1.6 ± 2.6	NS	1.0 ± 0.9	1.0 ± 1.1	NS
HIF1A	3.3 ± 3.3	3.8 ± 2.9	NS	2.2 ± 2.0	2.5 ± 1.9	NS	5.3 ± 4.4	4.6 ± 3.5	NS	3.1 ± 3.1	3.2 ± 2.8	NS
HMGB1	2.3 ± 3.3	2.0 ± 1.9	NS	1.7 ± 1.4	1.6 ± 1.7	NS	1.0 ± 0.9	1.0 ± 0.7	NS	2.8 ± 4.1	2.5 ± 2.1	NS
ICAM1	2.9 ± 2.6	3.1 ± 3.2	NS	2.1 ± 2.0	2.3 ± 1.9	NS	2.5 ± 2.6	2.7 ± 2.7	NS	3.3 ± 2.8	3.6 ± 3.7	NS
NFKB1	4.4 ± 3.4	4.6 ± 3.0	NS	3.5 ± 2.8	3.4 ± 2.9	NS	6.5 ± 3.8	5.2 ± 2.4	NS	4.1 ± 3.4	4.9 ± 3.1	0.04
P2RX7	3.7 ± 3.4	3.4 ± 3.3	NS	2.9 ± 2.9	2.7 ± 2.7	NS	4.0 ± 3.8	3.2 ± 4.3	NS	3.9 ± 3.5	3.7 ± 3.2	NS
PTX3	3.6 ± 4.4	4.1 ± 4.7	NS	4.3 ± 4.1	4.5 ± 4.1	NS	2.8 ± 3.3	2.7 ± 2.6	NS	3.6 ± 4.8	4.3 ± 5.3	NS
RELA	2.7 ± 2.5	2.7 ± 2.0	NS	4.7 ± 3.3	4.2 ± 2.3	NS	1.3 ± 1.2	1.3 ± 1.4	NS	2.4 ± 2.1	2.6 ± 1.7	NS
SELP	2.5 ± 2.4	2.7 ± 2.0	NS	2.8 ± 2.1	3.2 ± 2.2	NS	1.9 ± 1.1	2.0 ± 1.6	NS	2.5 ± 2.8	2.6 ± 2.1	NS
SOCS1	3.0 ± 2.6	2.7 ± 2.2	NS	3.1 ± 2.4	2.6 ± 1.9	NS	4.7 ± 3.2	4.0 ± 2.6	NS	2.5 ± 2.3	2.3 ± 2.1	NS
SOD2	1.7 ± 1.7	2.4 ± 3.2	NS	1.1 ± 0.9	1.1 ± 0.8	NS	1.1 ± 1.0	2.5 ± 2.1	0.007	2.1 ± 2.0	2.9 ± 3.8	NS
TLR2	2.5 ± 2.6	3.1 ± 3.9	NS	2.4 ± 3.5	2.0 ± 2.0	NS	2.7 ± 2.6	3.1 ± 3.2	NS	2.4 ± 2.3	3.5 ± 4.3	NS
TLR3	2.4 ± 2.6	2.4 ± 2.6	NS	2.0 ± 1.7	2.7 ± 2.0	NS	2.9 ± 4.0	2.9 ± 3.9	NS	2.5 ± 2.4	2.1 ± 2.3	NS
TLR4	2.2 ± 1.9	2.6 ± 3.2	0.02	2.5 ± 1.4	1.6 ± 1.1	0.02	2.8 ± 3.1	2.7 ± 2.6	NS	1.9 ± 1.5	3.0 ± 3.8	NS
VEGFA	1.5 ± 1.2	2.1 ± 2.7	NS	1.9 ± 1.6	2.0 ± 1.7	NS	1.7 ± 0.9	2.3 ± 1.3	NS	1.3 ± 1.1	2.0 ± 3.2	NS

Numbers indicate fold induction of gene expression relative to the reference genes, such as 18S and GAPDH

NS not statistically significant (p > 0.05), SD standard deviation

[a]Figures do not add up because one patient declared two pathologies simultaneously

[b]Mann-Whitney U Test p-value

[c]Difference statistically significant after Bonferroni adjustment for multiple comparisons (76 tests, cut-off is ≈ 0.0007)

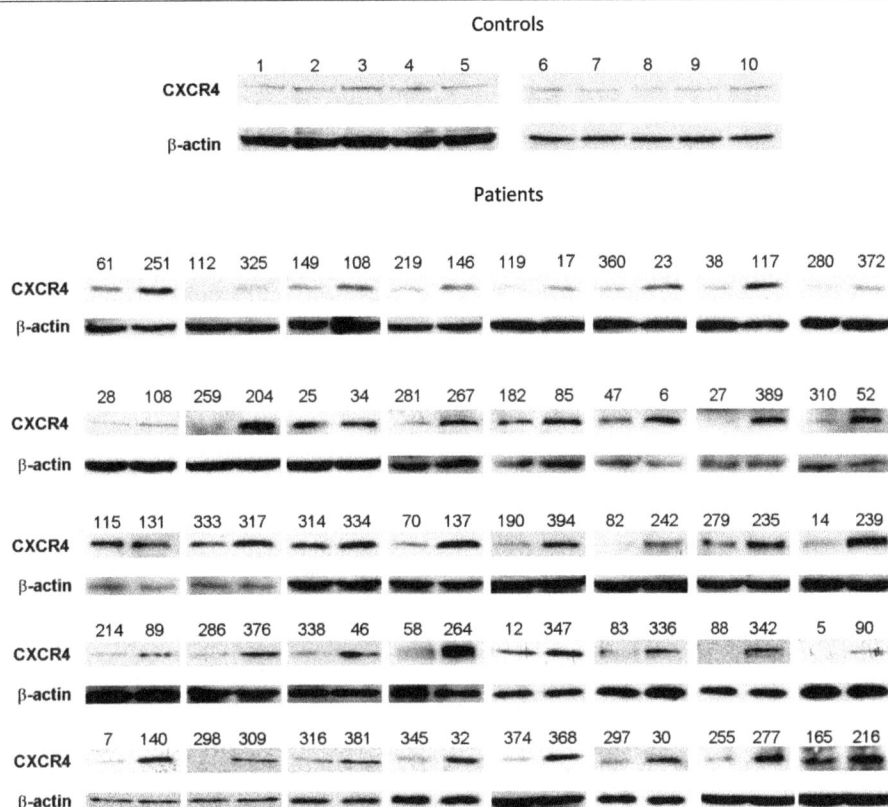

Fig. 3 Expression of inflammatory-reparative proteins in patients with chronic rhinitis, pharyngitis or sinusitis undergoing thermal water nasal inhalation and controls. Nasal epithelial cells from healthy subjects and from patients at time T0 and T1 were obtained and lysed as described under Methods. Proteins were separated by electrophoresis and expression of CXCR4 was measured by western blot in control subjects (upper panel) and in patients (lower panel). Each patient had two codes, one for time T0 (odd columns, e.g. 61 for the first patient, 112 for the second etc.) and one for T1 (even columns; e.g. 251 for the first patient, 325 for the second etc.). β-actin was used as loading control and for densitometric analysis

Table 4 CXCR4 protein and gene expression in patients undergoing thermal water nasal inhalation

	CXCR4 protein expression				CXCR4 gene expression			
	N	T0 Mean ± SD	T1 Mean ± SD	P - value[a]	N	T0 Mean ± SD	T1 Mean ± SD	P - value[a]
Controls	10	0.97 ± 0.51		NS[b]	10	0.66 ± 0.44	–	= 0.025[b]
All patients	40	1.0 ± 0.39	2.6 ± 0.66	< 0.0001[d]	143	1.2 ± 0.68	3.3 ± 1.2	< 0.0001[d]
Pathology[c]								
J30-J31.0 Rhinitis	10	1.2 ± 0.37	2.4 ± 0.66	< 0.0001[d]	34	1.1 ± 0.6	3.5 ± 1.2	< 0.0001[d]
J31.1-J31.2 Pharyngitis	7	1.2 ± 0.45	2.7 ± 0.6	= 0.0001[d]	37	1.2 ± 0.59	3.1 ± 1.3	= 0.0001[d]
J32 Sinusitis	24	0.96 ± 0.37	2.6 ± 0.69	< 0.0001[d]	77	1.1 ± 0.77	3.3 ± 1.1	< 0.0001[d]
Cigarette smoke								
Never smokers	23	0.99 ± 0.39	2.6 ± 0.66	< 0.0001[d]	68	1.2 ± 0.66	3.5 ± 1.2	< 0.0001[d]
Former smokers	13	1.0 ± 0.36	2.6 ± 0.50	< 0.0001[d]	56	1.1 ± 0.57	3.3 ± 1.2	< 0.0001[d]
Current smokers	4	1.4 ± 0.38	2.4 ± 1.2	NS	19	1.1 ± 0.98	2.7 ± 0.93	< 0.0001[d]

NS not statistically significant ($p > 0.05$), SD standard deviation
[a]Fisher's exact Test for difference T0 vs. T1
[b]Difference controls vs. T0
[c]Figures do not add up because some patients declared two pathologies simultaneously
[d]Difference statistically significant after Bonferroni adjustment for multiple comparisons (cut-off is ≈ 0.005)

13 (7.1%) reported other negative events (e.g. headache, fatigue).

Discussion

This is the largest study ever conducted on the efficacy and safety of thermal water nasal inhalation treatment for upper respiratory tract diseases in adult and elderly patients. The efficacy of the treatment was first demonstrated in terms of total symptom and clinical evaluation scores, while rhinomanometry gave more puzzling results. The possible mechanisms were then investigated at the molecular level, finding consistent increases in the expression of *CXCR4*, both as mRNA or as protein.

In addition to its large sample size, among the *pro* of the study is the inclusion of a substantial proportion of aged subjects (more than half of the sample), as it has been hypothesized that elderly patients affected by chronic diseases of the upper airways could represent a distinct population from adult patients, showing altered physiopathology and requiring different therapeutic approaches [2].

Other strengths are the evaluation of biomarkers of inflammation directly in nasal epithelial cells, the use of an epidemiologic questionnaire, which allowed to take into account the socio-economic profile and the lifestyle of patients (including smoking) who chose such a treatment, and the evaluation of different subsets of pathologies (rhinitis, pharyngitis, sinusitis), which may act as effect modifiers.

Patients who chose inhalation treatment showed a good compliance, as 90% completed their cycle of inhalations, despite the fact that it took time to reach the spa, which was located out of the town. Associated events or adverse effects were rare and not severe, in agreement with findings of a recently published meta-analysis [11]. Nearly 50% of the patients were retired and another 12% were housewife. Based on sensitivity analyses, it appeared that older subjects found it easier to comply with the protocol, because young age was the main obvious difference between dropouts or patients that could not strictly follow the protocol, and the others. We may speculate that time constraints linked to rigid work schedules most likely selected patients who chose the inhalation treatment. In addition, older patients may be more interested in non-pharmacological treatments, because they often take several drugs to control complex conditions.

A common limitation of studies on treatments with thermal water is the difficulty to extrapolate study results to the general population because of the strong selection of the subjects undergoing thermal treatments. To quantify this discrepancy, we compared basic statistics of our study group with the results of the population survey *Passi*, conducted in the period 2012–2015 in the same region where Terme di Genova spa is located [32, 33] The education level was similar, but several other endpoints confirmed as the population receiving inhalation treatment was extremely concerned about wellbeing. Our patients had a 50% lower prevalence of current smokers than the general population, ate much more fruit and vegetables (42% declared to eat 6 or more servings of fruit and vegetables every day vs 16% eating at least 5), and took dietary supplements such as vitamins or antioxidants in a considerable proportion (25% of patients).

Nasal inhalations with thermal water were perceived as an effective treatment by both the patients and the physicians. This feeling was supported by clinical results, which showed a general reduction of symptoms after treatment, much stronger for the more severe. Both total symptom and clinical evaluation scores dropped by more than 50% after treatment, with a statistically significant difference between T0 and T1. These results are in keeping with those of other published studies [14, 17, 34–36] confirming the beneficial effect of thermal water nasal inhalations. The present study was not designed to disentangle the therapeutic benefit from the placebo effect and therefore all clinical results should be interpreted with caution. Although clinical assessment was extremely careful, making more reliable and robust the assessment of the beneficial effects of treatment, we cannot exclude that our results were due to random chance, a placebo effect or the regression towards the mean.

Another strength of this study is the use of objective tools to assess clinical and biological endpoints. Among them we measured in all patients rhinomanometry, which is a standard diagnostic tool designed to objectively evaluate the nose respiratory function. Results from this exam were mixed, since resistance levels were higher after treatment than before. This trend was more evident among the patients with sinusitis. These results were in slight contrast with those of a meta-analysis including 6 studies with 347 patients (mostly affected by sinusitis [11]). Keller and coworkers found no statistically significant difference between nasal resistance at baseline and after 2 weeks of inhalations, aerosol or irrigations with thermal water from different sources. However, this parameter was diminished significantly after 30 days and remained at low levels at 90 days, in the subset of subjects who underwent rhinomanometric measurements at those time points. Patients treated with isotonic sodium chloride solution for reference had more than double nasal resistance levels after a 14 day treatment in comparison to baseline level ($p < 0.01$), falling at low levels after 30–90 days. The initial lack of effect followed by a significant improvement after 30 days shows as the kinetic of respiratory response to thermal water inhalation may vary, depending upon dose, chemical composition of the water and length of the follow up.

Among the most innovative contributions of the present study to the evidence concerning thermal water nasal inhalations is the effort to investigate the effect of treatment from a molecular point of view.

Few studies have shown a reduction of inflammatory cytokines such as TNF-α in nasal mucus samples and of serum IgE in patients with chronic rhinosinusitis, after treatment with thermal water [14, 36]. More recently, thermal water inhalation has been shown to modulate Th1 and Th2 cytokine expression and to increase IL-21 and IL-17 levels in blood samples of elderly and young patients with chronic upper respiratory tract infections [12]. In contrast with previous studies, the present research measured the expression of pro-inflammatory reparative molecules before and after thermal water inhalation directly in nasal cells, which may be subject to age-dependent variations in terms of epithelial proliferation, repair, and defenses [2].

Moreover, we measured both gene and protein expression, and validated our results in a large cohort of patients. In particular, by comparing the expression of 48 genes in a training set of 40 patients before (T0) and after (T1) thermal water nasal inhalations we could demonstrate that CXCR4, FLT1 and SOD2 were modulated in nasal epithelial cell by the treatment. In particular, CXCR4 showed a consistent increase in patients suffering from chronic rhinitis, pharyngitis or sinusitis and, in fact, the same trend was maintained when analyzing CXCR4 gene expression in the validation set represented by all 143 patients. This is an innovative finding, since no study has shown CXCR4 involvement during thermal water inhalation so far.

Due to the lack of previous studies, we can only speculate that thermal water chemical composition may contain elements that can activate CXCR4 transcription and translation, either directly or indirectly. Another possible explanation could be that thermal water exposure activates epigenetic changes in airway cells that, in turn, increase CXCR4 gene translation and protein expression.

However, independently from how thermal water causes CXCR4 expression it is also important to consider the effects of such an increase. In fact, CXCR4 is a well known membrane receptor whose ligand is represented by the cytokine called stromal derived factor 1 (SDF-1). CXCR4 is involved in recruiting stem cells into injured organs and, once activated, it transduces the molecular signal by activating multiple pathways to control cell migration, proliferation, survival, differentiation [24]. SDF-1/CXCR4 axis activation stimulates tissue repair after myocardial infarction [28] as well as in wound healing [29]. Therefore, it could be hypothesized that, in our system, increased expression of CXCR4 would activate repair of damaged mucosa as well as anti-inflammatory action of innate immune cells. In fact those cells can express high levels of CXCR4 and use it as chemotactic receptor to move towards the inflammatory site. Interestingly, it has been shown that CXCR4/SDF-1 axis is important for regulating migration, barrier maturation and integrity reconstitution of intestinal epithelial cells as well as activation of the innate host defense [37].

Impaired expression of CXCR4 in relation to ageing has been described in adipose-derived mesenchymal stem cells [38], in CD4(+) T cells [39], in cardiac tissue macrophages [40] and in mouse bone marrow mesenchymal stromal stem cells [41]. Such a decreased expression resulted in altered migration [38–40] and differentiation [40, 41], highlighting the importance of stimulating its expression, as we observed in elderly patients after inhalation treatment. Finally, CXCR4 increase was smaller in current smokers compared to the non smokers, suggesting an interference of smoking habit in the repairing pathway activated by CXCR4.

The present study evaluated the effect of thermal water nasal inhalations on different upper respiratory diseases in a large study group, with a comprehensive approach. Results show a remarkable and persistent clinical improvement of conditions and symptoms associated to the diseases evaluated. The key issue of establishing an objective evaluation of the therapeutical effects was addressed measuring resistance during normal inspiration and expiration through the nose with anterior rhinomanometry. Results from this assay were puzzling, suggesting that wellknown technical difficulties may have generated misclassification. As a matter of fact rhinomanometry is progressively dismissed by most otolaryngologists. Much more informative and technically robust was the evidence from gene and protein expression profiling of a set of candidate genes associated with inflammation. The use of a two steps procedure, based on a training set and a validation set, the large number of subjects evaluated, the evaluation of both gene and protein expression in the target tissue gives a solid support to the validity of results concerning the modulation of CXCR4 in patients treated with thermal water nasal inhalations.

Conclusions

These results confirm the clinical impact of thermal treatment on diseases of the upper respiratory tract, irrespective of the patients' age. Older patients may benefit greatly of this approach, as it may help to control symptoms and diminish drug use. In addition, our results offer a new player in the mechanisms regulating the interaction between thermal treatments and inflammation. New studies should be planned to further explore and validate the role of CXCR4 as a possible therapeutic target or a predictor of response in patients of all ages with chronic rhinitis, pharyngitis or sinusitis undergoing thermal water nasal inhalations.

Abbreviations

CES: Clinical evaluation score; SD: Standard deviation; TSS: Total symptom score

Acknowledgements

We thank Mrs. Martina Ottonello and Mr. Claudio Valle (Terme di Genova spa, Genoa, Italy) for their valuable help with data and sample management.

Funding

This work was supported by grants funded by FORST (Fondazione per la Ricerca Scientifica Termale), and University of Genoa.

Authors' contributions

MN: conception and design of the study; acquisition of data; analysis and interpretation of data; drafting the article; final approval of the version to be published. LS, LP: acquisition and interpretation of data; revising the article critically; final approval of the version to be published. AK: analysis of data; revising the article critically; final approval of the version to be published. EC, MAR: interpretation of data; revising the article critically; final approval of the version to be published. DU, MM: acquisition of data; revising the article critically; final approval of the version to be published. MT, SB: conception and design of the study; analysis and interpretation of data; drafting the article; final approval of the version to be published

Competing interests

The authors declare that they have no competing interests.

Author details

[1]Unit of Clinical and Molecular Epidemiology, IRCCS San Raffaele Pisana, Via di Val Cannuta, 247, 00166 Rome, Italy. [2]Department of Cellular and Molecular Pathology, IRCCS San Raffaele Pisana, Rome, Italy. [3]Department of Experimental Medicine, Sapienza University of Rome, Rome, Italy. [4]Terme di Genova, Genoa, Italy. [5]Terme di Acqui, AcquiTerme (AL), Italy. [6]Casa di Cura Villa Montallegro, Genova, Italy. [7]Consortium MEBIC, San Raffaele University, Rome, Italy. [8]Department of Internal Medicine, University of Genoa, Genoa, Italy. [9]Department of Human Sciences and Quality of Life Promotion, San Raffaele University, Rome, Italy.

References

1. Hastan D, Fokkens WJ, Bachert C, Newson RB, Bislimovska J, Bockelbrink A, et al. Chronic rhinosinusitis in Europe–an underestimated disease. A GA[2]LEN study. Allergy. 2011;66:1216–23.
2. Renteria AE, Mfuna Endam L, Desrosiers M. Do aging factors influence the clinical presentation and management of chronic rhinosinusitis? Otolaryngol Head Neck Surg. 2017;156:598–605.
3. Cardell LO, Olsson P, Andersson M, Welin KO, Svensson J, Tennvall GR, et al. TOTALL: high cost of allergic rhinitis-a national Swedish population-based questionnaire study. NPJ Prim Care Respir Med. 2016;26:15082.
4. Skoner DP. The tall and the short: repainting the landscape about the growth effects of inhaled and intranasal corticosteroids. Allergy Asthma Proc. 2016;37:180–91.
5. Chong LY, Head K, Hopkins C, Philpott C, Burton MJ, Schilder AG. Different types of intranasal steroids for chronic rhinosinusitis. Cochrane Database Syst Rev. 2016;4:CD011993.
6. Chong LY, Head K, Hopkins C, Philpott C, Glew S, Scadding G, et al. Saline irrigation for chronic rhinosinusitis. Cochrane Database Syst Rev. 2016;4: CD011995.
7. Chong LY, Head K, Hopkins C, Philpott C, Schilder AG, Burton MJ. Intranasal steroids versus placebo or no intervention for chronic rhinosinusitis. Cochrane Database Syst Rev. 2016;4:CD011996.
8. Head K, Chong LY, Hopkins C, Philpott C, Burton MJ, Schilder AG. Short-course oral steroids alone for chronic rhinosinusitis. Cochrane Database Syst Rev. 2016;4:CD011991.
9. Head K, Chong LY, Piromchai P, Hopkins C, Philpott C, Schilder AG, et al. Systemic and topical antibiotics for chronic rhinosinusitis. Cochrane Database Syst Rev. 2016;4:CD011994.
10. Head K, Chong LY, Hopkins C, Philpott C, Schilder AG, Burton MJ. Short-course oral steroids as an adjunct therapy for chronic rhinosinusitis. Cochrane Database Syst Rev. 2016;4:CD011992.
11. Keller S, König V, Mösges R. Thermal water applications in the treatment of upper respiratory tract diseases: a systematic review and meta-analysis. J Allergy (Cairo). 2014;2014:943824.
12. Magrone T, Galantino M, Di Bitonto N, Borraccino L, Chiaromonte G, Jirillo E. Effects of thermal water inhalation in chronic upper respiratory tract infections in elderly and young patients. Immun Ageing. 2016;13:18.
13. Passali D, De Corso E, Platzgummer S, Streitberger C, Lo Cunsolo S, Nappi G, et al. SPA therapy of upper respiratory tract inflammation. Eur Arch Otorhinolaryngol. 2013;270:565–70.
14. Passariello A, Di Costanzo M, Terrin G, Iannotti A, Buono P, Balestrieri U, et al. Crenotherapy modulates the expression of proinflammatory cytokines and immunoregulatory peptides in nasal secretions of children with chronic rhinosinusitis. Am J Rhinol Allergy. 2012;26:e15–9.
15. Ottaviano G, Marioni G, Giacomelli L, La Torre FB, Staffieri C, Marchese-Ragona R, et al. Smoking and chronic rhinitis: effects of nasal irrigations with sulfurous-arsenical-ferruginous thermal water: a prospective, randomized, double-blind study. Am J Otolaryngol. 2012;33: 657–62.
16. Pagani D, Galliera E, Dogliotti G, De Bernardi di Valserra M, Torretta S, et al. Carbon dioxide-enriched water inhalation in patients with allergic rhinitis and its relationship with nasal fluid cytokine/chemokine release. Arch Med Res. 2011;42:329–33.
17. Miraglia Del Giudice M, Decimo F, Maiello N, Leonardi S, Parisi G, Golluccio M, et al. Effectiveness of Ischia thermal water nasal aerosol in children with seasonal allergic rhinitis: a randomized and controlled study. Int J Immunopathol Pharmacol. 2011;24:1103–9.
18. Passali D, Lauriello M, Passali GC, Passali FM, Cassano M, Cassano P, et al. Clinical evaluation of the efficacy of Salsomaggiore (Italy) thermal water in the treatment of rhinosinusal pathologies. Clin Ter. 2008;159:181–8.
19. Benedetti F, Curreli S, Krishnan S, Davinelli S, Cocchi F, Scapagnini G, et al. Anti-inflammatory effects of H(2)S during acute bacterial infection: a review. J Transl Med. 2017;15:100.
20. Oppenheim JJ, Yang D. Alarmins: chemotactic activators of immune responses. Curr Opin Immunol. 2005;17:359–65.
21. Sabroe I, Parker LC, Dower SK, Whyte MK. The role of TLR activation in inflammation. J Pathol. 2008;214:126–35.
22. Ramasamy R, Vannucci SJ, Yan SS, Herold K, Yan SF, Schmidt AM. Advanced glycation end products and RAGE: a common thread in aging, diabetes, neurodegeneration, and inflammation. Glycobiology. 2005;15:16R–28R.
23. Lister MF, Sharkey J, Sawatzky DA, Hodgkiss JP, Davidson DJ, Rossi AG, et al. The role of the purinergic P2X7 receptor in inflammation. J Inflamm (Lond). 2007;4:5.
24. Ganju RK, Brubaker SA, Meyer J, Dutt P, Yang Y, Qin S, et al. The alpha-chemokine, stromal cell-derived factor-1alpha, binds to the transmembrane G-protein-coupled CXCR-4 receptor and activates multiple signal transduction pathways. J Biol Chem. 1998;273:23169–75.
25. Garlanda C, Bottazzi B, Bastone A, Mantovani A. Pentraxins at the crossroads between innate immunity, inflammation, matrix deposition, and female fertility. Annu Rev Immunol. 2005;23:337–66.
26. Curran EM, Judy BM, Duru NA, Wang HQ, Vergara LA, Lubahn DB, et al. Estrogenic regulation of host immunity against an estrogen receptor-negative human breast cancer. Clin Cancer Res. 2006;12:5641–7.
27. Solana R, Tarazona R, Gayoso I, Lesur O, Dupuis G, Fulop T. Innate immunosenescence: effect of aging on cells and receptors of the innate immune system in humans. Semin Immunol. 2012;24:331–41.
28. Huang C, Gu H, Zhang W, Manukyan MC, Shou W, Wang M. SDF-1/CXCR4 mediates acute protection of cardiac function through myocardial STAT3 signaling following global ischemia/reperfusion injury. Am J Physiol Heart Circ Physiol. 2011;301:H1496–505.
29. Bollag WB, Hill WD. CXCR4 in epidermal keratinocytes: crosstalk within the skin. J Invest Dermatol. 2013;133:2505–8.
30. Coccheri S, Gasbarrini G, Valenti M, Nappi G, Di Orio F. Has time come for a re-assessment of spa therapy? The NAIADE survey in Italy. Int J Biometeorol. 2008;52:231–7.

31. Nappi G. Medicina e clinica termale. Pavia: Selecta Medica ed; 2001.
32. Baldissera S, Campostrini S, Binkin N, Minardi V, Minelli G, Ferrante G, et al. Features and initial assessment of the Italian behavioral risk factor surveillance system (PASSI), 2007-2008. Prev Chronic Dis. 2011;8:A24.
33. Epicentro. Il portale dell'epidemiologia per la sanità pubblica. http://www.epicentro.iss.it/passi/default.asp. Accessed 20 Oct 2016.
34. Cantone E, Maione M, Di Rubbo V, Esposito F, Iengo M. Olfactory performance after crenotherapy in chronic rhinosinusitis in the elderly. Laryngoscope. 2015;125:1529–34.
35. Varricchio A, Giuliano M, Capasso M, Del Gaizo D, Ascione E, De Lucia A, et al. Salso-sulphide thermal water in the prevention of recurrent respiratory infections in children. Int J Immunopathol Pharmacol. 2013;26:941–52.
36. Salami A, Dellepiane M, Strinati F, Guastini L, Mora R. Sulphurous thermal water inhalations in the treatment of chronic rhinosinusitis. Rhinology. 2010; 48:71–6.
37. Smith JM, Johanesen PA, Wendt MK, Binion DG, Dwinell MB. CXCL12 activation of CXCR4 regulates mucosal host defense through stimulation of epithelial cell migration and promotion of intestinal barrier integrity. Am J Physiol Gastrointest Liver Physiol. 2005;288:G316–26.
38. Liu M, Lei H, Dong P, Fu X, Yang Z, Yang Y, et al. Adipose-derived mesenchymal stem cells from the elderly exhibit decreased migration and differentiation abilities with senescent properties. Cell Transplant. 2017; https://doi.org/10.3727/096368917X695416.
39. Cané S, Ponnappan S, Ponnappan U. Altered regulation of CXCR4 expression during aging contributes to increased CXCL12-dependent chemotactic migration of CD4(+) T cells. Aging Cell. 2012;11:651–8.
40. Pinto AR, Godwin JW, Chandran A, Hersey L, Ilinykh A, Debuque R, et al. Age-related changes in tissue macrophages precede cardiac functional impairment. Aging (Albany NY). 2014;6:399–413.
41. Guang LG, Boskey AL, Zhu W. Age-related CXC chemokine receptor-4-deficiency impairs osteogenic differentiation potency of mouse bone marrow mesenchymal stromal stem cells. Int J Biochem Cell Biol. 2013;45:1813–20.
42. International Standard Classification of Occupations. ISCO-2008. Geneva: International Labour Office; 2012.

Thymus and activation-regulated chemokine (TARC)/CCL17 and IgE are associated with elderly asthmatics

Kyung Mi Jo [1†], Hyo Kyung Lim [2†], Jae Woong Sull [1,3], Eugene Choi [4], Ji-Sook Lee [5], Mee Ae Cheong [1], Min Hwa Hong [1], Yoori Kim [1] and In Sik Kim [1,2*]

Abstract

Background: The pathogenesis of asthma, which is an allergic lung disease, is associated with a variety of allergens such as house dust mite, pollen, and mould, IgE containing serum IgE and allergen-specific-IgE, and inflammatory cytokines including thymus and activation-regulated chemokine (TARC)/CCL17. Because aging is an essential factor in the pathogenesis of asthma, we examined biomarkers related to asthmatic subjects depending on age.

Results: Physiological indices such as FEV1(forced expiratory capacity in 1 s), FEV1 (% predicted), and FEV1/FVC(forced vital capacity) (%) in asthmatic subjects were lower than those in normal subjects. Total IgE, Der p1 specific IgE, and Der f1 specific IgE were elevated in serum of asthmatics relative to normal individuals. Regulated on activation, normal T cell expressed and secreted (RANTES)/CCL5 in serum and interleukin 6 (IL-6), interleukin 8 (IL-8), monocyte chemoattractant protein (MCP)-1/CCL2, RANTES, and macrophage inflammatory protein (MIP)-1α/CCL3 in bronchoalveolar lavage fluid (BALF) of asthmatic subjects were higher than in normal individuals. Upon classification of experimental groups depending on age, physiological indices and Der p1-specific IgE (class) were decreased in middle aged adult and elderly adult groups relative to the young adult group. TARC levels in serum were strongly elevated in the elderly adult group relative to the young adult and the middle aged adult groups. TARC in serum was related to total IgE in serum in the elderly adult group.

Conclusions: Taken together, although TARC in serum and BALF is not different between normal and asthmatic individuals, TARC increases in serum of elderly asthmatic subjects. The level of TARC has a positive effect on the level of IgE in the elderly adult group. These findings may help us better understand the relationship of pathogenesis of allergic diseases and aging.

Keywords: Asthma, Aging, TARC, Allergen-specific IgE

Background

Asthma is an allergic disease in the respiratory tract that is characterized by lung inflammation and mucus secretion resulting in airway obstruction, as well as allergen-specific IgE [1, 2]. Asthma is caused by a variety of elements including environmental, genetic and immunological factors. House dust mites (HDMs), including

Dermatophagoides pteronissinus (DP) and *Dermatophagoides farinae* (DF), may be sources of many specific allergen proteins including Der p 1 and Der f 1 [3, 4]. More than half of asthmatics are sensitized to HDM and have elevated levels of HDM-specific IgE in their serum. Cytokine secretion, which is one of the most important allergic inflammatory responses, is increased by HDM via Toll-like receptor (TLR) and proteinase-activated receptor (PAR) [5, 6]. Cytokines including interleukin 4 (IL-4), interleukin 5 (IL-5), IL-6, IL-8, interleukin 10 (IL-10), monocyte chemoattractant protein (MCP)-1/CCL2, and thymus and activation-regulated chemokine (TARC)/

---

* Correspondence: orientree@eulji.ac.kr

†Equal contributors

[1]Department of Senior Healthcare, BK21 plus program, Graduate School, Eulji University, Daejeon 34824, Korea

[2]Department of Biomedical Laboratory Science, School of Medicine, Eulji University, 77, Gyeryoung-ro 771 beon-gil, Jung-Gu, Daejeon 34824, Republic of Korea

Full list of author information is available at the end of the article

CCL17 trigger secondary inflammatory events, aggravating asthma pathogenesis.

Aging is an unavoidable and complicated process characterized by progressive loss of functional activity, repair, and recovery. Interaction of the proinflammatory state with aging, which is very important, occurs via the inflamm-aging process [7, 8]. Aging studies have suggested that potential biomarkers containing proinflammatory cytokines, hypoxic indicators, and redox state may be related to inflammation-associated aging. Asthma in elderly subjects shows higher mortality than in younger members of the population, including children and younger adults, and is underdiagnosed by age-related alterations such as dyspnea, immunosenescence and decreased skin test sensitivity [9]. Although asthma in elderly subjects is associated with immunological and non-immunologic mechanisms, the exact interaction of aging and asthma has yet to be unveiled. In this study, we divided subjects into young adults, middle-aged adults, and elderly adults and studied the association of asthma and aging with biomarkers including cytokine and HDM-specific IgE in serum.

Methods

Study population

A total of 121 asthmatic subjects were randomly recruited from Konyang University Hospital according to the global initiative for asthma (GINA) guideline. The asthmatic subjects were classified as young adults (10–39 years), middle-aged adults (40–59 years), and elderly adults (≥ 60 years). Subjects were excluded if they had no history of smoking and other comorbidities. Additionally, 106 normal subjects were recruited as controls. The normal subjects had normal lung function, no history of asthma, and did not require medication.

Collection of serum and BALF

Blood samples were collected and then centrifuged, after which the supernatant was separated from the samples. Following local anesthesia with lignocaine, sterile phosphate-buffered saline (PBS) (5 × 20 mL) was administered to lungs of normal ($n = 9$) and asthmatic ($n = 39$) individuals, after which the fluid was gently aspirated, pooled and collected into a tube. Nucleated cells in BALF and blood were counted using a Neubauer hemocytometer. Differential cell counts were performed from cytospin slides. Serum and BALF were stored at −70 °C until used in this experiment.

Laboratory investigations

White blood cell differential counts, hemoglobin and hematocrit levels were determined directly using a Sysmex XE-5000 system (Sysmex Corporation, Kobe, Japan). For measurement of serum HDM-specific IgE,

serum was loaded into a Pharmacia Unicap 100 system (Pharmacia Unicap, Uppsala, Sweden). The DP or DF allergen covalently coupled to the cellulose solid-phase ImmunoCap and reacted with the specific IgE in the patient's serum specimen. After washing, enzyme-labeled antibodies against IgE were added to form a complex, after which the IgE concentration was measured by fluorescence. HDM (DP or/and DF)-specific IgE+ is defined as > 0.35kU/L; class 0, < 0.35 kUA/L; class 1, 0.35 − < 0.7 kUA/L; class 2, 0.70 − < 3.5 kUA/L; class 3, 3.50 − < 17.5 kUA/L; class 4, 17.5 −< 50 kUA/L; class 5, 50 − ≤100 kUA/L; and class 6, > 100 kUA/L. Pulmonary function tests such as FEV1, FEV1 (% predicted), FVC, and FEV1/FVC were measured to determine the state of lung obstruction.

Measurement of cytokine and chemokine concentrations

Concentrations of IL-4, IL-5, IL-6, IL-8, IL-10, MCP-1, tumor necrosis factor (TNF)-α, interferon (IFN)-γ, granulocyte macrophage colony simulation factor (GM-CSF), TARC, RANTES, and MIP-1α in serum were measured with a sandwich enzyme-linked immunosorbent assay (ELISA) using a cytokine measurement kit (BD Biosciences, San Diego, CA, USA; R&D Systems, Minneapolis, MN, USA) according to the manufacturer's instructions. Briefly, 96-well plates were coated with 100 µL/well of appropriate monoclonal antibodies in 0.1 M carbonate buffer and incubated overnight at 4 °C, after which the plates were washed with PBS solution containing 0.05% Tween-20 and blocked with PBS solution with 5% bovine serum albumin (BSA) for 30 min at room temperature. Next, serum was added to the plates and incubated for 2 h at room temperature. The plates were then washed three times, after which they were incubated with appropriate secondary antibodies for 2 h at room temperature. The plates were then washed three times and incubated with substrate solution. Finally, the reaction was blocked by adding stop buffer and the absorbance was read at 450 nm.

Statistical analysis

Data were presented as the means ± S.E.M. Statistical differences were analyzed using a Student's t test for two-group comparisons. ANOVA was used to compare the three investigated age groups. Multiple comparisons were performed with Tukey's post-hoc test. The Pearson correlation coefficient (R) was applied to present the strength of the relationship between variables. All analyses were conducted using the SPSS statistical software package (Version 20.0, Chicago, IL), with a $p < 0.05$ considered to be statistically significant.

Results
Characteristics of the study population
Physiology indices such as FEV1, FEV1 (% predicted) and FEV1/FVC in asthmatic subjects were decreased relative to normal subjects. Eosinophils in blood and BALF were increased in asthmatic subjects relative to normal subjects. Total IgE, Der p1-specific IgE and Der f1-specific IgE were increased in serum of asthmatic subjects relative to normal subjects (Table 1). Although Der p1-specific IgE (class) and Der f1-specific IgE (class) increased in the asthmatic group, the values did not differ significantly from those of the normal group. The level of MCP-1 and RANTES in serum and of IL-6, IL-8, MCP-1, RANTES and MIP-1α in BALF were significantly increased in the asthmatics relative to the normal subjects (Table 2).

Moreover, MIP-1α in serum of the asthmatic group was lower than in normal. Cytokines did not differ in serum and BALF between atopic and non-atopic asthmatic groups (Additional file 1: Table S1).

Different expression of measured parameters among normal and asthmatic age groups
The population of normal and asthmatic subjects was divided into three age groups, young adults (10–39 years), middle-aged adults (40–59 years) and elderly adults (60–83 years). Hb, Hct, ESR, Der p 1-specific IgE, and TARC were not significantly altered among three groups of normal (Additional file 1: Table S2). In asthmatic group, Hb and Hct were decreased in the elderly adult group, but ESR was increased in the elderly adult group relative to the young adult group. Indices such as FVC, FEV1 and FEV1/FVC were decreased in the elderly adult group relative to the young adult and middle-aged adult groups. The level of Der p1 IgE(class) in the middle-aged adult and elderly adult groups decreased significantly when compared to the young adult group. The level of serum TARC was markedly elevated in the elderly adult group relative to the young adult and the middle-aged adult groups (Table 3). The difference of TARC in each group between normal and asthmatic subjects is not significant (Additional file 1: Table S2).

Table 1 Characteristics of the study population

		Normal	Asthma
Number of subjects (female/male)		106(62/44)	121 (66/55)
Age (years)		45.3 ± 12.7(19~72)	50.8 ± 16.7 (15~84)
FEV1[§]		4.1 ± 0.9 (2.7~5.3)[**]	2.1 ± 0.8 (1~4)[**]
FEV1[§] (% predicted)		101.6 ± 11.9 (87.1~121.3)[*]	81.4 ± 22.2 (34~125)[*]
FVC[‖] (% predicted)		95.2 ± 11.5 (77.9~112.9)	91.3 ± 17.8 (40~140)
FEV1/FVC (%)		91.6 ± 4.9 (84.8~97.9)[**]	71.9 ± 14.2 (35~98)[**]
Blood cells	Neutrophils	55.3 ± 9.7 (28.5~75.4)	59.5 ± 14.3 (27~92)
	Lymphocytes	35.7 ± 9.3 (20~67.3)[**]	26.8 ± 11.0 (4~52)[**]
	Monocytes	6.7 ± 3.2 (2.0~19.0)[**]	7.0 ± 2.7 (1~17)[**]
	Eosinophils	2.0 ± 1.4 (0~6.0)[**]	5.7 ± 8.4 (0~55)[**]
	Basophils	0.3 ± 0.3(0~1.3)[*]	0.5 ± 0.5 (0~4)[*]
BALF cells	Neutrophils	2.0 ± 1.6 (0~5.1)[**]	16.6 ± 26.7 (0~90)[**]
	Lymphocytes	10.6 ± 8.4 (1.0~29.2)	16.9 ± 17.0 (0~69)
	Macrophage	86.2 ± 10.4 (62.0~99.0)[**]	59.9 ± 27.8 (3~95)[**]
	Eosinophils	0.2 ± 0.6 (0~1.9)	3.9 ± 8.5 (0~52)
	Basophils	0 ± 0 (0~0)	0.04 ± 0.1(0~1)
	Epithelial cells	0.8 ± 1.0 (0~2.5)	2.38 ± 9.6 (0~86)
	Total IgE	92.8 ± 143.4(2.2~694.2)[**]	376.4 ± 612.2 (2~3000)[**]
	Der p 1-specific IgE	0.8 ± 2.1(0~10.4)[*]	4.1 ± 15.3 (0~100)[*]
IgE	Der p 1-specific IgE (class)	0.4 ± 1.0(0~3)	0.62 ± 1.2 (0~5)
	Der f 1-specific IgE	1.5 ± 4.4(0~23.4)[**]	7.3 ± 19.5 (0~100)[**]
	Der f 1-specific IgE (class)	0.8 ± 1.2(0~4)	1.2 ± 1.5 (0~5)

FEV1[§]: forced expiratory volume in 1 second
FVC[‖]: forced vital capacity
Data are expressed as the means ± SD (the lowest value ~ the highest value)
*p < 0.05 and **p < 0.01 indicate statistically significant differences between the normal and asthma groups

Table 2 Measurement of cytokine concentration of the study population

		Normal	Asthma
Serum	IL-4	297.3 ± 1185.1 (0~ 7126.6)	342.0 ± 831.7 (0~ 4955)
	IL-5	136.2 ± 526.9 (0~ 2744.7)	189.7 ± 1184.7 (0~ 7399)
	IL-6	6.2 ± 22.2 (0~ 134.4)	11.0 ± 12.2 (0~ 50)
	IL-8	46.2 ± 234.8 (0~ 1460.9)	64.5 ± 155.5 (0~ 805)
	IL-10	29.9 ± 124.0 (0~ 723.2)	16.9 ± 77.6 (0~ 435)
	MCP-1	466.9 ± 860.4 (8.9~ 3032.4)[**]	2042.1 ± 1427.3 (246.9~ 8180.4)[**]
	TNF-α	87.2 ± 135.1 (8.5~ 884.3)[**]	9.5 ± 8.4 (0~ 38)[**]
	INF-γ	48.6 ± 161.8 (0~ 945.1)	52.6 ± 146.7(0~ 741)
	GM-CSF	31.1 ± 36.6 (13.1~ 185.1)	32.1 ± 5.1 (27.1~ 55.7)
	TARC	9.0 ± 23.9 (0~ 150.3)	4.9 ± 15.8 (0~ 64.7)
	RANTES	685.3 ± 56.6 (601.4~ 857.7)[**]	800.4 ± 98.0 (553.7~ 978.7)[**]
	MIP-1α	81.2 ± 91.5 (11.0~ 338.2)[**]	25.2 ± 43.7 (0~ 202.4)[**]
BALF	IL-4	26.8 ± 54.5 (0~ 144)	102.0 ± 191.2 (0~ 740)
	IL-5	0.0 ± 0.0 (0~ 0)	0.0 ± 0.0 (0~ 0)
	IL-6	1.7 ± 3.3 (0~ 8)[*]	11.2 ± 23.8 (0~ 89)[*]
	IL-8	470.9 ± 626.1 (0~ 2041)[**]	2682.1 ± 4417.5 (0~ 21,246)[**]
	IL-10	0.0 ± 0.0 (0~ 0)	0.0 ± 0.0 (0~ 0)
	MCP-1	197.7 ± 265.7 (0~ 701)[**]	936.7 ± 1268.5 (0~ 4452)[**]
	TNF-α	0.0 ± 0.0 (0~ 0)	0.0 ± 0.0 (0~ 0)
	INF-γ	9.0 ± 14.6 (0~ 39)	11.6 ± 15.6 (0~ 59)
	GM-CSF	0.0 ± 0.0 (0~ 0)	0.0 ± 0.0 (0~ 0)
	TARC	0.0 ± 0.0 (0~ 0)	2.7 ± 12.7 (0~ 73.1)
	RANTES	0.0 ± 0.0 (0~ 0)[**]	23.8 ± 40.1 (0~ 142.8)[**]
	MIP-1α	0.0 ± 0.0 (0~ 0)[**]	50.7 ± 84.9 (0~ 376.0)[**]

Correlation among measured parameters in the total group and the elderly adult group of asthmatic subjects

The correlations among measured parameters in the total and the elderly adult groups are shown in Table 4. The serum TARC showed a positive correlation with total IgE in asthmatic subjects and the elderly adult group based on Pearson's correlation coefficients. $(0.3 < r < 0.7)$. Serum IL-6 showed a negative correlation with Der p1 specific IgE (class) in the total asthmatic group based on Pearson's correlation coefficients $(-0.7 < r < -0.3)$. However, serum IL-6 was not significantly correlated with Der p1 IgE(class) in the elderly adult group.

Table 3 Different expression of the measured parameters among the asthmatic age groups

	Young adult group (N = 33,Ave 29.4 ± 6.7)	Middle-aged adult group (N = 49,Ave 50.1 ± 5.5)	Elderly adult group (N = 39,Ave 69.8 ± 5.9).	P value (Tukey HSD)
Hb	13.9 ± 2.0[$$]	13.6 ± 1.3	12.8 ± 1.3[$$]	0.007
Hct	41.2 ± 5.7[$]	40.1 ± 3.9	38.1 ± 4.0[$]	0.012
ESR	17.8 ± 17.3[$]	23.2 ± 24.3	34.7 ± 28.3[$]	0.036
Der p1-specific IgE(class)	1.12 ± 1.4[*$]	0.4 ± 1.1[*]	0.43 ± 1.1[$]	0.042, 0.050
FVC	3.6 ± 1.0[**$$]	2.9 ± 0.7[**]	2.4 ± 0.7[$$]	[$]0.000, [*]0.001
FEV1	3.0 ± 0.7[**$$]	2.1 ± 0.6[**##]	1.5 ± 0.5[$$##]	[$]0.000, [*]0.000, [#]0.001
FEV1/FVC	80.0 ± 9.6[$$]	73.2 ± 13.1[##]	63.6 ± 14.8[$$##]	[$]0.000, [#]0.004
Serum TARC	0.0 ± 0.0	0.0 ± 0.0[#]	12.9 ± 23.9[#]	[#]0.045

Data are expressed as the means ± SD

[*]p < 0.05 and [**]p < 0.01 indicate between the young adult group and middle-aged group

[#]p < 0.05 and [##]p < 0.01 indicate between the middle aged group and elderly group

[$]p < 0.05 and [$$]p < 0.01 indicate between the young adult group and elderly group

Table 4 Correlation among the measured parameters in the total group and the elderly adult group of asthmatic subjects

Total group	pb	Hct	ESR	FEV1/ FVC	Serum IL-6	Serum TARC
Total IgE	$R = 0.282$ $p = 0.004^{**}$	$R = 0.294$ $p = 0.004^{**}$	$R = -0.232$ $p = 0.050^{*}$	$R = 0.049$ $p = 0.653$	$R = -0.297$ $p = 0.111$	$R = 0.417$ $p = 0.022^{*}$
Der p1-specific gE	$R = -0.082$ $p = 0.388$	$R = -0.099$ $p = 0.298$	$R = 0.047$ $p = 0.667$	$R = -0.036$ $p = 0.713$	$R = -0.223$ $p = 0.173$	$R = -0.098$ $p = 0.553$
Der p1-specific IgE(class)	$R = -0.032$ $p = 0.734$	$R = -0.049$ $p = 0.611$	$R = -0.009$ $p = 0.932$	$R = 0.014$ $p = 0.884$	$R = -0.344$ $p = 0.032^{*}$	$R = -0.106$ $p = 0.519$
Der f1-specific IgE	$R = -0.041$ $p = 0.670$	$R = -0.058$ $p = 0.546$	$R = 0.013$ $p = 0.905$	$R = -0.048$ $p = 0.631$	$R = -0.218$ $p = 0.182$	$R = -0.099$ $p = 0.550$
Der f1-specific IgE(class)	$R = 0.033$ $p = 0.733$	$R = 0.030$ $p = 0.755$	$R = -0.114$ $p = 0.295$	$R = -0.015$ $p = 0.876$	$R = -0.160$ $p = 0.332$	$R = -0.042$ $p = 0.799$
Elderly adult group	Hb	Hct	ESR	FEV1/ FVC	S-IL-6	S-TARC
Total IgE	$R = 0.219$ $p = 0.229$	$R = 0.176$ $p = 0.336$	$R = -0.370$ $p = 0.069$	$R = 0.223$ $p = 0.246$	$R = -0.442$ $p = 0.173$	$R = 0.630$ $p = 0.038^{*}$
Der p1-specific IgE	$R = -0.090$ $p = 0.612$	$R = -0.119$ $p = 0.501$	$R = 0.066$ $p = 0.743$	$R = 0.143$ $p = 0.443$	$R = -0.073$ $p = 0.797$	$R = -0.006$ $p = 0.982$
Der p1-specific IgE(class)	$R = 0.128$ $p = 0.472$	$R = 0.094$ $p = 0.597$	$R = 0.049$ $p = 0.808$	$R = 0.185$ $p = 0.318$	$R = -0.304$ $p = 0.271$	$R = 0.186$ $p = 0.507$
Der f1-specific IgE	$R = 0.050$ $p = 0.780$	$R = 0.034$ $p = 0.849$	$R = 0.021$ $p = 0.917$	$R = 0.272$ $p = 0.139$	$R = 0.034$ $p = 0.906$	$R = -0.052$ $p = 0.853$
Der f1-specific IgE(class)	$R = 0.083$ $p = 0.643$	$R = 0.076$ $p = 0.668$	$R = -0.280$ $p = 0.157$	$R = 0.377$ $p = 0.037^{*}$	$R = -0.287$ $p = 0.300$	$R = 0.086$ $p = 0.760$

*correlation with $p < 0.05$
**correlation with $p < 0.01$

Discussion

Asthma, which is one of the most prevalent allergic diseases, is caused by a variety of pathophysiological mechanisms [10]. HDMs are a major source of allergic asthma and DP and DF are of the most common HDMs [11]. IgE is considered a clear sign of allergic disease including asthma [11]. Der p 1 and Der f 1, major allergens proteins of HDMs, have a high IgE reactivity [12], and total IgE and Der p 1- or Der f 1–specific IgE are elevated in asthma [13]. In our study, total IgE, Der p1-specific IgE, and Der f1-specific IgE were elevated in asthmatic subjects when compared to normal subjects (Table 1). In a previous study, asthmatic subjects showed significantly more eosinophils, neutrophils, and cytokines such as IL-5, IL-6, IL-8, granulocyte colony stimulation factor (G-CSF) and RANTES in BALF when compared to healthy control subjects [14, 15]. As shown in Tables 1 and 2, neutrophils, IL-6, IL-8, RANTES, MCP-1, and MIP-1α in BALF of asthmatic subjects were also elevated relative to normal subjects. Both IL-8 and RANTES are major factors in increasing migration and proliferation of neutrophils and bronchial smooth muscle cells. These cytokines may be involved in increases in immune cells, particularly neutrophils. Although we also measured IL-5 and GM-CSF in BALF and serum. The difference between normal and asthmatic subjects was not significant.

Aging is an unavoidable and complicated process characterized by progressive loss of functional activity, repair and recovery [16]. As shown in Table 2, hematological indices such as Hb and Hct in the elderly adult group decreased significantly when compared to the young adult group, and physiological indices such as FVC, FEV1 and FEV_1/FVC ratio in the elderly adult group showed stronger decreases than in the young adult group or middle-aged adult group. Aging is related to a progressive decline of lung function [17], and subjects with severe persistent asthma were much older than those with mild asthma [18]. Neutrophils were increased in the sputum of elderly asthma subjects. Therefore, neutrophilic airway inflammation is more common in elderly and severe asthma subjects [19, 20]. In our study, neutrophils in serum and BALF of asthmatic subjects were elevated when compared to normal subjects (Table 1). In the elderly adult group, neutrophils in serum and BALF were elevated as compared to the young adult and middle-aged adult groups, although this difference was not significant (data not shown). Accordingly, the relationship between neutrophils and aging after sub-classification should be analyzed further according to severity.

It is becoming recognized that the immune system declines with age via a process known as immunosenescence, which leads to a higher incidence of infections, neoplasia and autoimmune diseases [21]. The age-dependent decline in the immune system could be attributed to the functional activity of hematopoietic stem cells in older subjects [22]. Previous studies have reported that total serum IgE in the elderly adult group is lower than in the younger group and total IgE and allergen specific IgE have decreased with age in allergic patients as well as healthy members of the population [23]. In the present study, the level of total IgE in the elderly adult group was decreased relative to the young adult and middle-aged adult groups. However, this difference did not achieve statistical significance (data not shown). As shown in Table 3, Der p 1-specific IgE(class) was decreased in the middle-aged adult and the elderly adult groups relative to the young adult group. More than 31 allergens in the HDMs extracts have been reported to date, and specific IgE reactivity profiles to purified allergens vary in subjects from different countries [24]. Future investigations will need to be conducted to examine the association of other specific-IgEs with aging.

Although we could not detect statistically significant differences in serum TARC between normal subjects and asthmatic subjects, serum TARC was elevated in the elderly adult group relative to the young adult and the middle-aged adult groups, in which serum TARC was not detected (Table 3). Moreover, TARC was positively related to total IgE (Table 4). TARC plays a dominant role in Th$_2$-type disease conditions by recruiting Th$_2$ cells into inflammatory sites [25]. Several studies have demonstrated that there were elevated levels of TARC in patients with atopic dermatitis [26, 27] and asthma [28, 29]. The elevated TARC in asthma patients may be a reflection of increased TARC expression at inflammatory sites of the asthmatic airway [30]. The normal levels of serum TARC in healthy children and adults differ depending on age, with TARC levels being higher in children [31, 32].

However, in our study, the level only increased in the elderly adult group of the asthmatic subjects. It should be noted that this study had a few limitations. First, the asthmatic subjects included in this study show various allergic status (GINA 1–4). The relationship between severity and other parameters cannot be evaluated in this study. Second, we do not have any information regarding whether asthma found in elderly adult groups developed as a result of late onset asthma or was diagnosed in their childhood. Further study will be need to investigate these limitations.

Conclusion

TARC in serum of the elderly adult group was increased when compared to members of other younger groups, and was positively related to total IgE in the total and elderly adult asthma group. Cytokines such as IL-6, IL-8, MCP-1, RANTES, and MIP-1α were significantly altered in the elderly adult group. The results presented herein will help elucidate the pathogenesis of allergic diseases such as asthma, as well as to mining of biomarkers associated with age.

Abbreviations

BALF: Bronchoalveolar lavage fluid; BSA: Bovine serum albumin; DF: *Dermatophagoides farina*; DP: *Dermatophagoides pteronissinus*; ELISA: Enzyme linked immunosorbent assay; FEV1: Forced expiratory capacity in 1 s; FVC: Forced vital capacity; HDMs: House dust mites; MCP: Monocyte chemoattractant protein; PAR: Proteinase activated receptor; PBS: Phosphate buffered saline; TARC: Thymus and activation regulated chemokine; TLR: Toll like receptor

Acknowledgments

We thank normal volunteers and allergic patients to participate in this study.

Funding

This work was supported by the BK21 plus program through the National Research Foundation(NRF) funded by the Ministry of Education of Korea.

Authors' contributions

KMJ, HKL, and JWS conducted the experiments and the statistical analyses, EC, MHH and YK helped conducting the experiments with patients and performing immunoassays, ISK designed, supervised the project and the data analysis. All authors read and approved the final manuscript.

Competing interests

The authors declare that they have no competing interests.

Author details

[1]Department of Senior Healthcare, BK21 plus program, Graduate School, Eulji University, Daejeon 34824, Korea. [2]Department of Biomedical Laboratory Science, School of Medicine, Eulji University, 77, Gyeryoung-ro 771 beon-gil, Jung-Gu, Daejeon 34824, Republic of Korea. [3]Department of Biomedical Laboratory Science, College of Health Science, Eulji University, Seongnam 13135, Korea. [4]Department of Respiratory Internal Medicine, College of Medicine, Konyang University, Daejeon 35365, Korea. [5]Department of Clinical Laboratory Science, Wonkwang Health Science University, Iksan 54538, Republic of Korea.

References

1. Holgate ST. Pathogenesis of asthma. Clin Exp Allergy. 2008;38:872–97.
2. Gaffin JM, Phipatanakul W. The role of indoor allergens in the development of asthma. Curr Opin Allergy Clin Immunol. 2009;9:128–35.
3. Jacquet A. The role of innate immunity activation in house dust mite allergy. Trends Mol Med. 2011;17:604–11.
4. Kim DH, Choi E, Lee JS, et al. House dust mite allergen regulates constitutive apoptosis of normal and asthmatic neutrophils via toll-like receptor 4. PLoS One. 2015;10:e0125983.
5. Lee NR, Baek SY, Gu A, et al. House dust mite allergen suppresses neutrophil apoptosis by cytokine release via PAR2 in normal and allergic lymphocytes. Immunol Res. 2016;64:123–32.
6. Hammad H, Chieppa M, Perros F, et al. House dust mite allergen induces asthma via toll-like receptor 4 triggering of airway structural cells. Nat Med. 2009;15:410–6.
7. Xia S, Zhang X, Zheng S, et al. An update on inflamm-aging: mechanisms, prevention, and treatment. J Immunol Res. 2016;2016:8426874.
8. Zuo L, Pannell BK, Liu Z. Characterization and redox mechanism of asthma in the elderly. Oncotarget. 2016;7:25010–21.

9. Ventura MT, Scichilone N, Paganelli R, et al. Allergic diseases in the elderly: biological characteristics and main immunological and non-immunological mechanisms. Clin Mol Allergy. 2017;15:2.

10. Ahmad A, Obaidi AH, Mohamed A, et al. The predictive value of IgE as biomarker in asthma. J Asthma. 2008;45:654–63.

11. Jeong KY, Park JW, Hong CS. House dust mite allergy in Korea: the most important inhalant allergen in current and future. Allergy asthma. Immunol Res. 2012;4:313–25.

12. Arlian LG, Platts-Mills TA. The biology of dust mites and the remediation of mite allergens in allergic disease. J Allergy Clin Immunol. 2001;107:S406–13.

13. Abd Ella OH, Badawy EAM, Shahat M, et al. Allergy to *Dermatophagoides pteronyssinus* (Der p1) and *Dermatophagoides farina* (Der f1) in patients with atopic asthma. Int J Sci Res. 2015;4:1896–902.

14. Hosoki K, Ying S, Corrigan C, et al. Analysis of a panel of 48 cytokines in BAL fluids specifically identifies IL-8 levels as the only cytokine that distinguishes controlled asthma from uncontrolled asthma, and correlates inversely with FEV_1. PLoS One. 2015;10:e0126035.

15. Kuo PL, Hsu YL, Huang MS, et al. Bronchial epithelium-derived IL-8 and RANTES increased bronchial smooth muscle cell migration and proliferation by Kruppel-like factor 5 in areca nut-mediated airway remodeling. Toxicol Sci. 2011;121:177–90.

16. Rossi A, Ganassini A, Tantucci C, et al. Aging and the respiratory system. Aging Clin Exp Res. 1996;8:143–61.

17. Mathur SK. Allergy and asthma in the elderly. Semin Respir Crit Care Med. 2010;31:587–95.

18. Jatakanon A, Uasuf C, Maziak W, et al. Neutrophilic inflammation in severe persistent asthma. Am J Respir Crit Care Med. 1999;160:1532–9.

19. Thomas RA, Green RH, Brightling CE, et al. Influence of age on induced sputum differential cell counts in normal subjects. Chest. 2004;126:1811–4.

20. Mathur SK, Schwantes EA, Jarjour NN, et al. Age-related changes in eosinophil function in human subjects. Chest. 2008;133:412–9.

21. Pawelec G. Immunosenescence: impact in the young as well as the old? Mech Ageing Dev. 1999;108(1):1–7.

22. Aw D, Silva AB, Palmer DB. Immunosenescence: emerging challenges for an ageing population. Immunology. 2007;120:435–46.

23. De Amici M, Ciprandi G. The age impact on serum total and allergen-specific IgE. Allergy asthma. Immunol Res. 2013;5:170–4.

24. Weghofer M, Thomas WR, Kronqvist M, et al. Variability of IgE reactivity profiles among European mite allergic patients. Eur J Clin Investig. 2008;38:959–65.

25. Yoshie O. Immune chemokines and their receptors: the key elements in the genesis, homeostasis and function of the immune system. Springer Semin Immunopathol. 2000;22:371–91.

26. Fujisawa T, Fujisawa R, Kato Y, et al. Presence of high contents of thymus and activation-regulated chemokine in platelets and elevated plasma levels of thymus and activation-regulated chemokine and macrophage-derived chemokine in patients with atopic dermatitis. J Allergy Clin Immunol. 2002; 110:139–46.

27. Kakinuma T, Nakamura K, Wakugawa M, et al. Thymus and activation-regulated chemokine in atopic dermatitis: serum thymus and activation-regulated chemokine level is closely related with disease activity. J Allergy Clin Immunol. 2001;107:535–41.

28. Leung TF, Wong CK, Chan IH, et al. Plasma concentration of thymus and activation-regulated chemokine is elevated in childhood asthma. J Allergy Clin Immunol. 2002;110:404–9.

29. Reda SM, Hossny E, El-Fedawy S, El-Deen ME. Plasma concentration of thymus and activation-regulated chemokine in childhood asthma. Egypt J Pediatr Allergy Immunol. 2003;1:86–92.

30. Sekiya T, Yamada H, Yamaguchi M, et al. Increased levels of a TH2-type CC chemokine thymus and activation-regulated chemokine (TARC) in serum and induced sputum of asthmatics. Allergy. 2002;57(2):173–7.

31. Tamaki K, Saeki H, Kadono T, et al. Serum TARC/CCL17 levels as a disease marker of atopic dermatitis. Jap J Dermatol. 2006;116:27–39.

32. Fujisawa T, Nagao M, Hiraguchi Y, et al. Serum measurement of thymus and activation-regulated chemokine/CCL17 in children with atopic dermatitis: elevated normal levels in infancy and age-specific analysis in atopic dermatitis. Pediatr Allergy Immunol. 2009;20:633–41.

22

Vaccines for the elderly: current use and future challenges

Birgit Weinberger ⓘ

Abstract

Age-related changes of the immune system contribute to increased incidence and severity of infections in the elderly. Vaccination is the most effective measure to prevent infections and vaccination recommendations in most countries include specific guidelines for the elderly. Vaccination against influenza and *Streptococcus pneumoniae* is usually recommended for persons with underlying diseases and for the elderly with heterogeneous age limits between ≥ 50 years and ≥ 65 years. Some countries also recommend vaccination against herpes zoster. Several vaccines are recommended for all adults, such as regular booster shots against tetanus/diphtheria/pertussis/polio, or for specific groups, e.g. vaccination against tick-borne encephalitis in endemic areas or travel vaccines. These are also relevant for the elderly. Most currently used vaccines are less immunogenic and effective in the elderly compared to younger adults. Potential strategies to improve their immunogenicity include higher antigen dose, alternative routes of administration, and the use of adjuvants, which were all implemented for influenza vaccines, and induce moderately higher antibody concentrations. Research on universal vaccines against influenza and *S. pneumoniae* is ongoing in order to overcome the limitations of the current strain-specific vaccines. Respiratory syncytial virus causes significant morbidity in the elderly. Novel vaccines against this and other pathogens, for instance bacterial nosocomial infections, have tremendous potential impact on health in old age and are intensively studied by many academic and commercial organizations. In addition to novel vaccine developments, it is crucial to increase awareness for the importance of vaccination beyond the pediatric setting, as vaccination coverage is still far from optimal for the older population.

Keywords: Vaccine, Elderly, Aging, Immunosenescence, Influenza, Herpes zoster, *Streptococcus Pneumoniae*

Background

With increasing life expectancy, the global population ages, and the number of persons older than 60 years of age is expected to double by 2050, reaching 2.1 billion. The number of persons above 80 years is projected to increase even more dramatically from a worldwide total of 125 million in 2015 to 434 million in 2050 [1]. The severity of many infections is higher in the elderly compared to younger adults and infectious diseases are frequently associated with long-term sequelae such as impairments in activities of daily living, onset of frailty, or the loss of independence [2, 3]. This represents a serious challenge for public health systems, and the prevention of infectious disease is therefore an important measure to ensure healthy aging and improve the quality of life. The tremendous success of childhood vaccination is widely recognized, but the need for life-long vaccination programs and the importance of vaccination for the older population are frequently underestimated. This review summarizes current recommendations for developed countries, gives examples regarding immunogenicity and efficacy data for vaccines currently used for the elderly, and provides an outlook on novel vaccines developed specifically for this age group.

Vaccines specifically recommended for the elderly

Many countries have established vaccination recommendations for adults and most of these also include specific guidelines for older adults. Vaccination against influenza and *Streptococcus pneumoniae* is usually recommended for persons with underlying diseases and for the elderly with heterogeneous age limits between ≥ 50 years and ≥65 years. Some countries also recommend vaccination against herpes zoster for older adults. Table 1 summarizes current recommendations for Europe and the USA [4, 5].

Correspondence: birgit.weinberger@uibk.ac.at
Universität Innsbruck, Institute for Biomedical Aging Research, Rennweg 10, 6020 Innsbruck, Austria

Table 1 Vaccination recommendations for older adults in Europe and the US

	Influenza[a]	S. pneumoniae[b]	Herpes zoster[d]	Tetanus	Diphtheria[i]	Pertussis[j]
Austria	all adults	> 50; PCV + PPV[c]	> 50	every 5 years[e]	every 5 years[e]	every 5 years[e]
Belgium	> 65	> 65; PCV + PPV[c]		every 10 years	every 10 years	once[h]
Bulgaria	> 65	–	–	every 10 years	every 10 years	–
Croatia	> 65	–		once at 60	–	–
Cyprus	> 65	> 65; PPV		every 10 years	every 10 years	–
Czech Rep.	all adults	> 65; PCV + PPV[c]	> 50	every 10 years[f]	–	once at 65
Denmark	> 65	> 65; PCV or PPV		–	–	–
Estonia	> 65	–		every 10 years	every 10 years	–
Finland	> 65	> 65; PCV or PPV		every 10 years	every 10 years	–
France	> 65	–	65-75	every 10 years[g]	every 10 years[g]	once[h]
Germany	> 60	> 60; PPV		every 10 years	every 10 years	once[h]
Greece	> 60	> 65; PCV	> 60	every 10 years	every 10 years	once[h]
Hungary	> 60	> 50; PPV		–	–	–
Iceland	> 60	> 60; PPV		–	–	–
Ireland	> 65	> 65; PPV		–	–	–
Italy	> 65	> 65; PCV + PPV[c]	> 65	every 10 years	every 10 years	every 10 years
Latvia	> 65	–		every 10 years	every 10 years	–
Liechtenstein	> 65	–		every 10 years[g]	every 10 years[g]	every 10 years[g]
Lithuania	> 65	–		every 5-10 years	every 5-10 years	–
Luxembourg	> 65	> 60; PCV + PPV[c]		every 10 years	every 10 years	every 10 years
Malta	all adults	> 65; PCV		–	–	–
Netherlands	> 60	–		–	–	–
Norway	> 65	> 65; PPV		–	–	–
Poland	all adults	> 50; PCV		once[h]	once[h]	–
Portugal	> 65	–		every 10 years[g]	every 10 years[g]	–
Romania	> 65	–		–	–	–
Slovakia	> 60	> 60; PCV		every 15 years	every 15 years	–
Slovenia	all adults	> 65;PCV or PPV		every 10 years	every 10 years	once[h]
Spain	> 65	> 65; PPV		once at 65	once at 65	–
Sweden	–	> 65; PPV		every 20 years	every 20 years	–
UK	> 65	> 65; PPV	> 70	–	–	–
USA	all adults	> 65; PCV + PPV[c]	> 60	every 10 years	every 10 years	once[h]

Shown are recommendations for the general population for all countries listed by the European Centre for Disease Prevention and Control. Specific recommendations for risk groups (co-morbidities, health care personnel etc.) are available in most countries
[a]annual vaccination, inactivated trivalent vaccine
[b]recommendation for persons without prior vaccination against pneumococcal disease; no booster shots recommended for general population; recommendations may differ for persons with underlying medical conditions
[c]one dose of PCV13 (pneumococcal conjugate vaccine) followed by 1 dose of PPV23 (pneumococcal polysaccharide vaccine)
[d]one dose, contraindicated in immunosuppressed patients (live vaccine)
[e]for persons over 65 years; every 10 years for younger adults
[f]for persons over 65 years; every 10-15 years for younger adults
[g]for persons over 65 years; every 20 years for younger adults
[h]once during adulthood
[i]vaccine containing reduced diphtheria dose (d)
[j]vaccine containing acellular pertussis antigens

Influenza

Influenza causes approximately 100,000 hospitalizations and 36,000 deaths annually in the USA, which occur mainly in persons over the age 65 years [6, 7]. Vaccines against influenza usually contain three different strains (A/H1N1, A/H3N2, B) and the exact composition of the vaccine is determined each year by the World Health Organization (WHO) based on surveillance data.

Recently, quadrivalent vaccines became available, as two different B strains had circulated in parallel for several years [8, 9]. Annual vaccination against influenza is recommended, as the composition of the vaccine changes in order to reflect currently circulating virus strains.

Immunogenicity of influenza vaccines is usually measured by hemagglutination inhibition assay (HAI), which quantifies antibodies specific for the viral hemagglutinin. Many studies demonstrated that antibody concentrations after vaccination are lower in older compared to younger adults [10] and that co-morbidities and frailty further decrease responsiveness to vaccination [11, 12]. Clinical efficacy or effectiveness of influenza vaccines is difficult to analyze, as compilations of results from clinical studies are highly complex. Parameters such as study population (age distribution, co-morbidities, frailty etc.), epidemiological factors (transmission patterns e.g. in institutionalized cohorts, prevalence of the virus), and virological factors (virulence, mismatch between vaccine and circulating viral strains) are different for each study and each influenza season. In addition, various clinical read-out parameters for influenza disease such as influenza-like illness (ILI), laboratory confirmed influenza or hospitalization due to influenza are utilized. Meta-analyses have estimated clinical benefits of influenza vaccination, and it can be concluded that protection is lower in older than in young adults [13, 14]. Several strategies to improve influenza vaccines for the elderly led to the licensure of vaccines containing the oil-in-water emulsion adjuvant MF59 [15] or 60 µg instead of 15 µg of hemagglutinin protein per dose [16], and of a vaccine administered via the intradermal instead of the intramuscular route [17]. These vaccines elicit slightly higher antibody responses compared to the standard inactivated vaccine. Interestingly, MF59-adjuvanted vaccines induce substantially higher antibody responses against heterologous vaccine strains [18, 19], and this broader neutralizing activity probably contributes to the higher clinical efficacy observed with the adjuvanted vaccine. A large trial in Italy demonstrated that the risk of hospitalization for influenza or pneumonia was 25% lower for the adjuvanted vaccine compared to non-adjuvanted vaccine (relative risk 0.75, 95% CI 0.57-0.98) [20]. In a study including residents of long-term care facilities, the risk of ILI was higher in persons receiving standard TIV (OR 1.52, 95% CI 1.22-1.88) than in those who had received the adjuvanted vaccine. This effect was even more pronounced in patients with respiratory and cardiovascular disease [21].

Pneumococcal disease

Invasive pneumococcal disease (bacteremia, meningitis etc.) mainly affects young children and older adults [22, 23]. *S. pneumoniae* is also a common cause of community-acquired pneumonia (CAP) in the elderly [24]. A 23-valent polysaccharide vaccine has been used for many years for older adults, but polysaccharides induce IgM-dominated antibody responses without adequate immunological memory, as they are T cell-independent antigens. Conjugated vaccines have been developed for the vaccination of infants and very successfully reduced the burden of disease in children. A 13-valent conjugate vaccine has been introduced also for older adults. In a large randomized trial in persons over 65 years of age it was demonstrated that 45.6% (95.2% CI 21.8-62.5, $p < 0.001$) fewer first episodes of vaccine-type CAP requiring hospitalization and 75.0% (95% CI 41.4-90.8, $p < 0.001$) fewer first episodes of vaccine-type invasive pneumococcal disease occurred in the vaccine group compared to placebo [25]. Vaccination recommendations for *S. pneumoniae* are heterogeneous. Some countries still recommend the polysaccharide vaccine, while others recommend the conjugate vaccine alone or followed by the polysaccharide vaccine usually at least one year later. Details regarding the recommendations in European countries are published by the European Centre of Disease Prevention and Control. With the introduction of a 7-valent and a 10-valent conjugate vaccine for childhood vaccination around the year 2000 disease incidence and carriage of the serotypes included in the vaccines decreased in children. Consequently, transmission of these serotypes to older adults and therefore disease incidence in the older age group also decreased in the following years. However, serotype replacement was observed, which means that the incidence of pneumococcal disease caused by other serotypes, not included in the conjugated vaccines, increased both in children and older adults [26–28]. Similar effects have been observed for the 13-valent vaccine [29–31].

Herpes zoster

Almost all adults are latently infected with varicella zoster virus (VZV). The primary infection, which usually occurs in childhood, manifests as chickenpox and live-long latency is established afterwards. Partial reactivation of the virus probably occurs frequently throughout life, but is usually controlled by virus-specific T cell responses. In the absence of sufficient immunological control, e.g. due to immunosuppression or immunosenescence, viral reactivation can lead to herpes zoster (shingles) [32]. The incidence of herpes zoster increases with age and it has been estimated that up to 50% of all cases affect persons older than 85 years [33, 34]. In a fraction of the patients acute episodes of herpes zoster are followed by post-herpetic neuralgia (PHN), characterized by long-lasting severe pain after the resolution of the zoster rash. The incidence of this complication is higher in older zoster patients, where it occurs in approximately one third of the cases [35]. Particularly in older patients, PHN frequently leads to substantial impairment in activities of daily living or even loss of independence [36, 37]. A single-shot immunization with an attenuated live-vaccine against herpes zoster, which has been licensed for use in older adults in 2006, is recommended in some countries. This vaccine induces T cell and antibody responses [38]. It was shown to reduce the incidence of herpes zoster by 51.3% (95% CI 44.2-57.6) and the incidence of PHN by 66.5% (95% CI 44.5-79.2) compared to placebo in a large randomized trial including persons older than 60 years [39]. The protective effect of the vaccine was lower in the very old, and long-term follow-up studies showed that protection waned over time, dropping to 21.1% (95% CI 20.9-30.4) for the prevention of herpes zoster and 35.4% (95% CI 8.8-55.8%) for PHN in years 7-10 [40, 41]. Antibody responses to a second dose of the vaccine more than 10 years after the first dose were similar to the first response, but cellular immune responses were higher after the booster dose. These findings indicate that there was a residual effect of the first vaccination on cellular immunity more than 10 years later and that the second dose induced a booster response [42]. Repeated vaccination of older individuals at appropriate intervals could therefore be considered for future recommendations.

Vaccines recommended for all adults

Regular booster vaccinations against tetanus and diphtheria, in some cases combined with pertussis and/or polio, are recommended in many countries for all adults, including the elderly (summarized in Table 1). Regular vaccination against other pathogens is recommended in some countries, e.g. against tick-borne encephalitis in endemic areas. Most countries do not have specific recommendations for older adults, but e.g. in Austria, France, Liechtenstein and Portugal booster intervals are shortened for persons over 65 years.

Tetanus and diphtheria

Tetanus- and diphtheria-specific antibody concentrations are frequently below the levels considered to be protective for adults, and are even lower for the elderly [43–48]. We could show that approximately 10% of a healthy elderly cohort recruited in Austria did not develop protective antibodies against diphtheria after a single booster shot and that almost half of the participants did not have antibodies above protective levels 5 years later. A second booster shot at this time point did again not provide long-term protection [48, 49]. This could be due to insufficient priming earlier in life, inadequate boosters throughout adulthood or age-related defects of the immune system. Given the fact that tetanus-specific antibody concentrations were substantially higher in the same cohort, one could also speculate that the currently used combination vaccine, which contains a reduced amount of diphtheria toxoid, might not

be optimal. A more detailed overview of tetanus and diphtheria vaccination of the elderly has recently been published [50]. Antibody responses to booster vaccination against tick-borne encephalitis are also lower in old compared to young adults [51, 52].

Pertussis

Vaccination against pertussis is widely used and accepted in the pediatric setting, but epidemiological data show an increased incidence of pertussis in adults and particularly in the elderly, for whom the infection can be associated with severe symptoms and increased mortality [53–55]. Adults can also transmit the disease to newborn infants, who are too young to be vaccinated. Few countries recommend regular booster immunizations with combined vaccines containing tetanus, diphtheria and pertussis antigens, whereas some recommend only one dose of pertussis-containing vaccine during adulthood. Many countries, however, do not recommend booster vaccination against pertussis for adults. Booster doses of combined tetanus/diphtheria/pertussis vaccine are well tolerated and immunogenic when given periodically to young or older adults [56], but antibody concentrations 4 weeks after vaccination are lower in old compared to young adults [46].

Appropriate vaccination documentation is crucial to deliver booster vaccinations at the right time points. Unfortunately, this documentation is often fragmentary for older adults, and it is therefore difficult to reliably assess adequate primary vaccination in childhood and the number of booster immunizations received throughout life. Several studies on tetanus/diphtheria vaccination reported only incomplete immunization histories [45, 47, 48]. Launay et al. reported that the number of vaccine doses received in life decreases from 7.1 (95% CI 6.9-7.2) doses of tetanus vaccine in young adults, which corresponds well with recommendations of 5 doses during childhood/adolescence and 10 year-booster intervals afterwards, to only 5.7 (95% CI 4.6-6.8) doses for adults aged 50-60 years [47]. This indicates a lack of regular booster immunizations during adulthood for this age group. Vaccination strategies for the future should include regular and well-documented booster shots throughout life, as post-booster antibody concentrations correlate with pre-booster antibody concentrations [46].

Travel vaccines

Travel vaccines are becoming more important for older adults, as the number of older long-distance travelers increases due to improved health and mobility of this age group. Incidence and severity of typhoid fever and Japanese encephalitis are higher in older compared to younger adults [57, 58], highlighting the importance of travel vaccines for this age group. Vaccines against typhoid fever, Japanese encephalitis, rabies or yellow fever are neo-antigens for most older travelers and many older adults probably also never had contact with Hepatitis A and Hepatitis B. One hallmark of immunosenescence is the loss of naïve T cells and to a lesser extent of naïve B cells, which affects primary immune responses to these antigens. Impaired memory generation late in life has been demonstrated in animal models [59, 60] and therefore the success of primary vaccination late in life might be limited. Unfortunately, very few data are available regarding immune responses of the elderly to travel vaccines as most studies exclude older participants. Therefore, immunization guidelines rely primarily on studies with young adults. Antibody responses to Hepatitis A and B vaccines are already reduced in middle-aged adults compared to younger age groups [61, 62] and the percentage of non-responders without protective antibody concentrations against Hepatitis B increases with age [63]. Vaccination against Hepatitis B is not only relevant for older travels, but also for other risk groups, such as health care workers, household contacts of infected persons and hemodialysis patients, which also include older persons. Vaccination against yellow fever is mandatory for travelers to some South American and African countries. The live-attenuated yellow fever vaccine is highly immunogenic, but meta-analysis indicates that older adults have a higher risk for rare severe adverse events, such as e.g. yellow fever vaccine-associated viscerotropic disease, which mimics infection with the wild-type virus and has a high mortality of up to 60% [64].

New vaccines developed for the elderly
Next-generation vaccines against influenza, pneumococcal disease and herpes zoster

The current vaccines against influenza, *S. pneumoniae* and herpes zoster have several limitations. Vaccination against influenza has to be administered annually, as the vaccine provides protection only against the strains included in the formulation or closely related variants. Influenza virus strains are highly variable and new distinct strains circulate almost every year. A "universal" influenza vaccine inducing long-lasting immunity against all strains of influenza would solve the problem of annual revaccination and would probably improve compliance and vaccination coverage. Numerous candidate vaccines are investigated, which utilize various antigens, such as conserved regions of the surface proteins hemagglutinin and neuraminidase or internal viral proteins. Viral vectors, virus-like particles, DNA vaccines and the use of various adjuvants are discussed and tested as vaccine platforms in order to achieve potent $CD4^+$ and $CD8^+$ T cell responses, which are believed to be required for broad protection in addition to antibodies [65].

Universal pneumococcal vaccines would also be very useful, as there are approximately 100 serotypes of *S. pneumoniae*. Currently, vaccine manufacturers try to increase the number of serotypes included in conjugated vaccines, but antibody responses to polysaccharides will probably always be serotype-specific. Several pneumococcal proteins have been identified as potential vaccine candidates. They are highly conserved in all clinically relevant serotypes, and elicit potent immune responses in animal models. Additionally, whole-cell inactivated vaccines, live-attenuated vaccines and combinations of protein and polysaccharide components are investigated [66].

The incidence of herpes zoster is high not only in the elderly, but also in immunocompromised patients, such as after organ or stem cell transplantation, in HIV-positive individuals and in cancer patients, due a decline of cellular immunity. The current vaccine against herpes zoster contains live-attenuated virus and can therefore not be used for these patients due to safety issues [67, 68]. As described above, the efficacy of the vaccine is lower in the very old and wanes over time. Therefore, it is difficult to determine the optimal age for the vaccination, which is also reflected by differing age recommendations in the countries recommending the vaccine. Phase I/II studies demonstrated both the immunogenicity and safety of a novel inactivated vaccine containing the viral glycoprotein E in combination with the liposome-based AS01B adjuvant system (MPL and QS21) in older adults [69, 70] as well as in hematopoietic cell transplant recipients [71] and HIV-patients [72]. Large phase III randomized placebo-controlled trials demonstrated an overall clinical efficacy against herpes zoster of more than 90% with narrow confidence intervals. Remarkably, the vaccine efficacy was similar in all age groups, even in persons older than 80 years [73, 74]. This vaccine has recently been licensed in Canada and the US and might replace the live-attenuated herpes zoster vaccine in the future.

New targets for vaccine development

We still lack vaccines for many pathogens that are of clinical relevance in the elderly. Respiratory syncytial virus (RSV) is a major cause of severe respiratory infection in infants, but usually causes only mild or moderate symptoms in adults. However, older and particularly frail individuals and patients with underlying co-morbidities can experience severe RSV disease. In the UK, an estimated 18,000 hospitalizations and 8400 deaths per year – almost exclusively in the elderly - are caused by RSV and underlying co-morbidity further increases the risk of severe disease [75]. Research on RSV vaccines was slowed down in the past, because a first-generation vaccine used in the 1960s for vaccination of infants was associated with risk for disease enhancement. Several candidate vaccines against RSV based on recombinant proteins, virus-like particles, live-attenuated virus or viral vectors are now in clinical development. It is crucial that these novel vaccines are not only developed for the pediatric market, but also include adult and elderly target groups.

There are many more infections affecting the elderly and various vaccine candidates are in pre-clinical or clinical development. One group of pathogens, which attracted special attention over the last years are nosocomial infections. The risk for these infections is high in the elderly, due to more frequent hospitalization and invasive procedures in this age group. Vaccines against bacterial nosocomial infections are highly desirable, as antibiotic resistance is a growing problem, but no such vaccine is currently on the market. The most severe infections are caused by *Clostridium difficile*, which is the most common cause of nosocomial diarrhea and *Staphylococcus aureus*, which is responsible for infections of prostheses, catheters or surgical wounds. Two vaccine candidates against *S. aureus* have been clinically tested, but unfortunately did not provide protection [76, 77]. Novel vaccine candidates are now in early stages of development. Most vaccine candidates against *C. difficile* are based on bacterial toxins which are responsible for the clinical symptoms [78]. Vaccines against these and other nosocomial pathogens, such as *Klebsiella pneumoniae*, *Escherichia coli* and the fungal pathogen *Candida spp.* have the potential to substantially reduce healthcare costs and to save many lives [79].

Conclusion

Older adults are at high risk for infectious diseases and vaccination is an important preventive measure to facilitate healthy aging. Childhood vaccination programs are well-accepted and widely used, but unfortunately awareness for adult vaccination is by far less prominent. Several vaccines against influenza, *S. pneumoniae* and herpes zoster are available for the elderly and vaccines that are used throughout adulthood, such as tetanus, diphtheria and pertussis, are also relevant for the elderly. The first step towards optimal protection of the elderly is the comprehensive use of existing vaccines. Vaccination recommendations for adults and the elderly differ from country to country. Taking regional differences such as e.g. epidemiological parameters into account is of course necessary for optimal vaccine recommendations, but the diversity of recommendations e.g. throughout Europe can be confusing and might be interpreted as uncertainty. Therefore, increased efforts of harmonization would be desirable [80–82]. Nevertheless, without implementation strategies and sufficient vaccination coverage such guidelines provide only theoretical benefits. Vaccination coverage differs greatly between countries, and data are very difficult to obtain, as many countries do not have centralized databases collecting this information. The WHO goal of 75% influenza vaccination coverage for older adults (> 65 years)

until 2014/2015 was not reached by most countries. The UK and the Netherlands reported the highest vaccination rates in Europe (above 70%), but some other European countries did not even reach 10% coverage in this age group [83]. Vaccine uptake for other adult vaccinations is not sufficiently documented in most countries and e.g. data on adult vaccination coverage against tetanus and diphtheria is only available for 5 of 29 European countries [84]. Improved vaccines against influenza, pneumococcal disease and herpes zoster have been developed over the last years and continuous effort is put into further increasing their potential to provide broad and long-lasting protection. In addition, vaccines against additional pathogens such as RSV and nosocomial infections could substantially improve health in old age. For the rational design of optimized and novel vaccines for the elderly basic research to understand immunosenescence is essential, and it is of utmost importance that clinical development and testing includes also older age groups.

Abbreviations

C. difficile: *Clostridium difficile*; *Candida spp.*: *Candida species*; CAP: Community-acquired pneumonia; CI: Confidence interval; H: Hemagglutinin; HAI: Hemagglutination inhibition assay; IgM: Immunoglobulin M; ILI: Influenza-like illness; MPL: Monophosphoryl Lipid A; N: Neuraminidase; PCV: Pneumococcal conjugate vaccine; PHN: Post-herpetic neuralgia; PPV: Pneumococcal polysaccharide vaccine; RSV: Respiratory syncytial virus; *S. aureus*: *Staphylococcus aureus*; *S. pneumoniae*: *Streptococcus pneumoniae*; VZV: Varicella zoster virus; WHO: World Health Organization

Acknowledgements

Not applicable

Funding

This work was supported by the European Union's Seventh Framework Programme [FP7/2007-2013] under Grant Agreement No: 280873 ADITEC.

Authors' contributions

BW wrote the manuscript.

Competing interests

The author declares that she has no competing interests.

References

1. United Nations. World population prospects. 2017. http://esa.un.org/unpd/wpp. Accessed 30 July 2017.
2. Janssens JP. Pneumonia in the elderly (geriatric) population. Curr Opin Pulm Med. 2005;11:226–30.

3. Attal N, Deback C, Gavazzi G, Gorwood P, Labetoulle M, Liard F, et al. Functional decline and herpes zoster in older people: an interplay of multiple factors. Aging Clin Exp Res. 2015;27:757–65.

4. European Centre for Disease Prevention and Control: Vaccine schedule. 2017. http://vaccine-schedule.ecdc.europa.eu/Pages/Scheduler.aspx. Accessed 31 Oct 2017.

5. Kim DK, Riley LE, Harriman KH, Hunter P, Bridges CB. Advisory Commitee on immunization practices recommended immunization schedule for adults aged 19 years or older-United States, 2017. MMWR Morb Mortal Wkly Rep. 2017;66:136–8.

6. Thompson WW, Shay DK, Weintraub E, Brammer L, Cox N, Anderson LJ, et al. Mortality associated with influenza and respiratory syncytial virus in the United States. JAMA. 2003;289:179–86.

7. Thompson WW, Shay DK, Weintraub E, Brammer L, Bridges CB, Cox NJ, et al. Influenza-associated hospitalizations in the United States. JAMA. 2004;292: 1333–40.

8. Shaw MW, Xu X, Li Y, Normand S, Ueki RT, Kunimoto GY, et al. Reappearance and global spread of variants of influenza B/Victoria/2/87 lineage viruses in the 2000-2001 and 2001-2002 seasons. Virology. 2002;303:1–8.

9. Trucchi C, Alicino C, Orsi A, Paganino C, Barberis I, Grammatico F, et al. Fifteen years of epidemiologic, virologic and syndromic influenza surveillance: a focus on type B virus and the effects of vaccine mismatch in Liguria region, Italy. Hum Vaccin Immunother. 2017;13:456–63.

10. Goodwin K, Viboud C, Simonsen L. Antibody response to influenza vaccination in the elderly: a quantitative review. Vaccine. 2006;24:1159–69.

11. Mysliwska J, Trzonkowski P, Szmit E, Brydak LB, Machala M, Mysliwski A. Immunomodulating effect of influenza vaccination in the elderly differing in health status. Exp Gerontol. 2004;39:1447–58.

12. Yao X, Hamilton RG, Weng NP, Xue QL, Bream JH, Li H, et al. Frailty is associated with impairment of vaccine-induced antibody response and increase in post-vaccination influenza infection in community-dwelling older adults. Vaccine. 2011;29:5015–21.

13. Osterholm MT, Kelley NS, Sommer A, Belongia EA. Efficacy and effectiveness of influenza vaccines: a systematic review and meta-analysis. Lancet Infect Dis. 2012;12:36–44.

14. Beyer WE, McElhaney J, Smith DJ, Monto AS, Nguyen-Van-Tam JS, Osterhaus AD. Cochrane re-arranged: support for policies to vaccinate elderly people against influenza. Vaccine. 2013;31:6030–3.

15. De Donato S, Granoff D, Minutello M, Lecchi G, Faccini M, Agnello M, et al. Safety and immunogenicity of MF59-adjuvanted influenza vaccine in the elderly. Vaccine. 1999;17:3094–101.

16. DiazGranados CA, Dunning AJ, Kimmel M, Kirby D, Treanor J, Collins A, et al. Efficacy of high-dose versus standard-dose influenza vaccine in older adults. N Engl J Med. 2014;371:635–45.

17. Holland D, Booy R, de Looze F, Eizenberg P, McDonald J, Karrasch J, et al. Intradermal influenza vaccine administered using a new microinjection system produces superior immunogenicity in elderly adults: a randomized controlled trial. J Infect Dis. 2008;198:650–8.

18. DelGiudice G, Hilbert AK, Bugarini R, Minutello A, Popova O, Toneatto D, et al. An MF59-adjuvanted inactivated influenza vaccine containing a/Panama/ 1999 (H3N2) induced broader serological protection against heterovariant influenza virus strain a/Fujian/2002 than a subunit and a split influenza vaccine. Vaccine. 2006;24:3063–5.

19. Ansaldi F, Bacilieri S, Durando P, Sticchi L, Valle L, Montomoli E, et al. Cross-protection by MF59-adjuvanted influenza vaccine: neutralizing and haemagglutination-inhibiting antibody activity against a(H3N2) drifted influenza viruses. Vaccine. 2008;26:1525–9.

20. Mannino S, Villa M, Apolone G, Weiss NS, Groth N, Aquino I, et al. Effectiveness of adjuvanted influenza vaccination in elderly subjects in northern Italy. Am J Epidemiol. 2012;176:527–33.

21. Iob A, Brianti G, Zamparo E, Gallo T. Evidence of increased clinical protection of an MF59-adjuvant influenza vaccine compared to a non-adjuvant vaccine among elderly residents of long-term care facilities in Italy. Epidemiol Infect. 2005;133:687–93.

22. Kyaw MH, Christie P, Clarke SC, Mooney JD, Ahmed S, Jones IG, et al. Invasive pneumococcal disease in Scotland, 1999-2001: use of record linkage to explore associations between patients and disease in relation to future vaccination policy. Clin Infect Dis. 2003;37:1283–91.

23. Melegaro A, Edmunds WJ, Pebody R, Miller E, George R. The current burden of pneumococcal disease in England and Wales. J Inf Secur. 2006;52:37–48.

24. Centers for Disease Control and Prevention. Prevention of pneumococcal disease: recommendations of the Advisory Committee on Immunization Practices (ACIP). MMWR Recomm Rep. 1997;46:1-24.

25. Bonten MJ, Huijts SM, Bolkenbaas M, Webber C, Patterson S, Gault S, et al. Polysaccharide conjugate vaccine against pneumococcal pneumonia in adults. N Engl J Med. 2015;372:1114–25.

26. Dagan R. Serotype replacement in perspective. Vaccine. 2009;27(Suppl 3):C22–4.

27. Hanquet G, Kissling E, Fenoll A, George R, Lepoutre A, Lernout T, et al. Pneumococcal serotypes in children in 4 European countries. Emerg Infect Dis. 2010;16:1428–39.

28. Elberse KE, van der Heide HG, Witteveen S, van de Pol I, Schot CS, van der Ende A, et al. Changes in the composition of the pneumococcal population and in IPD incidence in The Netherlands after the implementation of the 7-valent pneumococcal conjugate vaccine. Vaccine. 2012;30:7644–51.

29. Esposito S, Principi N. Direct and indirect effects of the 13-valent pneumococcal conjugate vaccine administered to infants and young children. Future Microbiol. 2015;10:1599–607.

30. Waight PA, Andrews NJ, Ladhani SN, Sheppard CL, Slack MP, Miller E. Effect of the 13-valent pneumococcal conjugate vaccine on invasive pneumococcal disease in England and Wales 4 years after its introduction: an observational cohort study. Lancet Infect Dis. 2015;15:535–43.

31. Regev-Yochay G, Katzir M, Strahilevitz J, Rahav G, Finn T, Miron D, et al. The herd effects of infant PCV7/PCV13 sequential implementation on adult invasive pneumococcal disease, six years post implementation; a nationwide study in Israel. Vaccine. 2017;35:2449–56.

32. Oxman MN. Herpes zoster pathogenesis and cell-mediated immunity and immunosenescence. J Am Osteopath Assoc. 2009;109:S13–7.

33. Schmader K. Herpes zoster in older adults. Clin Infect Dis. 2001;32:1481–6.

34. Pinchinat S, Cebrian-Cuenca AM, Bricout H, Johnson RW. Similar herpes zoster incidence across Europe: results from a systematic literature review. BMC Infect Dis. 13:2013, 170.

35. Mallick-Searle T, Snodgrass B, Brant JM. Postherpetic neuralgia: epidemiology, pathophysiology, and pain management pharmacology. J Multidiscip Healthc. 2016;9:447–54.

36. Schmader K, Gnann JW Jr, Watson CP. The epidemiological, clinical, and pathological rationale for the herpes zoster vaccine. J Infect Dis. 2008; 197(Suppl 2):S207–15. S207-S215

37. Scott FT, Johnson RW, Leedham-Green M, Davies E, Edmunds WJ, Breuer J. The burden of herpes zoster: a prospective population based study. Vaccine. 2006;24:1308–14.

38. Levin MJ, Oxman MN, Zhang JH, Johnson GR, Stanley H, Hayward AR, et al. Varicella-zoster virus-specific immune responses in elderly recipients of a herpes zoster vaccine. J Infect Dis. 2008;197:825–35.

39. Oxman MN, Levin MJ, Johnson GR, Schmader KE, Straus SE, Gelb LD, et al. A vaccine to prevent herpes zoster and postherpetic neuralgia in older adults. N Engl J Med. 2005;352:2271–84.

40. Schmader KE, Oxman MN, Levin MJ, Johnson G, Zhang JH, Betts R, et al. Persistence of the efficacy of zoster vaccine in the shingles prevention study and the short-term persistence substudy. Clin Infect Dis. 2012;55:1320–8.

41. Morrison VA, Johnson GR, Schmader KE, Levin MJ, Zhang JH, Looney DJ, et al. Long-term persistence of zoster vaccine efficacy. Clin Infect Dis. 2015;60: 900–9.

42. Levin MJ, Schmader KE, Pang L, Williams-Diaz A, Zerbe G, Canniff J, et al. Cellular and Humoral responses to a second dose of herpes zoster vaccine administered 10 years after the first dose among older adults. J Infect Dis. 2016;213:14–22.

43. Bayas JM, Vilella A, Bertran MJ, Vidal J, Batalla J, Asenjo MA, et al. Immunogenicity and reactogenicity of the adult tetanus-diphtheria vaccine. How many doses are necessary? Epidemiol Infect. 2001;127:451–60.

44. Steger MM, Maczek C, Berger P, Grubeck-Loebenstein B, et al. Lancet. 1996; 348:762.

45. Van Damme P, Burgess M. Immunogenicity of a combined diphtheria-tetanus-acellular pertussis vaccine in adults. Vaccine. 2004;22:305–8.

46. Kaml M, Weiskirchner I, Keller M, Luft T, Hoster E, Hasford J, et al. Booster vaccination in the elderly: their success depends on the vaccine type applied earlier in life as well as on pre-vaccination antibody titers. Vaccine. 2006;24:6808–11.

47. Launay O, Toneatti C, Bernede C, Njamkepo E, Petitprez K, Leblond A, et al. Antibodies to tetanus, diphtheria and pertussis among healthy adults vaccinated according to the French vaccination recommendations. Hum Vaccin. 2009;5:341–6.

48. Weinberger B, Schirmer M, Matteucci GR, Siebert U, Fuchs D, Grubeck-Loebenstein B. Recall responses to tetanus and diphtheria vaccination are frequently insufficient in elderly persons. PLoS One. 2013;8:e82967.

49. Grasse M, Meryk A, Schirmer M, Grubeck-Loebenstein B, Weinberger B. Booster vaccination against tetanus and diphtheria: insufficient protection against diphtheria in young and elderly adults. Immun Ageing. 2016;13:26.

50. Weinberger B. Adult vaccination against tetanus and diphtheria: the European perspective. Clin Exp Immunol. 2017;187:93–9.

51. Weinberger B, Keller M, Fischer KH, Stiasny K, Neuner C, Heinz FX, et al. Decreased antibody titers and booster responses in tick-borne encephalitis vaccinees aged 50-90 years. Vaccine. 2010;28:3511–5.

52. Stiasny K, Aberle JH, Keller M, Grubeck-Loebenstein B, Heinz FX. Age affects quantity but not quality of antibody responses after vaccination with an inactivated flavivirus vaccine against tick-borne encephalitis. PLoS One. 2012;7:e34145.

53. Rendi-Wagner P, Tobias J, Moerman L, Goren S, Bassal R, Green M, et al. The seroepidemiology of Bordetella pertussis in Israel–estimate of incidence of infection. Vaccine. 2010;28:3285–90.

54. Ridda I, Yin JK, King C, Raina MC, McIntyre P. The importance of pertussis in older adults: a growing case for reviewing vaccination strategy in the elderly. Vaccine. 2012;30:6745–52.

55. Gil A, Oyaguez I, Carrasco P, Gonzalez A. Hospital admissions for pertussis in Spain, 1995-1998. Vaccine. 2001;19:4791–4.

56. Halperin SA, Scheifele D, de Serres G, Noya F, Meekison W, Zickler P, et al. Immune responses in adults to revaccination with a tetanus toxoid, reduced diphtheria toxoid, and acellular pertussis vaccine 10 years after a previous dose. Vaccine. 2012;30:974–82.

57. Taylor DN, Pollard RA, Blake PA. Typhoid in the United States and the risk to the international traveler. J Infect Dis. 1983;148:599–602.

58. Hennessy S, Liu Z, Tsai TF, Strom BL, Wan CM, Liu HL, et al. Effectiveness of live-attenuated Japanese encephalitis vaccine (SA14-14-2): a case-control study. Lancet. 1996;347:1583–6.

59. Haynes L. The effect of aging on cognate function and development of immune memory. Curr Opin Immunol. 2005;17:476–9.

60. Haynes L, Eaton SM, Burns EM, Randall TD, Swain SL. CD4 T cell memory derived from young naive cells functions well into old age, but memory generated from aged naive cells functions poorly. Proc Natl Acad Sci U S A. 2003;100:15053–8.

61. Stoffel M, Lievens M, Dieussaert I, Martin I, Andre F. Immunogenicity of Twinrix in older adults: a critical analysis. Expert Rev Vaccines. 2003;2:9–14.

62. Wolters B, Junge U, Dziuba S, Roggendorf M. Immunogenicity of combined hepatitis a and B vaccine in elderly persons. Vaccine. 2003;21:3623–8.

63. Fisman DN, Agrawal D, Leder K. The effect of age on immunologic response to recombinant hepatitis B vaccine: a meta-analysis. Clin Infect Dis. 2002;35:1368–75.

64. Rafferty E, Duclos P, Yactayo S, Schuster M. Risk of yellow fever vaccine-associated viscerotropic disease among the elderly: a systematic review. Vaccine. 2013;31:5798–805.

65. Wiersma LC, Rimmelzwaan GF, de Vries RD. Developing universal influenza vaccines: hitting the nail, not just on the head. Vaccines (Basel). 2015;3:239–62.

66. Feldman C, Anderson R. Review: current and new generation pneumococcal vaccines. J Inf Secur. 2014;69:309–25.

67. Harpaz R, Ortega-Sanchez IR, Seward JF. Prevention of herpes zoster: recommendations of the advisory committee on immunization practices (ACIP). MMWR Recomm Rep. 2008;57:1–30.

68. Hales CM, Harpaz R, Ortega-Sanchez I, Bialek SR. Update on recommendations for use of herpes zoster vaccine. MMWR Morb Mortal Wkly Rep. 2014;63:729–31.

69. Leroux-Roels I, Leroux-Roels G, Clement F, Vandepapeliere P, Vassilev V, Ledent E, et al. A phase 1/2 clinical trial evaluating safety and immunogenicity of a varicella zoster glycoprotein e subunit vaccine candidate in young and older adults. J Infect Dis. 2012;206:1280–90.

70. Chlibek R, Bayas JM, Collins H, de la Pinta ML, Ledent E, Mols JF, et al. Safety and immunogenicity of an AS01-adjuvanted varicella-zoster virus subunit candidate vaccine against herpes zoster in adults >=50 years of age. J Infect Dis. 2013;208:1953–61.

71. Stadtmauer EA, Sullivan KM, Marty FM, Dadwal SS, Papanicolaou GA, Shea TC, et al. A phase 1/2 study of an adjuvanted varicella-zoster virus subunit vaccine in autologous hematopoietic cell transplant recipients. Blood. 2014;124:2921–9.

72. Berkowitz EM, Moyle G, Stellbrink HJ, Schurmann D, Kegg S, Stoll M, et al. Safety and immunogenicity of an adjuvanted herpes zoster subunit candidate vaccine in HIV-infected adults: a phase 1/2a randomized, placebo-controlled study. J Infect Dis. 2015;211:1279–87.

73. Lal H, Cunningham AL, Godeaux O, Chlibek R, Diez-Domingo J, Hwang SJ, et al. Efficacy of an adjuvanted herpes zoster subunit vaccine in older adults. N Engl J Med. 2015;372:2087–96.

74. Cunningham AL, Lal H, Kovac M, Chlibek R, Hwang SJ, Diez-Domingo J, et al. Efficacy of the herpes zoster subunit vaccine in adults 70 years of age or older. N Engl J Med. 2016;375:1019–32.

75. Fleming DM, Taylor RJ, Lustig RL, Schuck-Paim C, Haguinet F, Webb DJ, et al. Modelling estimates of the burden of respiratory Syncytial virus infection in adults and the elderly in the United Kingdom. BMC Infect Dis. 2015;15:443.

76. Shinefield H, Black S, Fattom A, Horwith G, Rasgon S, Ordonez J, et al. Use of a Staphylococcus Aureus conjugate vaccine in patients receiving hemodialysis. N Engl J Med. 2002;346:491–6.

77. Fowler VG, Allen KB, Moreira ED, Moustafa M, Isgro F, Boucher HW, et al. Effect of an investigational vaccine for preventing Staphylococcus Aureus infections after cardiothoracic surgery: a randomized trial. JAMA. 2013;309:1368–78.

78. Swanson KA, Schmitt HJ, Jansen KU, Anderson AS. Adult vaccination. Hum Vaccin Immunother. 2015;11:150–5.

79. Cross AS, Chen WH, Levine MM. A case for immunization against nosocomial infections. J Leukoc Biol. 2008;83:483–8.

80. Michel JP, Chidiac C, Grubeck-Loebenstein B, Johnson RW, Lambert PH, Maggi S, et al. Advocating vaccination of adults aged 60 years and older in Western Europe: statement by the joint vaccine working Group of the European Union Geriatric Medicine Society and the International Association of Gerontology and Geriatrics-European Region. Rejuvenation Res. 2009;12:127–35.

81. Michel JP, Lang PO, Baeyens JP. Flu vaccination policy in old adults: need for harmonization of national public health recommendations throughout Europe. Vaccine. 2009;27:182–3.

82. Esposito S, Bonanni P, Maggi S, Tan L, Ansaldi F, Lopalco PL, et al. Recommended immunization schedules for adults: clinical practice guidelines by the Escmid vaccine study group (EVASG), European geriatric medicine society (EUGMS) and the world Association for Infectious Diseases and Immunological Disorders (WAidid). Hum Vaccin Immunother. 2016;12:1777–94.

83. European Centre for Disease Prevention and Control. Seasonal influenza vaccination in Europe. Vaccination recommendations and coverage rates in the EU member states for eight influenza seasons: 2007-2008 to 2014-2015. 2017. https://ecdc.europa.eu/sites/portal/files/documents/influenza-vaccination-2007%E2%80%932008-to-2014%E2%80%932015.pdf. Accessed 27 July 2017.

84. Kanitz EE, Wu LA, Giambi C, Strikas RA, Levy-Bruhl D, Stefanoff P, et al. Variation in adult vaccination policies across Europe: an overview from VENICE network on vaccine recommendations, funding and coverage. Vaccine. 2012;30:5222–8.

23

Immune response to influenza vaccination in the elderly is altered by chronic medication use

Divyansh Agarwal[1], Kenneth E. Schmader[2], Andrew V. Kossenkov[3], Susan Doyle[2], Raj Kurupati[3] and Hildegund C. J. Ertl[3*] (iD)

Abstract

Background: The elderly patient population is the most susceptible to influenza virus infection and its associated complications. Polypharmacy is common in the aged, who often have multiple co-morbidities. Previous studies have demonstrated that commonly used prescription drugs can have extensive impact on immune defenses and responses to vaccination. In this study, we examined how the dynamics of immune responses to the two influenza A virus strains of the trivalent inactivated influenza vaccine (TIV) can be affected by patient's history of using the prescription drugs Metformin, NSAIDs or Statins.

Results: We provide evidence for differential antibody (Ab) production, B-cell phenotypic changes, alteration in immune cell proportions and transcriptome-wide perturbation in individuals with a history of long-term medication use, compared with non-users. We noted a diminished response to TIV in the elderly on Metformin, whereas those on NSAIDs or Statins had higher baseline responses but reduced relative increases in virus-neutralizing Abs (VNAs) or Abs detected by an enzyme-linked immunosorbent assay (ELISA) following vaccination.

Conclusion: Collectively, our findings suggest novel pathways that might underlie how long-term medication use impacts immune response to influenza vaccination in the elderly. They provide a strong rationale for targeting the medication-immunity interaction in the aged population to improve vaccination responses.

Keywords: Influenza vaccine, Metformin, NSAIDs, Statin, Immune response

Background

The trivalent inactivated influenza vaccine (TIV) protects against severe influenza by inducing the production of virus neutralizing Abs. According to recent estimates by the Center for Disease Control & Prevention (CDC), between October 1, 2017 and February 3, 2018, clinical laboratories tested more than 600,000 specimens for influenza virus, approximately 125,000 of which tested positive [1]. Among individuals who tested positive, the majority had influenza A, subtypes H3N2 and H1N1. More than a third of these cases were patients ≥65 years old, who experienced more severe illness than other age groups. Not only did they account for more than half of

the influenza-associated hospitalizations, their mortality rates were also highest.

Recent studies have demonstrated that in people over 65 years of age, the vaccine efficacy against influenza A viruses is less than 20% [2, 3]. Vaccine effectiveness in the elderly is variable, secondary to a variety of reasons such as ethnic background, inflammatory responses at baseline, timing of vaccination, gender and prior vaccination history [2–5]. Furthermore, primary B-cell responses in the elderly are commonly low and short-lived, resulting in Abs with low affinity [6]. A decrease in germinal center formation and decline of the B and T lymphocyte attenuator (BTLA) expression on B cells during immunosenescence also contribute to lack of sustained Ab responses in the aged [7]. Imperfectly matching antibodies due to antigenic sin may further result in poor responses to the influenza vaccine and

* Correspondence: ertl@wistar.org
[3]The Wistar Institute, Philadelphia, PA 19104, USA
Full list of author information is available at the end of the article

suboptimal pathogen control in the aged population. The 'original antigenic sin' concept refers to the impact of the first encounter with antigens of an influenza virus on lifelong immunity [8]. When a virus strain undergoes antigenic drift, some epitopes remain conserved, and pre-existing antibodies to such epitopes cross-react to the drifted strain. This in turn suppresses antigen levels through epitope masking and Fc-mediated mechanisms. Consequently, pre-existing influenza virus-specific antibody responses are boosted while the diversity of the overall response is diminished. This becomes increasingly pronounced in the aged who are typically exposed multiple times to different influence A virus variants. Additionally, it has been shown that the defects in B-cell responses in the elderly are related to a decline of helper functions from CD4$^+$ T-cells [9], and reduced expression of costimulatory receptors, such as CD28 and CD40L, which are essential for B-cell activation and germinal center formation [10].

Although our understanding of the complex biological processes that regulate vaccine responses in the elderly has evolved over the past decade, it is yet unclear how long-term medication use in individuals with chronic diseases affects immune responses to vaccination. While some vaccine–drug interactions, such as influenza–warfarin, have been reported, it is likely that many others remain unrecognized. A non-specific mechanism underlying the interaction between the influenza vaccine and medicines such as warfarin, phenytoin and theophylline is suggested to be due to the vaccine's ability to inactivate the hepatic cytochrome P-450 system, thereby reducing drug clearance [11]. More recently, studies have found that virus neutralizing Ab (VNA) titers to influenza A (H1N1 and H3N2), and B strains were lower in subjects receiving chronic Statin therapy, compared with those not receiving this drug and that vaccine effectiveness against the H1N1 strain was reduced [12, 13] . Relatedly, it has been shown that a Type 2 Diabetes (T2D) medication, Metformin, increases the proportion of circulating switched memory B-cells, decreases the fraction of exhausted memory B-cells, and reduces B-cell-intrinsic inflammation [14]. Consequently, higher VNA titers in response to influenza vaccination have been associated with Metformin use in patients [14]. These observations have underscored the importance of examining the effects of chronic drug use on vaccine responses in order to both better understand how the drugs alter immunity in the aged, as well as design supplementary therapeutic approaches for the elderly who are vulnerable to influenza virus infections, and comprise the largest customer segment for medications prescribed for chronic conditions.

We sought to examine this question in a 5-year study of TIV responses in the healthy, community-dwelling elderly (≥65 years of age) by (i) collecting prior drug-use data on each patient, (ii) testing each individual's Ab responses to the two influenza A viruses of the vaccine, H1N1 and H3N2, (iii) measuring proportions and phenotypes of different B-cell subsets, and (iv) performing genome-wide gene expression analysis of whole-blood. These immunological and clinical parameters were recorded at baseline (pre-vaccination) and on days 7 and 14 or 28 after vaccination, which allowed us to examine longitudinal trends. The overall aim of our study was to analyze how chronic drug use of commonly prescribed medicines in the elderly might affect responses to the influenza vaccine. We wanted to correlate post-vaccination changes in the immune system with the patient's prior history of drug use. These associations would allow us to assess the impact of polypharmacy on how the aging human body responds to the influenza vaccine. By providing a more complete picture of how the medication–immunity interaction changes vaccination responses, this study may help guide the development of alternative strategies to promote long-lasting immunity and better protect the at-risk, aging population.

Results

Patient characteristics

Between 2011 and 2016, we recorded 164 vaccinations in 80 individuals. Of these, data for thirteen patients was filtered out upon initial quality control because either they had missing values for Ab measurements or several B-cell phenotypic parameters, or we were unable to obtain reliable micro-array data on their transcriptome. Thus, for subsequent analyses, we examined data from patients for whom complete datasets were available, which included 131 vaccinations in 67 individuals with a mean age of 76.3 years (Table 1: Summary of Patient Characteristics). Some individuals were enrolled repeatedly during the 5-year study period. Each vaccination was considered as independent and identically distributed (iid) data, an assumption necessary to conduct statistical inference on the dataset. We defined the "elderly" population as individuals ≥65 years of age. The maximum age in our cohort was 89 years. The majority of the human subjects in our study were White/Caucasians (91.6%), followed by African-Americans (5.3%) and others (3.1%). We recorded prior clinical history of drug use for each patient, and converted this information to a binary variable: 1, if the patient had one year or greater of medication use and was using the drug at the time of assessment, and 0 otherwise. We divided the patient cohort into two categories for each of the three drugs — Metformin, Non-Steroidal Anti-inflammatory Drugs (NSAIDs) and Statins. Fifty-two percent of our observations corresponded to chronic NSAIDs users. In contrast, only 32% and 8% of the enrolled elderly used Statin and Metformin, respectively. Females comprised

Table 1 Summary of Patient Characteristics

Mean Age		76.3 years
	# Visits	%
Total	131	
Female	86	65.6
Male	45	34.4
Vaccinated in AM	85	64.9
Vaccinated in PM	46	35.1
Race		
Caucasian	120	91.6
Black	7	5.3
Others	4	3.1
Metformin-Users	11	8.4
Female	8	72.7
Male	3	27.3
NSAIDS-Users	68	51.9
Female	47	69.1
Male	21	30.9
Statin-Users	42	32.1
Female	22	52.4
Male	20	47.6

most of the subjects in our study, 65.6%. Sixty-five percent of the vaccinations were also performed before noon and the others were done in the afternoon.

VNA titer and Ig ab levels provide evidence for drug–immunity interaction

We determined the VNA titers and quantified immunoglobulin (Ig) isotypes to H1N1 and H3N2 at baseline (Day 0, visit 1), and at one (visit 2) and two or four weeks (visit 3) after vaccination. Based on a comparison of absolute values, we found that at all three time points, Metformin users had significantly lower VNA titer to H1N1 compared with non-users. This difference became more pronounced after vaccination, when by visit 3 Metformin users were found to have significantly lower titers (840 international units [IU] versus 2065 IU in non-users (Fig. 1a), p-value < 0.05). When the visit 1 and 2 titer levels were normalized by baseline levels, the poor responses in Metformin users became more apparent – at visit 2, they witnessed a 3-fold increase in H1N1 VNA titers, compared with a 20-fold increase in non-users (p-value =0.002), and at visit 3, the latter cohort experienced a 37-fold increase in titers compared with a mere 5-fold increase in the Metformin users (p = 0.003). Similarly, we found that Metformin users tend to have lower H3N2 VNA titers at all time points of the study. At baseline, the users had a mean titer of 625 IU compared with 4749 IU in non-users (p-value $=2 \times 10^{-4}$). This

significant difference was maintained with samples collected at visits 2 and 3 (Fig. 1d).

NSAIDs users had higher VNA titers to H1N1 and H3N2 at baseline, although increases in titers were comparable between users and non-users. (Fig. 1b, e). At subsequent visits 2 and 3, NSAIDs users had higher absolute titers compared with non-users. Individuals on Statin therapy also tended to have higher baseline VNA titers compared with non-users although this difference did not reach the threshold for statistical significance. Interestingly, the degree of fold-change in titers was similar between the Statin users and non-users (Fig. 1c, f).

In addition to VNA titer differences, we observed that individuals on long-term Metformin therapy had significantly lower IgA, IgG and IgM responses to the H1N1 strain after vaccination. Compared with non-users, they exhibited a diminished IgM Ab response up to visit 3 (Fig. 2a). Similarly, we observed diminished IgA and IgM Ab production against the H3N2 strain in Metformin users at visit 2. After an additional week, the IgA Ab levels in Metformin users were significantly lower compared with non-users (Fig. 2b; p-value < 0.05). No significant differences in Ig-Ab responses were noticeable in the NSAIDs cohort (data not shown). Individuals with a history of long-term Statin use displayed reduced IgG and IgM levels against both strains of the influenza vaccine. They had significantly lower IgG levels to the H3N2 strain, and considerably lower IgM and IgG levels against the H1N1 strain at visits 2 and 3 (see Additional file 1: Figure S1).

B-cell phenotypic markers provide insight into the effects of chronic medication use on vaccine response

Encouraged by our preliminary results of differential responses to the influenza vaccine conditional on the medication use history among the elderly, we sought to examine the underlying mechanisms, which might explain those differences. Using flow cytometry, we defined five subsets of B-cells, viz., transitional, mature naïve, non-switched memory, switched memory and Ab secreting cells (ASCs), and then tested for the expression of B-cell phenotypic or metabolic markers. B and T lymphocyte attenuator (BTLA), Programmed cell death protein (PD) 1, Programmed death-ligand (PD-L) 1 and 2, mitochondrial reactive oxygen species (ROS), B-cell lymphoma (Bcl)-6, Octamer transcription factor (Oct)-2 and Sirtuin (Sirt) 1 showed differences in mean florescence intensity (MFI) levels in drug users. These markers were chosen based on their role in regulating different physiological aspects of B-cell differentiation and metabolism. BTLA and PD1 are immunoinhibitors, which interact with the herpes virus entry mediator or PD-L1/L2 respectively [15, 16]. They also play a role in interactions between B-cells and follicular T-helper cells.

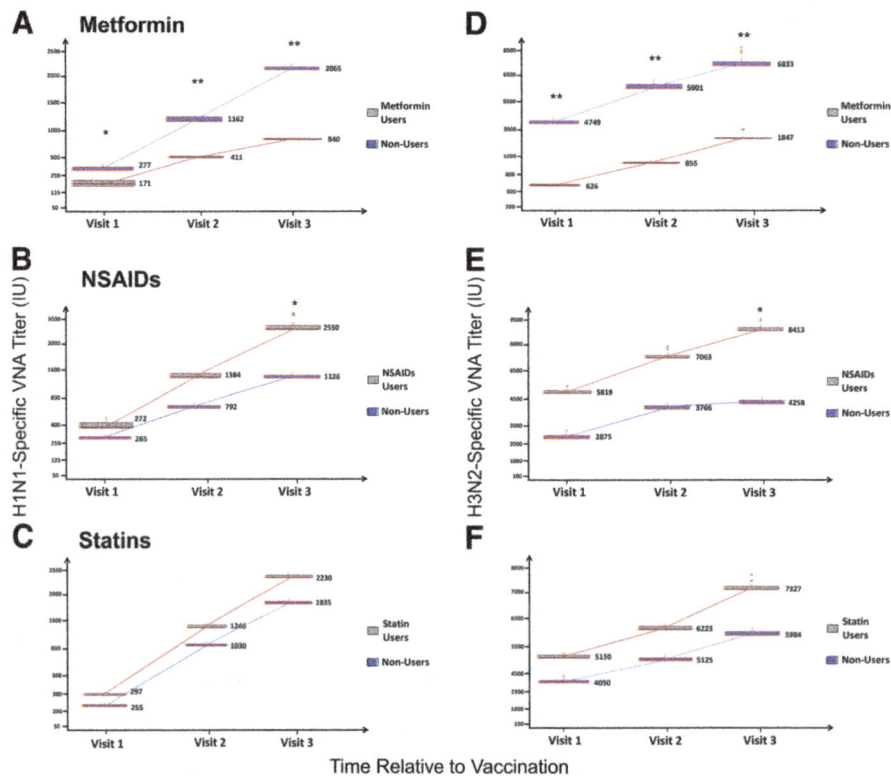

Fig. 1 Influenza virus-specific VNA titers: Virus neutralizing antibody (VNA) responses are summarized between drug-users and non-users for each of the three drug categories examined. The line within the box plots show medians (the values are written adjacent to the boxes), and the boxes show the interquartile range for the titer levels of H1N1- (a-c) and H3N2-specific (d-f) VNAs in sera. Top panels a, d show VNA titers for 11 samples from individuals on chronic Metformin use compared with 120 samples from non-users. Middle panels b, e show the titers for 68 and 63 samples, respectively, from individuals with or without a history of NSAIDs use and the bottom panels c, f show the titers for 42 samples from Statin users, compared with 89 samples from non-users. Pair-wise differences between the two cohorts in each of the six panels were performed using the non-parametric Mann-Whitney U Test. Stars above boxes indicate significant differences * p-value ≤0.05, ** p-value ≤0.005

Bcl-6 plays a pivotal role in germinal center maturation of B-cells [17], while the transcription factor Oct-2 sponsors differentiation of B-cells into Ab secreting plasma cells [18]. As B-cell differentiation is also driven by metabolic cues we tested for a number of markers indicative of pathways of energy production. An increase in ROS is observed in cells that enhance energy production through mitochondrial oxidative phosphorylation [19]. Sirt1, a nuclear energy sensor that becomes activated by NAD^+, increases fatty acid oxidation and gluconeogenesis [20]. Sirt1 reduces inflammatory reactions through inhibition of NF-κB, enhances insulin secretion and glucose tolerance and regulates circadian rhythm [20, 21]. Sirt1 also inhibits regulatory T (T_{reg}) cell formation, and enhances Th17 cell generation [22]. In B-cells, it promotes cytokine production [23]. Its activity also increases upon caloric restriction as well as in response to DNA damage that occurs during B-cell class switching reactions. Depending on the type of DNA damage, Sirt1 promotes cell survival and affects overall lifespan [24, 25].

We found numerous B-cell markers that were significantly altered in the cohort of individuals using either of

the mediations under study, when compared with their corresponding non-drug user cohorts using two-sample t-tests. Among the Metformin users, we found significantly elevated MFI levels of Oct-2 in transitional, mature naïve and non-switched memory B-cells (Fig. 3a). We also found elevated levels of Sirt1 in mature naïve B-cells, although non-switched memory B-cells and ASCs in Metformin users had decreased levels of Sirt1 compared to non-users (Fig. 3b). Additionally, we detected elevated levels of BTLA and PD1 in the mature naïve B-cells among the Metformin users (see Additional file 2: Figure S2).

Among the individuals who were long-term users of NSAIDs, the switched memory B-cell subset was found to have significantly higher MFI levels of mitochondrial reactive oxygen species (MROS) and diminished levels of Bcl-6 (see Additional file 3: Figure S3). Similarly, the mature naïve B-cells in the NSAIDs user group exhibited dramatically greater intensity of BTLA and PD1 (see Additional file 2: Figure S2); p-value < 0.005, for each pair-wise comparison). When examining the individuals on long-term Statin therapy, levels of PD-L1 were found

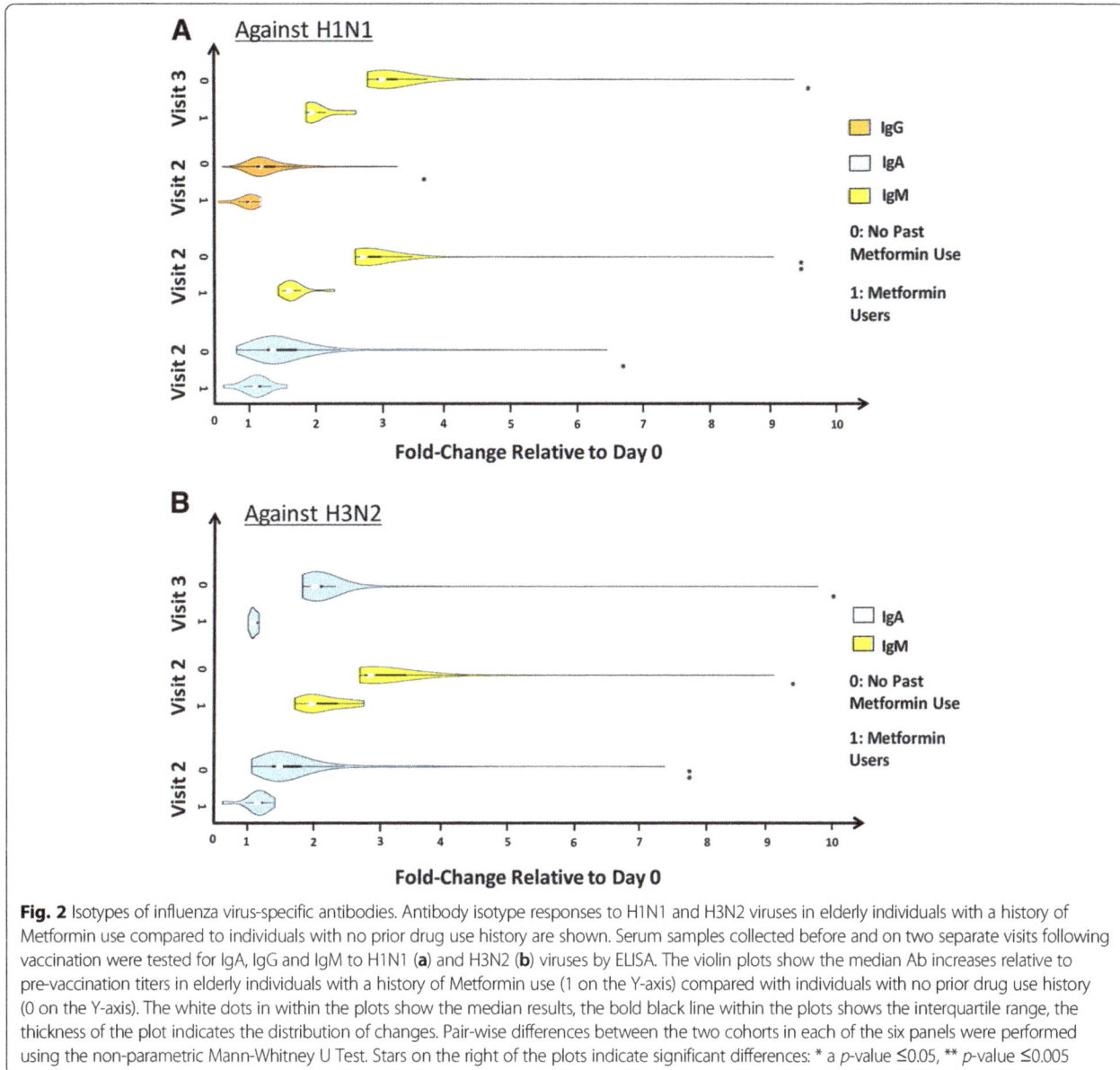

Fig. 2 Isotypes of influenza virus-specific antibodies. Antibody isotype responses to H1N1 and H3N2 viruses in elderly individuals with a history of Metformin use compared to individuals with no prior drug use history are shown. Serum samples collected before and on two separate visits following vaccination were tested for IgA, IgG and IgM to H1N1 (**a**) and H3N2 (**b**) viruses by ELISA. The violin plots show the median Ab increases relative to pre-vaccination titers in elderly individuals with a history of Metformin use (1 on the Y-axis) compared with individuals with no prior drug use history (0 on the Y-axis). The white dots in within the plots show the median results, the bold black line within the plots shows the interquartile range, the thickness of the plot indicates the distribution of changes. Pair-wise differences between the two cohorts in each of the six panels were performed using the non-parametric Mann-Whitney U Test. Stars on the right of the plots indicate significant differences: * a p-value ≤0.05, ** p-value ≤0.005

to be raised in transitional B-cells, mature naïve B-cells and ASCs (Fig. 3c). ASCs and switched memory B-cells in Statin users were also observed to have much lower MFI of Bcl-6 compared with non-users (Fig. 3d).

Whole-transcriptome analysis and pathway-level alterations
Whole blood gene expression profiles obtained at baseline and at visit 2 after vaccination showed differential expression of 51 genes (FDR < 10%) in individuals receiving Metformin compared to the non-users; the majority of these genes were downregulated in the Metformin-user group and coded for extracellular exosomal proteins, as well as enzymes involved in protein digestion, histamine biosynthesis and the LPS/IL-1-mediated inhibition of RXR function ((see Additional file 4: Figure S4); Table 2).

In the elderly taking NSAIDs, gene expression analysis showed significant differences for 42 probes (FDR < 10%) (Fig. 4). Notably, DAVID identified many of those genes as being involved in antiviral defense, mainly by inhibiting viral genome replication, and mediating innate immunity and the type-1 interferon signaling pathway (Table 1). For example, the gene RSAD2, which encodes Viperin, showed a 1.6-fold increase in NSAIDs users. Viperin disrupts the lipid rafts on cell plasma membranes and inhibits influenza viral budding and release [26]. Its upregulation in NSAIDs users, who were found to have more pronounced Ab production and better VNA titers against H1N1, suggests a possible mechanism by which NSAIDs could alter immune response to the influenza vaccine. Similarly, 39 genes were found to

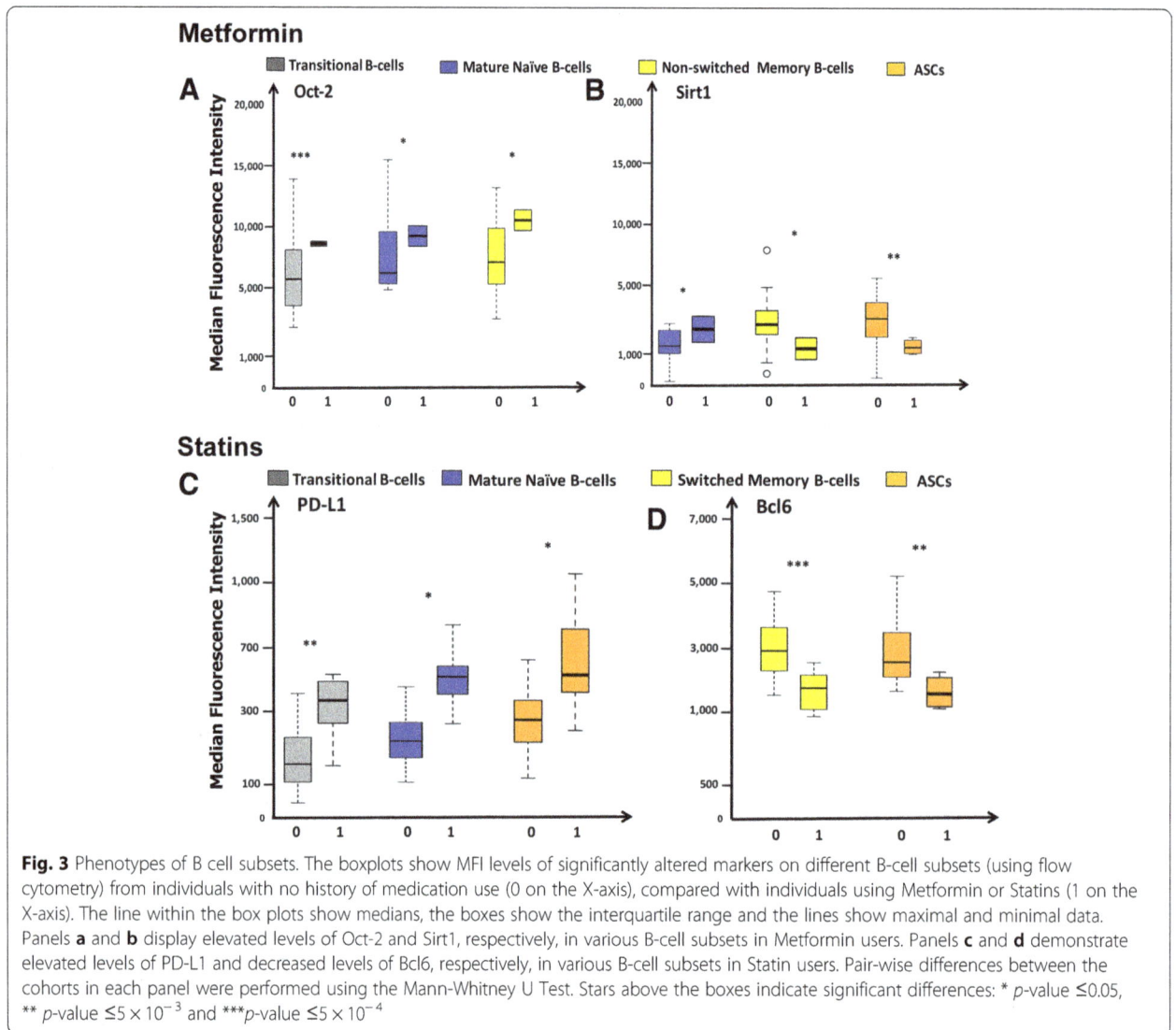

Fig. 3 Phenotypes of B cell subsets. The boxplots show MFI levels of significantly altered markers on different B-cell subsets (using flow cytometry) from individuals with no history of medication use (0 on the X-axis), compared with individuals using Metformin or Statins (1 on the X-axis). The line within the box plots show medians, the boxes show the interquartile range and the lines show maximal and minimal data. Panels **a** and **b** display elevated levels of Oct-2 and Sirt1, respectively, in various B-cell subsets in Metformin users. Panels **c** and **d** demonstrate elevated levels of PD-L1 and decreased levels of Bcl6, respectively, in various B-cell subsets in Statin users. Pair-wise differences between the cohorts in each panel were performed using the Mann-Whitney U Test. Stars above the boxes indicate significant differences: * p-value ≤ 0.05, ** p-value $\leq 5 \times 10^{-3}$ and *** p-value $\leq 5 \times 10^{-4}$

have statistically significant differential expression (FDR < 10%) in the cohort using Statins when compared with non-users (see Additional file 5: Figure S5). Several of these genes encode for proteins that are known to affect major immune-regulatory pathways, such as the OX40 signaling pathway, B cell development, and CD28 and iCOS-iCOSL Signaling in T Helper cells (Table 1).

Differences in the proportion of immune cells in the drug-using cohorts

We assessed cell distribution by deconvoluting the gene expression data using CIBERSORT [27]. The most remarkable changes were in the proportion of CD8+ T-cells in individuals using Metformin. At baseline, we found that individuals with a history of long-term Metformin use tend have a 25% higher proportion of CD8+ T-cells. One week after influenza vaccination, there appeared to be minimal changes in the proportion of CD8+ T-cells in

non-users, whereas metformin users had a 41% higher proportion (Fig. 5). Additionally, at visit 2, Metformin users were found to have a 60% lower proportion of resting mast cells. Moreover, when we examined the cell type proportions in individuals with a history of NSAIDs use versus those who were non-users, we found the former group to have a significantly lower quantity of γ-δ T-cells. At visit 2, although this difference was no longer statistically significant, the NSAID group was now found to have a 39% greater fraction of memory B-cells compared to the non-NSAIDs users. We also noted individuals with a history of long-term use of Statins tend to have significantly lower proportions T_{reg} cells, both at baseline and at visit 2 after vaccination. At visit 1, Statin users had on average 25% lower proportion of T_{reg} cells. Although at visit 2, both groups saw an absolute increase of 0.2% in the T_{reg} proportion, Statin users continued to have a 25% lower fraction of T_{reg} cells (Fig. 5).

Table 2 Signature Pathways Altered Between the Drug-User and Non-User Cohorts based on the significant DE genes. Pathway enrichments were assessed using the Laboratory of Immunopathogenesis and Bioinformatics resource, DAVID. Only Pathway associations with a *p*-value < 0.05 and an FDR < 10% were considered statistically noteworthy

Top Canonical Pathways associated with DE genes	FDR (%)	*p*-value
METFORMIN		
Extracellular Exosome	6.2	$2.5 \times 10-3$
LPS/IL-1 Mediated Inhibition of RXR Function	8.1	$1.1 \times 10-3$
Histamine Biosynthesis	8.1	$2.0 \times 10-3$
Protein Digestion	8.5	$2.8 \times 10-4$
NSAIDS		
Antiviral Defense	$2 \times 10-2$	$5.6 \times 10-7$
Cell Division and Chromosome Partitioning	$9.8 \times 10-2$	$6.6 \times 10-6$
type I interferon signaling pathway	0.16	$3.2 \times 10-6$
Inhibition of Viral Genome Replication	2.2	$3.5 \times 10-5$
Innate Immunity	5.7	$4.7 \times 10-4$
STATIN		
Antigen Presentation Pathway	$1 \times 10-3$	$1.5 \times 10-7$
Interferon-gamma-mediated signaling pathway	$1.9 \times 10-3$	$2.9 \times 10-8$
Regulation of interleukin-10 secretion	$5.1 \times 10-3$	$2 \times 10-9$
OX40 Signaling Pathway	$8.7 \times 10-3$	$5.2 \times 10-6$
Regulation of interleukin-4 production	$1 \times 10-2$	$7.8 \times 10-9$
B Cell Development	$1.5 \times 10-2$	$1.2 \times 10-5$
Cdc42 Signaling	$3.4 \times 10-2$	$5.7 \times 10-5$
Nur77 Signaling in T Lymphocytes	$3.4 \times 10-2$	$5.7 \times 10-5$
Th1 and Th2 Activation Pathway	$4.3 \times 10-2$	$8.7 \times 10-5$
Dendritic Cell Maturation	$4.6 \times 10-2$	$1 \times 10-4$
iCOS-iCOSL Signaling in T Helper Cells	0.17	$5.1 \times 10-4$
CD28 Signaling in T Helper Cells	0.19	$6.3 \times 10-4$
Phagosome Maturation	0.26	$8.7 \times 10-4$
PKCtheta Signaling in T Lymphocytes	0.3	$1.1 \times 10-3$
Role of NFAT in Regulation of the Immune Response	0.46	$1.7 \times 10-3$
Role of JAK family kinases in IL-6-type Cytokine Signaling	7.1	$3.1 \times 10-2$

Discussion

The current study systematically examined the effects of three commonly used medications on the immune system's response of the aged to influenza vaccination. We corroborated the differences observed in VNA titer or Ab levels with focused B-cell marker studies as well as global blood transcriptomic analyses. The drugs we analyzed included Metformin, NSAIDs and Statins. Metformin activates AMPK and inhibits mTOR and STAT3 activation [28]. It also activates IKKα/β, reduces ROS production and blunts the secretion of pro-inflammatory cytokines [29]. Metformin increases oxidative phosphorylation and fatty acid catabolism and thereby promotes memory formation of T cells instead of their differentiation into effector cells, which preferentially use glycolysis for energy and biomass production [30, 31]. B cells also switch to glycolysis upon activation and drugs that promote pathways of energy production other than glycolysis might reduce B cell proliferation [32]. Metformin similar to DNA breaks, which occur during immunoglobulin class switch reactions, inactivates the CREB Regulated Transcription Coactivator 2, which in turn promotes B cell differentiation [33]. It is currently unknown how Metformin affects different steps of plasma cell developments; the drug's effects on glycolysis may dampen while its role on transcriptional regulation may promote antibody responses.

NSAIDs function through inhibition of prostaglandin synthesis and cyclooxygenases 1 and 2 (Cox-1 and Cox-2), two components of the respiratory chain that catalyzes the reduction of oxygen to water [34]. Cox-2 is upregulated in activated human B lymphocytes and is

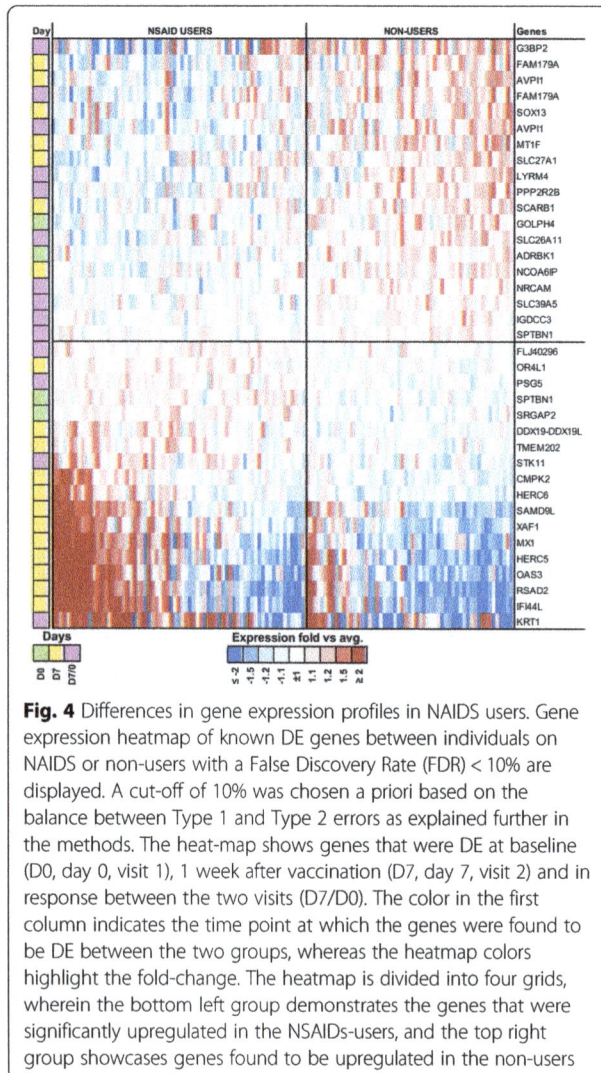

Fig. 4 Differences in gene expression profiles in NAIDS users. Gene expression heatmap of known DE genes between individuals on NAIDS or non-users with a False Discovery Rate (FDR) < 10% are displayed. A cut-off of 10% was chosen a priori based on the balance between Type 1 and Type 2 errors as explained further in the methods. The heat-map shows genes that were DE at baseline (D0, day 0, visit 1), 1 week after vaccination (D7, day 7, visit 2) and in response between the two visits (D7/D0). The color in the first column indicates the time point at which the genes were found to be DE between the two groups, whereas the heatmap colors highlight the fold-change. The heatmap is divided into four grids, wherein the bottom left group demonstrates the genes that were significantly upregulated in the NSAIDs-users, and the top right group showcases genes found to be upregulated in the non-users

required for optimal Ab synthesis. It has been found that NSAIDs blunt antibody production in stimulated human peripheral blood mononuclear cells (PBMCs) [35] by reducing the expression of Blimp-1 a transcription factor that is crucial for plasma cell differentiation [36]. It also suppresses T-cell activation by inhibiting p38 MAPK induction.

Statins inhibit HMG-CoA reductase and thereby the mevalonate pathway, which leads to production of cholesterol and heme; the latter plays a role in B-cell differentiation and class switching [37]. Statins in part through reduction of intracellular cholesterol, which is an essential cell wall component needed to for dividing cells, reduces cell proliferation [38]. It inhibits cytokine induced increases in MHC class II expression [39] and thereby affects antigen-driven stimulation of $CD4^+$ T cells. Statins also impede the production of coenzyme Q10, an electron carrier in the electron transport chain, which shifts the balance from mitochondrial energy

production towards glycolysis. They have been shown to decrease CD40/CD40L expression, inhibit T-cell activation as well as diminish Ab production [40].

Previous studies have found correlations between drug use and dysregulation of the immune system. For instance, Metformin use has been shown to promote fatty acid metabolism and increase $CD8^+$ memory T-cell formation, thus supporting development of immunological memory [41]. In addition to having lower baseline VNA titers to the H1N1 and H3N2 influenza virus strains, we found that individuals on Metformin also had suppressed Ab responses following vaccination combined with lower expression of metabolic phenotypic markers, such as Sirt1 on Ab secreting and non-switched memory B-cells. Metformin may thus have inhibited formation of ASCs by reducing the metabolic switch to glycolysis, which is a hallmark of lymphocytes undergoing activation and which is essential to provide rapid energy and biomass for proliferating cells. Moreover, we find compelling evidence that both at baseline and a week after vaccination, Metformin users exhibited a significantly higher proportion $CD8^+$ T-cells. The majority of the genes involved in the LPS/IL-1—mediated inhibition of RXR function canonical pathway were also downregulated in Metformin users. RXR is a ligand-dependent nuclear receptor that affects transcriptional receptors, and LPS/IL-1 mediated inhibition of RXR function impairs metabolism, transport and biosynthesis of lipids and cholesterol [42], which are essential for membrane formation by proliferating cells. Thus, our results are consistent with previous associations between Metformin's effects on immunity through metabolic dysregulation. Still yet, these observations propose an overarching mechanism explaining how Metformin potentially inhibits RXR, alters the utilization of fatty acids by lymphocytes and weakens their ability to proliferate. It should be pointed out though that our results of reduced antibody responses to influenza vaccination in Metformin users are in contrast to a previous study, which showed that in individuals with T2D Metformin increases responses [14]. We assume that the contrasting results reflect that in this study patients were younger than our cohorts and Metformin users were compared to diabetic individuals, who had not yet initiated treatment.

Our results show that although absolute VNA titers were higher in individuals receiving NSAIDs, relative to their pre-vaccination baseline there was no statistically significant difference in vaccine responses between users and non-users. This observation is in line with previous studies [43, 44] which have suggested that influenza vaccination effectiveness is likely not reduced in patients taking NSAIDs. In our study, individuals on NSAIDs also had increased levels of BTLA on their naïve mature B-cells, which as we reported previously is linked to

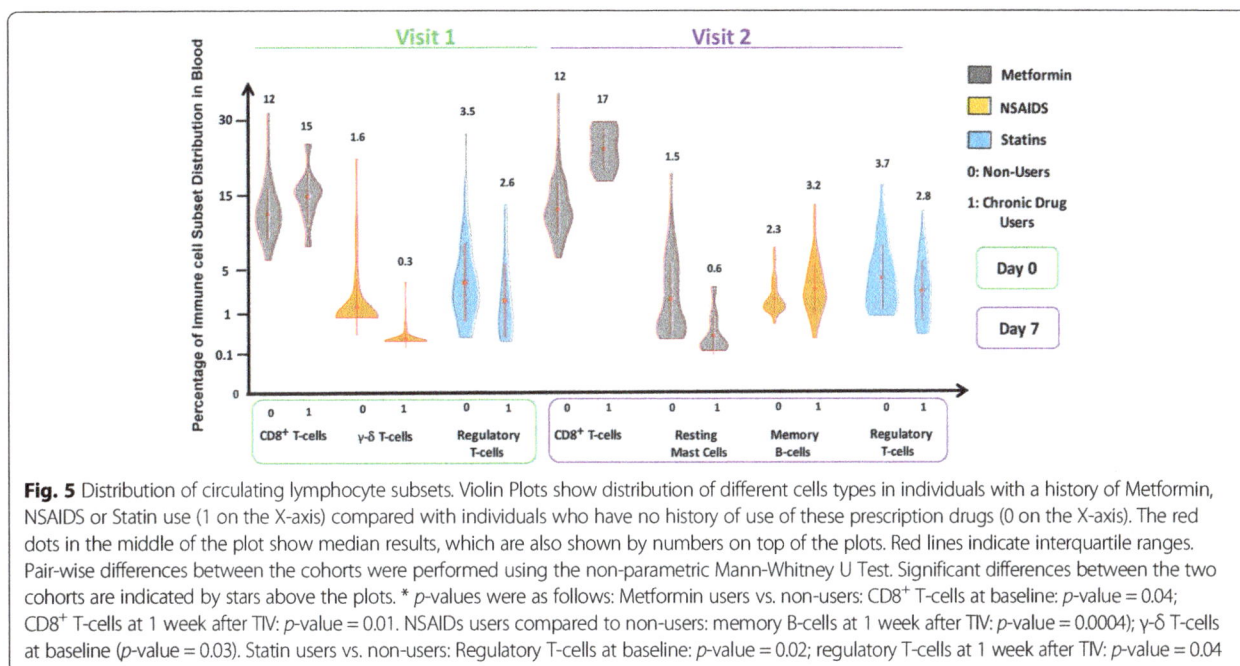

Fig. 5 Distribution of circulating lymphocyte subsets. Violin Plots show distribution of different cells types in individuals with a history of Metformin, NSAIDS or Statin use (1 on the X-axis) compared with individuals who have no history of use of these prescription drugs (0 on the X-axis). The red dots in the middle of the plot show median results, which are also shown by numbers on top of the plots. Red lines indicate interquartile ranges. Pair-wise differences between the cohorts were performed using the non-parametric Mann-Whitney U Test. Significant differences between the two cohorts are indicated by stars above the plots. * p-values were as follows: Metformin users vs. non-users: CD8+ T-cells at baseline: p-value = 0.04; CD8+ T-cells at 1 week after TIV: p-value = 0.01. NSAIDs users compared to non-users: memory B-cells at 1 week after TIV: p-value = 0.0004); γ-δ T-cells at baseline (p-value = 0.03). Statin users vs. non-users: Regulatory T-cells at baseline: p-value = 0.02; regulatory T-cells at 1 week after TIV: p-value = 0.04

higher and more sustained Ab responses to influenza vaccination [7]. One week after vaccination, NSAIDs users had elevated proportion of memory B-cells (Fig. 5). These findings corroborate previous reports and help provide the missing link between NSAIDs, memory B-cells and a possible mechanism by which NSAIDs might exert affect vaccine response in the aged. Recently, it has been found that activated γ-δ T-cells can regulate the organization of B-cells within follicles of lymphoid tissues; they are also crucial in the induction of vaccine-mediated immunity in various animal models [45, 46]. Interestingly, we noted that at baseline, NSAIDs users had a significantly lower proportion of γ-δ T-cells.

Long-term Statin therapy has been associated with a reduced response to the influenza vaccine in elderly individuals [12] and increases in medically attended acute respiratory diseases as well as influenza related office visits or hospitalizations in vaccinated individuals [13, 47]. It has been reported that this is due to its action on the transcription factor Foxp3, which in turn affects differentiation of CD4+ T-cells into T_{reg} cells and alters the migration of CD4+CD25+ T_{regs} [48]. In accordance with previous studies, we found that Statin users have enfeebled IgG and IgM responses against both H1N1 and H3N2 strains of the influenza virus. Although we observed modestly higher baseline VNA titers in Statin users compared with non-users, the rate of titer increase at visits 2 and 3 was comparable between the two cohorts. Higher absolute titers could likely be due to better induction of long-term ASCs in individuals with long-term Statin use. Using deconvolution on microarrays obtained from individuals before vaccination and

one week post-vaccination, we demonstrated that Statin users have significantly lower proportion of circulating T_{regs} at both time points. Furthermore, reduced responses were linked to reduced expression of Bcl-6 on both switched memory B-cells and ASCs. Bcl-6 is crucial for germinal cell formation and inhibits terminal differentiation of B-cells into plasma cells. On the other hand, PD-L1, which facilitates interactions between B-cells and follicular T helper cells, was increased on transitional and naïve B-cells as well as ASCs from a Statin user.

The fundamental limitation of a correlative analytic approach like ours is that establishment of perfect causal order is not always possible. Our findings are thus not meant to settle the issues of drug-vaccination interaction in the elderly, but rather contribute to a dialogue that has only recently commenced. These observations are all the more stimulating because the three drugs under investigation in this study are widely and commonly used by the aged, who are also the most vulnerable population to the complications of an influenza infection. Other limitations of our study include its modest sample size, which might explain why many of the Ab and VNA titer differences observed between Statin/NSAIDs users and non-users did not reach statistical significance. Due to the limited number of human subjects enrolled in the study, we also did not consider drug-drug interaction because less than 10% of the individuals were on multiple drugs, and such a sample size would drastically limit the power to detect any meaningful differences as well as limit our confidence in the biological validity of the results. Additionally, most of the individuals in the study were Caucasian women because of geographical and patient recruitment reasons. Sex and race differences in immunity have been well-documented, and in general, women have been shown to develop higher Ab responses than males [3], although we failed to confirm this trend in our studies. Other potential limitations are that additional factors, which could potentially influence immune responses, such as overall fitness, levels of daily physical activity, underlying chronic diseases, use of other prescription drugs, diet and weight, and others, were not taken into account. Thus, caution must be taken when interpreting our results across individuals from different ethnic/racial backgrounds, and we encourage future research to look at the epistasis between a patients' history of medication use and other factors such as sex and gender. Since we followed 67 individuals over 5 years and used their data to evaluate four conditions. i.e., Metformin use, NSAIDs use, Statin use and no medication use, our conclusions are affected by both Type 1 and Type 2 errors. Nonetheless, our study addresses a fundamental gap in knowledge regarding a clinically relevant topic of how chronic drug use affects vaccine response in the aged, and opens the door for future studies to replicate our preliminary findings in larger, diverse cohorts.

Conclusions

We show that compared with non-users, Metformin users exhibit significantly lower increases in VNA titers and Abs tested for by an ELISA after influenza vaccination, while individuals using NSAIDs and Statins developed absolute higher responses but as their baseline titers tended to be higher, their overall increases in influenza virus-specific Abs following vaccination were also attenuated. We correlated these observations with differences in B cell phenotypes, whole transcriptome analyses and inferred immune cell distribution based on deconvolution. Subsequent pathway analysis reveals mechanistic routes underlying the medication-immunity interaction in response to vaccination. We conclude that chronic medication use in the aged population significantly impacts immune responses to vaccination, and greater emphasis must be placed on medication history while considering alternate protective strategies for the elderly to reduce influenza-associated mortality. Overall, our results are important in two ways: first, they offer an important step in the ongoing effort to explain the differential responses to the influenza vaccine in the exposed elderly population. Second, they provide a partial road map to vaccine researchers and immunologists who can begin the transition from documenting the effects of long term medication use on immunosenescence to explaining how medication use can be exploited or countered to ensure that the elderly are adequately protected by the influenza vaccine. In summary, we generate novel data to explain how chronic medication use in the elderly affects their immune system, and in turn alter their responsiveness to vaccination.

Methods
Human subjects and study design
Blood was collected in the Duke Clinical Research Unit (DCRU) after informed consent from community dwelling persons in the Durham-Raleigh-Chapel Hill area of North Carolina (USA). Eighty healthy individuals, $\geq$ 65 years of age, who did not meet the criteria for age-related frailty, were included in the study. Subjects with acute febrile infections or underlying diseases or therapies that affect the immune system were not enrolled. Subjects with contraindication to the influenza vaccination, such as anaphylactic hypersensitivity to eggs or to other components of the vaccine, or acute illness with or without fever, or a history of Guillain-Barré Syndrome within 6 weeks following a previous dose of influenza vaccine were not enrolled. Demographic data and medical history including medical diagnoses, medications, past vaccination, and history of influenza or influenza-like diseases during the last 5 years were recorded. Subjects were bled and vaccinated with TIV. Subjects were bled again on days 7 and 14 or 28, following the injection of TIV.

Virus strains
The egg-adapted influenza A vaccine strains, H1N1 and H3N2, present in the vaccines during our study were obtained from the Center for Disease Control and Prevention (CDC), Atlanta, Georgia. The same H1N1 strain i.e., A/California/7/2009, was used throughout the entire period. The H3N2 stain was changed throughout the study period: 2011/12: A/Perth/16/2009, 2–12/2013/2014: A/Victoria/361/2011; 2014/15: A/Texas/50/2012; 2015/16: A/Switzerland/9715293/2013. Viruses were expanded in 10-day-old, pathogen-free embryonated eggs. Cleared allantoic fluids were purified by fractionation over 10–55% sucrose density gradients at 25,000 rpm for 2 h. Mean tissue culture infective doses ($TCID_{50}$) were determined by titration on Madin-Darby Canine Kidney (MDCK) cells after 3 days of infection by screening for cytopathic effects (CPE).

Blood and serum samples
Blood was collected from the enrolled individuals. The blood samples for the gene expression analyses were collected in PaxGene tubes to immediately stabilize RNA for analysis as described previously [49]. Samples were shipped overnight from the point of collection in the DCRU to The Wistar Institute in Philadelphia, PA (USA). Sera were isolated and frozen at – 20 °C until further use. Sera were heat-inactivated by a 30-min incubation at 56 °C prior to testing.

Micro-neutralization assay

Two-fold serially diluted (1:20 to 1:10240) heat-inactivated human sera were tested for neutralizing Abs to influenza A virus strains by micro-neutralization assays [50]. Briefly, equal volume of 100 $TCID_{50}$ per well of the titrated virus was added to the diluted serum in 96-well plates and incubated at 37 °C. After 1 h, serum-virus mixtures were added to MDCK cells that had been washed twice with serum-free Dulbecco's Modified Eagles Medium (DMEM). The cells were incubated for two hours at 37 °C with 5% CO_2. The cells were washed and re-incubated with DMEM supplemented with L – 1-Tosylamide-2-phenyl-ethyl chloromethyl ketone (TPCK) trypsin for 3 days. CPEs were scored under a microscope. Neutralization titers were defined as the dilution of the serum that resulted in 50% inhibition of CPE formation.

Enzyme-linked immunosorbent assay (ELISA)

H1N1- and H3N2-specific binding Ab isotypes were measured by ELISA. Briefly, wells of Nunc Maxisorp™ plate were coated with 10 µg/ml of influenza H1N1 or H3N2 virus along with isotype standards for IgA1, IgG and IgM (Athens Research & Technology, Inc., Georgia, USA) in bicarbonate buffer overnight at 4 °C. The plates were blocked with 3% BSA in phosphate-buffered saline (PBS) and incubated for 2 h. at room temperature with heat-inactivated sera of subjects at a dilution of 1/250. The plates were washed 4X with PBS containing 0.05% PBS-tween (PBST) and incubated for 1 h. at room temperature with alkaline phosphatase conjugated mouse anti-human IgA1 at 1:1000, IgG at 1:3000 and IgM at 1:1000 dilutions (Southern Biotech, Alabama, USA). Following the incubation, plates were washed 4X with PBST and developed using alkaline phosphatase substrate containing pNPP tablets (Sigma Aldrich, Missouri, USA) dissolved in DEA buffer. Adsorbance values were recorded at 405 nm and plotted against standard curves from each plate for every isotype. Ab concentrations were determined, and expressed in µg/ml.

B cell detection by flow cytometry

Peripheral blood mononuclear cells (PBMCs) were isolated as previously described [7]. Each subject's PBMC sample was initially treated with Human TruStain FcX Fc Receptor Blocking solution (BioLegend, San Diego, CA) for 30 min, washed with PBS at 1500 rpm for 5 min and then stained with fluorochrome-conjugated Abs. Multi-parametric flow cytometry was performed on the PBMCs using a panel to detect B cell subsets by identifying mature naïve B cells ($CD19^+CD20^+IgD^+CD27^-CD38^-$), transitional B cells ($CD19^+CD20^+IgD^+CD27^{+/-}CD38^{+/-}$), non-switched memory B cells ($CD19^+CD20^+IgD^+CD27^+CD38^-$), switched memory B cells ($CD19^+CD20^{+/-}IgD^-CD27^+CD38^-$), double-negative B cells ($CD19^+CD20^+IgD^-CD27^-CD38^-$) and ASCs ($CD19^+CD20^-IgD^-CD27^{++}CD38^{++}$). PBMCs were stained with Ab conjugates for the following surface markers: CD3-Pacific Blue (UCHT1, Biolegend, San Diego, CA), CD14-Pacific Blue (M5E2, Biolegend), CD19-BV650 (HIB19, Biolegend), CD20-BV570 (2H7, Biolegend), CD27-BV785 (O323, Biolegend), CD38-BV711 (HIT2, Biolegend), IgD-PerCP/Cy5.5 (IA6–2, Biolegend), BTLA-PE (MIH26, Biolegend), PD1-PE/Cy7 (EH12.2H7, Biolegend), and Live/Dead Fixable Aqua Dead Cell Stain (Life Technologies, Carlsbad, CA) for 30 min at 4 °C.

Cells were washed twice with cell staining buffer (Biolegend), and fixed using Cytofix/Cytoperm (BD Biosciences). Intracellular antigens were detected by staining for IgG-BV605 (G18–145, BD Biosciences, San Jose, CA) and IgM-APC/Cy7 (MHM-88, Biolegend) for 30 min at 4 °C. The stained samples were analyzed in a LSRII flow cytometer (BD Biosciences, San Jose, CA) using FlowJo (Tree Star, Ashland, OR).

Microarray data analysis and statistical inference

PAXgene tubes were stored at – 80 °C until RNA extraction. RNA was extracted using the PAXgene Blood RNA Kit IVD for isolation and purification of intracellular RNA according to the manufacturer's directions. RNA integrity (RIN) was assessed using a bioanalyzer and only samples with a RIN score of > 7.5 were processed for arrays. A constant amount (400 ng) of total RNA was amplified, as recommended by Illumina, and hybridized to the Illumina H12-v4 human whole genome bead arrays. All arrays were processed in the Wistar Institute Genomics Facility. Illumina GenomeStudio software was used to export expression levels and detection p-values for each probe of each sample. From individual hybridizations, data normalization and transformation to make meaningful comparisons of expression levels and select genes for further analysis and data mining was done as previously described [51]. Signal intensity data was quantile normalized and log2 transformed. Expression level comparisons between two groups were done using two-sample t-test and the Benjamini-Hochberg (BH) correction for multiple testing was performed [52]. A False Discovery Rate (FDR) < 10% was used as a significance threshold. We decided the cut-off of 10% a priori based on a balance of tolerance for Type 1 vs. Type 2 errors. An FDR of 0.1 ensures that majority of the genes detected as differentially expressed likely represent true biological differences, yet it provides us with an optimum tolerance of false positives to maximize the discovery of real biological signals.

Additionally, we used the gene-expression data to estimate the abundances of different immune cell types in the mixed blood cell population. The deconvolution was performed using CIBERSORT, a support vector regression based model [27]. We then compared the differences in cell type composition in the samples collected from individuals who were on a given medication versus those who were not, using the Mann-Whitney U Test. Gene set enrichment analysis for biological functions and canonical pathways was also performed using the Database for Annotation, Visualization and Integrated Discovery (DAVID) *v*6.8 [53]. All statistical analyses were conduction using the statistical language *R v*3.4.3. Results with BH corrected *p*-values < 0.05 were considered significant unless noted otherwise.

Additional files

Additional file 1: Figure S1. Serum samples collected on two separate visits following vaccination were tested for IgA, IgG and IgM to H1N1 and H3N2 viruses by ELISA. The violin plots as described in legend to Fig. 2 show the median Ab levels between the two groups. Pair-wise differences between the two cohorts in each of the six panels were performed using the Mann-Whitney U Test, * *p*-values ≤0.05 and ** *p*-values ≤

Additional file 2: Figure S2. The boxplots show MFI levels of significantly altered markers, PD1 and BTLA, on different B-cell subsets from individuals with no history of medication use, compared with individuals using Metformin, NSAIDs or Statins as described in legend to Fig. 3. The B-cell subsets were identified using flow cytometry. Pair-wise differences between the cohorts in each panel were performed using the Mann-Whitney U Test. Significant differences are indicted by stars: * *p*-values ≤0.05, ** *p*-values ≤5 × 10^{-3}, *p*-value ≤5 × 10^{-4}

Additional file 3: Figure S3. The boxplots show MFI levels of significantly altered markers, Bcl-6, MROS and PD-L2, on different B-cell subsets from individuals with no history of medication use, compared with individuals using NSAIDs. as described in legend to Fig. 3. Pair-wise differences between the cohorts in each panel were performed using the Mann-Whitney U Test, Significant differences are indicted by stars: * *p*-value ≤0.05, ** *p*-value ≤5 × 10^{-3}, *** *p*-value ≤5 × 10^{-4}

Additional file 4: Figure S4. Differentially expressed (DE) genes in the chronic Metformin-user cohort compared with non-users. Gene expression heatmap of known DE genes between the two cohorts with a False Discovery Rate (FDR) of < 10% are displayed. The heat-map indicates genes that were DE at baseline (D0, day 0, visit 1), 1 week after vaccination (D7, day 7, visit 2)

Additional file 5: Figure S5. Differentially expressed (DE) genes in the chronic Statin-user cohort compared with non-users. Gene expression heatmap of known DE genes between the two cohorts with a False Discovery Rate (FDR) of < 10% are displayed. The heat-map indicates genes that were DE at baseline (D0, day 0, visit 1), 1 week after vaccination (D7, day 7, visit 2) and in

Abbreviations

Ab: Antibody; ASCs: Ab secreting cells; Bcl6: B-cell lymphoma 6; BH: Benjamini-Hochberg; BTLA: B and T lymphocyte attenuator; CD: Cluster of Differentiation; CDC: Centers for Disease Control and Prevention; Cox: Cyclooxygenase; CPE: Cytopathic effects; DAVID: Database for Annotation, Visualization and Integrated Discovery; DCRU: Duke Clinical Research Unit; DMEM: Dulbecco's Modified Eagles Medium; ELISA: Enzyme-linked immunosorbent assay; Ig: Immunoglobulin; MDCK: Madin-Darby Canine Kidney; MFI: Mean Florescence Intensity; MROS: Mitochondrial Reactive Oxygen Species; NSAIDs: Non-steroidal anti-inflammatory drugs; Oct2: Octamer transcription factor 2; PBMC: Peripheral blood mononuclear cell; PBS: Phosphate Buffered saline; PD1: Programmed cell death protein 1; PD-L: Programmed death-ligand; RIN: RNA integrity; ROS: Reactive Oxygen Species; Sirt1: Sirtuin 1; TCID: Tissue culture infective dose; TIV: Trivalent inactivated influenza vaccine; TPCK: Tosylamide-2-phenylethyl chloromethyl ketone; Treg: Regulatory T-cells; VNA: Virus-neutralizing Ab

Funding

This work was supported by the National Institutes of Health, National Institute of Allergy and Infectious Disease (NIAID) Contract [BAA 26620050030] to HCJE. KES also received support from the National Institute on Aging (NIA), Duke Pepper Older Americans Independence Center Grant P30AG028716.

Authors' contributions

HCJE, RK, and AK designed and organized the study. KES and SD oversaw the clinical study. DA and AK analyzed the data. DA wrote the first draft of the paper. All authors read and approved the final manuscript.

Competing interests

The authors declare that they have no competing interests.

Author details

[1]Genomics and Computational Biology, Perelman School of Medicine, University of Pennsylvania, Philadelphia, PA 19104, USA. [2]Division of Geriatrics, Duke University Medical Center; Geriatric Research, Education, and Clinical Center, Durham VA Medical Center, Durham, NC 27705, USA. [3]The Wistar Institute, Philadelphia, PA 19104, USA.

References

1. Budd AP. Update: Influenza Activity — United States, October 1, 2017–February 3, 2018. MMWR Morb Mortal Wkly Rep. 2018;67. Available from: https://www.cdc.gov/mmwr/volumes/67/wr/mm6706a1.htm. [cited 2018 Aug 1]
2. Nakaya HI, Hagan T, Duraisingham SS, Lee EK, Kwissa M, Rouphael N, et al. Systems analysis of immunity to influenza vaccination across multiple years and in diverse populations reveals shared molecular signatures. Immunity. 2015;43:1186–98.
3. Giefing-Kröll C, Berger P, Lepperdinger G, Grubeck-Loebenstein B. How sex and age affect immune responses, susceptibility to infections, and response to vaccination. Aging Cell. 2015;14:309–21.
4. Kannan S, Kossenkov A, Kurupati RK, Xiang JZ, Doyle SA, Schmader KE, et al. A shortened interval between vaccinations with the trivalent inactivated influenza vaccine increases responsiveness in the aged. Aging (Albany NY). 2015;7:1077–85.
5. Kurupati RK, Kossenkoff A, Kannan S, Haut LH, Doyle S, Yin X, et al. The effect of timing of influenza vaccination and sample collection on antibody titers and responses in the aged. Vaccine. 2017;35:3700–8.
6. Frasca D, Blomberg BB. Effects of aging on B cell function. Curr Opin Immunol. 2009;21:425–30.
7. Kannan S, Kurupati RK, Doyle SA, Freeman GJ, Schmader KE, Ertl HCJ, et al. BTLA expression declines on B cells of the aged and is associated with low responsiveness to the trivalent influenza vaccine. Oncotarget. 2015;6:19445–55.
8. Vatti A, Monsalve DM, Pacheco Y, Chang C, Anaya J-M, Gershwin ME. Original antigenic sin: a comprehensive review. J Autoimmun. 2017;83:12–21.
9. Herati RS, Reuter MA, Dolfi DV, Mansfield KD, Aung H, Badwan OZ, et al. Circulating CXCR5+PD-1+ response predicts influenza vaccine antibody responses in young adults but not elderly adults. J Immunol. 2014;193:3528–37.
10. Moro-García MA, Alonso-Arias R, Lopez-Larrea C. When Aging Reaches CD4 + T-Cells: Phenotypic and Functional Changes. Front Immunol. 2013;4. Available from: https://www.ncbi.nlm.nih.gov/pmc/articles/PMC3650461/. [cited 2018 Aug 1]
11. D'Arcy PF. Vaccine-drug interactions. Drug Intell Clin Pharm. 1984;18:697–700.
12. Black S, Nicolay U, Del Giudice G, Rappuoli R. Influence of statins on influenza vaccine response in elderly individuals. J Infect Dis. 2016;213:1224–8.
13. McLean HQ, Chow BDW, VanWormer JJ, King JP, Belongia EA. Effect of Statin use on influenza vaccine effectiveness. J Infect Dis. 2016;214:1150–8.

14. Diaz A, Romero M, Vazquez T, Lechner S, Blomberg BB, Frasca D. Metformin improves in vivo and in vitro B cell function in individuals with obesity and Type-2 diabetes. Vaccine. 2017;35:2694–700.

15. Lasaro MO, Tatsis N, Hensley SE, Whitbeck JC, Lin S-W, Rux JJ, et al. Targeting of antigen to the herpesvirus entry mediator augments primary adaptive immune responses. Nat Med. 2008;14:205–12.

16. Lages CS, Lewkowich I, Sproles A, Wills-Karp M, Chougnet C. Partial restoration of T-cell function in aged mice by in vitro blockade of the PD-1/PD-L1 pathway. Aging Cell. 2010;9:785–98.

17. Zhang T-T, Gonzalez DG, Cote CM, Kerfoot SM, Deng S, Cheng Y, et al. Germinal center B cell development has distinctly regulated stages completed by disengagement from T cell help. Elife. 2017;6. https://doi.org/10.7554/eLife.19552.

18. Emslie D, D'Costa K, Hasbold J, Metcalf D, Takatsu K, Hodgkin PO, et al. Oct2 enhances antibody-secreting cell differentiation through regulation of IL-5 receptor α chain expression on activated B cells. J Exp Med. 2008;205:409–21.

19. Zorov DB, Juhaszova M, Sollott SJ. Mitochondrial reactive oxygen species (ROS) and ROS-induced ROS release. Physiol Rev. 2014;94:909–50.

20. Rahman S, Islam R. Mammalian Sirt1: insights on its biological functions. Cell Communication and Signaling. 2011;9:11.

21. Yuan Y, Cruzat VF, Newsholme P, Cheng J, Chen Y, Lu Y. Regulation of SIRT1 in aging: roles in mitochondrial function and biogenesis. Mech Ageing Dev. 2016;155:10–21.

22. Lim HW, Kang SG, Ryu JK, Schilling B, Fei M, Lee IS, et al. SIRT1 deacetylates RORγt and enhances Th17 cell generation. J Exp Med. 2015;212:973.

23. Wang Q, Yan C, Xin M, Han L, Zhang Y, Sun M. Sirtuin 1 (Sirt1) overexpression in BaF3 cells contributes to cell proliferation promotion, apoptosis resistance and pro-inflammatory cytokine production. Med Sci Monit. 2017;23:1477–82.

24. Boily G, Seifert EL, Bevilacqua L, He XH, Sabourin G, Estey C, et al. SirT1 regulates energy metabolism and response to caloric restriction in mice. PLoS One. 2008;3:e1759.

25. Bordone L, Cohen D, Robinson A, Motta MC, van Veen E, Czopik A, et al. SIRT1 transgenic mice show phenotypes resembling calorie restriction. Aging Cell. 2007;6:759–67.

26. Wang X, Hinson ER, Cresswell P. The interferon-inducible protein Viperin inhibits influenza virus release by perturbing lipid rafts. Cell Host Microbe. 2007;2:96–105.

27. Newman AM, Liu CL, Green MR, Gentles AJ, Feng W, Xu Y, et al. Robust enumeration of cell subsets from tissue expression profiles. Nat Methods. 2015;12:453–7.

28. Sukumar M, Liu J, Ji Y, Subramanian M, Crompton JG, Yu Z, et al. Inhibiting glycolytic metabolism enhances CD8⁺ T cell memory and antitumor function. J Clin Invest. 2013;123:4479–88.

29. Rena G, Hardie DG, Pearson ER. The mechanisms of action of metformin. Diabetologia. 2017;60:1577–85.

30. Ravera S, Cossu V, Tappino B, Nicchia E, Dufour C, Cavani S, et al. Concentration-dependent metabolic effects of metformin in healthy and Fanconi anemia lymphoblast cells. J Cell Physiol. 2018;233:1736–51.

31. Prlic M, Immunology BMJ. A metabolic switch to memory. Nature. 2009;460:41–2.

32. Doughty CA, Bleiman BF, Wagner DJ, Dufort FJ, Mataraza JM, Roberts MF, et al. Antigen receptor–mediated changes in glucose metabolism in B lymphocytes: role of phosphatidylinositol 3-kinase signaling in the glycolytic control of growth. Blood. 2006;107:4458–65.

33. Sherman MH, Kuraishy AI, Deshpande C, Hong JS, Cacalano NA, Gatti RA, et al. AID-induced genotoxic stress promotes B cell differentiation in the germinal center via ATM and LKB1 signaling. Mol Cell. 2010;39:873–85.

34. Tsurufuji S, Sugio K, Sato H, Ohuchi K. A review of mechanism of action of steroid and non-steroid anti-inflammatory drugs. Inflammation: mechanisms and treatment. Dordrecht: Springer; 1980. p. 63–78. Available from: https://link.springer.com/chapter/10.1007/978-94-010-9423-8_7. [cited 2018 Aug 1]

35. Bancos S, Bernard MP, Topham DJ, Phipps RP. Ibuprofen and other widely used non-steroidal anti-inflammatory drugs inhibit antibody production in human cells. Cell Immunol. 2009;258:18–28.

36. Bernard MP, Phipps RP. Inhibition of cyclooxygenase-2 impairs the expression of essential plasma cell transcription factors and human B-lymphocyte differentiation. Immunology. 2010;129:87–96.

37. Mehrbod P, Omar AR, Hair-Bejo M, Haghani A, Ideris A. Mechanisms of Action and Efficacy of Statins against Influenza. BioMed Research International. 2014. Available from: https://www.hindawi.com/journals/bmri/2014/872370/. [cited 2018 Aug 1]

38. Warita K, Warita T, Beckwitt CH, Schurdak ME, Vazquez A, Wells A, et al. Statin-induced mevalonate pathway inhibition attenuates the growth of mesenchymal-like cancer cells that lack functional E-cadherin mediated cell cohesion. Sci Rep. 2014;4:7593.

39. Kwak B, Mulhaupt F, Myit S, Mach F. Statins as a newly recognized type of immunomodulator. Nat Med. 2000;6:1399–402.

40. Bu D, Griffin G, Lichtman AH. Mechanisms for the anti-inflammatory effects of statins. Curr Opin Lipidol. 2011;22:165.

41. Pearce EL, Walsh MC, Cejas PJ, Harms GM, Shen H, Wang L-S, et al. Enhancing CD8 T-cell memory by modulating fatty acid metabolism. Nature. 2009;460:103–7.

42. Klaassen CD, Aleksunes LM. Xenobiotic, Bile Acid, and Cholesterol transporters: function and regulation. Pharmacol Rev. 2010;62:1–96.

43. Jackson ML, Bellamy A, Wolff M, Hill H, Jackson LA. Low-dose aspirin use does not diminish the immune response to monovalent H1N1 influenza vaccine in older adults. Epidemiol Infect. 2016;144:768–71.

44. Epperly H, Vaughn FL, Mosholder AD, Maloney EM, Rubinson L. Nonsteroidal anti-inflammatory drug and aspirin use, and mortality among critically ill pandemic H1N1 influenza patients: an exploratory analysis. Jpn J Infect Dis. 2016;69:248–51.

45. Hogg AE, Worth A, Beverley P, Howard CJ, Villarreal-Ramos B. The antigen-specific memory CD8+ T-cell response induced by BCG in cattle resides in the CD8+γ/δTCR–CD45RO+ T-cell population. Vaccine. 2009;27:270–9.

46. Zaidi I, Diallo H, Conteh S, Robbins Y, Kolasny J, Orr-Gonzalez S, et al. γδ T cells are required for the induction of sterile immunity during irradiated Sporozoite vaccinations. J Immunol. 2017;199:3781–8.

47. Omer SB, Phadke VK, Bednarczyk RA, Chamberlain AT, Brosseau JL, Orenstein WA. Impact of statins on influenza vaccine effectiveness against medically attended acute respiratory illness. J Infect Dis. 2016;213:1216–23.

48. Mascitelli L, Goldstein MR. How regulatory T-cell induction by statins may impair influenza vaccine immunogenicity and effectiveness. J Infect Dis. 2016;213:1857.

49. Rainen L, Oelmueller U, Jurgensen S, Wyrich R, Ballas C, Schram J, et al. Stabilization of mRNA expression in whole blood samples. Clin Chem. 2002;48:1883–90.

50. Laurie KL, Engelhardt OG, Wood J, Heath A, Katz JM, Peiris M, et al. International laboratory comparison of influenza microneutralization assays for a(H1N1)pdm09, a(H3N2), and a(H5N1) influenza viruses by CONSISE. Clin Vaccine Immunol. 2015;22:957–64.

51. Quackenbush J. Microarray data normalization and transformation. Nat Genet. 2002;32:496–501.

52. Green GH, Diggle PJ. On the operational characteristics of the Benjamini and Hochberg false discovery rate procedure. Stat Appl Genet Mol Biol. 2007;6:Article27.

53. Huang DW, Sherman BT, Lempicki RA. Systematic and integrative analysis of large gene lists using DAVID bioinformatics resources. Nat Protoc. 2009;4:44–57.

Antibodies against 1940s era a/H1N1 influenza strains a/Weiss/43 and a/FM/1/47 and heterotypic responses after seasonal vaccination of an elderly Spanish population

Ivan Sanz[1,2]*, Silvia Rojo[1,2], Sonia Tamames[3], Jose María Eiros[1,4] and Raúl Ortiz de Lejarazu[1,2]

Abstract

Background and methods: Elderly people have experienced several influenza natural infections and seasonal vaccinations during their lives. The aim of this work was to evaluate in an elderly Spanish population the presence of antibodies (Abs) against some 1940s era A/H1N1 influenza viruses and some new influenza viruses. We also evaluated the homologous and heterotypic responses after seasonal influenza vaccination. We collected pre- and post-vaccination serum samples from 174 elderly people (≥65 years) who were vaccinated with seasonal influenza vaccines during the 2006–2007, 2008–2009, 2009–2010, and 2010–2011 northern hemisphere influenza campaigns. The presence of Abs against the 1940s era A/Weiss/43 and A/FM/1/47 strains of the A/H1N1 influenza virus was evaluated by using hemagglutination inhibition assays.

Results: Pre-vaccination Abs against the A/Weiss/43 and A/FM/1/47 strains were present at protective titres (≥1/40) in 43. 7% and 20.1% of the study population respectively. Seasonal influenza vaccination induced heterotypic seroconversion against A/Weiss/43 in 16.1% of the individuals and against A/FM/1/47 in 13.2% of the individuals. The seroprotection rate for the study population after seasonal vaccination was 63.2% against A/Weiss/43 and 31.0% against A/FM/1/47. The heterotypic response did not satisfy the European Medicament Agency criteria for people aged ≥60 years.

Conclusions: A moderate percentage of elderly people had Abs against the 1940s era A/Weiss/43 and A/FM/1/47 strains of the A/H1N1 influenza subtype. Seasonal influenza vaccination induced a low but significant heterotypic response against both 1940s era influenza strains, reaching a high seroprotection rate for the A/Weiss/43 strain. Seasonal influenza vaccination can increase, within certain limitations, the Abs titres against old influenza strains not included in the composition of the vaccine itself.

Background

Influenza A/H1N1 subtype viruses have been circulating intermittently for 82 of the 100 years since the 1918 Spanish Influenza pandemic [1]. This subtype has been extinguished two times during its existence. The first time was in 1957 at the emergence of the A/H2N2 pandemic subtype [2], after which it re-emerged in 1977 as the A/USSR/90/1977 strain [3]. The second time was in 2009 after the emergence of the A/H1N1pdm09 pandemic subtype [4]. The drift experienced by A/H1N1 subtypes since 1918 has caused slight antigenic and genetic differences among the viruses circulating between the first decades of the twentieth century and the first decade of the twenty-first century [5].

It is likely that people born before 2009 have been in contact with different strains of A/H1N1 during their life. Thus, while elderly people have had more experiences with A/H1N1 viruses and can still have protective antibodies (Abs) against the different strains, it is probable that younger people

---

* Correspondence: isanzm@saludcastillayleon.es
[1]Valladolid National Influenza Centre, Avenida Ramón y Cajal s/n, 47005 Valladolid, Spain
[2]Microbiology and Immunology Unit, Hospital Clínico Universitario de Valladolid, Avenida Ramón y Cajal s/n, 47005 Valladolid, Spain
Full list of author information is available at the end of the article

are not protected against the 1940s era influenza strains. The ability of the Abs present in elderly people to protect other age groups against possible re-emergence of older strains is uncertain. It is probable that within 30–40 years there will be no persons with Abs against the 1940s era influenza strains such as A/Weiss/43 or A/FM/1/47. Thus, the existing herd immunity will be gradually phased out. This may pose a risk of re-emergence of any of these viruses [2, 6].

Vaccination is still the best method to avoid influenza and to limit the severity of these infections [7]. Vulnerability and immune-senescence processes [8, 9] make elderly people one of the main targets for seasonal influenza vaccination [10]. Although the elderly population is not the age group with the highest prevalence of flu infection, they usually register the highest rates of mortality and of clinical complications [11]. Because of that, it is of special interest to identify the particular requirements of elderly people for increasing the efficacy of seasonal influenza vaccination in this age group.

One of the most relevant aspects of elderly susceptibility to influenza infection and associated morbidity is the high number of contacts with different influenza viruses that they have experienced by natural infections and vaccinations during their life. Elderly people have been in contact with very old influenza viruses, such as those circulating during the 1940 decade, or even others phylogenetically close to the 1918 Spanish Flu virus. It is probable that these people currently have Abs against the 1940s era influenza viruses. On the other hand, current seasonal vaccines could help to increase the titre of pre-existing Abs by means of heterotypic responses, as has been shown in other studies against other influenza viruses [12]. These heterotypic responses are based on antigenic and genetic homology between the different types and subtypes of influenza viruses [13, 14] and are extremely important for the design of universal influenza vaccines.

The ability of current seasonal influenza vaccines to increase Abs against influenza viruses that are not specifically targeted for the current expected strains is not well known. Recent history has taught us that the re-emergence of certain subtypes of influenza, especially A/H1N1, is not frequent, but it presents significant public health problems when it happens [3]. Thus, it is of high importance to know what the Ab levels are to older influenza strains and how

current vaccines can help maintain them at a high level. The aim of this study was to describe in a ≥ 65-year-old population the presence of pre-vaccination Abs against two different 1940s era A/H1N1 strains, A/Weiss/43 and A/FM/1/47, and also to assess the heterologous response against those strains after seasonal influenza vaccination.

Methods

Patient recruitment

Pre- and post-vaccination sera were analysed from 174 healthy individuals ≥65-years who were recruited in vaccination programs run by primary health care centres during the Influenza Vaccine Campaigns (IVCs) of 2006–2007 ($n_1 = 45$), 2008–2009 ($n_2 = 43$), 2009–2010 ($n_3 = 43$), and 2010–2011 ($n_4 = 43$). The sera were obtained by clinicians of the Influenza Sentinel Surveillance Network of Castile and Leon (Spain). The samples were stored at – 20 °C before sending to the Valladolid National Influenza Centre for analysis. Pre-vaccination sera were sampled immediately before influenza vaccination, and post-vaccination sera were obtained 28 days after seasonal vaccination. The administered trivalent influenza seasonal vaccines contained the A and B influenza strains recommended by the World Health Organization (WHO) for the northern hemisphere in each IVC. Thus, the A/H1N1 and A/H1N1pdm09 vaccine components were administered: in winter 2006–2007 the A/New Caledonia/20/99 strain, in winters 2008–2009 and 2009–2010 the A/Brisbane/59/2007 strain, and the A/California/07/2009 strain in winter 2010–2011 [15–18].

Informed consent was obtained, and the recruitment of the patients was done following Spanish Organic Law for Data Protection, patient's rights and obligations for clinical documents (BOE n°298 of 14th December of 1999, Law 41/2002). This research was performed according to the Declaration of Helsinki.

Influenza a/H1N1 viruses used for serological assays

The viruses that we selected for analysis (Table 1) included two of the most representative influenza A/H1N1 strains, A/Weiss/43 and A/FM/1/47 [19, 20], that circulated during the 1940 decade. It also included the strains A/New Caledonia/20/99 (A/H1N1 subtype), A/Brisbane/59/2007 (A/H1N1

Table 1 Influenza A/H1N1 and A/H1N1pdm09 strains included in the study

Viruses tested			
Subtype	Strain	Origin	Type of Ab evaluation
A/H1N1	A/Weiss/43	WHO Collaborating Centre Francis Crick Institute, London, UK	Heterotypic
A/H1N1	A/FM/1/47	WHO Collaborating Centre Francis Crick Institute, London, UK	Heterotypic
A/H1N1	A/New Caledonia/20/99	WHO Collaborating Centre Francis Crick Institute, London, UK	Homologous/Heterotypic
A/H1N1	A/Brisbane/59/2007	WHO Influenza Reagent Kit for Identification of Influenza Isolates	Homologous/Heterotypic
A/H1N1pdm09	A/California/07/2009	GSK, Brentford, UK	Homologous/Heterotypic

WHO World Health Organization

subtype), and A/California/07/2009 (A/H1N1pdm09 subtype). The presence of antibodies and the heterologous responses after seasonal vaccination were evaluated against both the 1940s era influenza A/H1N1 strains, i.e., A/Weiss/43 and A/FM/1/47. Also, the presence of antibodies and the homologous responses after vaccination were evaluated against the strains A/New Caledonia/20/99 in the IVC 2006–2007, A/Brisbane/59/2007 in the 2008–2009 and 2009–2010 IVCs, and A/California/07/2009 in the 2010–2011 IVC. The heterologous responses in those seasons in which the strains were not included in the seasonal vaccine were also evaluated.

Hemagglutination inhibition assay
The presence of anti-hemagglutination (HA) Abs was analysed in pre- and post-vaccination sera by the hemagglutination inhibition assay (HIA). Following the protocol published by WHO and the Influenza Surveillance Network for the surveillance of influenza viruses and vaccine efficacy [21, 22], nonspecific inhibitors of the HIA were remove by combining 100 μl of serum with 300 μl of receptor destroying enzyme (RDE, Denka Seiken, Japan). The RDE-serum combination was incubated at 37 °C in a water bath for 18 h and then inactivated at 56 °C for 1 h. Serial double dilutions of 50 μl of each serum sample were performed in 96-V-microwells plates. After that, 50 μl of a standard containing 4 haemagglutinin units was added to each well and the plates were incubated for 30 min at room temperature. Hens erythrocytes (0.75%, 50 μl) were added and incubated for another 30 min. The Ab titre was determined as the highest dilution that caused complete hemagglutination inhibition.

Phylogenetic analysis
We performed a phylogenetic analysis of the HA gene of old A/H1N1 strains, vaccine strains, and A/H1N1pdm09 subtype (A/Weiss/43-EPI_ISL_66107; A/FM/1/47-EPI_ISL_69263; A/New Caledonia/20/99-EPI_ISL_22227; A/Brisbane/59/2007-EPI_ISL_154502; A/California/07/2009-EPI_ISL_227813). In this analysis it was also included the A/South Carolina/1/18 strain of 1918 Spanish Influenza virus (EPI_ISL_1213), A/PR/8/34 strain (EPI_ISL_14962) and also the A/USSR/90/1977 strain (EPI_ISL_243351). Because HIAs identify only specific epitopes of the globular head domain of haemagglutinin proteins [23], the genetic analysis was only performed for the haemagglutinin 1 (HA1) subunit. HA1 DNA sequences were aligned using the ClustalW algorithm of Bioedit 7.2.3 software. The best model for the phylogenetic analysis was predicted using the Best-Fit tool of Mega 5.2 software (MegaSoftware, Tempe, AZ, USA). The general time reversible model, with gamma-distributed rates, produced the highest Bayesian information criterion score. Thus, we used this model for constructing a phylogenetic tree based on the

aligned DNA sequences of the HA1 gene subunit. The reproducibility of the phylogenetic tree was guaranteed by a bootstrap analysis of 1000 replications. We also constructed a distance matrix for the HA1 subunit, using the maximum composite likelihood algorithm. The results of this matrix were inversely transformed and expressed as a percentage of genetic homology (% of similarity/100).

Statistical analysis
The results were analysed using the classic serological European Medicament Agency (EMA) criteria for the evaluation of vaccine efficacy [24]. The criteria establish different parameters for analysing the vaccine efficacy in people ≥60 years. The criteria included a seroprotection rate (SPR) ≥60%, a seroconversion rate (SCR) ≥30%, and a geometric mean titre (GMT) increase ≥2.0. The GMT increase was calculated as the rate between post- and pre-vaccination serum GMT [25]. Negative results obtained in the HIA were assumed to be half of the detection value (1/10) for the calculation of the GMT. For this study, a titre ≥1/40 was considered to be protective [25]. Although some studies suggest that higher protective titres may be used for evaluating seroprotection in ≥65 years [26], the current consensus maintains that 1/40 is a protective titre; therefore we decided to comply with that criterion. Seroconversion was defined as a titre increase of at least four-fold between the pre- and post-vaccination sera. Additionally, seroconversion was considered to have occurred in negative pre-vaccination titres that reached ≥1/40 after vaccination. Different statistical parametric and non-parametric tests were used, such as the Bonferroni test and McNemar test, using SPSSV20 (IBM, Armonk, NY, USA). Statistical significance was taken at the $p < 0.05$ value.

Results
Population characteristics
The mean age of the study population was 75.9 years (95% confidence interval [CI95%]:74.9–77.0), and 57.5% were males ($n = 100$). The mean age of individuals recruited during the 2006–2007 IVC was 74.7 years (CI95%:72.9–77.0), 79.2 during the 2008–2009 IVC (CI95%:76.7–81.4), 74.8 in the 2009–2010 IVC (CI95%:72.7–76.8), and 75.3 in the 2010–2011 IVC (CI95%:72.8–77.7). The mean age was significantly higher in 2008–09 IVC than in the rest of IVCs (Bonferroni = 3.678; $p = 0.013$). The percentage of men in each IVC was 64.4% ($n_1 = 29$) in the 2006–2007 IVC, 46.5% ($n_2 = 20$) in the 2008–2009 IVC, 62.8% ($n_3 = 27$) in the 2009–2010 IVC, and 55.8% ($n_4 = 24$) in the 2010–2011 IVC.

Presence of pre-vaccination antibodies against 1940s era a/H1N1 viruses and against new a/H1N1 viruses
Within the entire study population of elderly subjects, pre-vaccination Abs against either or both of the 1940s era influenza strains, A/Weiss/43 and A/FM/1/47, were present

in 89.7% of the individuals. Among these, 58.6% had pre-vaccination Abs against both of the 1940s era influenza strains, 20.7% against only the A/Weiss/43 strain, and 10.3% against only the A/FM/1/47 strain. Among the subjects, 88.5% had pre-vaccination Abs against the A/H1N1 subtype strains A/Brisbane/59/2007 and A/New Caledonia/20/99, and 20.7% against the A/H1N1pdm09 subtype.

The percentages of individuals having protective pre-vaccination Abs during the full study period and in each IVC are described in Fig. 1. Of all the study population individuals who expressed Abs prior to seasonal vaccinations, 43.7% had protective Ab titres ($\geq 1/40$) against A/Weiss/43, 20.1% against A/FM/1/47, 39.1% against A/H1N1 A/New Caledonia/20/99 and the A/Brisbane/59/2007 vaccine strains, and 3.4% against the A/H1N1pdm09 subtype. Before vaccinations in each IVC, almost all subjects had protective Ab titres against all of the viral strains. The only exception was against the A/H1N1pdm09 subtype during the 2006–2007 IVC.

Abs response after seasonal vaccination

After seasonal vaccination, 97.1% of the entire study population had Abs against the A/Weiss/43 or A/FM/1/47 strains, though not all of the titres were sufficiently high to provide protection. Among the subjects, 74.1% had Abs against both 1940s era A/H1N1 strains, 17.2% against only the A/Weiss/43 strain, and 5.8% against only the A/FM/1/47 strain. Most individuals, 98.9%, had Abs against the A/H1N1 subtype strains A/New Caledonia/20/99 and A/Brisbane/59/2007 and 70.1% against the A/H1N1pdm09 subtype. After seasonal vaccination, 63.2% of the study population had protective levels of Abs against the A/Weiss/43 strain, 31.0% against the A/FM/1/47 strain, 73.0% against the A/H1N1 subtype

strains A/New Caledonia/20/99 and A/Brisbane/59/2007, and 35.6% against the A/H1N1pdm09 subtype.

The 2006–2007, 2008–2009, and 2009–2010 IVCs volunteers were vaccinated against A/New Caledonia/20/99 and A/Brisbane/59/2007 strains (A/H1N1 subtypes). These vaccinations induced a significant heterotypic seroconversion against the A/Weiss/43 strain (McNemar, $p < 0.05$) (Table 2). The 2010–2011 IVC volunteers was vaccinated against the A/California/07/2009 (A/H1N1pdm09 subtype), which induced a significant heterotypic seroconversion against the A/FM/1/47 strain (McNemar; $p < 0.05$). During the 2006–07, 2008–09, and 2009–10 IVCs, vaccination with the A/H1N1 strains also induced significant heterotypic seroconversion against A/H1N1pdm09 (McNemar; $p < 0.05$). Finally, vaccination with the A/H1N1pdm09 subtype during the 2010–2011 IVC also induced heterotypic seroconversion against the A/Brisbane/59/2007 strain of the A/H1N1 subtype (McNemar; $p < 0.05$).

These data show that seasonal vaccination induced a significant homologous seroconversion against A/H1N1 vaccine strains in all IVCs vaccinated against this subtype (McNemar; $p < 0.05$). Also, seasonal vaccination induced a significant homologous seroconversion against the A/H1N1pdm09 subtype in the 2010–11 IVC (McNemar; $p < 0.05$). The number of seroconversions and the SCR induced by influenza seasonal vaccination in the whole study period and in each IVC are summarized in Table 2.

Heterotypic and homologous responses to seasonal vaccination according to EMA requirements

Analysis of the seasonal influenza vaccination efficacy for the whole study period and each IVC was assessed by applying the classical EMA criteria for people ≥ 60 years. The pre- and

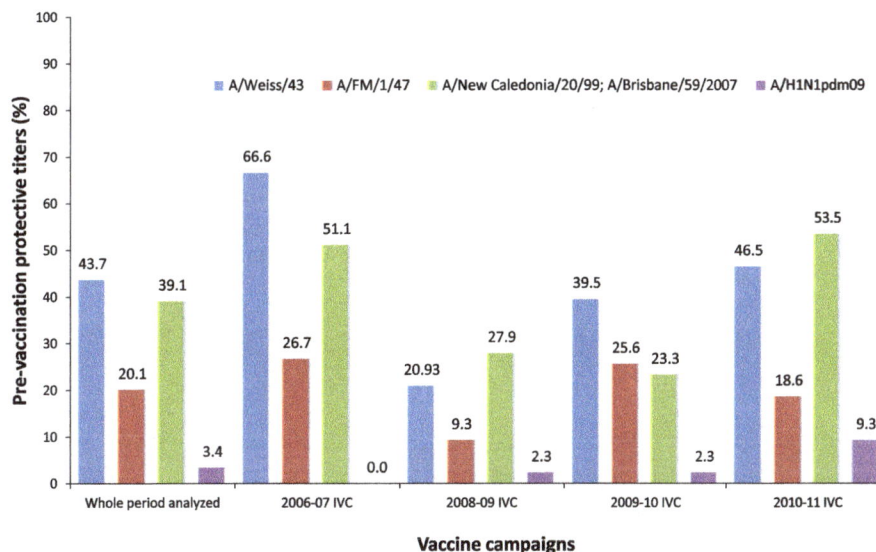

Fig. 1 Percentage of individuals showing pre-vaccination protective Abs against 1940s era A/H1N1 strains, A/H1N1 vaccine strains, and the A/H1N1pdm09 subtype during the whole study period and in each IVC (influenza vaccine campaign)

Table 2 Number of seroconversions and seroconversion rate against 1940s era A/H1N1 strains, A/H1N1 vaccine strains, and A/H1N1pdm09 subtype

Vaccinated cohorts (strain included in seasonal vaccine)	A/Weiss/43		A/FM/1/47		A/H1N1		A/H1N1pdm09	
	SCn[a]	SCR[b]	SCn	SCR	SCn	SCR	SCn	SCR
Whole period analysed (N = 174)	28	16.1	23	13.2	59	33.9	55	31.6
2006–2007 (A/New Caledonia/20/99) (n1 = 45)	11	24.4	5	11.1	19	42.2	6	13.3
2008–2009 (A/Brisbane/59/2007) (n2 = 43)	6	14.0	2	4.7	26	60.5	6	14
2009–2010 (A/Brisbane/59/2007) (n3 = 43)	7	16.4	3	7.0	7	16.3	9	20.9
2010–2011 (A/California/07/2009) (n4 = 43)	4	9.3	13	30.2	7	16.3	34	79.1

[a]Number of seroconversions
[b]Seroconversion rate

post-vaccination GMT, GMT increase, SPR, and SCR values are described in Table 3. Within the entire study population, the SPR was higher than 60% against the A/Weiss/43 strain (63.2%) and against the A/H1N1subtype strains A/New Caledonia/20/99 and A/Brisbane/59/2007 (73.0%). The SCR after seasonal vaccination was higher than 30% against the A/H1N1subtype strains A/New Caledonia/20/99 and A/Brisbane/59/2007 (33.9%) and against the A/H1N1pdm09 subtype (31.6%). The GMT increase was higher than 2.0 against all viruses except the A/FM/1/47 strain.

For each IVC, the SPR was higher than 60% against the A/Weiss/43 strain in 2006–2007 and 2009–2010 IVCs

Table 3 Pre- and post-vaccination GMT values, GMT increase, seroprotection, and seroconversion rates in each IVC against all analysed A/H1N1 and A/H1N1pdm09 viruses

Strain/Subtype	Input Vaccine strain	Whole period analyzed	Vaccinated cohorts			
			2006-2007 A/New Caledonia/20/99	2008-2009 A/Birsbane/59/2007	2009-2010 A/Birsbane/59/2007	2010-2011 A/California/07/2009
A/Weiss/43						
	Pre-vaccine GMT[a](CI95%)	18.3 (13.5-23.1)	38.4 (23.6-63.3)	8.2 (5.1-13.7)	18.7 (11.0-31.4)	19.0 (10.2-32.9)
	Post-vaccine GMT(CI95%)	44.2 (33.6-52.8)	83.8 (50.8-143.1)	24.5 (16.6-37.3)	45.8 (28.8-73.7)	39.4 (21.0-68.0)
	GMT increase	2.4	2.2	3.0	2.4	2.1
	SPR[b]	63.2	84.4	46.5	65.1	55.8
	SCR[c]	16.1	24.4	14.0	16.3	9.3
A/FM/1/47						
	Pre-vaccine GMT(CI95%)	7.8 (6.3-9.8)	7.8 (4.9-13.0)	3.4 (2.2-5.1)	12.5 (8.7-18.1)	11.3 (7.6-16.7)
	Post-vaccine GMT(CI95%)	13.6 (10.6-17.4)	20.5(13.7-31.0)	4.6 (2.9-7.1)	15.3 (10.4-22.6)	23.1 (13.6-37.0)
	GMT increase	1.7	2.6	1.4	1.2	2.0
	SPR	31.0	35.6	14	30.2	44.2
	SCR	13.2	11.1	4.7	7	30.2
A/New Caledonia/20/99						
A/Brisbane/59/2007						
	Pre-vaccine GMT(CI95%)	20.9 (16.6-25.1)	34.5 (27.6-51.2)	13.6 (8.3-21.1)	13.2 (8.6-19.8)	29.8 (21.7-39.8)
	Post-vaccine GMT(CI95%)	63.8 (53.1-77.6)	112.3(69.7-145.8)	103.5 (72.3-147.4)	27.8 (19.5-37.4)	50.1 (37.9-66.7)
	GMT increase	3.1	3.3	7.6	2.1	1.7
	SPR	73.0	82.2	83.7	58.1	67.4
	SCR	33.9	42.2	60.5	16.3	16.3
A/H1N1pdm09						
	Pre-vaccine GMT(CI95%)	1.8 (1.5-2.1)	1.5 (1.2-1.9)	1.6 (1.1-2.3)	1.9 (1.3-2.6)	2.4 (1.7-3.7)
	Post-vaccine GMT(CI95%)	12.7 (9.5-17.2)	5.4 (3.4-8.7)	7.5 (4.8-11.2)	7.2 (4.2-11.9)	93.0 (54.3-150.0)
	GMT increase	7.1	3.6	4.7	3.8	38.8
	SPR	35.6	13.3	20.9	23.3	86
	SCR	31.6	13.3	14	20.9	79.1

[a]Geometric mean titers; [b]Seroprotection rate; [c]Seroconversion rate

(84.4% and 65.1% respectively), but the SCR was lower than 30% in all IVCs. The GMT increase against the A/Weiss/43 strain was higher than 2.0 in all IVCs except 2010–2011. The SCR for the A/FM/1/47 strain after seasonal vaccination was higher than 30% only in the 2010–2011 IVC (30.2%), but the SPR was not ≥60% in any of the IVCs analysed. The GMT increase against A/FM/1/47 strain was higher than 2.0 in 2006–2007 IVC (2.6) and 2010–2011 IVC (2.0). The SPR was higher than 60% for the A/H1N1subtype strains A/New Caledonia/20/99 and A/Brisbane/59/2007 in all IVCs except for the volunteers of the 2009–2010 IVC (58.1%) that was vaccinated against the A/Brisbane/59/2007 strain. The SCR for the A/H1N1subtype strains A/New Caledonia/20/99 and A/Brisbane/59/2007 was higher than 30% in the 2006–2007 IVC (42.2%) with vaccination against A/New Caledonia/20/99 strain, and in the 2008–2009 IVC (60.5%) with vaccination against the A/Brisbane/59/2007 strain. The GMT increase was higher than 2.0 against both A/H1N1 strains in all IVCs analysed excepting 2010–2011. Both SPR and SCR were higher than 60% and 30% respectively for the A/H1N1pdm09 subtype only in the 2010–11 IVC (86.0% and 79.1% respectively). GMT increase was higher than 2.0 against A/H1N1pdm09 subtype in all IVCs analysed.

Phylogenetic analysis

The homology (% of similarity/100) between the different A/H1N1 and A/H1N1pdm09 strains analysed in this work is described in Table 4. The mean genetic homology between the HA1 subunit of the HA gene between all viruses was 0.833 (83.3%, CI95%: 0.795–0.867). The highest homology was between the A/New Caledonia/20/1999 and A/Brisbane/59/2007 strains (96.7%), and the lowest was between the A/Brisbane/59/2007 and A/California/07/2009 strains (64.2%). The phylogenetic tree constructed using the DNA sequences of the HA genes is shown in Fig. 2.

Discussion

The year 2018 marks 100 years since the Great Pandemic of 1918 caused by the Spanish Flu virus. This pandemic affected over 500 million people and caused the death of over 50 million, representing a mortality rate over 2.5% [1]. The large period of circulation of A/H1N1 subtypes since their emergence has caused a moderate intrasubtypic antigenic and genetic drift. The A/H1N1 viruses phylogenetically close to those circulating in 1918 are slightly different from the A/H1N1 viruses circulating during the first decades of this century [5]. This makes it likely that very young people will not be protected against the 1940s era viruses. Thus, all of the protection available for younger individuals against these strains of influenza resides in the antibodies present in older individuals.

Our data show that before vaccination, a high proportion of the elderly population had Abs that recognized the 1940s era A/H1N1 strains. Many of these Abs where found at protective titres. The detection of these Abs after a prolonged time lapse without any documented circulation of these strains is relevant. The results of our work demonstrate that serologic protection against influenza viruses can persists for many years. Consistent with other reports [27, 28], our data suggest that past infections could protect a large part of the population throughout their lives.

The origin of these Abs is uncertain. The mean age of the populations analysed was high, so it is possible that these Abs could have been induced by multiple exposures of the elderly study population with A/H1N1 viruses since their childhood, some of them even with Spanish influenza. On the other hand, because elderly people are a risk group with a specific recommendation for seasonal influenza vaccination [10], they are likely to have been vaccinated several times during their lives. These vaccinations could have induced previous heterotypic or cross-immune reactions against viruses not included in the vaccine composition, but that are phylogenetically related to the vaccine strains. Because we do not know the previous vaccination history of the elderly people in the study population, it is difficult to ascertain with certainty the origin of the observed Abs.

The phylogenetic analysis conducted in our work showed that the mean genetic homology between the HA1 subunits

Table 4 Similarity values expressed as a percentage of genetic homology (% of similarity/100) between A/H1N1 and A/H1N1pdm09 viruses

Influenza A/H1N1 strains	A/South Carolina/1/18	A/PR/8/34	A/Weiss/43	A/FM/1/1947	A/USSR/90/1977	A/New Caledonia /20/1999	A/Brisbane /59/2007	A/California /07/2009
A/South Carolina/1/18	1.000	–	–	–	–	–	–	–
A/PR/8/34	0.891	1.000	–	–	–	–	–	–
A/Weiss/43	0.873	0.929	1.000	–	–	–	–	–
A/FM/1/1947	0.864	0.912	0.934	1.000	–	–	–	–
A/USSR/90/1977	0.840	0.891	0.916	0.952	1.000	–	–	–
A/New Caledonia/20/1999	0.796	0.844	0.860	0.886	0.913	1.000	–	–
A/Brisbane/59/2007	0.780	0.824	0.841	0.864	0.888	0.967	1.000	–
A/California/07/2009	0.771	0.711	0.704	0.709	0.679	0.651	0.642	1.000

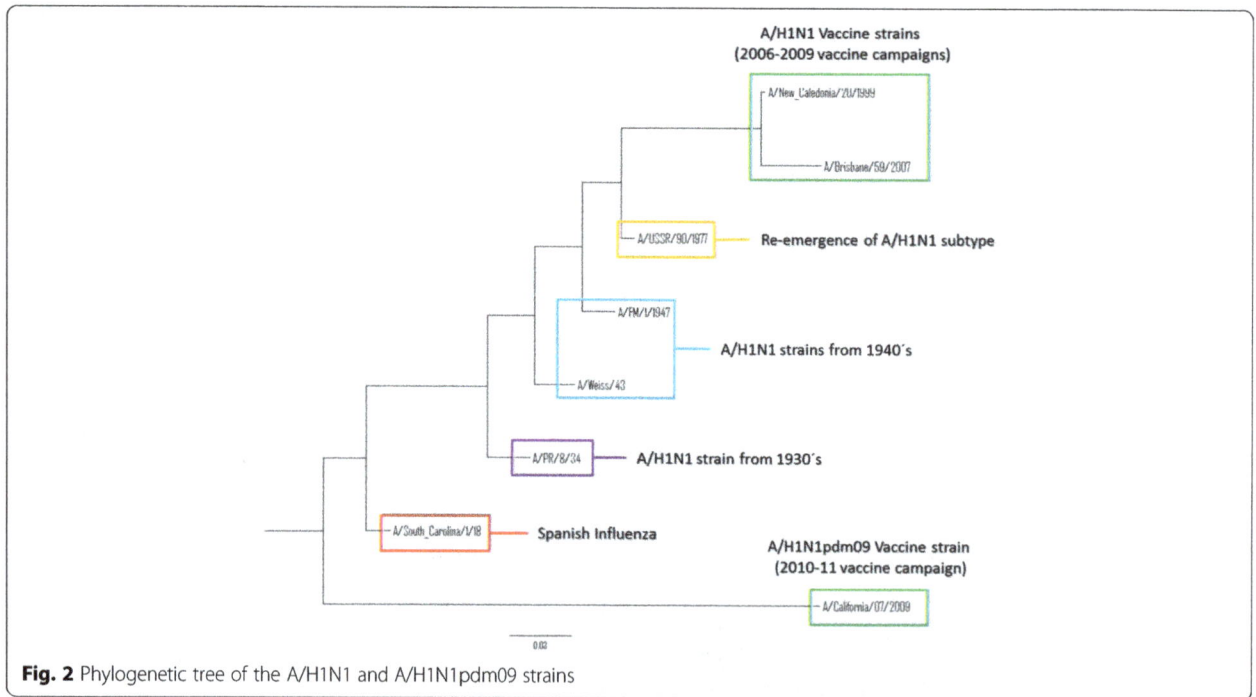

Fig. 2 Phylogenetic tree of the A/H1N1 and A/H1N1pdm09 strains

of the A/H1N1 strains that we analysed is high (> 80%). Influenza A type viruses share specific antigenic epitopes that can be recognized by a wide range of Abs [13, 14]. Cross-immune reactions between different influenza subtypes and strains are frequent and have been documented by different authors [14, 29]. These types of results are the reason for the high interest and hope for a universal influenza vaccine [30, 31]. Our data also showed the presence of pre-vaccination Abs against the A/H1N1pdm09 subtype in a small percentage of the elderly people before the emergence of the 2009 pandemic. This issue was documented previously with different percentages among different countries [32–34]. It was probably responsible for the lower incidence of A/H1N1pdm09 subtype in elderly people compared to younger groups during the 2009 pandemic [34, 35].

The lower percentage of individuals having pre-vaccination protective Abs against both of the 1940s era A/H1N1 influenza strains, i.e., A/Weiss/43 and A/FM/1/47, in the 2008–09 IVC is surprising. The population recruited during 2008–09 IVC had a significantly higher mean age than the rest of the groups, so these people were born 10 to 15 years before the circulation of A/Weiss/43 and A/FM/1/47 strains. It is probable that the 2008–09 IVC was primed with older strains than those circulated during the 1940 decade, and this population seems to have generated a lower humoral response against the A/H1N1 viruses that circulated later. This issue can be caused by the so called "Original Antigenic Sin" [36–38], and it marks the importance of the first contacts with influenza viruses in a person's life. Unfortunately, a weakness of our work is that we were not able to analyse the presence of

heterotypic Abs against other A/H1N1 strains older than those circulated during the 1940 decade, e.g., A/PR/8/34, so this issue cannot be tested with certainty.

Despite the high genetic homology present between both old A/H1N1 strains (93.4%), a lower percentage of individuals showed pre-vaccination Abs against the A/FM/1/47 strain than the A/Weiss/43 strain in all IVCs. This was probably caused by events that occurred during the emergence of the A/FM/1/47 strain. According to some authors, this strain emerged because of a more pronounced intrasubtypic drift than in previous years [20]. However, other authors suggest that this strain was separated from the strains circulating during the early years of the 1940 decade and did not produce epidemics until 1947 [19]. The spread of this strain throughout the world was fast during 1947, and it produced an unusually high number of cases but without an increase in the mortality rates of previous epidemics [20]. Repeated infections with minor variants of the same influenza subtype decreased the humoral response against the new strains that were phylogenetically close [39]. While this effect has not been well documented, some authors suggest that this phenomenon induced a lower immune response against influenza viruses that were different from the virus that primed each individual [40–42]. The lower response was likely to be harmful for the host. More people than in a normal epidemic were infected during 1947, and the humoral response in them was lower than in a normal epidemic due to the phylogenetic proximity of the strain to previously circulated strains. This hypothesis is consistent with our data, explaining the lower percentage of people with pre-vaccination protective Abs against the A/FM/1/47 strain.

After influenza seasonal vaccination, 63.2% of elderly people showed protective Abs against the A/Weiss/43 strain, 31.0% against A/FM/1/47 strain, 73.0% against the A/H1N1subtype strains A/New Caledonia/20/99 and A/Brisbane/59/2007, and 35.6% against the A/H1N1pdm09 subtype. Our results showed that seasonal vaccination induced a low but significant heterotypic response against the A/Weiss/43 strain when the elderly people were vaccinated against the A/New Caledonia/20/99 and A/Brisbane/59/2007 strains. Thus, this heterotypic response against the A/Weiss/43 strain was higher when this population was vaccinated with the A/New Caledonia/20/99 strain. Vaccination with A/H1N1 strains did not induce a significant heterotypic response against the A/FM/1/47 virus, while vaccination with the A/H1N1pdm09 subtype induced a moderate and significant heterotypic response against the 1947 strain.

As previously described, genetic homology between the 1940s era A/H1N1 strains is high, 93.4%, and it is also high between the 1940s era strains and the A/H1N1 vaccine strains included in seasonal vaccines, 84–87%. However, vaccination with the A/H1N1pdm09 subtype induced a higher than expected heterotypic response to the A/FM/1/47 strain, 30.2%, compared to the closely related A/Weiss/43 strain, 9.3%. This surprising observation lead us to hypothesize that despite the close genetic homology between the A/FM/1/47 and A/Weiss/43 strains, the epitopes formed by A/H1N1pdm09 subtype were more similar to those formed by the A/FM/1/47 strain than the A/Weiss/43 strain. This has been documented in other influenza viruses before [43]. Further research is needed to discover the cause of the divergent heterotypic responses of the A/H1N1pdm09 subtype vaccine in the production of Abs to the A/FM/1/47 and A/Weiss/43 epitopes.

Influenza seasonal vaccination induced a significant homologous response against A/H1N1 vaccine strains in all IVCs in which these subtypes were used. Also, we observed a significant heterotypic response against A/H1N1 subtypes when elderly people were vaccinated against A/H1N1pdm09 (2010–2011 IVC). Seasonal vaccination against A/H1N1 vaccine strains also induced a significant heterotypic response against the A/H1N1pdm09 subtype in all IVC (from 2006 till 2009). This heterotypic response was observed in at least 20% of the individuals the 2009–2010 IVCs. The results of our study demonstrate that seasonal vaccination with an A/H1N1 subtype seroprotected a low-to-moderate percentage of the elderly population against the 2009 pandemic virus before its emergence. These kinds of heterotypic responses after vaccination, and those induced by natural infections, may be responsible for the lower incidence of A/H1N1pdm09 subtype in the elderly population during the 2009 pandemic [34, 35].

The homologous response to influenza A/H1N1 strains was moderate, but sufficient to achieve high seroprotection rates in those older than 65 years. However, in the 2009–2010 IVC, there was a very low seroconversion rate, only 16.3%. In that IVC, the new pandemic subtype A/H1N1pdm09 emerged and was very actively circulated in Spain during the 2009–2010 IVC. We hypothesize that a certain percentage of the individuals vaccinated during that campaign were already infected or were in contact with this subtype during their window period. This could have negatively affected the humoral response. Further research is needed to clarify the true reasons for the low homologous response to the subtype A/H1N1 this IVC. The homologous response was very high in the season vaccinated with the A/H1N1pdm09 subtype. Our data show the complexity of the response to vaccination, which is influenced not only by the strains introduced in the vaccine, but also by the characteristics of the viruses, the target populations, the scheduling of the vaccination programs, and probably many other variables.

According to classical EMA criteria for vaccine efficacy evaluation in individuals ≥60-years old [24], the seasonal influenza vaccine was not effective in inducing a heterotypic humoral response against any of the 1940s era A/H1N1 strains that we analysed. The heterotypic response against the A/Weiss/43 strain was limited in most of the IVCs. However, the moderate percentage of individuals with pre-vaccination protective titres was likely responsible for the 48–85% of the elderly population that was seroprotected after vaccination against a subtype that had not been in circulation for more than 60 years. This issue has interesting implications for the protection of the population against re-emerging viruses. Despite the fact that there is only a low risk of re-emergence of old A/H1N1 strains, we are not exempt from biological incidents like the one that triggered the emergence of the A/USS/90/1977 strain during 1977 [3]. The Abs observed in a large percentage of the elderly population represent a moderate-to-high herd immunity that may protect other populations in the case of re-emergence of any of the cited A/H1N1 strains [44, 45]. More research is needed to understand the seasonal vaccine responses to old influenza strains in adults and children and the natural presence of antibodies in naïve people.

One of the limitations of this study is that the methodology did not allow the evaluation of the presence of heterotypic Abs against the HA2 subunit of haemagglutinin, which is the most conserved part of this protein. To know more about the nature of the heterotypic reactions observed in this work, it will be necessary to extend this study using other methodologies such as microneutralization or prior adsorption of sera with seasonal viruses before testing them against older viruses. It will also be instructive to perform these experiments with other old strains from other decades such as A/PR/8/34 or A/USSR/90/1977. For a wider view of seroprotection, these studies need to be conducted with adults in other age groups and with children that never have been in contact with the 1940s era A/

H1N1 strains. The results of our study show that seasonal vaccines can increase the Ab titres against already extinct strains. This may provide a better understanding of the cross-immunity phenomena that is necessary to achieve a truly universal vaccine against influenza.

Conclusions

In summary, seasonal influenza vaccination is useful in elderly people for strengthening seroprotection and increasing the Ab titres against older A/H1N1 influenza viruses. However, we do not know the exact role of immune memory in the presence of these Abs before vaccination. Protective Abs are present in a moderate percentage of the elderly population, and they may contribute to herd immunity that can prevent the re-emergence of extinguished influenza viruses. The results of our study provide data regarding cross-immune responses between different influenza viruses and how seasonal vaccines can be useful against other viruses not included in the vaccine composition. Our results also support the need for increasing the seasonal influenza vaccine coverage in the elderly.

Acknowledgments
Not applicable.

Funding
This work did not receive any funding.

Authors' contributions
IS, SR and ROL designed the study. IS and SR performed the experiments. IS, SR and ST wrote the manuscript. IS, SR, ST, JME and ROL revised the manuscript. All authors approved the final version of this manuscript.

Competing interest
The authors declare that they have no competing interests.

Author details
[1]Valladolid National Influenza Centre, Avenida Ramón y Cajal s/n, 47005 Valladolid, Spain. [2]Microbiology and Immunology Unit, Hospital Clínico Universitario de Valladolid, Avenida Ramón y Cajal s/n, 47005 Valladolid, Spain. [3]Epidemiology Unit, Consejería de Sanidad, Junta de Castilla y León, Paseo de Zorrilla 1, 47007 Valladolid, Spain. [4]Microbiology Unit, Hospital Universitario Río Hortega, Calle Dulzaina 2, 47012 Valladolid, Spain.

References
1. Taubenberger JK, Morens DM. 1918 influenza: the mother of all pandemics. Emerg Infect Dis. 2006;12:15–22.
2. Kilbourne ED. Influenza pandemics of the 20th century. Emerg Infect Dis. 2006;12:9–14.
3. Kozlov JV, Gorbulev VG, Kurmanova AG, Bayev AA, Shilov AA, Zhdanov VM. On the origin of the H1N1 (a/USSR/90/77) influenza virus. J Gen Virol. 1981; 56:437–40.
4. Del Rio C, Guarner J. The 2009 influenza a (H1N1) pandemic: what have we learned in the past 6 months. Trans Am Clin Climatol Assoc. 2010;121:128–40.
5. Liu M, Zhao X, Hua S, Du X, Peng Y, Li X, et al. Antigenic patterns and evolution of the human influenza a (H1N1) virus. Sci Rep. 2015;5:14171.
6. Smith GJD, Bahl J, Vijaykrishna D, Zhang J, Poon LLM, Chen H, et al. Dating the emergence of pandemic influenza viruses. Proc Natl Acad Sci U S A. 2009;106:11709–12.
7. Cotter CR, Jin H, Chen Z. A single amino acid in the stalk region of the H1N1pdm influenza virus HA protein affects viral fusion, stability and infectivity. PLoS Pathog. 2014 Jan;10:e1003831.
8. Haq K, McElhaney JE. Immunosenescence: influenza vaccination and the elderly. Curr Opin Immunol. 2014;29:38–42.
9. Pera A, Campos C, López N, Hassouneh F, Alonso C, Tarazona R, et al. Immunosenescence: implications for response to infection and vaccination in older people. Maturitas. 2015;82:50–5.
10. ECDC. Priority risk groups for Influenza vaccination [Internet]. [cited 2017 Oct 15]. Available from: http://ecdc.europa.eu/en/healthtopics/seasonal_influenza/vaccines/Pages/influenza_vaccination.aspx#riskgroups
11. Glezen WP, Keitel WA, Taber LH, Piedra PA, Clover RD, Couch RB. Age distribution of patients with medically-attended illnesses caused by sequential variants of influenza a/H1N1: comparison to age-specific infection rates, 1978-1989. Am J Epidemiol. 1991;133:296–304.
12. Sanz I, Rojo S, Tamames S, Eiros JM, Ortiz de Lejarazu R. Heterologous humoral response against H5N1, H7N3, and H9N2 avian influenza viruses after seasonal vaccination in a European elderly population. Vaccine. 2017 Jul 17;5(3)
13. Staneková Z, Varečková E. Conserved epitopes of influenza a virus inducing protective immunity and their prospects for universal vaccine development. Virol J. 2010;7:351.
14. Epstein SL, Price GE. Cross-protective immunity to influenza a viruses. Expert Rev Vaccines. 2010;9:1325–41.
15. WHO. Recommendations for Influenza Vaccine Composition: Northern hemisphere: 2006–2007 [Internet]. 2006 [cited 2016 Nov 18]. Available from: www.who.int/entity/influenza/vaccines/2007northreport.pdf
16. WHO. Recommended composition of influenza virus vaccines for use in the 2008–2009 influenza season [Internet]. 2008 [cited 2017 Oct 20]. Available from: www.who.int/entity/influenza/vaccines/recommended_compositionFeb08FullReport.pdf
17. WHO. Recommended composition of influenza virus vaccines for use in the 2009–2010 influenza season [Internet]. 2009 [cited 2017 Oct 20]. Available from: www.who.int/entity/influenza/vaccines/200902_recommendation.pdf
18. WHO. Recommended viruses for influenza vaccines for use in the 2010–11 northern hemisphere influenza season [Internet]. 2010 [cited 2017 Oct 20]. Available from: www.who.int/entity/influenza/vaccines/virus/recommendations/201002_Recommendation.pdf
19. Nakajima S, Nishikawa F, Nakajima K. Comparison of the evolution of recent and late phase of old influenza a (H1N1) viruses. Microbiol Immunol. 2000;44:841–7.
20. Kilbourne ED, Smith C, Brett I, Pokorny BA, Johansson B, Cox N. The total influenza vaccine failure of 1947 revisited: major intrasubtypic antigenic change can explain failure of vaccine in a post-world war II epidemic. Proc Natl Acad Sci U S A. 2002;99:10748–52.
21. WHO. Recommendations and laboratory procedures for detection of avian influenza A(H5N1) virus in specimens from suspected human cases [Internet]. 2007 [cited 2017 Sep 24]. Available from: http://www.who.int/influenza/resources/documents/RecAIlabtestsAug07.pdf.
22. WHO Global Influenza, Surveillance Network. Manual for the laboratory diagnosis and virological surveillance of influenza. 2011.
23. He W, Mullarkey CE, Miller MS. Measuring the neutralization potency of influenza a virus hemagglutinin stalk/stem-binding antibodies in polyclonal preparations by microneutralization assay. Methods San Diego Calif. 2015;90:95–100.
24. EMA. Note for guiadance on harmonisation of requirements for influenza vaccines (CPMP/BWP/214/96) [Internet]. 1997 [cited 2017 Oct 20]. Available from: http://www.ema.europa.eu/docs/en_GB/document_library/Scientific_guideline/2009/09/WC500003945.pdf
25. Trombetta CM, Perini D, Mather S, Temperton N, Montomoli E. Overview of serological techniques for influenza vaccine evaluation: past, present and future. Vaccine. 2014;2:707–34.
26. Petrie JG, Ohmit SE, Johnson E, Truscon R, Monto AS. Persistence of antibodies to influenza hemagglutinin and neuraminidase following one or two years of influenza vaccination. J Infect Dis. 2015 Dec 15;212(12):1914–22.
27. Dou Y, Fu B, Sun R, Li W, Hu W, Tian Z, et al. Influenza vaccine induces intracellular immune memory of human NK cells. PLoS One. 2015;10: e0121258.

28. Bonduelle O, Carrat F, Luyt C-E, Leport C, Mosnier A, Benhabiles N, et al. Characterization of pandemic influenza immune memory signature after vaccination or infection. J Clin Invest. 2014;124:3129–36.

29. Laurie KL, Carolan LA, Middleton D, Lowther S, Kelso A, Barr IG. Multiple infections with seasonal influenza a virus induce cross-protective immunity against a(H1N1) pandemic influenza virus in a ferret model. J Infect Dis. 2010;202:1011–20.

30. Chen C-J, Ermler ME, Tan GS, Krammer F, Palese P, Hai R. Influenza a viruses expressing intra- or intergroup chimeric hemagglutinins. J Virol. 2016;90:3789–93.

31. Ermler ME, Kirkpatrick E, Sun W, Hai R, Amanat F, Chromikova V, et al. Chimeric hemagglutinin constructs induce broad protection against influenza B virus challenge in the mouse model. J Virol. 2017;91

32. Chen Y, Zheng Q, Yang K, Zeng F, Lau S-Y, Wu WL, et al. Serological survey of antibodies to influenza a viruses in a group of people without a history of influenza vaccination. Clin Microbiol Infect. 2011;17(9):1347.

33. Chi CY, Liu CC, Lin CC, Wang HC, Cheng YT, Chang CM, et al. Preexisting antibody response against 2009 pandemic influenza H1N1 viruses in the Taiwanese population. Clin Vaccine Immunol. 2010;17:1958–62.

34. Hancock K, Veguilla V, Lu X, Zhong W, Butler EN, Sun H, et al. Cross-reactive antibody responses to the 2009 pandemic H1N1 influenza virus. N Engl J Med. 2009;361:1945–52.

35. Miller E, Hoschler K, Hardelid P, Stanford E, Andrews N, Zambon M. Incidence of 2009 pandemic influenza a H1N1 infection in England: a cross-sectional serological study. Lancet. 2010;375:1100–8.

36. Ortiz de Lejarazu R, Landínez R. Importancia epidemiológica de la nueva variante de virus gripal A/USSR/90/77. Laboratorio. 1978;66:339–50.

37. Kim JH, Skountzou I, Compans R, Jacob J. Original antigenic sin responses to influenza viruses. J Immunol. 2009;183:3294–301.

38. Thomas Francis, Jr. On the doctrine of original antigenic sin. Proc Am Philos Soc 1960;104:572–578.

39. Davenport FM, Hennessy AV. A serologic recapitulation of past experiences with influenza a; antibody response to monovalent vaccine. J Exp Med. 1956;104:85–97.

40. Kim JH, Davis WG, Sambhara S, Jacob J. Strategies to alleviate original antigenic sin responses to influenza viruses. Proc Natl Acad Sci U S A. 2012;109:13751–6.

41. Morens DM, Burke DS, Halstead SB. The wages of original antigenic sin. Emerg Infect Dis. 2010;16:1023–4.

42. null F d SG, Webster RG. Disquisitions of original antigenic sin. I. Evidence in man. J Exp Med. 1966;124:331–45.

43. Peeters B, Reemers S, Dortmans J, de Vries E, de Jong M, van de Zande S, et al. Genetic versus antigenic differences among highly pathogenic H5N1 avian influenza a viruses: consequences for vaccine strain selection. Virology. 2017 Mar;503:83–93.

44. Plans-Rubió P. The vaccination coverage required to establish herd immunity against influenza viruses. Prev Med. 2012;55:72–7.

45. Mooring EQ, Bansal S. Increasing herd immunity with influenza revaccination. Epidemiol Infect. 2016;144:1267–77.

The baseline levels and risk factors for high-sensitive C-reactive protein in Chinese healthy population

Ying Tang[1,2†], Peifen Liang[1,2†], Junzhe Chen[1,2†], Sha Fu[1,2], Bo Liu[1,2], Min Feng[1,2], Baojuan Lin[1,2], Ben Lee[5], Anping Xu[1,2*] and Hui Y. Lan[3,4*]

Abstract

Background: Recent studies show that C-reactive protein (CRP) is not only a biomarker but also a pathogenic mediator contributing to the development of inflammation and ageing-related diseases. However, serum levels of CRP in the healthy ageing population remained unclear, which was investigated in the present study.

Methods: Serum levels of high sensitive C-reactive protein (hs-CRP), glucose (Glu), triglyceride (TG), cholesterol (CHOL), high-density lipoprotein cholesterol (HDL-c), low-density lipoprotein cholesterol (LDL-c), superoxide dismutase (SOD), serum creatinine (SCr), serum uric acid (SUA) were measured in 6060healthy subjects (3672 male and 2388 female, mean age:45.9 years) who received routine physical examination at Sun Yat-sen Memorial Hospital, Guangzhou, China.

Results: In total of 6060 healthy people, serum levels of hs-CRP were significantly increased with ageing ($P < 0.05$), particularly in those with age over 45-year-old (1.31[0.69–2.75] vs 1.05[0.53–2.16]mg/L, $P < 0.001$). Interestingly, levels of serum hs-CRP were significantly higher in male than female population (1.24[0.65–2.57] vs 1.07[0.53–2.29]mg/L, $P < 0.001$). Correlation analysis also revealed that serum levels of hs-CRP positively correlated with age and SUA, but inversely correlated with serum levels of HDL-c and SOD (all $P < 0.05$).

Conclusions: Baseline levels of serum hs-CRP are increased with ageing and are significantly higher in male than female healthy population. In addition, elevated serum levels of hs-CRP are also associated with increased SUA but decreased HDL-c and SOD. Thus, serum levels of hs-CRP may be an indicator associated with ageing in healthy Chinese population.

Keywords: Hs-CRP, Ageing, Inflammation, Risk factor

Background

Ageing is a natural phenomenon characterized by gradual deterioration of the body structure and function with important social, public health, and economic implications. Increasing evidence shows that inflammation is one of the key mechanisms associated with many ageing-related diseases, including cancer, atherosclerosis, hypertension, diabetes mellitus, ischemic heart disease, cirrhosis, Alzheimer's disease and other dementias and chronic diseases [1, 2].Therefore, disentangling age-related low grade inflammation may slow or delay ageing process [2]. Many inflammatory effector molecules and biomarkers, especially C-reactive protein (CRP), interleukin-6 (IL-6) and tumor necrosis factor-alpha (TNF-α), have been considered as important factors associated with ageing, ageing-related diseases or disability [3]. CRP, an acute phase protein, is primarily produced and secreted by the liver in response to IL-6.Serum levels of CRP can be measured by a high sensitivity immunoturbidometric assay termed high-sensitive CRP (hs-CRP). Many studies have shown that elevated levels of serum hs-CRP are associated with ageing and ageing-related diseases including cardiovascular disease (CVD), hypertension, diabetes mellitus, and kidney disorders [4–8].However, there is still a lack of evidence

---

* Correspondence: anpxu@163.com; hylan@cuhk.edu.hk
†Ying Tang, Peifen Liang and Junzhe Chen contributed equally to this work.
[1]Department of Nephrology, Sun Yat-sen Memorial Hospital, Sun Yat-sen University, Guangzhou, China
[3]Department of Medicine and Therapeutics, Li KaShing Institute of Health Sciences, the Chinese University of Hong Kong, Hong Kong, SAR, China
Full list of author information is available at the end of the article

for the relationship between the baseline levels of hs-CRP and the ageing progress in general healthy population, which was investigated in this study. In addition, although many inflammatory mediators including dyslipidemia, insulin resistance, oxidative stress, and serum uric acid (SUA) have also been shown to contribute to high levels of serum hs-CRP under various disease conditions [9–16]. The link between hs-CRP and these factors in the healthy population remains unknown, which was also analyzed in this study.

Methods
Study population
This was a retrospective study in the healthy Chinese population who underwent routine health examination carried out between April 1st, 2009 and May 1st, 2017 at Sun Yat-sen Memorial Hospital, Sun Yat-sen University, Guangzhou, China. As described previously [17–19], the population enrolled into this study included the healthy subjects aged 18–89 years old without evidence of acute infection, cardiovascular disease, chronic kidney disease, cancer, diabetes, gout, obstructive pulmonary disease and Alzheimer's disease based on the previous medical record in Sun Yat-sen Memorial Hospital. Those with various diseases and abnormal medical laboratory tests such as eGFR less than 60 ml/min/1.73m^2 were excluded from this study. The study protocol was approved by the Institutional Review Boards of the Sun Yat-sen Memorial Hospital and waived the need for informed consent and conducted in accordance with the principles embodied in the Declaration of Helsinki (2013).

Methods
Serum levels of glucose (Glu), triglyceride (TG), high-density lipoprotein cholesterol (HDL-c), low-density lipoprotein cholesterol (LDL-c), superoxide dismutase (SOD), serum creatinine (SCr), SUA, hs-CRP in fasting blood samples were measured by automated biochemical Analyzer 5800 (BECKMAN) or 7600 (HITACHI). The normal references of serum hs-CRP levels were set at 0–3.0 mg/L. The value of estimated glomerular filtration rate (eGFR) was calculated using the North American Chronic Kidney Disease Epidemiology (CKD-EPI) Collaboration equation.

Statistical analysis
The baseline characteristics of healthy population and subgroups were analyzed by using SPSS version 19 (IBM Corporation, Armonk, New York, USA). For continuous variables with symmetric distribution, mean data were expressed as mean±standard deviations (SD), whereas median and interquartile range (IQR) was used for those with asymmetric distribution and examined by Student's t-test, analysis of variance (ANOVA), chi-square test. Factors found to be statistically significant from univariate analysis

($P < 0.05$) were then tested in multivariate analysis using Linear regression analysis modeling. The correlations between hs-CRP and other risk factors were shown in the scatter plots with linear regression line and P-value of < 0.05 from two-sided tests was considered statistically significant.

Results
Baseline characteristics of healthy population
A total of 6060 healthy people who underwent routine health check were included in this study. Of them, 3672 cases (60.4%) were male and 2388 (39.4%) were female, and the age ranged from 18 to 89 years old with the mean age of45-year-old. Since age of 45 years old is known to be one of the risks for the development of atherosclerotic cardiovascular diseases in men and is the mean menopause age in women with declining steroid hormones and increasing pro-inflammatory markers [3], therefore the age of 45-year-old was stratified as a subgroup for the risk factor of hs-CRP. As shown in Fig. 1, serum levels of hs-CRP were increased with ageing. Compared to male, female population exhibited higher levels of HDL-c and eGFR ($P < 0.05$) but lower levels of hs-CRP, TG, CHOL, LDL-c, SOD, Glu and SUA ($P < 0.05$).The population with age > 45-year-old had higher levels of hs-CRP, TG, CHOL, LDL-c and Glu ($P < 0.05$), but lower levels of eGFR and SOD ($P < 0.05$) compared to age between 18 and 45. There were no differences in levels of SUA and HDL-c ($P > 0.05$) between these two groups (Table 1).

Risk factors of hs-CRP in the overall healthy population
As shown in Table 2, the univariate linear regression analysis showed that age and levels of SUA and Glu were positively correlated with levels of serum hs-CRP ($P < 0.05$), whereas, serum levels of HDL-c and SOD were negatively correlated with levels of serum hs-CRP ($P < 0.05$). The multivariate linear regression analysis further identified significant correlations between hs-CRP and age ($\beta = 0.033$, $P = 0.012$), the levels of HDL-c ($\beta = -0.062$, $P < 0.001$), SOD ($\beta = -0.100$, $P < 0.001$) and SUA ($\beta = 0.033$, $P = 0.015$).

Risk factors of hs-CRP in healthy population stratified by gender
Considering the possible effects of gender on serum hs-CRP levels, we analyzed the risk factor of hs-CRP in male and female respectively. In the male subgroup, the multivariate linear regression analysis showed that serum levels of hs-CRP correlated significantly with the age ($\beta = 0.037$, $P = 0.026$) and SUA ($\beta = 0.034$, $P = 0.042$), but negatively correlated with the levels of HDL-c ($\beta = -0.041$, $P = 0.014$) and SOD ($\beta = -0.086$, $P < 0.001$) (Additional file 1: Table S1).The correlations between hs-CRP and these

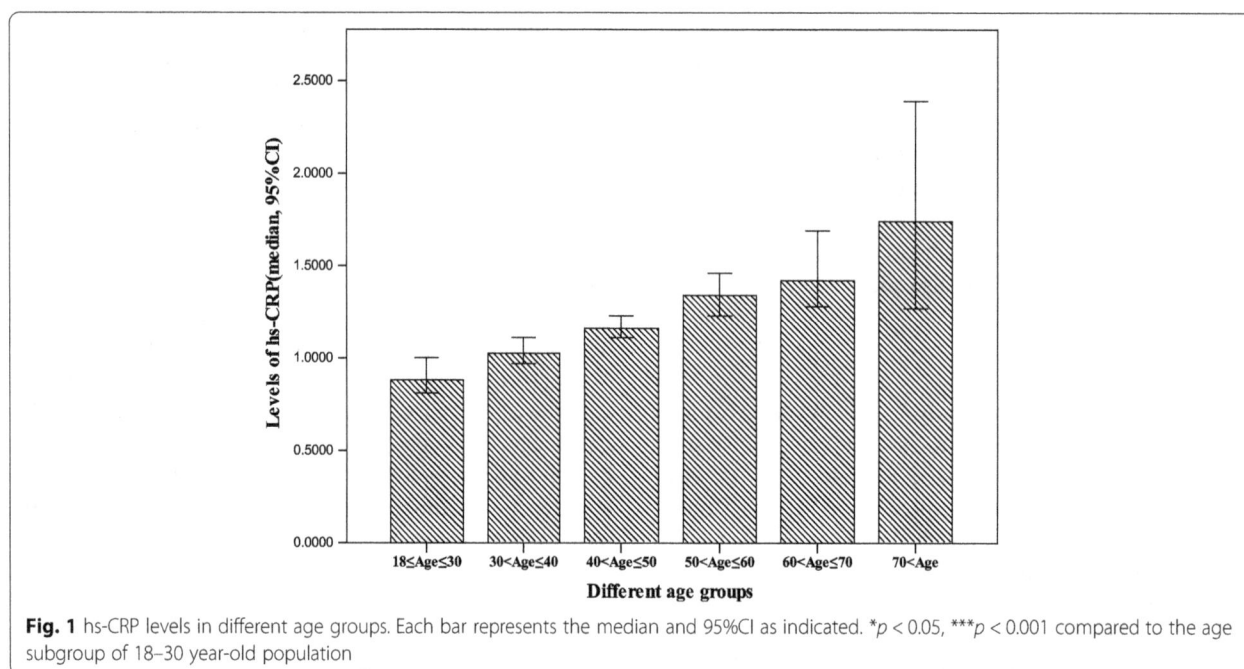

Fig. 1 hs-CRP levels in different age groups. Each bar represents the median and 95%CI as indicated. *$p < 0.05$, ***$p < 0.001$ compared to the age subgroup of 18–30 year-old population

factors in the male population were shown in Figure 2. Similarly, in the female subgroup, results from the multivariate linear regression analysis were generally consistent with the male subgroup (Additional file 1: Table S1). Figure 3 showed the correlations between hs-CRP and these factors in the female population.

Risk factors of hs-CRP in healthy population stratified by age and gender

A higher level of hs-CRP was associated with ageing and male in 6060 healthy population (Table 1), further

analysis was performed to identify the co-risk factors for hs-CRP in healthy people stratified by the mean age and gender. In healthy population with age of less than 45-year-old, the univariate linear regression analysis showed that levels of hs-CRP positively correlated with SUA($P < 0.05$), but negatively with levels of HDL-c and SOD ($P < 0.05$) in both genders, which were further confirmed by the multivariate linear regression analysis (Tables 3 and 4). Similar results were also found in those with age more than 45-year-old subpopulation (Tables 3 and 4).

Table 1 Baseline characteristics of healthy population

	Overall ($n = 6060$)	Sex subgroup			Age subgroup		
		Male ($n = 3672$)	Female ($n = 2388$)	P	18 ≤ Age ≤ 45 ($n = 3046$)	45 < Age ($n = 3014$)	P
Age, y	45.90 ± 11.16	45.40 ± 10.97	46.67 ± 11.41	< 0.001	36.98 ± 6.06	54.92 ± 7.18	< 0.001
hs-CRP, mg/L	1.18(0.60, 2.47)	1.24(0.65,2.57)	1.07(0.53,2.29)	< 0.001	1.05(0.53,2.16)	1.31(0.69,2.75)	< 0.001
TG, mmol/L	1.33(0.93, 1.99)	1.53(1.07,2.27)	1.08(0.80,1.57)	< 0.001	1.26(0.87,1.97)	1.39(0.99,2.02)	< 0.001
CHOL, mmol/L	5.35 ± 1.11	5.39 ± 1.13	5.28 ± 1.08	< 0.001	5.19 ± 1.09	5.50 ± 1.11	< 0.001
HDL-c, mmol/L	1.35 ± 0.33	1.26 ± 0.29	1.49 ± 0.34	< 0.001	1.35 ± 0.32	1.36 ± 0.34	0.204
LDL-c,mmol/L	3.35 ± 0.85	3.42 ± 0.85	3.25 ± 0.85	< 0.001	3.24 ± 0.84	3.47 ± 0.85	< 0.001
SOD, U/mL	158.67 ± 32.55	161.33 ± 36.06	154.57 ± 25.72	< 0.001	162.81 ± 21.05	154.48 ± 40.59	< 0.001
eGFR,ml/min.1.73m^2	83.89 ± 15.04	82.50 ± 14.50	86.02 ± 15.60	< 0.001	88.55 ± 15.77	79.18 ± 12.63	< 0.001
SUA, μmol/L	369.00(307.00,436.75)	409.00[358.00,466.00]	305.00[263.00,353.00]	< 0.001	370.00[303.00,444.00]	367.50(310.00,429.00)	0.184
Glu, mmol/L	5.50 ± 1.58	5.65 ± 1.82	5.28 ± 1.09	< 0.001	5.26 ± 1.31	5.74 ± 1.78	< 0.001

hs-CRP High sensitive C-reactive protein, *TG* Triglyceride, *HDL-c* High-density lipoprotein cholesterol, *LDL-c* Low-density lipoprotein cholesterol, *SOD* Superoxide dismutase, *eGFR* Estimated glomerular filtration rate, *SUA* Serum uric acid, *Glu* Glucose

Table 2 The relationship between hs-CRP and biomarkers in healthy population ($N = 6060$)

| | Linear regression analysis | | | |
| | Univariate analysis | | Multivariate analysis | |
	β	P	β	P
Age	0.046	< 0.001	0.033	0.012
TG	0.005	0.698		
CHOL	−0.004	0.729		
LDL-c	0.002	0.901		
HDL-c	−0.061	< 0.001	−0.062	< 0.001
SOD	−0.096	< 0.001	−0.100	< 0.001
eGFR	−0.007	0.576		
SUA	0.045	< 0.001	0.033	0.015
Glu	0.027	0.034		

Discussion

The present cross-sectional study revealed that serum levels of hs-CRP were increased with ageing and higher in male than female in Chinese healthy population. Our results showed that higher serum levels of hs-CRP were strongly associated with higher levels of SUA, lower levels of HDL-c and enzymatic antioxidants SOD. These results suggested that elevated serum levels of SUA might trigger CRP production, whereas serum HDL-c and SOD might have an opposite effect. Thus, serum levels of hs-CRP may be a useful indicator for ageing in healthy population.

Ageing is thought to be related to the inflammatory processes. Numerous studies have shown that levels of several cytokines, especially IL-6, TNF alpha and CRP, increase with age in the absence of acute infection [20, 21]. In the present study, we found that elevated levels of hs-CRP levels were correlated with ageing. Interestingly, consistent with previous population-based studies [22, 23], we also found that high serum levels of CRP were significantly correlated with elevated levels of SUA

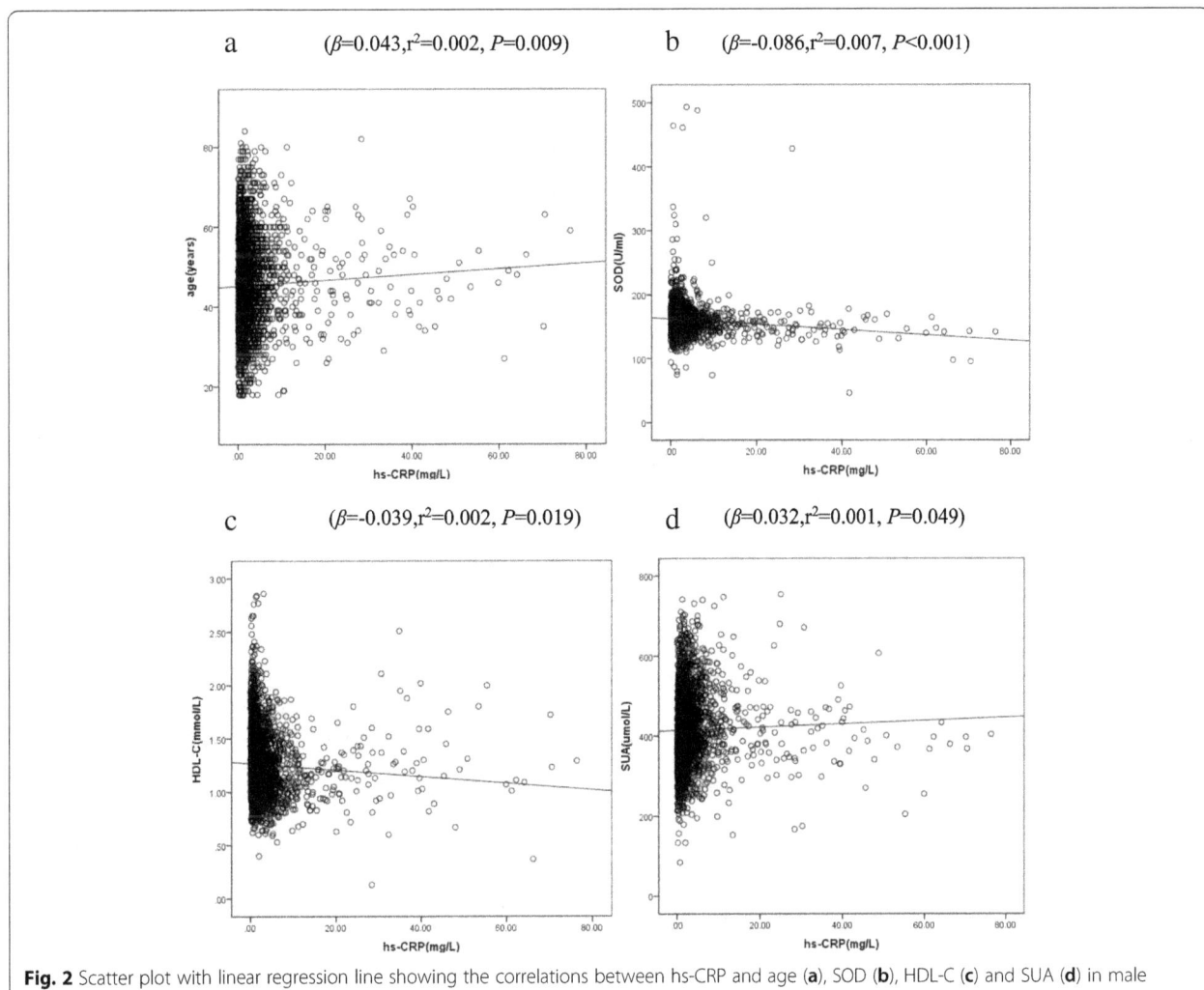

Fig. 2 Scatter plot with linear regression line showing the correlations between hs-CRP and age (**a**), SOD (**b**), HDL-C (**c**) and SUA (**d**) in male

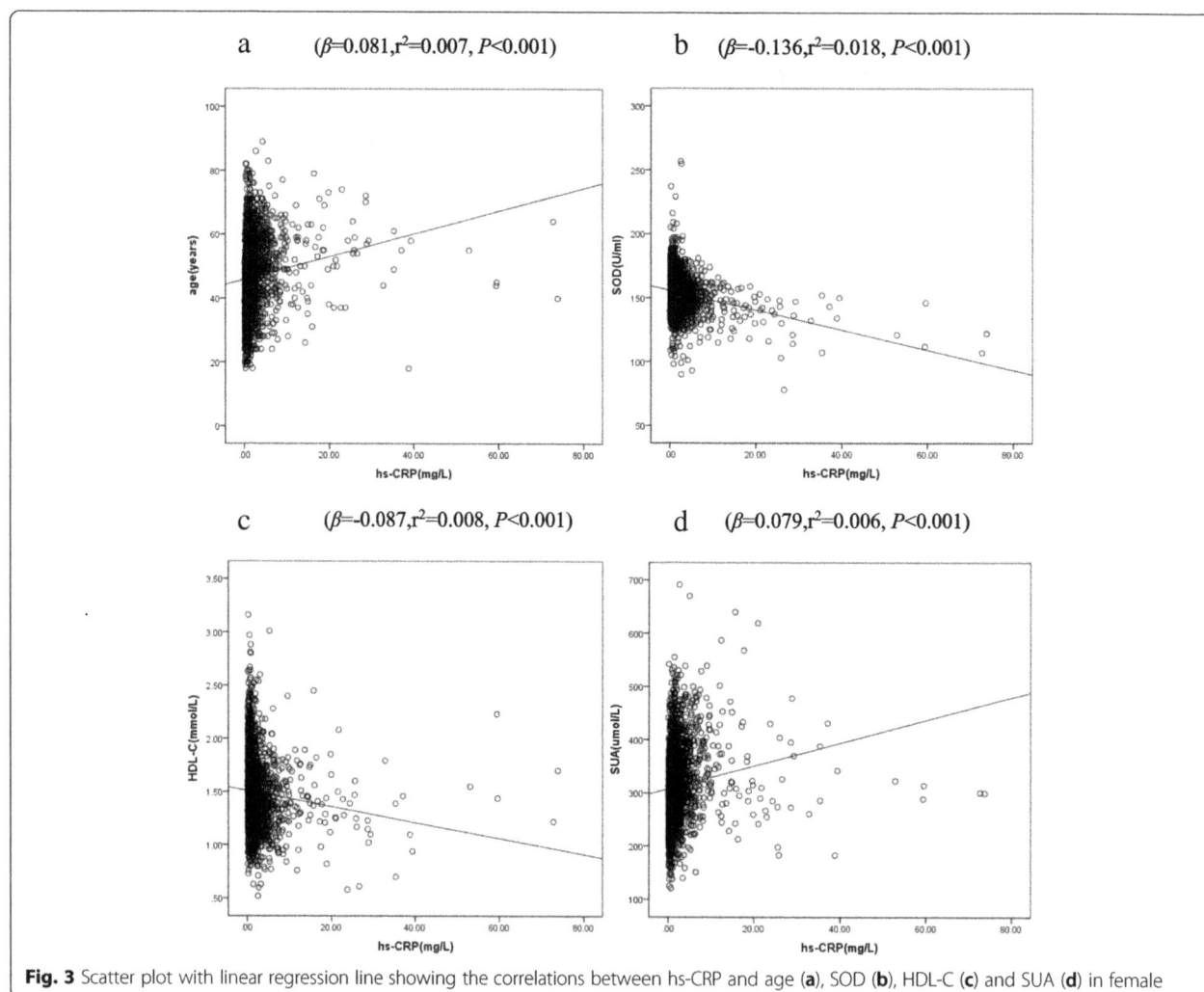

a (β=0.081, r^2=0.007, P<0.001)

b (β=-0.136, r^2=0.018, P<0.001)

c (β=-0.087, r^2=0.008, P<0.001)

d (β=0.079, r^2=0.006, P<0.001)

Fig. 3 Scatter plot with linear regression line showing the correlations between hs-CRP and age (**a**), SOD (**b**), HDL-C (**c**) and SUA (**d**) in female

but low levels of HDL-c and SOD. Hyperuricemia has been shown to contribute to the development of hypertension, chronic kidney disease, cardiovascular diseases, type 2 diabetes mellitus and the metabolic syndrome by inducing endothelial dysfunction and pathologic vascular remodeling [24–27]. Thus, SUA and CRP may share common features in vascular remodeling, and it is possible that SUA may trigger CRP expression. Currently, evidence from experimental studies has shown that mitogen-activated protein kinases (MAPK) signaling is a

Table 3 The relationship between hs-CRP and biomarkers in healthy male population

| | Linear regression analysis(18 ≤ age ≤ 45) (n = 1945) | | | | Linear regression analysis(age > 45)(n = 1727) | | | |
| | Univariate analysis | | Multivariate analysis | | Univariate analysis | | Multivariate analysis | |
	β	P	β	P	β	P	β	P
Age	0.004	0.846			0.023	0.346		
TG	0.004	0.847			−0.018	0.461		
CHOL	−0.005	0.811			−0.037	0.120		
LDL-C	−0.002	0.935			−0.039	0.108		
HDL-C	−0.064	0.005	−0.060	0.008	−0.081	0.001	−0.081	0.001
SOD	−0.140	< 0.001	−0.143	< 0.001	− 0.065	0.007	− 0.074	0.002
eGFR	−0.012	0.594			0.004	0.860		
UA	0.078	0.001	0.065	0.004	0.055	0.021	0.049	0.041
Glu	0.031	0.177			0.010	0.671		

Table 4 The relationship between hs-CRP and biomarkers in healthy female population

| | Linear regression analysis($18 \leq$ age ≤ 45) ($n = 1101$) | | | | Linear regression analysis(age > 45)($n = 1287$) | | | |
| | Univariate analysis | | Multivariate analysis | | Univariate analysis | | Multivariate analysis | |
	β	P	β	P	β	P	β	P
Age	0.016	0.596			0.079	0.005		
TG	0.027	0.374			0.023	0.410		
CHOL	0.034	0.256			−0.002	0.937		
LDL-C	0.041	0.179			0.017	0.547		
HDL-C	−0.110	< 0.001	−0.112	< 0.001	−0.129	< 0.001	−0.120	< 0.001
SOD	−0.165	< 0.001	−0.169	< 0.001	−0.139	< 0.001	−0.140	< 0.001
eGFR	0.043	0.154			−0.029	0.297		
UA	0.084	0.005	0.062	0.037	0.142	< 0.001	0.109	< 0.001
Glu	0.006	0.852			0.045	0.103		

common pathway by which uric acid triggers CRP production in vascular smooth muscle cells and vein endothelial cells [28–30]. It has also been shown that the addition of UA is able to stimulate the expression of CRP by activating the proinflammatory NF-κB signaling cascade [31]. Also, we recently revealed the pathogenic role for CRP in acute and chronic kidney diseases via a NF-κB-dependent mechanism [32–34]. Furthermore, changes of hs-CRP have been applied as a biomarker clinically as evidenced by the lowering of serum CRP in response to various treatments under disease conditions [35–39].Taken together, results from the present study suggested that CRP might not only be a biomarker and mediator for inflammatory disease, but also as a sensitive indicator for the healthy ageing.

The gender difference with respect to the serum levels of CRP has not been fully clarified. Previous studies have shown a higher prevalence of high hs-CRP concentrations in Inuit or Pakistan women populations than that in men [40, 41]. In our study, we found that higher levels of hs-CRP were more prevalent in male than female individuals. This maybe partly attributed to the higher level of SUA but lower level of HDL-c. Previous studies also reported that circulating levels of CRP in elderly subjects were positively correlated with levels of blood glucose and HbA1c, but inversely correlated with renal dysfunction [42–45]. However, in this population-based study, we could not find any relationship between hs-CRP and Glu or eGFR. This may be largely due to the normal levels of Glu and eGFR in the healthy population.

There are some limitations in this study. First, since this study was retrospectively based on the healthy population who underwent routine healthy examination at clinic, we are unable to acquire data regarding BMI, smoking habit, and other information that are potentially associated with the occurrence of inflammation and their consequences [3]. Second, since CRP was

co-existing with other inflammatory conditions, our retrospective data may not be able to exclude those with minor acute inflammation, although the enrolled subjects were apparently healthy. Finally, since the majority of our study subjects were limited to those with age between 30 and 60 years old, the study outcomes may be more generalized to young and middle-aged healthy people, despite the fact that high serum levels of CRP were found in the population with age more than 65 years old.

Conclusions

This retrospective study shows that serum levels of hs-CRP are increased with ageing, particularly in male than female healthy population. Furthermore, elevated serum levels of hs-CRP are associated with high levels of SUA, but low levels of HLD-c and SOD, suggesting that the inflammatory status may also contribute to ageing in the healthy population.

Abbreviations
ANOVA: Analysis of variance; CHOL: Cholesterol; CRP: C-reactive protein; CVD: Cardiovascular disease; eGFR: Estimated glomerular filtration rate; Glu: Glucose; HDL-c: High-density lipoprotein cholesterol; hs-CRP: High sensitive C-reactive protein; IL-6: Interleukin-6; IQR: Interquartile range; LDL-c: Low-density lipoprotein cholesterol; SCr: Serum creatinine; SD: Standard deviation; SOD: Superoxide dismutase; SUA: Serum uric acid; TG: Triglyceride

Acknowledgements
We would like to thank Professor Li Ling and Dr. Cheng Gong for the assistance in statistical analysis and data interpretation and Thomas Mak for English editing.

Funding
This study was supported by grants from National Natural Scientific Foundation of China (81500512); and the Fundamental Research Funds for the Central Universities(17ykjc19); the LuiChe Woo Institute of Innovative Medicine (CARE program); Research Grants Council of Hong Kong (GRF 14121816,C7018-16G, TRS T12–402/13 N); and Health and Medical Research Fund of Hong Kong (HMRF 03140486, 14152321).

Authors' contributions

Study design: YT. Data analysis and interpretation: YT, JZ C, PF L, SF, Ben L. Data collection: JZ C, PF L, SF, BL, MF, BJ L, Ben L. Manuscript preparation: YT, PF L, JZ C, SF, BL, HY L, AP X. Manuscript revision: YT, JZ C, HY L, AP X. Statistical analysis: JZ C, SF, BL. All authors read and approved the final manuscript.

Competing interests

The authors declare that they have no competing interests.

Author details

[1]Department of Nephrology, Sun Yat-sen Memorial Hospital, Sun Yat-sen University, Guangzhou, China. [2]Guangdong Provincial Key Laboratory of Malignant Tumor Epigenetics and Gene Regulation, Sun Yat-sen Memorial Hospital, Sun Yat-sen University, Guangzhou, China. [3]Department of Medicine and Therapeutics, Li KaShing Institute of Health Sciences, the Chinese University of Hong Kong, Hong Kong, SAR, China. [4]Lui Che Woo Institute of Innovative Medicine, the Chinese University of Hong Kong, Hong Kong, SAR, China. [5]Guangzhou Deling Software Technology Co., Ltd, Guangzhou, China.

References

1. Franceschi C, Bonafè M, Valensin S, Olivieri F, De Luca M, Ottaviani E, et al. Inflamm-aging. An evolutionary perspective on immunosenescence. Ann N Y AcadSci. 2000;908:244–54.
2. Candore G, Caruso C, Jirillo E, Magrone T, Vasto S. Low grade inflammation as a common pathogenetic denominator in age-related diseases: novel drug targets for anti-ageing strategies and successful ageing achievement. Curr Pharm Des. 2010;16(6):584–96.
3. Singh T, Newman AB. Inflammatory markers in population studies of aging. Ageing Res Rev. 2011;10(3):319–29.
4. Tang Y, Fung E, Xu A, Lan HY. C-reactive protein and ageing. Clin Exp Pharmacol Physiol. 2017;4 https://doi.org/10.1111/1440-1681.12758.
5. Hamer M, Chida Y. Associations of very high C-reactive protein concentration with psychosocial and cardiovascular risk factors in an ageing population. Atherosclerosis. 2009;206(2):599–603.
6. Sujarwoto S, Tampubolon G. Inflammatory markers and physical performance in middle-aged and older people in Indonesia. Age Ageing. 2015;44(4):610–5.
7. Buffière C, Mariotti F, Savary-Auzeloux I, Migné C, Meunier N, Hercberg S, et al. Slight chronic elevation of C-reactive protein is associated with lower aerobic fitness but does not impair meal-induced stimulation of muscle protein metabolism in healthy old men. J Physiol. 2015;593(5):1259–72.
8. Sousa AC, Zunzunegui MV, Li A, Phillips SP, Guralnik JM, Guerra RO. Association between C-reactive protein and physical performance in older populations: results from the international mobility in aging study (IMIAS). Age Ageing. 2016;45(2):274–80.
9. Tsioufis C, Kyvelou S, Dimitriadis K, Syrseloudis D, Sideris S, Skiadas I, et al. The diverse associations of uric acid with low-grade inflammation, adiponectin and arterial stiffness in never-treated hypertensives. J Hum Hypertens. 2011;25(9):554–9.
10. Latourte A, Soumaré A, Bardin T, Perez RF, Debette S, Richette P. Uric acid and incident dementia over 12 years of follow-up: a population-based cohort study. Ann Rheum Dis. 2017;28 https://doi.org/10.1136/annrheumdis-2016-210767.
11. Mirhafez SR, Ebrahimi M, Saberi KM, Avan A, Tayefi M, Heidari BA, et al. Serum high-sensitivity C-reactive protein as a biomarker in patients with metabolic syndrome: evidence-based study with 7284 subjects. Eur J ClinNutr. 2016;70(11):1298–304.
12. Agirbasli M, Tanrikulu A, Acar SB, Azizy M, Bekiroglu N. Total cholesterol-to-high-density lipoprotein cholesterol ratio predicts high-sensitivity C-reactive protein levels in Turkish children. J ClinLipidol. 2015;9(2):195–200.
13. Lodovici M, Bigagli E, Luceri C, Mannucci E, Rotella CM, Raimondi L. Gender-related drug effect on several markers of oxidation stress in diabetes patients with and without complications. Eur J Pharmacol. 2015;766:86–90.
14. Caccamo G, Bonura F, Bonura F, Vitale G, Novo G, Evola S, et al. Insulin resistance and acute coronary syndrome. Atherosclerosis. 2010;211(2):672–5.
15. Liu Q, Han L, Du Q, Zhang M, Zhou S, Shen X. The association between oxidative stress, activator protein-1, inflammatory, total antioxidant status and artery stiffness and the efficacy of olmesartan in elderly patients with mild-to-moderate essential hypertension. Clin Exp Hypertens. 2016;38(4):365–9.

16. Peng C, Wang X, Chen J, Jiao R, Wang L, Li YM, et al. Biology of ageing and role of dietary antioxidants. Biomed Res Int. 2014;831841 https://doi.org/10.1155/2014/831841.
17. Bousquet J, Malva J, Nogues M, Mañas LR, Vellas B, Farrell J, MACVIA Research Group. Operational Definition of Active and Healthy Aging (AHA): The European Innovation Partnership(EIP) on AHA Reference Site Questionnaire: Montpellier October 20–21, 2014, Lisbon July 2, 2015. J Am Med Dir Assoc. 2015;16(12):1020–6.
18. Malik R, Aneni EC, Shahrayar S, Freitas WM, Ali SS, Veledar E, et al. Elevated serum uric acid is associated with vascular inflammation but not coronary artery calcification in the healthy octogenarians: the Brazilian study on healthy aging. Aging Clin Exp Res. 2016;28(2):359–62.
19. Cicero AF, Rosticci M, Cagnati M, Urso R, Scapagnini G, Morbini M, et al. Serum uric acid and markers of low-density lipoprotein oxidation in nonsmoking healthy subjects: data from the Brisighella heart study. Pol Arch Med Wewn. 2014;124(12):661–8.
20. Ferrucci L, Corsi A, Lauretani F, Bandinelli S, Bartali B, Taub DD, et al. The origins of age-related proinflammatory state. Blood. 2005;105(6):2294–9.
21. Fagiolo U, Cossarizza A, Scala E, Fanales BE, Ortolani C, Cozzi E, et al. Increased cytokine production in mononuclear cells of healthy elderly people. Eur J Immunol. 1993;23(9):2375–8.
22. Fröhlich M, Imhof A, Berg G, Hutchinson WL, Pepys MB, Boeing H, et al. Association between C-reactive protein and features of the metabolic syndrome: a population-based study. Diabetes Care. 2000;23(12):1835–9.
23. Ruggiero C, Cherubini A, Ble A, Bos AJ, Maggio M, Dixit VD, et al. Uric acid and inflammatory markers. Eur Heart J. 2006;27(10):1174–81.
24. Tsai WC, Huang YY, Lin CC, Li WT, Lee CH, Chen JY, et al. Uric acid is an independent predictor of arterial stiffness in hypertensive patients. Heart Vessel. 2009;24(5):371–5.
25. Kanbay M, Yilmaz MI, Sonmez A, Turgut F, Saglam M, Cakir E, et al. Serum uric acid level and endothelial dysfunction in patients with nondiabetic chronic kidney disease. Am J Nephrol. 2011;33(4):298–304.
26. Ma QQ, Yang XJ, Yang NQ, Liu L, Li XD, Zhu K, et al. Study on the levels of uric acid and high-sensitivity C-reactive protein in ACS patients and their relationships with the extent of the coronary artery lesion. Eur Rev Med Pharmacol Sci. 2016;20(20):4294–8.
27. Dehghan A, Van HM, Sijbrands EJ, Hofman A, Witteman JC. High serum uric acid as a novel risk factor for type 2 diabetes. Diabetes Care. 2008;31(2):361–2.
28. Kang DH, Park SK, Lee IK, Johnson RJ. Uric acid-induced C-reactive protein expression: implication on cell proliferation and nitric oxide production of human vascular cells. J Am SocNephrol. 2005;16(12):3553–62.
29. Johnson RJ, Rodriguez-Iturbe B, Kang DH, Feig DI, Herrera-Acosta J. A unifying pathway for essential hypertension. Am J Hypertens. 2005;18(3):431–40.
30. Kanellis J, Watanabe S, Li JH, Kang DH, Li P, Nakagawa T, Wamsley A, Sheikh-Hamad D, Lan HY, Feng L, Johnson RJ. Uric acid stimulates monocyte chemoattractant protein-1 production in vascular smooth muscle cells via mitogen-activated protein kinase and cyclooxygenase-2. Hypertension. 2003;41(6):1287–93.
31. Spiga R, Marini MA, Mancuso E, Di FC, Fuoco A, Perticone F, et al. Uric acid is associated with inflammatory biomarkers and induces inflammation via activating the NF-κB signaling pathway in HepG2 cells. Arterioscler Thromb Vasc Biol. 2017;37(6):1241–9.
32. Lai W, Tang Y, Huang XR, Ming-Kuen Tang P, Xu A, Szalai AJ, et al. C-reactive protein promotes acute kidney injury via Smad3-dependent inhibition of CDK2/cyclinE. Kidney Int. 2016;90(3):610–26.
33. Liu F, Chen HY, Huang XR, Chung AC, Zhou L, Fu P, et al. C-reactive protein promotes diabetic kidney disease ina mouse model of type 1 diabetes. Diabetologia. 2011;54(10):2713–23.
34. Li Z, Chung AC, Zhou L, Huang XR, Liu F, Fu P, et al. C-reactive protein promotes acute renal inflammation and fibrosis in unilateral ureteral obstructive nephropathy in mice. Lab Investig. 2011;91(6):837–51.
35. El-Sheakh AR, Ghoneim HA, Suddek GM, Ammar ES. Attenuation of oxidative stress, inflammation, and endothelial dysfunction inhypercholesterolemic rabbits by allicin. Can J Physiol Pharmacol. 2016;94(2):216–24.
36. Lu YX, Zhang Q, Li J, Sun YX, Wang LY, Cheng WM, Hu XY. Antidiabetic effects of total flavonoids from Litsea Coreana leve on fat-fed, streptozotocin-induced type 2 diabetic rats. Am J Chin Med. 2010;38(4):713–25.
37. Bian GX, Li GG, Yang Y, Liu RT, Ren JP, Wen LQ, Guo SM, Lu QJ. Madecassoside reduces ischemia-Reperfusioninjury on regional ischemia induced heartinfarction in rat. Biol Pharm Bull. 2008;31(3):458–63.

The baseline levels and risk factors for high-sensitive C-reactive protein in Chinese healthy...

247

38. Wang D, Zhang X, Li D, Hao W, Meng F, Wang B, Han J, Zheng Q. Kaempferide protects against myocardial ischemia/reperfusion injury through activation of the PI3K/Akt/GSK-3β pathway. Mediat Inflamm 2017; 5278218. doi: https://doi.org/10.1155/2017/5278218.

39. El-Awady MS, Nader MA, Sharawy MH. The inhibition of inducible nitric oxide synthase and oxidative stress by agmatine attenuates vascular dysfunction in rat acute endotoxemicmodel. Environ Toxicol Pharmacol. 2017;10(55):74–80.

40. Labonté ME, Dewailly E, Chateau DM, Couture P, Lamarche B. Population-based study of high plasma C-reactive protein concentrations among the Inuit of Nunavik. Int J Circumpolar Health. 2012:71. https://doi.org/10.3402/ijch.v71i0.19066.

41. Riaz M, Fawwad A, Hydrie MZ, Basit A, Shera AS. Is there any association of serum high-sensitivity C-reactive protein with various risk factors for metabolic syndrome in a healthy adult population of karachi, Pakistan? Metab Syndr Relat Disord. 2011;9(3):177–82.

42. Wijsman CA, Mooijaart SP, Westendorp RG, Maier AB. Responsiveness of the innate immune system and glucose concentrations in the oldest old. Age (Dordr). 2012;34(4):983–6.

43. Costello WR, Ryff CD, Coe CL. Aging and low-grade inflammation reduce renal function in middle-aged and older adults in Japan and the USA. Age (Dordr). 2015;37(4):9808.

44. Liu W, Yu F, Wu Y, Fang X, Hu W, Chen J, et al. A retrospective analysis of kidney function and risk factors by chronic kidney disease epidemiology collaboration (CKD-EPI) equation in elderly Chinese patients. Ren Fail. 2015; 37(8):1323–8.

45. Keller CR, Odden MC, Fried LF, Newman AB, Angleman S, Green CA, et al. Kidney function and markers of inflammation in elderly persons without chronic kidney disease: the health, aging, and body composition study. Kidney Int. 2007;71(3):239–44.

26

Interventions to restore appropriate immune function in the elderly

Richard Aspinall[1,3*] and Pierre Olivier Lang[2,3]

Abstract

Advanced age is one indicator of likely immune dysfunction. As worldwide, the global population contains progressively more and more older individuals there is likelihood of an increased prevalence and incidence of infectious diseases due to common and emergent pathogens. The resultant increase in mortality and morbidity would be matched by the risk of functional decline and disability. Maintaining immune function at a plateau throughout life may therefore be associated with considerable cost savings. The aim of improving immune function in older individuals may be achieved through considering a therapeutic approach to rejuvenate, stimulate or support the indigenous immune system to perform in a more optimal manner. In terms of cost effectiveness a therapeutic approach may prove difficult because of issues associated with; identifying those who would benefit the most from this treatment, identifying the type of treatment which would suit them and identifying whether the treatment was successful. The alternative of supporting or providing a stronger stimulus through vaccination, whilst more cost effective, may be a more valuable option in the short term. Both approaches will be addressed in this review.

Background

The slow and inexorable increase in the number of older individuals worldwide over the next few decades will have a considerable impact on healthcare services and also on the epidemiology of transmissible and non transmissible diseases. The latter are expected to reach unprecedent rates [1, 2]. Those over the age of 65 currently travel more frequently and more widely than either their parents or grandparents [3]. They are also physically more active than their counterparts a few decades ago and these factors will play a role in changing the epidemiology of disease. Another factor contributing to the problem is the way the globe is now so closely networked that any individual or any pathogen may cross the planet within hours, as has been reported recently with H5N1, H1N1, MERS, SRAS, Chikungunya, and other emerging pathogens outbreaks [4, 5]. Also we must include into this algorithm the increased vulnerability in part, due to the decline in immune functioning in this older group. All together, these factors will contribute to shift in the pattern of common and emerging infectious diseases.

* Correspondence: richard.aspinall@anglia.ac.uk
[1]Rivock Ltd, Bury St Edmunds, UK
[3]Anglia Ruskin University, Cambridge, UK
Full list of author information is available at the end of the article

Pre-emptive action is required to preserve this growing sector of the general population and to keep them functionally independent in their daily lives. Whilst vaccination is one of the most effective medical interventions ever introduced and prevents millions of cases of infections worldwide every year, vaccines are often thought to be less effective in providing protection in this older section of society. One major reason for this statement is again the decline seen in effective immunity in this population. Studies from several countries have reported that the immune system declines with age indicating the global nature of this problem, but there are fewer studies which have sought the solution to this problem. One approach has been to try to restore immunity within this population to something akin to that seen in younger individuals. Another has been to take a more practical approach believing that a weaker immune system may be provoked into providing a response if the stimulus is considerably strengthened and enhanced. Both approaches will be discussed in this review.

Recipients

Identification of individuals who would receive specific therapy to restore their immune function is very challenging. The main issue is to how to recognise an individual who is not immune competent enough to deal with new and/or common antigens but who still seems healthy. This has been approached in a very pragmatic manner by some policy makers. To the outsider, it would appear that decisions have been made in the following way

(i) Immune senescence or immune insufficiency is associated with old age.
(ii) Individuals are considered old when they reach a specific age, frequently thought of as around 60-65 in developed and developing countries because after this age people receive benefits and concessions.
(iii) Since individuals who are over 65 are old they must have dysfunctional immune systems.
(iv) So everyone over 65 should be offered vaccines which are supplemented with adjuvants or increased amounts of antigen to compensate for immune decline.

Our issue with such a dogmatic approach is with the idea of using precisely defined criteria, which in this case is age, with immune dysfunction which is imprecisely defined and only weakly linked with the ageing process. What we believe to be required is a means of grading immune functioning quantitatively and qualitatively [6].

Appropriate immune functioning

One of the problems with the immune system is that its action is invisible and hence not easy to quantify. The immune system provides protection from a series of potential pathogens which we may encounter daily. Their failure to cause disease is neither recognised nor perceived. We have no way of counting the rate of our exposure to pathogenic organisms and we only become aware of the role of the immune system in our survival when it is lacking or through the incidence of some specific diseases. Of course, individuals who are immune deficient show an increased susceptibility to opportunistic pathogens, poorer responses to vaccination, and greater likelihood of morbidity and mortality associated with infections. However, infections are not restricted to those individuals, and healthy people with normal functioning immunity also suffer from viral, bacteria, fungal and parasitic infections.

As a consequence, and in comparison to organs such as the skin where there is greater visibility of age-related changes and methods for measuring them, neither device nor method exists for assessing an individual's overall immune capacity and its rate of change. People can be identified after vaccination with for example influenza antigen whose responses are less than adequate making them liable to infection with the corresponding virus strains. But this is one of a few cases following vaccination where immunity is associated with an a priori defined amount of specific antibody. Clinicians wishing to

measure immune competency may call for full blood counts, T and B cell counts including their subsets, the quantity of immunoglobulin in the serum and the presence of specific antibodies. Whilst this provides a general overview of some of the elements of the immune system it does not provide a functional measure of the capacity of an individual to respond to a specific threat unless values are well below the normal boundaries. An older individual with immune parameters within the normal levels who may have immune dysfunction would thus not be easily identified. So any attempt to restore immunity in older individuals first requires that simple methods of assessment are derived to determine the effectiveness of the process as a whole. These assessment methods must (i) be function related; (ii) must be relatively rapid in providing results; (iii) must be relatively non-invasive; and (iv) require relatively simple forms of equipment.

In view of these guidelines it becomes apparent that such measures as improved responses to vaccination (against for example untreated age matched controls) or reduction in the incidence of infection may be acceptable as measures in the long-term but in the short-term there needs to be some more immediate indicators.

Contributing factors to immune decline

Change in the fat content of tissues varies between individuals and over the life course. Overall, the body composition changes with age and there is a gradual loss of lean body mass combined with the accumulation of fatty tissue at different locations [7, 8]. Nowhere is this more apparent than in the primary lymphoid organs where the increase in adipocyte numbers leads to macroscopic changes in the colour of these tissues, and the loss of cellular niches and a gradual decline in their overall function as primary generator of lymphocytes. Reduction in the active area of thymus through fat accumulation leads to a loss of an adequate productive environment for thymocyte development and a consequent reduction in the thymic output [9–11]. Similarly the increase in the amount fat in the bone marrow with age as shown by its change in colour from red to yellow alters the ability of the marrow to provide a supportive framework for the production of B cells [12]. In addition to change in the rate of production of new lymphocytes, immune decline may also be linked to the longevity of specific lymphocyte clones. This is a complex process; since lymphocytes have a limited replicative lifespan and the faster more of them reach the limit through responding to antigen the more rapidly will be the onset of functional holes in the repertoire and an inability to respond to a specific challenge.

Adipose tissue expansion with age is also thought of as a major source of inflammation that has a marked influence on systemic metabolism and contributes to the onset of devastating conditions such as insulin resistance, type-2 diabetes, and cardiovascular disorders [13]. However, during the development of diet-induced obesity or age-associated adiposity, immunocompetent cells infiltrate and proliferate in the adipose tissue. Cells of the adaptive immune system, including T and B cells, thus contribute significantly to generate chronic and lowgrade inflammation. Lymphocytes regulate recruitment of innate immune cells into fat tissue, and hence produce a large panel of pro-inflammatory cytokines [14]. This influences the helpful-to-harmful inflammatory balance that, in turn, contributes to the age-associated functional decline in the immune system and the onset of conditions affecting health and well-being [15].

Approaches to restoration or stimulating immune function

In considering older individuals we may choose to improve their immunity specifically, non-specifically in the periphery, or consider rejuvenating their immune system through the reversal of the decline observed in their primary lymphoid organs. Each of these will be dealt with in turn.

Restoration through enhanced stimulation or metabolic manipulation

Nutrition

One of the issues which is often overlooked is the considerable amount of energy required to undertake an immune response. Naïve T cells which are normally in a close to quiescent state must shift to activation by changing their metabolism after encountering antigen. Successful activation is followed by an increased uptake of nutrients, increased mitochondrial oxidative phosphorylation and the cells metabolism becomes predominantly glycolytic. This shift presages the demand for energy and cell components precursors required for proliferation [16]. For many older individuals the necessary energy to make a successful immune response may be lacking because of either an inadequate diet or the change in the permeability of the gut to specific elements. Insufficient energy to deliver an immune response which is adequate may be due to a number of simple reasons. For example one previous study indicated a significant association between inadequate calorie intake and being underweight in older people with deficient or poorly functioning dentition [17]. Studies in which the diet of older individuals was supplemented, with an energy source and trace elements revealed that treated individuals could produce a greater response to influenza [18–21] and pneumococcal vaccination [22, 23]. Changes in the permeability of the gut alter the uptake of trace elements such as zinc. The critical role of zinc for the immune system comes from studies on zinc deficient individuals who may have

thymic atrophy, lymphopenia and recurrent infection [24] however studies on zinc supplementation of the diet of older individuals has failed to provide a conclusive result which would be beneficial to vaccine practitioners [25]. The immunomodulatory role and the potential immune enhancer property of vitamin D have been highlighted recently. Studies which have looked at ability of vitamin D supplements to improve the effectiveness of vaccines provide conflicting information [26].

Rapamycin

The fungus *Streptomyces hygroscopicus* found in a soil sample from Easter Island was shown to produces a macrolide compound named rapamycin which was subsequently found to inhibit proliferation of mammalian cells and to possess immunosuppressive properties. These properties led to it being approved by the Food and Drug Administration in the United States for cancer therapy such as renal cell carcinoma. The normal oral dose for cancer patients would be in the region of 10 mg a day. Later experiments in mouse models suggested that at lower doses rapamycin could improve response to influenza antigen possibly by inhibiting the formation of germinal centres thus reducing the production of high affinity antibodies but permitting the production of lower affinity antibody and increasing the presence of influenza-specific IgM antibodies [27]. These results prompted trials in humans where recipients received 0.5 mg daily, or 5 or 20 mg weekly or placebo. After a six-week course and a two-week gap the recipients were vaccinated with the trivalent influenza vaccine. Those in the treatment group showed considerable and significant improvement in their immune response when compared to those in the placebo group [28].

Adjuvants

One approach to restoring an effective immune response to a vaccine antigen in older individuals and to ensure adequate levels of protection has been to introduce an adjuvant in the vaccine composition [29]. The classic adjuvant containing aluminium salts has more recently been replaced by oil in water emulsions which have been used with great effect to promote a response to a zoster subunit vaccine for example. However success with adjuvants is a double edged sword. In one study of those who received the adjuvanted herpes zoster subunit vaccine 81.5% showed injection site reactions and 66.1% showed systemic reactions [30]. The mechanisms of action of adjuvants are not entirely clear yet. It is thought that they may in part act as depots of antigen prolonging it presence in the periphery, or interact with pattern recognition elements on accessory cells, or stimulate a local inflammatory response so bringing more cells to the area [29]. Whilst adjuvants have been shown to be effective in improving vaccine related responses in older adults their use may be limited to vaccines which are given infrequently. For example it may not be wise to vaccinate an older individual every year for 30 years (from age 65 to 95) with an influenza vaccine supplemented with adjuvant. Used in such a way this may drive all specific clones of responding cells to reach their replicative limit sooner which may prove counterproductive.

Increased amounts of antigen

Increasing the amount of antigen within the dose of vaccine has been also shown to improve the response in older individuals, but not in a directly correlative manner. So, giving for example ten times the antigen dose will not produce a ten-fold increase in the immune response to the corresponding vaccine antigen. Vaccines with increased amounts of antigen include the influenza vaccine with four times the amount of antigen than the standard-dose vaccine (60 μg instead of 15 μg of haemagglutinin antigen for each of the three influenza A/H1N1, A/H3N2 and B strains) and Zostavax a live attenuated varicella zoster virus vaccine administered only to seniors, which contains more than 14 times the number of plaque forming units than the standard varicella vaccine recommended for children. This latter vaccine boosts immunity to the varicella zoster virus in older individuals and significantly reduces the incidence of herpes zoster and post-herpetic neuralgia [31].

Specific rejuvenation
Adoptive transfer of specific clones

One of the issues which is often considered to be a major problem in older people is latent virus infections. Control of these viruses is present throughout life but as we age this control begins to wain as seen with those harbouring the varicella zoster virus (human herpes virus 3 or HHV-3) who become susceptible to increased bouts of shingles the disease associated with herpes zoster and an increase in the prevalence of post herpetic neuralgia with age. Control of cytomegalovirus (CMV or HHV-5) has also been shown to decline with age with the appearance of detectable virus in the urine of older people [32]. Studies using the adoptive transfer of CMV specific CD8 T cells showed that overt disease could be controlled in individuals post-transplant [33, 34]. Whilst this treatment is still at an early phase and unlikely to be offered to older individuals in the near future more recent work suggests that virus specific T cells could be generated from autochthonous stem cells [35].

Non-specific rejuvenation
Blood transfusion

Heterochronic parabiosis; the surgical joining of two animals of different ages such that they have a common

blood circulation has been used successfully in the past to identify means of ameliorating age related changes in the cardiac system [36] and in cognitive function [37]. Experiments to modify the immune system of the older partner of the parabiont by an extrinsic factor from the younger parabiont revealed that whilst pre-T cells from either parabiont could seed the opposing thymus and undergo thymopoiesis there was no reversal of thymic atrophy suggesting that the defect was in the thymic environment [38, 39]. Immune rejuvenation by a serum based factor is therefore ruled out as an option but the idea of rejuvenating the peripheral immune system by the adoptive transfer of blood from younger to older individuals has a long history. In the early 1920's Prof A.A. Bogdanov tested the hypothesis that the transfusion of blood from young into older individuals may rejuvenate the latter. He experimented on himself, accepting transfused blood on up to 11 occasions, before the 12th transfusion killed him in 1928 [40].

Half a litre of blood (500 ml) is the amount normally donated for transfusion and this amount of blood will contain approximately 7.5×10^8 T cells. In individuals aged 20 to mid 30's approximately 50% or more of these cells will be naïve and the rest memory cells. It would seem feasible to collect this amount of blood and extract the leukocytes on a regular basis and then store them in ampoules in liquid nitrogen until the individual becomes much older. The memory cells will have a repertoire dependent on the pathogens and antigens already encountered and so should be slightly more restricted in terms of its diversity than the naïve T cell population. The latter should contain recent thymic emigrants and so have a diverse receptor repertoire.

In older individuals age related changes in both the peripheral T and B pool of cells include the presence of holes in the antigen specific receptor repertoire which consequently is diminished and the presence of lymphocytes at or close to their limit of replication. Re-transfusion of leukocytes at a later stage of life could provide a means of combatting both of these problems. There are of course issues around how many cells to transfuse back into a recipient, whether this number would integrate easily into the indigenous population and whether the receptors for specific pathogens would be present in the transfused lymphocytes. Preliminary answers to these questions have been provided by animal work [41], but more work is needed on human volunteers to determine these parameters. Despite this, several companies have grown up offering a service for individuals to collect their leukocytes early in their lifespan and store them in lymphocytes in liquid nitrogen for a prolonged period so that they can be reinfused at later date.

Interleukin 7

Interleukin 7 (IL-7) is a type 1 short chain cytokine produced by the stromal cells of primary and secondary lymphoid organs which binds to a cell surface receptor composed of an IL-7 specific alpha chain (CD127) and a common gamma chain (CD132). The latter is termed common since it is used as one of the receptor chains for cytokines IL-2, 4, 9, 15 and 21 [42]. Expression of CD127 and CD132 together are found at several stages of the T cell development pathway from early progenitors to memory cells. At the early intrathymic stages of the T cell pathway the IL-7:IL-7R interaction is responsible for ensuring cell survival [43] may be responsible for generating T cell receptor diversity [44] and is associated with clonal expansion of mature thymocytes prior to their export to the naïve T cell pool [45]. In peripheral T cells the IL-7 ligand receptor interaction is mainly associated with clonal maintenance through ensuring cell survival and proliferation in both the naïve and memory T cell pools [46]. The potential for IL-7 to act as an immune rejuvenating agent came from initial studies by Bhatia et al. [47] on young mice treated for prolonged periods with anti-IL-7 antibody. These mice showed severe thymic atrophy and a decline in thymic cellularity similar to that seen in older animals. Treatment of old mice with IL-7 could reverse age-related atrophy of the thymus, leading to a restoration of thymic output and an improvement in peripheral T cell function [43, 48]. One striking feature of using IL-7 to reverse thymic atrophy was the importance of the quantity of IL-7 present in the thymus as shown by experiments in which three lines of transgenic mice were generated in which the IL-7 gene was placed under the control of an lcx promoter. Each line produced different amounts of IL-7 and the line which produced the most (termed TgB) showed lower levels of thymocytes numbers when compared with wild type controls and were found to have a bottleneck in differentiation at the early stage of T cell development [49]. Later work suggest that high levels of IL-7 antagonise Notch signalling and as such impact on the choice of T versus B cell lineage by stem cells in the thymus [50]. Rejuvenation of immunity in old female rhesus macaques treated with recombinant simian IL-7 prior to vaccination with influenza showed an increase in thymic output and higher haemagglutinin titres in treated animals compared to saline treated controls [51]. The first clinical trial using IL-7 examined the therapeutic effects of IL-7 administered to humans with metastatic cancer [52]. A more recent placebo controlled double blind phase IIa trial in patients with lymphopaenic metastatic breast cancer [53], some of whom received recombinant IL-7 as part of their treatment regimen reported encouraging results with IL-7 inducing a significant increase in T cell numbers when delivered before chemotherapy. In another study on HIV infected patients who were also receiving antiviral therapy the data suggest that repeated cycles of recombinant human IL-7

were tolerated quite well by the recipients and sustained T cell restoration was seen in the majority of the participants of the study [53]. To date no trial has reported on the treatment of healthy older individuals who have received IL-7 therapy.

Surgical or chemical castration

Early work on rodents showed that surgical castration could lead to reversal of the age associated atrophy seen in the thymus [54, 55] although this has been reported to be transitory [56]. Chemical castration using luteinizing hormone releasing hormone agonists have been shown to be effective in inducing thymic regrowth in old rodents [57] and in old primates [58] through a mechanism which may involve the upregulation of Delta-like 4 a Notch ligand crucial for T cell differentiation [59]. Experiments in humans suggest that this might be an attractive approach to improve immunity in older males [60, 61], however the side effects associated with the treatment may mitigate against this choice of approach.

Keratinocyte growth factor

Keratinocyte Growth Factor (KGF) is a member of the fibroblast growth factor family, a family which contains secreted proteins which signal to receptor tyrosine kinases and intracellular non-signalling proteins which act as co-factors for voltage gated calcium channels [62]. KGF is the 7th member of this family and a secreted signalling molecule which interacts with its receptor expressed on thymic epithelial cells and induces the proliferation of thymic epithelial cell progenitors and mature epithelial cells in fetal thymic organ cultures [63]. Early experiments in murine system suggested that the subcutaneous administration of KGF to mice for 3 consecutive days at 5 mg/Kg per day enhanced thymopoeisis for almost 2 months. Moreover the treatment restored thymopoeisis in old mice [64]. These results prompted experiments in primates which were reconstituted with CD34$^+$ peripheral blood progenitor cells after irradiation. Animals receiving treatment with KGF showed increased frequencies of naïve T cells in their lymph nodes compared with controls and more cells recognised as recent thymic emigrants. In addition, KGF treated animals preserved their thymic architecture up to at least 12 months after the reconstitution [65].

Palifermin is a recombinant form of KGF of bacterial origin which has been used to treat patients receiving chemotherapy or radiation therapy to stimulate the growth of cells in the mucosal barrier. The positive non-human primate results prompted experiments using Palifermin on patients with HIV-1 infection who were receiving antiretroviral therapy. The hypothesis was that poor CD4 levels in these patients was due to reduced thymic function and treatment with Palifermin should improve the blood profile of CD4 cells in these patients. However a randomised double blind placebo controlled trial in HIV infected patients receiving ART [66] revealed no significant change in either the numbers of recent thymic emigrants, naïve cell numbers or thymic size. The dose range used in these studies was from 20 to 60µg/Kg which is considerable less than the 5 mg/Kg given to the mice in the original model and may be the reason why no change was seen alternatively it is possible that the structure of the thymus was such that it was irreparable within the time frame of the experiment.

Methods of assessment

To illustrate the problems associated with assessing overall immunity let us consider the example of blood pressure management. Years of gathering and analysing data from blood pressure measurement has enabled physicians to derive a normal range for blood pressure values for specific ages and/or specific health status. Thus different thresholds have been tailored according to the best risk/benefit ratio to initiate lowering blood pressure drugs for robust, frail and terminally ill individuals. Specific target values under treatment have been also personalized [67]. No such scheme currently exists for the immune system. Moreover, the challenge to face with the immune system is it's degree of complexity and predicting individual immune capacity and responsiveness to specific antigen using a single and robust method able to distinguish between a robust, frail and deficient system would be very challenging [68].

Using vaccine response as a direct method of assessment

The assessment of an individual immune responsiveness by confronting the immune system with common or new vaccine antigens and hence quantifying the quality of the immune functioning in its whole is a desirable challenge. For example, the response to influenza vaccine is blunted in older people so one method of determining the effectiveness of a rejuvenation/restoration therapy has been to carry out randomised clinical trials comparing a treated aged group with a placebo treated control group and assessing the difference in the titre of the hemagglutination inhibition antibody levels. This approach was used successfully in the rapalogue trials [28], but has the drawback that large numbers of individuals have to be recruited for each arm to ensure statistically significant results are achieved.

Longitudinal studies in which the same individual is followed and tested before and after treatment may appear more preferable but has the problem in that if vaccination is used as an assay system it would have to be given before and the after the treatment. This may prove a problem especially when the repeat vaccination is against previously used strains because high pre-vaccination hemagglutination antibody inhibition titres because the history of previously encountered influenza subtypes impacts the ensuing immune response [69–71].

Equally well, with other vaccines such as pneumococcal polysaccharides vaccines subsequent repetitive vaccination would fail to show benefit because of the hyporesponsiveness [72] seen on revaccination. Another option is to choose to issue the participants with illness diaries which monitor the number of infections during the period of the study and also their duration [73]. Compliance is often a factor with this approach as is veracity. Subjective assessment whilst sometimes necessary may not be optimal which is why many have chosen a more objective approach and taken to using indirect methods of assessment.

Indirect methods of assessment

Clinicians can have access to a large battery of biological tests. They include complete blood counts, lymphocyte subsets, serum immunoglobulin levels and the presence of specific antibodies, none of which could be used to assess immune rejuvenation satisfactorily. This is principally because these values can be similar in individuals who are immune competent and those who provide a less than adequate response. Approaches to identifying improvements in global immunity have included measuring change in the numbers of recent thymic emigrants [51], the presence of increased numbers of naïve lymphocytes or changes in subsets cells at different stages of differentiation [74], cutaneous skin responses [75] or changes in the parameters [76] of the immune risk phenotype [77].

Conclusion

The issue at the core of the question about whether we can rejuvenate the immune response is one of measurement. We currently have no method of measuring the overall immune capacity of an individual. Often this measure is through clinical observation that the patient has infections which are unusual, persistent, or alternatively which have become recurrent or have progressed to becoming systemic. These are often subjective assessments and there are no objective laboratory based tests which provide a measure of overall immune capacity. This despite a long history of assays which quantify a response to an antigen through demonstrating the antibody titre or assessing an individual T cell specific response to a viral glycoprotein. We only know the level of response associated with protection from a disease for a small handful of pathogens.

There is no normal range for immune activity and until we can provide a method for measuring this activity we have firstly no means of determining whether an individual is in need of therapy and secondly what the effect of that rejuvenation therapy may be. The complexity of the problem is also added to by the identification that a successful immune response is not only dependant on producing enough specific antibody of effector T cells. Susceptibility to disease is also reliant on a number of innate immune system barriers, such as the integrity of the skin, the flushing action of tears, saliva or urine, the action of ciliated epithelium and mucous as well as the response from neutrophils, macrophages and natural killer cells.

Funding

Not applicable.

Authors' contributions

RA and POL participated in drafting the manuscript. Both authors read and approved the final manuscript.

Competing interests

The authors declare that they have no competing interests.

Author details

[1]Rivock Ltd, Bury St Edmunds, UK. [2]Geriatric and Geriatric Rehabilitation Division, Department of Medicine, University Hospital of Lausanne, Lausanne, Switzerland. [3]Anglia Ruskin University, Cambridge, UK.

References

1. Fulop T, et al. Aging, frailty and age-related diseases. Biogerontology. 2010; 11:547–63. https://doi.org/10.1007/s10522-010-9287-2.

2. Lang PO, Mitchell WA, Lapenna A, Pitts D, Aspinall R. Immunological pathogenesis of main aged-related disease and frailty: role of immunosenescence. Eur Geriatric Med. 2010;1:9.

3. Cliff A, Haggett P. Time, travel and infection. Br Med Bull. 2004;69:87–99. https://doi.org/10.1093/bmb/ldh011.

4. Lang, P. O., Loulergue, P. & Aspinall, R. Chikungunya Virus Infection: Why Should U.S. Geriatricians Be Aware of It? J Am Geriatr Soc. 2017. https://doi.org/10.1111/jgs.15104.

5. Yin Y, Wunderink RG. MERS, SARS and other coronaviruses as causes of pneumonia. Respirology. 2017; https://doi.org/10.1111/resp.13196.

6. Aspinall R, Lang PO. Vaccination choices for older people, looking beyond age specific approaches. Expert Rev Vaccines. 2018;17:23-30. https://doi.org/10.1080/14760584.2018.1411197.

7. Lang PO, Trivalle C, Vogel T, Proust J, Papazian JP. Markers of metabolic and cardiovascular health in adults: comparative analysis of DEXA-based body composition components and BMI categories. J Cardiol. 2015;65:42–9. https://doi.org/10.1016/j.jjcc.2014.03.010.

8. Lang PO, et al. Is obesity a marker of robustness in vulnerable hospitalized aged populations? Prospective, multicenter cohort study of 1 306 acutely ill patients. J Nutr Health Aging. 2014;18:66–74. https://doi.org/10.1007/s12603-013-0352-9.

9. Dixit VD. Thymic fatness and approaches to enhance thymopoietic fitness in aging. Curr Opin Immunol. 2010;22:521–8. https://doi.org/10.1016/j.coi.2010.06.010.

10. Yang H, et al. Obesity accelerates thymic aging. Blood. 2009;114:3803–12. https://doi.org/10.1182/blood-2009-03-213595.

11. Yang H, Youm YH, Dixit VD. Inhibition of thymic adipogenesis by caloric restriction is coupled with reduction in age-related thymic involution. J Immunol. 2009;183:3040–52. https://doi.org/10.4049/jimmunol.0900562.

12. Siegrist CA, Aspinall R. B-cell responses to vaccination at the extremes of age. Nat Rev Immunol. 2009;9:185–94. https://doi.org/10.1038/nri2508.

13. Bharath LP, Ip BC, Nikolajczyk BS. Adaptive immunity and metabolic health: harmony becomes dissonant in obesity and aging. Compr Physiol. 2017;7: 1307–37. https://doi.org/10.1002/cphy.c160042.

14. Choi CHJ, Cohen P. Adipose crosstalk with other cell types in health and disease. Exp Cell Res. 2017;360:6–11. https://doi.org/10.1016/j.yexcr.2017.04.022.

15. Calder PC, et al. Health relevance of the modification of low grade inflammation in ageing (inflammageing) and the role of nutrition. Ageing Res Rev. 2017;40:95–119. https://doi.org/10.1016/j.arr.2017.09.001.

16. Johnson MO, Siska PJ, Contreras DC, Rathmell JC. Nutrients and the microenvironment to feed a T cell army. Semin Immunol. 2016;28:505–13. https://doi.org/10.1016/j.smim.2016.09.003.

17. Seman K, Abdul Manaf H, Ismail AR. Association between functional dentition with inadequate calorie intake and underweight in elderly people living in "Pondok" in Kelantan. Arch Orofac Sci. 2007;2(1):10-9.

18. Langkamp-Henken B, et al. Nutritional formula improved immune profiles of seniors living in nursing homes. J Am Geriatr Soc. 2006;54:1861–70. https://doi.org/10.1111/j.1532-5415.2006.00982.x.

19. Akatsu H, et al. Enhanced vaccination effect against influenza by prebiotics in elderly patients receiving enteral nutrition. Geriatr Gerontol Int. 2016;16: 205–13. https://doi.org/10.1111/ggi.12454.

20. Vidal K, et al. Immunomodulatory effects of dietary supplementation with a milk-based wolfberry formulation in healthy elderly: a randomized, double-blind, placebo-controlled trial. Rejuvenation Res. 2012;15:89–97. https://doi.org/10.1089/rej.2011.1241.

21. Girodon F, et al. Impact of trace elements and vitamin supplementation on immunity and infections in institutionalized elderly patients: a randomized controlled trial. MIN VIT AOX Geriatr Netw Arch Intern Med. 1999;159:748–54.

22. Freeman SL, et al. Dairy proteins and the response to pneumovax in senior citizens: a randomized, double-blind, placebo-controlled pilot study. Ann N Y Acad Sci. 2010;1190:97–103. https://doi.org/10.1111/j.1749-6632.2009.05264.x.

23. Moriguti JC, Ferriolli E, Donadi EA, Marchini JS. Effects of arginine supplementation on the humoral and innate immune response of older people. Eur J Clin Nutr. 2005;59:1362–6. https://doi.org/10.1038/sj.ejcn.1602247.

24. Pae M, Meydani SN, Wu D. The role of nutrition in enhancing immunity in aging. Aging Dis. 2012;3:91–129.

25. Braga CB, et al. Effect of zinc supplementation on serological response to vaccination against streptococcus Pneumoniae in patients undergoing chemotherapy for colorectal cancer. Nutr Cancer. 2015;67:926–32. https://doi.org/10.1080/01635581.2015.1053497.

26. Lang PO, Aspinall R. Vitamin D status and the host resistance to infections: what it is currently (not) understood. Clin Ther. 2017;39:930–45. https://doi.org/10.1016/j.clinthera.2017.04.004.

27. Keating R, et al. The kinase mTOR modulates the antibody response to provide cross-protective immunity to lethal infection with influenza virus. Nat Immunol. 2013;14:1266–76. https://doi.org/10.1038/ni.2741.

28. Mannick, J. B. et al. mTOR inhibition improves immune function in the elderly. Science translational medicine 6, 268ra179, https://doi.org/10.1126/scitranslmed.3009892 (2014).

29. Lefebvre JS, Haynes L. Vaccine strategies to enhance immune responses in the aged. Curr Opin Immunol. 2013;25:523–8. https://doi.org/10.1016/j.coi.2013.05.014.

30. Cunningham AL, et al. Efficacy of the herpes zoster subunit vaccine in adults 70 years of age or older. N Engl J Med. 2016;375:1019–32. https://doi.org/10.1056/NEJMoa1603800.

31. Levin MJ. Immune senescence and vaccines to prevent herpes zoster in older persons. Curr Opin Immunol. 2012;24:494–500. https://doi.org/10.1016/j.coi.2012.06.002.

32. Stowe RP, et al. Chronic herpesvirus reactivation occurs in aging. Exp Gerontol. 2007;42:563–70. https://doi.org/10.1016/j.exger.2007.01.005.

33. Cobbold M, et al. Adoptive transfer of cytomegalovirus-specific CTL to stem cell transplant patients after selection by HLA-peptide tetramers. J Exp Med. 2005;202:379–86. https://doi.org/10.1084/jem.20040613.

34. Neuenhahn, M. et al. Transfer of minimally manipulated CMV-specific T cells from stem cell or third-party donors to treat CMV infection after allo-HSCT. Leukemia : official journal of the Leukemia Society of America, Leukemia Research Fund, U.K 31, 2161-2171, https://doi.org/10.1038/leu.2017.16 (2017).

35. Dave H, et al. Toward a rapid production of multivirus-specific T cells targeting BKV, adenovirus, CMV, and EBV from umbilical cord blood. Mol Ther Methods Clin Dev. 2017;5:13–21. https://doi.org/10.1016/j.omtm.2017.02.001.

36. Loffredo FS, et al. Growth differentiation factor 11 is a circulating factor that reverses age-related cardiac hypertrophy. Cell. 2013;153:828–39. https://doi.org/10.1016/j.cell.2013.04.015.

37. Villeda SA, et al. Young blood reverses age-related impairments in cognitive function and synaptic plasticity in mice. Nat Med. 2014;20:659–63. https://doi.org/10.1038/nm.3569.

38. Davies J, Pulko V, Thompson H, Nikolich-Zugich J. Hetero.Chronic parabiosis: allowing the dissection of the aged immune system. J Immunol. 2015;194:1.

39. Pishel I, et al. Accelerated aging versus rejuvenation of the immune system in heterochronic parabiosis. Rejuvenation Res. 2012;15:239–48. https://doi.org/10.1089/rej.2012.1331.

40. Huestis D, Alexander W. Bogdanov: the forgotten pioneer of blood transfusion. Transfus Med Rev. 2007;21:337–40. https://doi.org/10.1016/j.tmrv.2007.05.008.

41. Aspinall R, Govind S, Lapenna A, Lang PO. Dose response kinetics of CD8 lymphocytes from young animals transfused into old animals and challenged with influenza. Immun Ageing : I & A. 2013;10:34. https://doi.org/10.1186/1742-4933-10-34.

42. Mackall CL, Fry TJ, Gress RE. Harnessing the biology of IL-7 for therapeutic application. Nat Rev Immunol. 2011;11:330–42. https://doi.org/10.1038/nri2970.

43. Andrew D, Aspinall R. Il-7 and not stem cell factor reverses both the increase in apoptosis and the decline in thymopoiesis seen in aged mice. J Immunol. 2001;166:1524–30.

44. Muegge K, Vila MP, Durum SK. Interleukin-7: a cofactor for V(D)J rearrangement of the T cell receptor beta gene. Science. 1993;261:93–5.

45. Lundstrom W, Fewkes NM, Mackall CL. IL-7 in human health and disease. Semin Immunol. 2012;24:218–24. https://doi.org/10.1016/j.smim.2012.02.005.

46. Fry TJ, Mackall CL. The many faces of IL-7: from lymphopoiesis to peripheral T cell maintenance. J Immunol. 2005;174:6571–6.

47. Bhatia SK, Tygrett LT, Grabstein KH, Waldschmidt TJ. The effect of in vivo IL-7 deprivation on T cell maturation. J Exp Med. 1995;181:1399–409.

48. Henson SM, Snelgrove R, Hussell T, Wells DJ, Aspinall R. An IL-7 fusion protein that shows increased thymopoietic ability. J Immunol. 2005;175:4112–8.

49. El Kassar N, et al. A dose effect of IL-7 on thymocyte development in Blood. 2004;104:1419–27. https://doi.org/10.1182/blood-2004-01-0201.

50. El-Kassar N, et al. High levels of IL-7 cause dysregulation of thymocyte development. Int Immunol. 2012;24:661–71. https://doi.org/10.1093/intimm/dxs067.

51. Aspinall R, et al. Old rhesus macaques treated with interleukin-7 show increased TREC levels and respond well to influenza vaccination. Rejuvenation Res. 2007;10:5–17. https://doi.org/10.1089/rej.2006.9098.

52. Rosenberg SA, et al. IL-7 administration to humans leads to expansion of CD8+ and CD4+ cells but a relative decrease of CD4 T-regulatory cells. J Immunother. 2006;29:313–9. https://doi.org/10.1097/01.cji.0000210386.55951.c2.

53. Tredan O, et al. ELYPSE-7: a randomized placebo-controlled phase IIa trial with CYT107 exploring the restoration of CD4+ lymphocyte count in lymphopenic metastatic breast cancer patients. Ann Oncol. 2015;26:1353–62. https://doi.org/10.1093/annonc/mdv173.

54. Goldberg GL, et al. Sex steroid ablation enhances lymphoid recovery following autologous hematopoietic stem cell transplantation. Transplantation. 2005;80:1604–13.

55. Heng TS, et al. Effects of castration on thymocyte development in two different models of thymic involution. J Immunol. 2005;175:2982–93.

56. Min H, Montecino-Rodriguez E, Dorshkind K. Reassessing the role of growth hormone and sex steroids in thymic involution. Clin Immunol. 2006;118:117–23. https://doi.org/10.1016/j.clim.2005.08.015.

57. Greenstein BD, Fitzpatrick FT, Kendall MD, Wheeler MJ. Regeneration of the thymus in old male rats treated with a stable analogue of LHRH. J Endocrinol. 1987;112:345–50.

58. Scalea JR, et al. The rejuvenating effects of leuprolide acetate on the aged baboon's thymus. Transpl Immunol. 2014;31:134–9. https://doi.org/10.1016/j.trim.2014.09.001.

59. Velardi E, et al. Sex steroid blockade enhances thymopoiesis by modulating notch signaling. J Exp Med. 2014;211:2341–9. https://doi.org/10.1084/jem.20131289.

60. Velardi E, Dudakov JA, van den Brink MR. Sex steroid ablation: an immunoregenerative strategy for immunocompromised patients. Bone Marrow Transplant. 2015;50(Suppl 2):S77–81. https://doi.org/10.1038/bmt.2015.101.

61. Sutherland JS, et al. Activation of thymic regeneration in mice and humans following androgen blockade. J Immunol. 2005;175:2741–53.

62. Ornitz DM, Itoh N. Fibroblast growth factors. Genome Biol. 2001;2(3): REVIEWS3005. Epub 2001 Mar 9.

63. Berzins SP, et al. Thymic regeneration: teaching an old immune system new tricks. Trends Mol Med. 2002;8:469–76.

64. Min D, et al. Sustained thymopoiesis and improvement in functional immunity induced by exogenous KGF administration in murine models of aging. Blood. 2007;109:2529–37. https://doi.org/10.1182/blood-2006-08-043794.

65. Seggewiss R, et al. Keratinocyte growth factor augments immune reconstitution after autologous hematopoietic progenitor cell transplantation in rhesus macaques. Blood. 2007;110:441–9. https://doi.org/10.1182/blood-2006-12-065623.

66. Jacobson JM, et al. A randomized controlled trial of palifermin (recombinant human keratinocyte growth factor) for the treatment of inadequate CD4+ T-lymphocyte recovery in patients with HIV-1 infection on antiretroviral therapy. J Acquir Immune Defic Syndr. 2014;66:399–406. https://doi.org/10.1097/QAI.0000000000000195.

67. Benetos A, et al. Polypharmacy in the aging patient: Management of Hypertension in octogenarians. JAMA. 2015;314:170–80. https://doi.org/10.1001/jama.2015.7517.

68. Lang PO, Govind S, Aspinall R. Reversing T cell immunosenescence: why, who, and how. Age. 2013;35:609–20. https://doi.org/10.1007/s11357-012-9393-y.

69. Lang PO, et al. Effectiveness of influenza vaccine in aging and older adults: comprehensive analysis of the evidence. Clin Interv Aging. 2012;7:55–64. https://doi.org/10.2147/CIA.S25215.

70. Pica N, et al. Hemagglutinin stalk antibodies elicited by the 2009 pandemic influenza virus as a mechanism for the extinction of seasonal H1N1 viruses. Proc Natl Acad Sci U S A. 2012;109:2573–8. https://doi.org/10.1073/pnas.1200039109.

71. Lang PO, Bonduelle O, Benhabiles N, Combadiere B. Prior contact with the 2000-2003 seasonal vaccines extends the 2009 pandei a/H1N1 vaccine specific immune protection to non-numoral compartments. Eur Geriatric Med. 2014;5:2.

72. Musher DM, et al. Safety and antibody response, including antibody persistence for 5 years, after primary vaccination or revaccination with pneumococcal polysaccharide vaccine in middle-aged and older adults. J Infect Dis. 2010;201:516–24. https://doi.org/10.1086/649839.

73. Percival SS. Aged garlic extract modifies human immunity. J Nutr. 2016;146: 433S–6S. https://doi.org/10.3945/jn.115.210427.

74. Moro-Garcia MA, et al. Oral supplementation with lactobacillus delbrueckii subsp. bulgaricus 8481 enhances systemic immunity in elderly subjects. Age. 2013;35:1311–26. https://doi.org/10.1007/s11357-012-9434-6.

75. Akbar AN, et al. Investigation of the cutaneous response to recall antigen in humans in vivo. Clin Exp Immunol. 2013;173:163–72. https://doi.org/10.1111/cei.12107.

76. Ndumbi P, Gilbert L, Tsoukas CM. Comprehensive evaluation of the immune risk phenotype in successfully treated HIV-infected individuals. PLoS One. 2015;10:e0117039. https://doi.org/10.1371/journal.pone.0117039.

77. Pera A, et al. Immunosenescence: implications for response to infection and vaccination in older people. Maturitas. 2015;82:50–5. https://doi.org/10.1016/j.maturitas.2015.05.004.

27

Chlorinative stress in age-related diseases

Marco Casciaro[1], Eleonora Di Salvo[2], Elisabetta Pace[2], Elvira Ventura-Spagnolo[3], Michele Navarra[4] and Sebastiano Gangemi[1*]

Abstract

Aging is an agglomerate of biological long-lasting processes that result being inevitable. Main actors in this scenario are both long-term inflammation and oxidative stress. It has been proved that oxidative stress induce alteration in proteins and this fact itself is critically important in the pathophysiological mechanisms leading to diseases typical of aging. Among reactive species, chlorine ones such as hypochlorous acid (HOCl) are cytotoxic oxidants produced by activated neutrophils during chronic inflammation processes. HOCl can also cause damages by reacting with biological molecules. HOCl is generated by myeloperoxidase (MPO) and augmented serum levels of MPO have been described in acute and chronic inflammatory conditions in cardiovascular patients and has been implicated in many inflammatory diseases such as atherosclerosis, neurodegenerative conditions, and some cancers. Due to these data, we decided to conduct an up-to-date review evaluating chlorinative stress effects on every age-related disease linked; potential anti-oxidant countermeasures were also assessed. Results obtained associated HOCl generation to the aging processes and confirmed its connection with diseases like neurodegenerative and cardiovascular pathologies, atherosclerosis and cancer; chlorination was mainly linked to diseases where molecular (protein) alteration constitute the major suspected cause: i.e. inflammation, tissue lesions, DNA damages, apoptosis and oxidative stress itself. According data collected, a healthy lifestyle together with some dietary suggestion and/or the administration of nutracetical antioxidant integrators could balance the effects of chlorinative stress and, in some cases, slow down or prevent the onset of age-releated diseases.

Keywords: Oxidative stress, Myeloperoxidase, Chlorine, Chlorinative stress, Chlorination, Aging, Age, Protein damage, Hypochlorous acid, Inflammation

Background

Aging is an agglomerate of biological long-lasting processes that result being inevitable. It is correlated to gradual and autonomous biochemical and physiological changes, which often leads to an increased diseases susceptibility. The key players in this scenario are both long-term inflammation and oxidative stress [1]. The aging process is dynamic and characterized by a continuous remodelling. DNA repair, apoptosis, immune response, oxidative stress and inflammation contribute to this dynamic process [2]. The natural deduction is that oxidative stress and aging are strictly connected.

Reactive oxygen species (ROS) are a critical class of DNA detrimental agents and, unfortunately, they are constantly produced in human cells in response to toxicant either generated from our own metabolism and/or exposure to environmental agents [3–5]. ROS include different chemical species such as superoxide anion radical (O2-), hydrogen peroxide (H2O2), hydroxyl radical (·OH), and singlet oxygen (O2). Mitochondrion and NADPH oxidases are contemplated major sources of ROS generation in cells. In mitochondria, electrons slipping from the electron transport chain, in the course of mitochondrial respiration, can combine with oxygen in generating O2; O2 itself could subsequently be converted to H2O2 by superoxide dismutase (SOD) [6]. The oxidative process could affect many redox-sensitive biological molecules (i.e. amino acids) depending on the site of ROS production [5, 6]. Inflammatory cells, recruited after a chemical, physical or biological damage,

* Correspondence: gangemis@unime.it
[1]School and Division of Allergy and Clinical Immunology, Department of Clinical and Experimental Medicine, Azienda Ospedaliera Universitaria Policlinico "G. Martino", University of Messina, Messina, Italy
Full list of author information is available at the end of the article

promote the activation or the induction of different oxidant-generating enzymes. These enzymes generate high levels of reactive oxygen, nitrogen, and halogen species on site of the inflammation process. Some of these species are i.e. superoxide anion, nitric oxide, peroxynitrite, hydrogen peroxide, hypochlorous acid, and hypobromous acid. Their main objective is neutralizing invading pathogens, but often their action could lead to the DNA damage of host cells as side effect [5, 6]. It has been proved that oxidative stress induce alteration in proteins and this fact itself is critically important in the pathophysiological mechanisms leading to diseases typical of aging, extending from atherosclerosis to neurodegenerative disorders [7] as well as other inflammatory and immunological diseases [8, 9].

The maintenance of optimal conditions in an organism in order to contrast aging is accomplished by a complex network of longevity assurance processes that are controlled by Vitagenes, a group of genes aimed at preserving cellular homeostasis during stressful conditions; in particular Vitagenes encode the genes for the formation of Hsp (heat shock proteins), useful to counteract the formation of miticondrial ROS and thus, the progression of unsuccessful aging [10]. Vitagens have also been studied in diseases typical of the old age such as neurodegenerative ones [11]. In recent years, many scientific researches were aimed to refine new techniques based on proteomics, which lead to the discovery of new proteins and molecules having a key role in oxidative stress and aging processes, and for the identification of selected proteins to be used in a specific therapeutic targets [12].

Among the above cited reactive species, chlorine ones such as hypochlorous acid (HOCl) are cytotoxic oxidants produced by activated neutrophils during chronic inflammation processes [13]. Neutrophils and some monocyte-macrophage line cells generate HOCl by the myeloperoxidase (MPO) enzyme intervention. HOCl is a powerful cytotoxic oxidant acting a main role in fighting microbial pathogens. By the way it can also cause damages by reacting with biological molecules (i.e. amino acids, lipids, nucleic acids) sustaining its inflammation. Proteins are the most common targets of HOCl and for this reason changes induced in their sub-elements (peptides and amino acids) have been largely examined [5, 6, 13]. HOCl oxidizes cysteine and methionine, leading to the production of disulfides, oxyacids, sulfoxides, and molecules where sulfur is linked to nitrogen. Other reactive species could generate oxygenated sulfur products too, but they are useless as biomarkers for HOCl-induced damage [14].

HOCl is generated by the heme enzyme myeloperoxidase [15]. MPO is a glycosylated heme-enzyme stored in neutrophils and macrophages azurophilic granules; these granules have a powerful bactericidal action which is mediated by the production of hypochlorous acid from hydrogen peroxide and chloride ions. MPO could be secreted in the extracellular space; augmented serum levels of MPO have been described in acute and chronic inflammatory conditions in cardiovascular patients and have been implicated in many inflammatory diseases such as atherosclerosis, neurodegenerative conditions, and some cancers [16–20]. Due to these data, we decided to search literature trying to delineate a complete and up to date overview about hypochlorous acid and chlorinative stress effects in aging and in all the age related diseases linked. Moreover, potential anti-oxidant countermeasures were also assessed.

Methods

This literature review was conducted employing MEDLINE database. On this database, we searched for articles from inception to march 2017 using key terms related to aging and chlorinative stress.

It was decided to read the abstract of articles whose titles indicated that they might have examined HOCl involvement and the role of chlorinative stress in age-related diseases. The entire article was read if the abstract indicated that the article potentially met the inclusion criteria. Lastly, we reviewed and searched references of the selected articles. Articles were included in the present review according to the following inclusion criteria: English language, publication in peer reviewed journals, research paper. Articles were excluded by title, abstract or full text for irrelevance to the topic in question. Two authors (MC, EDS) performed the initial search and independently reviewed and selected the references based on the inclusion and exclusion criteria. Principal outcomes of interest included original studies concerning HOCl involvement and/or chlorinative stress in age-related diseases.

Chlorinative stress and cardiovascular diseases

Due to well-known HOCl generation by myeloperoxidase, Daugherty et al. in 1994. studied atherosclerotic lesions where they detected the enzyme MPO; their data sustained that MPO induced LDL oxidation by pathways involving HOCl and promoting atherogenesis [21]. These data were studied thoroughly by Hazen et al. which demonstrated that HOCl produced by the system myeloperoxidase-H_2O_2-Cl oxidated LDL l-tyrosine. Oxidated LDL were known to have a main role in converting macrophages into foam cells and in forming atherosclerotic lesions typical of aged people [22]. In a successive paper, they also demonstrated that 3-chlorotyrosine was a marker of chlorination at sites of inflammation [7]. Also the eosinophil peroxidase (EPO) was thought being implicated in provoking oxidative tissue damage in many conditions (i.e. asthma, allergic inflammatory disorders, cancer, infections). But Wu et al. reported that EPO generated reactive nitrogen species by direct oxidation of NO 2 and not by secondary oxidation of NO 2 by HOCl [23]. Every paper reported seemed to address the chlorinating stress as responsible of cardiovascular-age related damage so next step was demonstrating if oxidative stress HOCl-related could induce endothelial dysfunction by interfering with the NO synthetic pathway. Zhang et al. noticed that a treatment with HOCl caused the inhibition of aortic relaxation correlated to HOCl concentration. In their experiments, they also dosed endothelial NO synthase (NOS III) after the administration of HOCl then supplemented rats with L-arginine and reported a complete inversion of HOCl inhibitory effect vessel relaxation [24]. As Oxidized lipoproteins act a main role in atherosclerosis and high levels of 3-chlorotyrosine were demonstrated being in atherosclerotic lesion, Bergt et al. studied how activated phagocytes chlorinated specific region in HDL by mass spectrometry. Results obtained demonstrated how HOCl selectively targeted tyrosine residues nearby primary amino-groups in proteins. This oxidation process performed by phagocytes lead to damage host tissue during inflammatory diseases (i.e. atherosclerosis) [14]. As demonstrated by Cook et al., SERCA activity is fundamental in human homeostasis; it is blocked by oxidant agents and deregulated in aged tissues and cardiovascular pathologies. They reported that HOCl targeted thiols and provoked cellular impairment. They speculated that HOCl could inhibit SERCA activity by thiol oxidation and generated cytosolic Ca2+ augmented levels in artery endothelial cells [17]. Ismael et al. shown that exposure of macrophages to HOCl and HOSCN or to LDL already modified by these chlorinative stress agents caused a compromised lysosomal enzyme function reducing both proteolytic capacity and decrease cholesteryl ester hydrolysis; according the authors these events could conduct to the accumulation of protein and lipids in the arterial wall fundamental for the development of atherosclerosis [25].

Therefore, Wang et al. in vivo studies demonstrated that damaged LV-tissue by the induction of an acute myocardial infarction lead to the recruitment and activation of neutrophils and concomitant increase in MPO-activity and consequently of the HOCl; the 3-Cl-Tyr formed by the HOCl modification of the heme protein Mb impaired the protein's affinity for binding oxygen in the myocardium [26].

From other studies emerged that MPO augmented activity during inflammatory processes could worsen diseases such as atherosclerosis and reperfusion injury; in fact, an increased release of hypochlorite contributed to the damage observed in these pathologies [24, 27–30]. On these basis Sand et al. evaluated the effects of hypochlorite and H2O2 on 1-adrenoceptor, ET-1 receptors and M2 receptors processes on mice. They concluded that formation of hypochlorite provoked the amplification of the oxidative capabilities of H2O2 enhancing the damage of endothelial physiology. Hypochlorite also interfered with the normal transduction of the 1-adrenoceptor by altering the coupling of the muscarinic M2 receptor to the G-proteins favouring the progression of inflammation-associated pathologies in the cardiovascular system [31].

Chlorinative stress and other aging conditions

On the other hand it was also important understanding the inflammatory mechanisms HOCl - associated, so Raftery et al. demonstrated that HOCl produced by myeloperoxidase and H2O2 and by phorbol 12-myristate 13-acetate stimulated and activated neutrophils. HOCl oxidation during inflammation caused the formation of sulfamide monomers having chemotactic activity for neutrophils in inflammation. These changes in human proteins could, according Raftery et al. potentially play a critical role in physiological and pathological processes fundamental in aging and age-related diseases [32]. In a rat hepatocytes experiment, Mallis et al. reported that HOCl generated in a non-reversible way oxidized forms of carbonic anhydrase III in case of low doses or absence of glutathione (GSH). As it is known that there is a physiological reduction of glutathione in aged animals, these condition may together with other mechanisms favourite a higher irreversible protein oxidation [33]. Strosovà et al. 2005., studied the effects of HOCl in rabbit skeletal sarcoplasmic reticulum (SR) speculating an aging model. It was found that HOCl blocked Ca^{2+}-ATPase activity. It also oxidated SH groups and formed protein carbonyls. On the other side they tested and demonstrated the antioxidant effect of stobadine (at least as much as lipoic acid), trolox and Pycnogenol [34]. Hazell et al., wanted to determine if HOCl could be involved in protein modifications associated to age-related eye disease such as nuclear cataract. In the human lens samples analysed no chlorotyrosine derivates could be detected and no myeloperoxidase activity trace could be found either [35].

In the attempt to report the role of neutrophils as source of oxidative stress in rheumatoid arthritis (RA), Baskol et al. 2006., described how advanced oxidation protein products (AOPP) are formed by the interaction of HOCl/HOCl and proteins. In the samples analysed the protein oxidative damage corresponded to increased levels of AOPP and nominated them as marker of oxidative stress. According their data, neutrophils, which produce great quantities of chlorinated oxidants by MPO, could augment serum AOPP levels and play a fundamental role in the pathogenesis of RA by generating pro-inflammatory mediators [36]. Although its known induction of oxidant intermediates Leung et Al. decided to study skin and NF-kB effects of topical application of HOCl. They reported HOCl capacity to block NF-kB signalling and to attenuate NF-kB related disease as acute radiation dermatitis and skin aging process [37].As regards the young and the elderly's immune system, many years ago it emerged that neutrophil extracellular traps (NETs) are part of the defensive mechanism of neutrophils; their formation requires reactive oxygen species presence. Hazeldine et al. demonstrated that NET generation in response to HOCl was lower only in aged patients. A deficit on NET formation could contribute to a higher incidence of infection in older adults [38]. Superoxide (O2-) and hydrogen peroxide (H2O2) are consequences of hyperglycemia; during last years was clarified their role in the apoptosis of endothelial cells and in causing diabetic vascular injury. This damage is the result of endothelial dysfunction and vascular complications. As NADPH oxidase-derived ROS and vascular-bound MPO are increased in diabetic vessels, MPO/NADPH oxidase/H2O2/HOCl could constitute a main path in diabetic vascular damages. According Tian et al. blocking the MPO-NADPH oxidase-HOCl pathway could be a novel therapeutic strategy for the prevention and the recovery of vascular diseases [39].

MPO and its consequent product HOCl resulted involved in the pathophysiology of neurodegenerative diseases. In fact, MPO is expressed with increased levels in the cerebral tissue of patients affected by Alzheimer disease (AD) and this enzyme appears being catalytically active [40]. Not present in normal brains of old patients, MPO was detectable in amyloid plaques of AD patients. It was speculated a model where MPO expression in astrocytes promoted a HOCl related damage, contributing to neuronal damage and cognitive impairment [40, 41].

Discussion

It has always been known that oxidation of proteins was a detrimental process leading to the damage of human tissues. Both inflammation and the consequent cellular damage are two of the most threatening causes of the unsuccessful aging process. Oxidative stress has always been designated as an inflammatory source leading to many aging diseases and the stress caused by hypochlorous acid is a consistent part of it. Since 1991 with the first studies involving MPO, it appeared to be quite clear the importance of one of myeloperoxidase "normal" products, the HOCl, in the above cited oxidation process. The word "chlorination" was used to describe the modification induced in molecules by HOCl intervention; "chlorinative stress" expression was chosen to define the sum of HOCl pathological interaction in a physiological organism [14, 21, 42, 43]. Several of the diseases induced by this stress either favourite or provoke age-related diseases. The generation of HOCl was demonstrated to interfere with lipoproteins with a consequent oxidation resulting in the conversion of macrophages in foam cells and in the acceleration of the atherosclerotic process [7, 14, 21, 22]. HOCl also induced endothelial dysfunction by interfering with the NO synthetic pathway. This event blocked vessel relaxation and together with the pro-atherosclerotic effect

above described could generate the basis for many heart diseases [23, 24]. Chlorination could also augment inflammation at damage sites by recruiting neutrophils and induce muscle-associated pathologies by irreversibly blocking carbonic anhydrase III, creating so a vicious circle involving also calcium balance and smooth muscle contraction [17, 32–34]. MPO-dependent chlorinating stress it was demonstrated to be also related to the presence of ANCA antibodies; in fact, MPO can be individuated by MPO-ANCA, and in consequence neutrophils burst and degranulation are enhanced with a subsequent HOCl MPO-dependent generation [44–47]. It also emerged that neutrophils recruitment and consequent HOCl production in myocardium after IMA could modify heme proteins and compromise the post-infarction recovery contributing to the progression of heart failure [26]. By literature analysis other than heart-related diseases, HOCl seemed also to favourite the production of pro-inflammatory mediators in AR by forming AOPP agents [36]. Recently hypochlorous acid emerged to be not so effective in older people in generating neutrophils inflammatory response as in younger ones [38].

Although HOCl was shown being detrimental, studies conducted during last years exonerated it from being a cataract causing-agent and from generating reactive nitrogen species via EPO [23, 35]. HOCl topic application could even prevent skin aging [37]. Novel data supported outdated results and confirmed the hypothesis of a serious endothelial damage induced by chlorinative stress; above all, authors deepened the detrimental effects induced by hyperglycaemia and by neutrophils intervention immediately after an acute myocardial injury [26, 39]. During last years, it emerged also the role of hypoclorous acid produced by MPO in causing neuronal apoptosis and damages [40, 41].

These findings associated HOCl generation to aging processes and confirmed its connection with some diseases such as neurodegenerative and cardiovascular pathologies, atherosclerosis and cancer (Fig. 1); chlorination was mainly linked to diseases where molecular alterations constituted the major suspected cause: i.e. inflammation, tissue lesions, DNA damages, apoptosis and oxidative stress itself [17].

Novel, preventive and, in some cases, therapeutic approaches should be planned in order to contrast aging effects and the development of the above cited diseases. A specific low chlorine diet, rich in natural and endogenous antioxidant foods could favourite this prevention [48]. For example, Taurine was demonstrated to be a physiological primary scavenger of HOCl; since serum and urine taurine levels in elderly patients with chronic inflammatory disorders were found to be reduced, an adequate level of the amino acid inside the body may be useful in order to prevent age-related diseases [49].

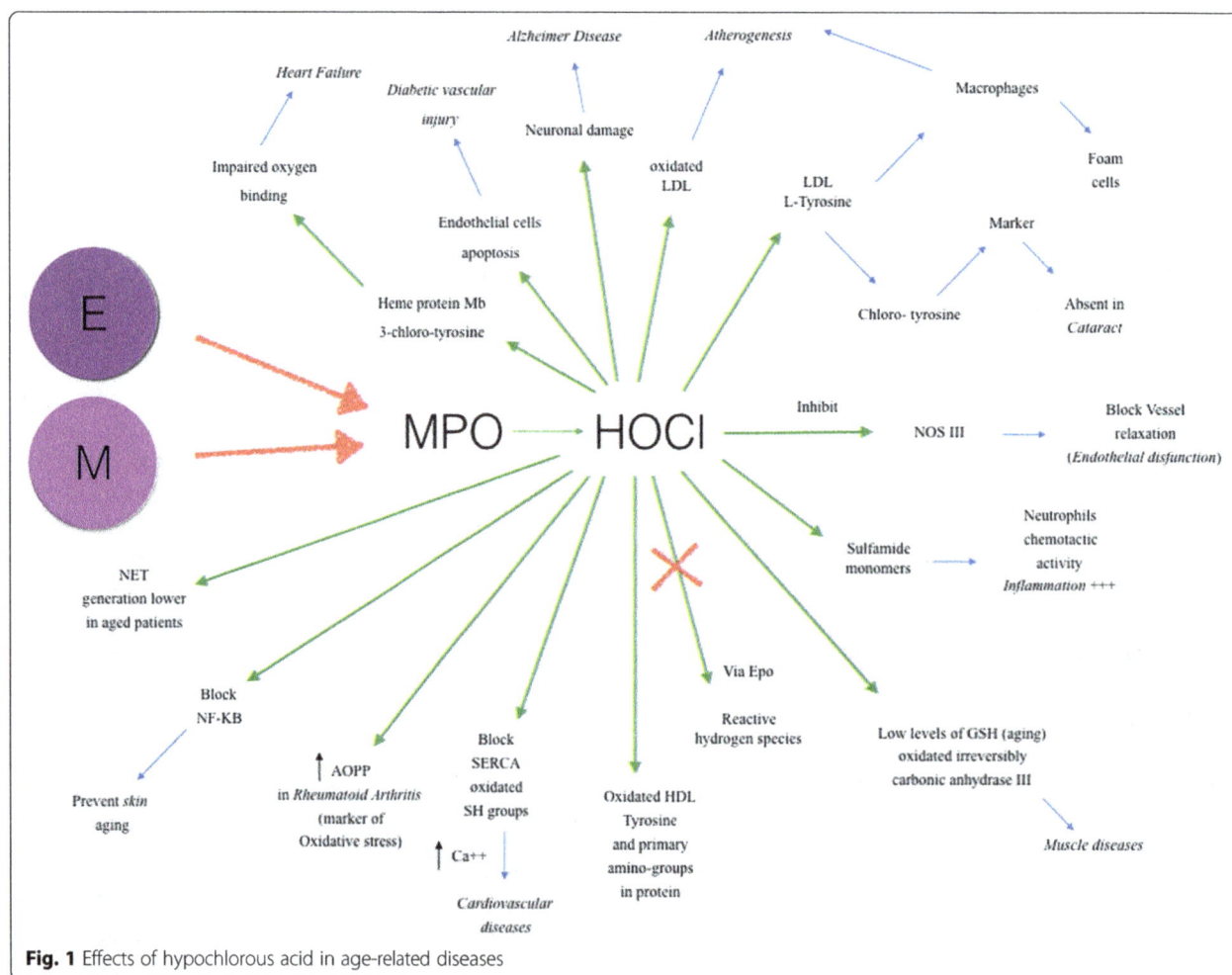

Fig. 1 Effects of hypochlorous acid in age-related diseases

Another innovative therapeutic approach could be provided by the administration natural antioxidants such as Resveratrol, Green Tea, Curcumin and Ferulic Acid; their intervention could be protective versus several diseases capable of causing tissue damage and the generation of free radical (i.e. neurodegeneration) [50].

Recent advances in the nutraceutical field highlighted the importance of some dietary integrator in aging-related pathologies. Some of these integrators such as ascorbic acid, docosahexaenoic acid (DHA) and in general low molecular weight antioxidant, associated with an adequate diet and sport could efficiently contrast ROS formation [51].

One of the most interesting molecules observed in the studies was 3-chlorotyrosine and according us should be studied in depth. Using 3-chlorotyrosine as serum and urine chlorination marker could be useful in monitoring neutrophils and macrophages activity (as major MPO sources) in some pathological phases; clarifying their involvement and diminishing their activity could finally lead to the down-regulation of HOCl production.

Conclusion

A healthy lifestyle together with some dietary suggestion and/or the administration of nutracetical antioxidant integrators could balance the effects of chlorinative stress and, in some cases, slow down or prevent the onset of age-releated diseases.

Once understood that ROS formation is in part responsible for cell damages and senescence, the next step will be focusing on studies of neurogenetics, proteomic and concerning the identification of new biomarkers. In order to contrast the most severe diseases, probably, the development of more specific ligands targeting the molecules involved in oxidative stress should have the priority. In accordance of what described above, one of these eligible targets could be the leading actor of this review, the product of MPO: hypoclorous acid [52].

Acknowledgements
Not applicable.

Funding
Not applicable.

Authors' contributions

SG designed the study. SG and MN made data analysis and interpretation, and revised the manuscript. MC and EDS carried out the bibliographic search, wrote and coordinated the draft of the manuscript. EP, EVS made data interpretation and contributed to the figure. All authors read and approved the final manuscript.

Competing interests

The authors declare that they have no competing interest.

Author details

[1]School and Division of Allergy and Clinical Immunology, Department of Clinical and Experimental Medicine, Azienda Ospedaliera Universitaria Policlinico "G. Martino", University of Messina, Messina, Italy. [2]IBIM-CNR Institute of Biomedicine and Molecular Immunology, National Research Council, 90100 Palermo, Italy. [3]Legal Medicine Section, Department for Health Promotion and Mother-Child Care, University of Palermo, Via del Vespro, 129, 90127 Palermo, Italy. [4]Department of Chemical, Biological, Pharmaceutical and Environmental Sciences, University of Messina, Messina, Italy.

References

1. Sharma S, Ebadi M. Significance of metallothioneins in aging brain. Neurochem Int. 2014;65:40–8.
2. Minciullo PL, et al. Inflammaging and anti-Inflammaging: the role of cytokines in extreme longevity. Arch Immunol Ther Exp. 2016;64(2):111–26.
3. D'Autreaux B, Toledano MB. ROS as signalling molecules: mechanisms that generate specificity in ROS homeostasis. Nat Rev Mol Cell Biol. 2007;8(10):813–24.
4. Krause KH. Aging: a revisited theory based on free radicals generated by NOX family NADPH oxidases. Exp Gerontol. 2007;42(4):256–62.
5. Brieger K, et al. Reactive oxygen species: from health to disease. Swiss Med Wkly. 2012;142:w13659.
6. Yu Y, et al. Occurrence, biological consequences, and human health relevance of oxidative stress-induced DNA damage. Chem Res Toxicol. 2016;29(12):2008–39.
7. Hazen SL, et al. Mass spectrometric quantification of 3-chlorotyrosine in human tissues with attomole sensitivity: a sensitive and specific marker for myeloperoxidase-catalyzed chlorination at sites of inflammation. Free Radic Biol Med. 1997;23(6):909–16.
8. Di Lorenzo G, et al. Differences in the behavior of advanced glycation end products and advanced oxidation protein products in patients with allergic rhinitis. J Investig Allergol Clin Immunol. 2013;23(2):101–6.
9. Gangemi S, et al. Oxidative stress markers are increased in patients with mastocytosis. Allergy. 2015;70(4):436–42.
10. Calabrese V, et al. Cellular stress responses, hormetic phytochemicals and vitagenes in aging and longevity. Biochim Biophys Acta. 2012;1822(5):753–83.
11. Calabrese V, et al. Major pathogenic mechanisms in vascular dementia: roles of cellular stress response and hormesis in neuroprotection. J Neurosci Res. 2016;94(12):1588–603.
12. Calabrese V, et al. Analytical approaches to the diagnosis and treatment of aging and aging-related disease: redox status and proteomics. Free Radic Res. 2015;49(5):511–24.
13. Whiteman M, et al. Do mitochondriotropic antioxidants prevent chlorinative stress-induced mitochondrial and cellular injury? Antioxid Redox Signal. 2008;10(3):641–50.
14. Bergt C, et al. Lysine residues direct the chlorination of tyrosines in YXXK motifs of apolipoprotein A-I when hypochlorous acid oxidizes high density lipoprotein. J Biol Chem. 2004;279(9):7856–66.
15. Marcinkiewicz J, et al. Antimicrobial and cytotoxic activity of hypochlorous acid: interactions with taurine and nitrite. Inflamm Res. 2000;49(6):280–9.

16. Sharma RN, Goel S. Chlorinated drinking water, cancers and adverse health outcomes in Gangtok, Sikkim, India. J Environ Sci Eng. 2007;49(4):247–54.
17. Cook NL, et al. Myeloperoxidase-derived oxidants inhibit sarco/endoplasmic reticulum Ca^{2+}–ATPase activity and perturb Ca^{2+} homeostasis in human coronary artery endothelial cells. Free Radic Biol Med. 2012;52(5):951–61.
18. Straface E, et al. Does oxidative stress play a critical role in cardiovascular complications of Kawasaki disease? Antioxid Redox Signal. 2012;17(10):1441–6.
19. Cabassi A, et al. Myeloperoxidase-related chlorination activity is positively associated with circulating Ceruloplasmin in chronic heart failure patients: relationship with Neurohormonal, inflammatory, and nutritional parameters. Biomed Res Int. 2015;2015:691493.
20. Ray RS, Katyal A. Myeloperoxidase: bridging the gap in neurodegeneration. Neurosci Biobehav Rev. 2016;68:611–20.
21. Daugherty A, et al. Myeloperoxidase, a catalyst for lipoprotein oxidation, is expressed in human atherosclerotic lesions. J Clin Invest. 1994;94(1):437–44.
22. Hazen SL, Heinecke JW. 3-Chlorotyrosine, a specific marker of myeloperoxidase-catalyzed oxidation, is markedly elevated in low density lipoprotein isolated from human atherosclerotic intima. J Clin Invest. 1997;99(9):2075–81.
23. Wu W, Chen Y, Hazen SL. Eosinophil peroxidase nitrates protein tyrosyl residues. Implications for oxidative damage by nitrating intermediates in eosinophilic inflammatory disorders. J Biol Chem. 1999;274(36):25933–44.
24. Zhang C, et al. Endothelial dysfunction is induced by proinflammatory oxidant hypochlorous acid. Am J Physiol Heart Circ Physiol. 2001;281(4):H1469–75.
25. Ismael FO, et al. Role of Myeloperoxidase oxidants in the modulation of cellular Lysosomal enzyme function: a contributing factor to macrophage dysfunction in atherosclerosis? PLoS One. 2016;11(12):e0168844.
26. Wang XS, et al. Neutrophils recruited to the myocardium after acute experimental myocardial infarct generate hypochlorous acid that oxidizes cardiac myoglobin. Arch Biochem Biophys. 2016;612:103–14.
27. Okabe E, et al. The effect of hypochlorous acid and hydrogen peroxide on coronary flow and arrhythmogenesis in myocardial ischemia and reperfusion. Eur J Pharmacol. 1993;248(1):33–9.
28. Raschke P, et al. Postischemic dysfunction of the heart induced by small numbers of neutrophils via formation of hypochlorous acid. Basic Res Cardiol. 1993;88(4):321–39.
29. Mian KB, Martin W. Hydrogen peroxide-induced impairment of reactivity in rat isolated aorta: potentiation by 3-amino-1,2,4-triazole. Br J Pharmacol. 1997;121(4):813–9.
30. Jaimes EA, Sweeney C, Raij L. Effects of the reactive oxygen species hydrogen peroxide and hypochlorite on endothelial nitric oxide production. Hypertension. 2001;38(4):877–83.
31. Sand C, et al. Effects of hypochlorite and hydrogen peroxide on cardiac autonomic receptors and vascular endothelial function. Clin Exp Pharmacol Physiol. 2003;30(4):249–53.
32. Raftery MJ, et al. Novel intra- and inter-molecular sulfinamide bonds in S100A8 produced by hypochlorite oxidation. J Biol Chem. 2001;276(36):33393–401.
33. Mallis RJ, et al. Irreversible thiol oxidation in carbonic anhydrase III: protection by S-glutathiolation and detection in aging rats. Biol Chem. 2002;383(3–4):649–62.
34. Strosova M, Skuciova M, Horakova L. Oxidative damage to Ca^{2+}–ATPase sarcoplasmic reticulum by HOCl and protective effect of some antioxidants. Biofactors. 2005;24(1–4):111–6.
35. Hazell LJ, et al. Is hypochlorous acid (HOCl) involved in age-related nuclear cataract? Clin Exp Optom. 2002;85(2):97–100.
36. Baskol G, et al. Investigation of protein oxidation and lipid peroxidation in patients with rheumatoid arthritis. Cell Biochem Funct. 2006;24(4):307–11.
37. Leung TH, et al. Topical hypochlorite ameliorates NF-kappaB-mediated skin diseases in mice. J Clin Invest. 2013;123(12):5361–70.
38. Hazeldine J, et al. Impaired neutrophil extracellular trap formation: a novel defect in the innate immune system of aged individuals. Aging Cell. 2014;13(4):690–8.
39. Tian R, et al. Myeloperoxidase amplified high glucose-induced endothelial dysfunction in vasculature: role of NADPH oxidase and hypochlorous acid. Biochem Biophys Res Commun. 2017;484(3):572–8.

40. Lu N, et al. Inhibition of myeloperoxidase-mediated oxidative damage by nitrite in SH-SY5Y cells: relevance to neuroprotection in neurodegenerative diseases. Eur J Pharmacol. 2016;780:142–7.

41. Maki RA, et al. Aberrant expression of myeloperoxidase in astrocytes promotes phospholipid oxidation and memory deficits in a mouse model of Alzheimer disease. J Biol Chem. 2009;284(5):3158–69.

42. Marcinkiewicz J, et al. Enhancement of immunogenic properties of ovalbumin as a result of its chlorination. Int J BioChemiPhysics. 1991;23(12):1393–5.

43. Guo Y, Schneider LA, Wangensteen OD. HOCl effects on tracheal epithelium: conductance and permeability measurements. J Appl Physiol (1985). 1995;78(4):1330–8.

44. Foote CS, Goyne TE, Lehrer RI. Assessment of chlorination by human neutrophils. Nature. 1983;301(5902):715–6.

45. Falk RJ, et al. Anti-neutrophil cytoplasmic autoantibodies induce neutrophils to degranulate and produce oxygen radicals in vitro. Proc Natl Acad Sci U S A. 1990;87(11):4115–9.

46. Xu PC, et al. Influence of myeloperoxidase-catalyzing reaction on the binding between myeloperoxidase and anti-myeloperoxidase antibodies. Hum Immunol. 2012;73(4):364–9.

47. Wang J, et al. Deglycosylation influences the oxidation activity and antigenicity of myeloperoxidase. Nephrology (Carlton). 2016. doi:10.1111/nep.12926.

48. Arrigo T, et al. Role of the diet as a link between oxidative stress and liver diseases. World J Gastroenterol. 2015;21(2):384–95.

49. Yamori Y, et al. Fish and lifestyle-related disease prevention: experimental and epidemiological evidence for anti-atherogenic potential of taurine. Clin Exp Pharmacol Physiol. 2004;31(Suppl 2):S20–3.

50. Calabrese V, et al. The hormetic role of dietary antioxidants in free radical-related diseases. Curr Pharm Des. 2010;16(7):877–83.

51. Capó X, et al. Effects of almond- and olive oil-based Docosahexaenoic- and vitamin E-enriched beverage dietary supplementation on inflammation associated to exercise and age. Nutrients. 2016;8(10):619.

52. Calabrese V, et al. Hormesis, cellular stress response and neuroinflammation in schizophrenia: early onset versus late onset state. J Neurosci Res. 2017; 95(5):1182–93.

A comprehensive characterization of aggravated aging-related changes in T lymphocytes and monocytes in end-stage renal disease: the iESRD study

Yen-Ling Chiu[1,2,3], Kai-Hsiang Shu[1,4], Feng-Jung Yang[2,5], Tzu-Ying Chou[1], Ping-Min Chen[1], Fang-Yun Lay[1], Szu-Yu Pan[1], Cheng-Jui Lin[6], Nicolle H R Litjens[7], Michiel G H Betjes[7], Selma Bermudez[8], Kung-Chi Kao[4], Jean-San Chia[4], George Wang[9], Yu-Sen Peng[1] and Yi-Fang Chuang[8,10,11*]

Abstract

Background: Patients with end-stage renal disease (ESRD) exhibit a premature aging phenotype of the immune system. Nevertheless, the etiology and impact of these changes in ESRD patients remain unknown.

Results: Compared to healthy individuals, ESRD patients exhibit accelerated immunosenescence in both T cell and monocyte compartments, characterized by a dramatic reduction in naïve CD4+ and CD8+ T cell numbers but increase in CD8+ T_{EMRA} cell and proinflammatory monocyte numbers. Notably, within ESRD patients, aging-related immune changes positively correlated not only with increasing age but also with longer dialysis vintage. In multivariable-adjusted logistic regression models, the combination of high terminally differentiated CD8+ T cell level and high intermediate monocyte level, as a composite predictive immunophenotype, was independently associated with prevalent coronary artery disease as well as cardiovascular disease, after adjustment for age, sex, systemic inflammation and presence of diabetes. Levels of terminally differentiated CD8+ T cells also positively correlated with the level of uremic toxin *p*-cresyl sulfate.

Conclusions: Aging-associated adaptive and innate immune changes are aggravated in ESRD and are associated with cardiovascular diseases. For the first time, our study demonstrates the potential link between immunosenescence in ESRD and duration of exposure to the uremic milieu.

Keywords: Immunosenescence, Aging, CVD, Inflammation, ESRD

Background

Patients with end-stage renal disease (ESRD) exhibit many physiological changes reminiscent of accelerated aging processes and have an increased mortality and susceptibility to diseases when compared to chronological age-matched individuals [1]. Impaired physical functions, muscle wasting, cognitive function decline, accelerated vascular disease and increased risks of death are among the many aging-related complications increased in

frequency in ESRD [2]. The immune system of ESRD patients also exhibits significant changes from that of healthy individuals. For example, while a low grade-inflammation can be observed during normal aging [3], it is significantly enhanced by uremia [4]. Accompanying low-grade inflammation, immune cells develop different phenotypic markers and functions during normal aging. These changes are are collectively called "immunosenescence" and are considered to contribute to various aging-related morbidities, including increased risks for infectious events and cardiovascular diseases [5–7].

During normal aging, lymphocytes and monocytes experience dramatic changes. The subset distribution in the CD8+ T cell compartment is different between young

* Correspondence: chuangy@ym.edu.tw
[8]International Health Program, National Yang Ming University School of Public Health, Taipei, Taiwan
[10]Institute of Public Health, National Yang Ming University School of Public Health, Taipei, Taiwan
Full list of author information is available at the end of the article

and old people; with progressive terminal differentiation [8], loss of co-stimulatory molecules, shortening of telomeres and impaired response toward infectious pathogens and vaccinations [9, 10] occur during aging. CD4+ T cells also exhibit aging-related changes. For example, naïve CD4 T cells from aged animals show reduced IL-2 production, proliferation, helper function, effector generation and memory function [11]. Premature aging of the T cell compartment has been observed in ESRD patients, characterized by decreased thymic output of naïve cells and increased susceptibility toward apoptosis [12]. We had previously reported that higher levels of CD4+ CD28- cells can be found in ESRD patients [13] and CD4+ T cells activation is affected in ESRD patients in an age-dependent manner [14]. Recently, it has been reported that elderly kidney transplant patients also exhibit more advanced T cell differentiation compared to younger patients [15]. Besides lymphocytes, CD14++CD16+ intermediate monocytes as well as the CD14+ CD16++ non-classical monocytes also increase in numbers during aging [16] and are further increased in ESRD patients [17]. CD14++CD16+ intermediate monocytes are of particular interest because these cells produce high levels of TNF-α and IL-6 upon activation and are involved in many infectious and pathogenic inflammatory diseases [18, 19].

As a result, enhanced aging-related immune changes can be considered as one characteristic of the premature aging phenotype of renal failure. However, it remains unclear how mechanistically the immune system suffers from these enhanced aging-related changes in renal failure patients. In addition, previous studies attempted to characterize the immune system of ESRD patients were frequently based on small numbers of patient and did not include both monocyte and lymphocyte panels at the same time. We hypothesize that if ESRD patients have accelerated aging, exposure of immune cells to the uremic milieu will also have an impact on immunosenescence, independent of chronological age. In addition, profiling both adaptive and innate immune subsets should be performed simultaneously to better understand the overall effects of uremia on aging-related immune responses.

We thus initiated the *Immunity in ESRD study*, or the iESRD study to comprehensively characterize the immune changes in ESRD. The iESRD study is an on-going longitudinal cohort study with the ultimate goal to investigate if immune changes are associated with long-term clinical outcomes. Here, we present the findings from analyzing the baseline data of this study based on 412 hemodialysis patients.

Methods

Study participants
The immunity in ESRD study (iESRD) is a multicenter study which recruited ESRD patients undergoing regular hemodialysis with age > 20 years at two academic teaching hospitals in Taiwan: the Far Eastern Memorial Hospital and the National Taiwan University Hospital Yun Lin branch. A total 432 patients signed informed consent and were screened for eligibility. Those with recent hospitalization within three months, active infection, incomplete blood test results or poor blood samples quality were excluded, making only 412 patients included in the final study (198 from Far Eastern Memorial Hospital and 214 from National Taiwan University Hospital).

CMV serostatus in all individuals were determined using the Roche Elecsys assay. All methods were carried out in accordance with relevant guidelines and regulations. All experimental protocols were approved by the Research Ethics Committee of both institutions (FEMH 103084-E and NTUYL 201511092 RINA). Informed consent was obtained from all participants and/or their legal guardians.

Data collection
Biochemical data were collected on the same day of peripheral blood mononuclear cells (PBMCs) sampling. Blood samples were collected before start of a hemodialysis session in the middle of week. Diagnosis of coronary artery disease (CAD) was defined as either 1) > 50% stenosis of at least one coronary artery on coronary angiography or 2) documented reperfusion defect on stressed nuclear medicine scan. Peripheral arterial occlusive disease and stroke were based on medical chart review. Cardiovascular disease (CVD) is defined by the medical history of either CAD, peripheral arterial occlusive disease or stroke.

T cell and monocyte differentiation panel
On the day of blood sampling, PBMCs were isolated by Ficoll-Paque PLUS gradient centrifugation following the manufacturer's protocol (GE Healthcare). Freshly isolated PBMCs were immediately stained with antibody cocktails and processed for flow cytometer reading and analysis as previously described [12, 17]. The gating strategy is shown in Additional file 1: Figure S1. Briefly, singlets were identified by forward scatter area and height. Lymphocytes were subsequently gated by forward and side scatter characteristics, and anti-CD3-AF700 (clone UCHT1, Biolegend) was used to identify CD3+ T cells. CD4+ and CD8+ T cells, determined by anti-CD4-PerCP-Cy5.5 (clone OKT4, Biolegend) and anti-CD8-APC-Cy7 (clone SK1, Biolegend), were further analyzed by their surface anti-CCR7-APC (clone G043H7, Biolegend) and anti-CD45RA-Alexa488 (clone HI100, Biolegend) expression to separate into the CCR7+ CD45RA+ T_{NAIVE} subset, the CCR7+ CD45RA-T_{CM} subset, the CCR7-CD45RA-T_{EM} subset and the CCR7-CD45RA +T_{EMRA} subset. CD28-PE-Cy5 (clone CD28.2, eBioscience) and CD95-PE (clone DX2, eBioscience) were used to further

define stem cell memory T cells (Tscm) from the T_{NAIVE} subset.

Anti-CD86-PE (clone IT2.2, eBioscience) was used to gate the CD86+ monocytes. By anti-CD14-FITC (clone M5E2, Biolegend) and anti-CD16-APC (clone 3G8, eBioscience), monocytes were further classified as classical (Mon1, CD14++CD16-), intermediate (Mon2, CD14++CD16+), and non-classical (Mon3, CD14 + CD16++) monocytes. We used a clinical complete blood count (CBC) analyzer Beckman Coulter LH 780 to determine the absolute lymphocyte and monocyte counts for each sample and subset cell numbers were subsequently enumerated. All the experiments were performed in Far Eastern Memorial Hospital and analyzed using a Beckman Coulter MoFlo™-XDP multicolor flow cytometer.

Measurements of uremic toxin p-cresyl sulfate and indoxyl sulfate

Serum p-cresyl sulfate (PCS) and indoxyl sulfate (IS) were measured with liquid chromatography-mass spectrometry (4000 QTRAP, USA). In brief, serum samples were prepared and deproteinised by heat denaturation. The concentrations of IS and PCS were measured in serum ultrafiltrates, obtained by using Microcon YM-30 separators (Millipore, Billerica, MA, USA). HPLC was performed at room temperature using a dC18 column (3.0 × 50 mm, Atlantis, Waters). The sensitivity of this assay was 1 μg/L for PCS and 1 μg/L for IS.

Statistical analyses

Baseline characteristics were described as mean ± standard deviation for continuous variables, and frequency for categorical variables. Spearman's correlation was applied to evaluate the correlation of immunological markers with age and biochemical data. Partial regression plots were used to analyze the relationships between immune cell subset percentages and age adjusting for dialysis vintage, or between immune cell subset percentages and dialysis vintage adjusting for age. CAD and CVD were analyzed separately as in most cardiovascular outcome studies.

The R corrplot package was used to draw the correlogram to visualize the relationships between immune cell subsets (Freely available at http://www.sthda.com/english/wiki/visualize-correlation-matrix-using-correlogram). A p value of more than 0.05 was considered insignificant and only significant results are shown on the correlogram.

Logistic regression models, adjusted for age, gender, albumin, hemoglobin, diabetes mellitus, and hs-CRP, were used to evaluate the independent relationship between immunophenotype and the presence of CAD or CVD. All statistical tests were two-tailed, and a p value of less than 0.05 was considered be significant. The statistical analyses were performed with STATA version 13.1.

Results

Aggravated aging-related immune changes in ESRD patients

First, we compared the immune cell subsets in the peripheral blood between 412 ESRD patients and 57 age-matched healthy individuals using multicolor flow cytometry (representative staining, Additional file 1: Figure S1). The demographic and biochemical data of the iESRD participants are summarized in Table 1. Main causes of ESRD were diabetes (37.3%), chronic glomerulonephritis (27.6%), hypertension (14.3%) and others (20.8%). Because cytomegalovirus (CMV) infection profoundly affects human immune system homeostasis, we first tested CMV seropositivity frequency among participants. All healthy individuals ($n = 57$; 100% seropositive) were CMV seropositive and only 4 out of 412 ESRD patients were seronegative for CMV (99% seropositive). Despite the majority of our study samples was CMV seropositive, we detected many immune subsets differences between healthy versus ESRD (Table 2). For both CD4+ and CD8+ T cells, ESRD patients demonstrated lower percentages of T_{NAIVE} cells but increased percentages of memory stem T_{SCM} cells, which are the considered to be the least differentiated memory T cells in humans and plays an important role in immune protection upon pathogen rechallenge [20]. Interestingly, these antigen-experienced, naïve phenotype T cells recently were reported to increase during aging [21]. CD8 + Effector memory T_{EM} and terminally differentiated T_{EMRA} cells, both memory T cells with higher levels of differentiation, were increased in percentages in ESRD patients. Besides these distributional changes, ESRD

Table 1 Demographic data of iESRD participants

Variable	Mean (SD)
Age (years)	61.7 (12.2)
Male (%)	50.7
Diabetes (%)	44.6
Malignancy (%)	12.1
Dialysis vintage (years)	6.2 (5.1)
Albumin (g/dL)	4.0 (0.4)
Hemoglobin (g/dL)	10.9 (1.4)
T-cholesterol (mg/dL)	152.2 (37.3)
Triglyceride (mg/dL)	147.1 (95.4)
intact-PTH (pg/mL)	374.5 (423.6)
Calcium (mg/dL)	9.3 (0.8)
Phosphate (mg/dL)	4.9 (1.4)
Kt/V (Gotch)	1.4 (0.2)

The complete demographic data of 412 iESRD participants is shown

Table 2 Comparisons of immune cell subsets between ESRD and controls

Cell subset percentage	Healthy (57)	ESRD (412)	P value
CD4+ T cells	62.8 (10.3)	56.8 (13.3)↓	0.001*
Naïve T cells	41.6 (15.6)	28.5 (12.9)↓	< 0.001*
Stem Memory T cells	3.18 (2.01)	7.50 (6.24)↑	< 0.001*
Central Memory T cells	30.7 (9.6)	41.6 (11.1)↑	< 0.001*
Effector Memory T cells	27.0 (14.7)	28.3 (12.9)	0.47
Terminally Differentiated T cells	1.80 (2.24)	2.36 (2.72)	0.13
CD8+ T cells	26.5 (8.97)	29.2 (10.1)	0.051
Naïve T cells	32.9 (16.6)	21.8 (16.1)↓	< 0.001*
Stem Memory T cells	4.78 (5.26)	7.66 (6.20)↑	0.002*
Central Memory T cells	6.30 (3.58)	7.02 (7.91)	0.50
Effector Memory T cells	29.1 (11.7)	34.1 (16.6)↑	0.023*
Terminally Differentiated T cells	32.9 (14.4)	38.1 (16.7)↑	0.025*
Monocytes			
Classical Monocytes	64.1 (12.7)	56.9 (11.7)↓	< 0.001*
Intermediate Monocytes	6.25 (4.91)	10.1 (6.55)↑	< 0.001*
Non-Classical Monocytes	14.1 (10.8)	19.9 (9.7)↑	< 0.001*
Absolute cell number	Healthy (57)	ESRD (412)	P value
CD4+ T cells	530 (307)	523 (232)↓	0.02*
Naïve T cells	247 (199)	164 (112)↓	< 0.001*
Stem Memory T cells	17.2 (15.5)	11.5 (9.1)↓	< 0.001*
Central Memory T cells	188 (114)	229 (116)	0.65
Effector Memory T cells	89.0 (49.5)	120 (86.4)↑	0.006*
Terminally Differentiated T cells	5.76 (7.59)	9.25 (11.7)	0.10
CD8+ T cells	277 (270)	275 (180)↓	0.012*
Naïve T cells	103 (97.7)	54.5 (61.9)↓	< 0.001*
Stem Memory T cells	13.7 (17.6)	4.63 (5.50)↓	< 0.001*
Central Memory T cells	11.6 (9.22)	12.1 (13.9)	0.47
Effector Memory T cells	92.9 (58.0)	102 (83.6)	0.26
Terminally Differentiated T cells	70.2 (53.9)	105 (95.2)↑	0.013*
Monocytes			
Classical Monocytes	248 (91.2)	264 (141)	0.13
Intermediate Monocytes	19.2 (21.9)	40.3 (33.9)↑	0.001*
Non-Classical Monocytes	18.4 (12.0)	56.3 (38.2)↑	< 0.001*

Percentages and absolute numbers (per μl blood) of naïve (T_{NAIVE}), stem cell memory (T_{SCM}), central memory (T_{CM}), effector memory (T_{EM}), terminally differentiated (T_{EMRA}) subsets and three monocyte subsets (classical monocytes, intermediate monocytes, non-classical monocytes) were shown as mean (SD) and were compared between healthy controls and ESRD patients. The inter-group differences were analyzed by Student's t-test
*P value < 0.05

patients exhibit a dramatic 40–50% reduction in CD4+ and CD8+ naïve T cell numbers and especially have a significant increase in their CD8+ T_{EMRA} cell numbers. For CD4+ T cells, although percentages of T_{EM} and T_{EMRA} subsets were not significantly increased, the absolute cell number of T_{EM} cells was increased in ESRD patients.

Significant differences in the monocyte differentiation status were also found (Table 2). ESRD patients exhibited higher percentages of intermediate and non-classical monocytes and lower percentages of classical monocytes in their peripheral blood. In absolute cell number terms, the intermediate and non-classical monocytes were both significantly increased. Similar to T_{EMRA} cells, levels of intermediate monocytes and non-classical monocytes are known to increase during aging [16]. Overall, our observations confirmed that many immunological changes observed in ESRD are reminiscent of immunosenescence observed during normal aging.

We next tested whether T cell compartment changes and monocyte compartment changes are related. As shown in Additional file 1: Figure S2, we performed correlogram analyses in both healthy and ESRD individuals using either cell type percentage or absolute cell numbers. We found that monocyte subset distribution and T cell differentiation are not significantly correlated, but cells of the same lineage tend to be significantly correlated in absolute number.

Dialysis vintage positively associates with immunosenescence

Although ESRD patients clearly exhibit aggravated immune aging, the etiology of aggravated immune aging remains unclear. We hypothesize, if the uremia milieu affects immune cell homeostasis, duration of ESRD or dialysis treatment (dialysis vintage years) should have a significant impact on the severity of observed aging phenotype, independent from the effect of age. We next interrogated the relationship between percentage of each immune cell subset with age and dialysis vintage in multivariable-adjusted regression models. The complete regression analysis results are shown in Table 3 and key representative plots are shown in Fig. 1. Because longer dialysis vintage was associated with the progressive decrease in total T cell counts (significant for both CD4+ and CD8+ T cells, data not shown), for this analysis we used subset percentages to reflect premature aging of each cell compartment instead of absolute cell counts. As shown in Table 3, age profoundly affected the T cell differentiation status by decreasing the percentage of T_{NAIVE} cells and increasing the percentage of T_{EM} and T_{EMRA} cells. Both CD4+ and CD8+ T_{NAIVE} cells decrease in percentage with aging, but effects of age on T_{EMRA} cells were more pronounced in the CD8+ compartment than CD4+ cells. Consistent with a previous study made in non-renal failure population [16], we also found that age positively associated with the percentage of intermediate monocytes. When we further adjusted etiology of ESRD in the model, the relationships between age and immune cell subsets did not change (data not shown). Longer dialysis vintage years robustly associated

Table 3 Independent effects of age and dialysis vintage on immune cell aging

Cell Subset (percentage)	Age		Dialysis Vintage	
	β	P value	β	P value
CD4+ T cells				
Naïve T cells	−0.22	< 0.001*	0.20	0.095
Stem Memory T cells	0.08	0.029*	0.03	0.72
Central Memory T cells	−0.05	0.24	−0.60	< 0.001*
Effector Memory T cells	0.26	< 0.001*	0.41	0.001*
Terminally Differentiated T cells	0.02	0.12	0.02	0.46
CD8+ T cells				
Naïve T cells	−0.56	< 0.001*	0.14	0.31
Stem Memory T cells	0.12	0.002*	0.001	0.91
Central Memory T cells	−0.01	0.61	0.11	0.16
Effector Memory T cells	0.16	0.014*	−0.67	< 0.001*
Terminally Differentiated T cells	0.42	< 0.001*	0.47	0.002*
Monocytes				
Classical Monocytes	0.02	0.72	−0.32	0.005*
Intermediate Monocytes	−0.03	0.21	0.27	< 0.001*
Non-Classical Monocytes	−0.02	0.64	0.06	0.56

To separate the effects of age from dialysis vintage on immune changes, we tested the independent effects of age and dialysis vintage on cell subset percentages. In a multivariable-adjusted regression model (using subset percentage as the independent variable), the independent associations between immune cell percentage and age as well as the independent associations between immune cell percentage and vintage are shown
*P value < 0.05

with higher percentages of CD8+ T_{EMRA} cells (β = 0.47, p = 0.002). Importantly, dialysis vintage also positively associated with percentages of intermediate monocytes and negatively associated with the percentages of classical monocytes. To further confirm the effects of dialysis vintage on immune changes, ESRD patients were separated into tertiles based on vintage years for trend analysis and were also analyzed by robust regression to eliminate the concern of outliers (Additional file 1: Table S1). CD4+ CD28null cells are important aging-related T cell subset that had been reported to increase during aging. Although CD4+ CD28null cells were also increased in dialysis patients, neither percentages nor absolute counts of CD4+ CD28null cells in dialysis patients were correlated with dialysis vintage (data not shown). Overall, the dialysis vintage, after statistical adjustment for age, significantly associated with both immunosenescent T cell differentiation (especially in CD8+ T cells) and higher levels of intermediate monocytes.

Aging-related immune changes correlate with cardiovascular risk factors and systemic inflammation

It is well-known that ESRD patients exhibit a dramatic increased risk for cardiovascular disease when compared to age-matched healthy individuals [22]. In the literature,

inflammation is responsible for increased risk of atherosclerotic diseases and mortality in ESRD because ESRD patients also exhibit high level of chronic inflammation [23, 24]. Since immunosenescence contributes to atherosclerotic diseases in the elderly without renal diseases [25], we studied the correlation between parameters of immunosenescence with traditional as well as non-traditional cardiovascular risk factors in the iESRD cohort. We selected CD8+ T_{NAIVE}, CD8+ T_{EMRA} and intermediate monocytes as key immunosenescence parameters to perform further analysis in the current study because both adaptive and innate immunity were implicated in previous studies on atherosclerotic vascular diseases [26] and these subsets were closely associated with age and/or dialysis vintage. As shown in Additional file 1: Table S2, these immune changes were associated with traditional and non-traditional cardiovascular risk factors. Most importantly, systemic inflammation as measured by high-sensitivity C-reactive protein was associated with decreased CD8+ T_{NAIVE} and increase in intermediate monocyte numbers. The presence of diabetes, another important cardiovascular risk factor, has little impact on the extent of immunosenescence (Additional file 1: Table S3).

ESRD patients with concurrent cardiovascular disease display more severe immunosenescence

To test the impact of aging-related immune changes on cardiovascular health, percentages and cell numbers of CD8+ T_{NAIVE}, CD8+ T_{EMRA} cells and intermediate monocytes were further compared between patients with and without coronary artery disease (CAD) and between patients with and without cardiovascular disease (CVD). Among 412 patients, 106 patients had history of coronary artery disease determined by history of myocardial infarction, positive coronary angiography or positive thallium scan; 132 patients had cardiovascular disease defined by the history of either coronary artery disease as defined in the method section, stroke, or peripheral arterial occlusive disease. As shown in Additional file 1: Table S4, patients with CAD or CVD had lower percentages of CD8+ naive T cells and higher percentages of CD8+ T_{EMRA} cells. Patients with CVD also had significant higher percentages of intermediate monocytes.

The high-CD8+T_{EMRA}/high-intermediate monocyte immunophenotype independently associates with existing cardiovascular diseases

Although patients with concurrent cardiovascular disease had higher percentages of CD8+ T_{EMRA} cells and CD14++CD16+ intermediate monocytes in their peripheral blood, the differences between groups were relatively small regarding a given immune subset. These findings prompted us to create a composite immunophenotype based on both cell subsets. To date, no study has studied

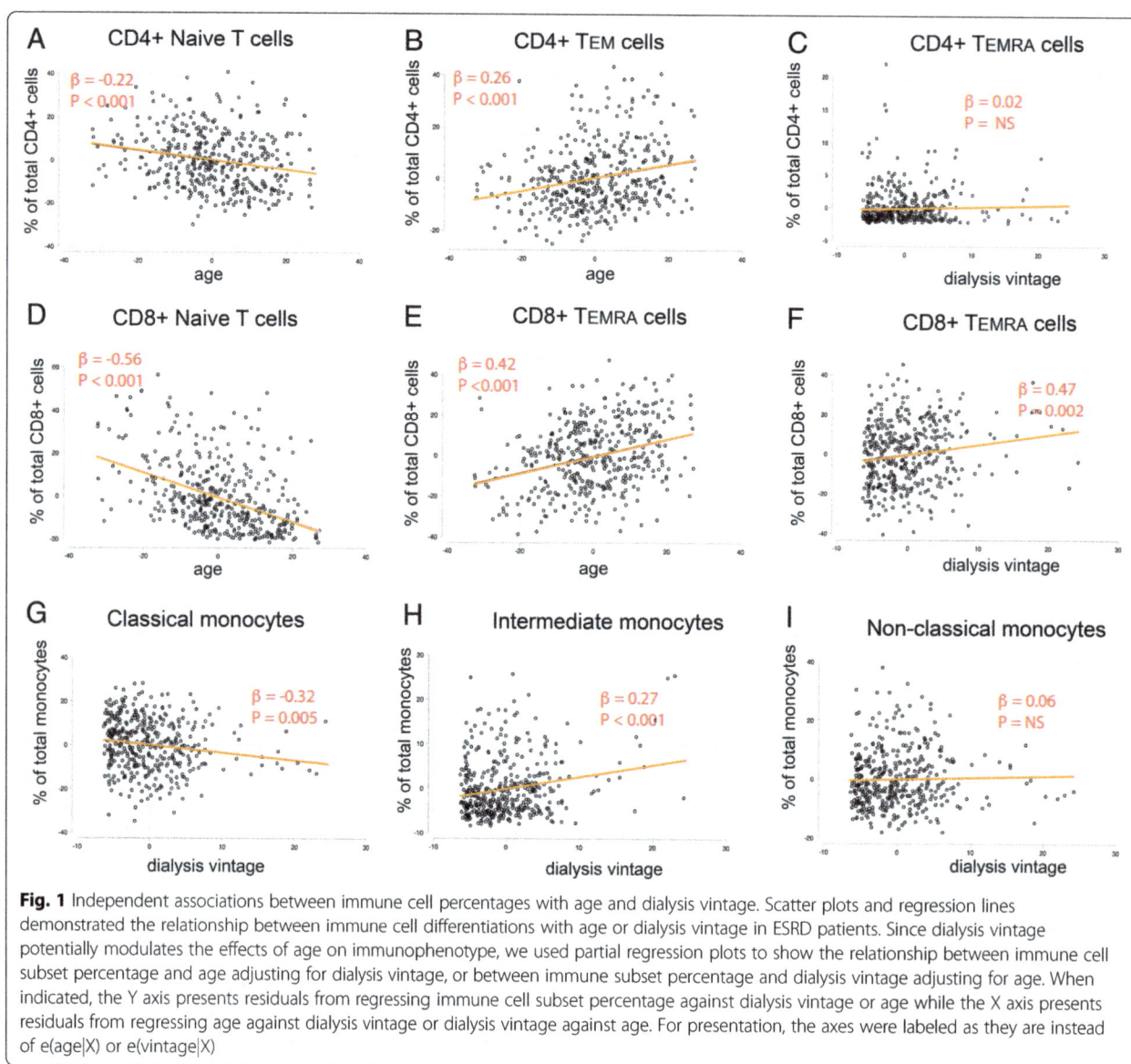

Fig. 1 Independent associations between immune cell percentages with age and dialysis vintage. Scatter plots and regression lines demonstrated the relationship between immune cell differentiations with age or dialysis vintage in ESRD patients. Since dialysis vintage potentially modulates the effects of age on immunophenotype, we used partial regression plots to show the relationship between immune cell subset percentage and age adjusting for dialysis vintage, or between immune subset percentage and dialysis vintage adjusting for age. When indicated, the Y axis presents residuals from regressing immune cell subset percentage against dialysis vintage or age while the X axis presents residuals from regressing age against dialysis vintage or dialysis vintage against age. For presentation, the axes were labeled as they are instead of e(age|X) or e(vintage|X)

both adaptive and innate immune cells simultaneously to investigate whether aging-related immune changes in ESRD patients (or even individuals with normal renal function) are related to atherosclerotic complications. To characterize a clinically useful phenotype based on both cell types, we tested the use of medium-split of each variable and defined immunophenotypes based on expression levels of CD8+ T_{EMRA} and intermediate monocyte. We found that all the iESRD participants can be separated into four groups: high CD8+ T_{EMRA}/high intermediate monocytes, high CD8+ T_{EMRA}/low intermediate monocytes, low CD8+ T_{EMRA}/high intermediate monocytes and the low CD8+ T_{EMRA}/low intermediate monocytes. We then tested the independent associations of immunophenotypes with the concomitant presence of CAD and CVD. We found that the "high CD8+ T_{EMRA}/high intermediate

monocyte" phenotype is independently associated with the presence of CAD and CVD (Table 4). We performed the likelihood ratio test to compare models with and without immunophenotype in the presence of age, DM, CRP and Hb, and the result was significant (p value = 0.0137). This suggests that immunophenotype as a whole results in a statistically significant improvement in model fit. When cell percentages instead of cell numbers were used in the model, the associations between immunophenotype and CAD or CVD remains statistically significant (Additional file 1: Table S5).

Uremic toxin *p*-cresyl sulfate positively correlated with levels of CD8+ T_{EMRA} cells

In renal failure patients, retention of uremic toxins is a key mechanism underlying the generation of oxidative

Table 4 A combinatorial aging-associated immunophenotype independently associates with coronary artery disease and cardiovascular disease

	OR (95% CI)	P value
Variables in model (independent variable: CAD)		
Immunophenotype		
High CD8+ T_{EMRA} High Mon$_{INT}$	2.40 (1.18–4.90)	0.016*
High CD8+ T_{EMRA} Low Mon$_{INT}$	1.56 (0.74–3.28)	0.24
Low CD8+ T_{EMRA} High Mon$_{INT}$	1.01 (0.46–2.16)	0.99
Low CD8+ T_{EMRA} Low Mon$_{INT}$	1.00	
Age	1.03 (1.01–1.06)	0.003*
Gender (Male)	1.28 (0.79–2.08)	0.31
Diabetes	3.26 (1.99–5.33)	< 0.001*
Albumin (g/dL)	1.21 (0.56–2.21)	0.62
hs-CRP (mg/dL)	1.49 (1.17–1.89)	0.001*
Hemoglobin (g/dL)	1.10 (0.93–1.30)	0.28
Variables in model (independent variable: CVD)		
Immunosenescence		
High CD8+ T_{EMRA} High Mon$_{INT}$	2.39 (1.21–4.70)	0.012*
High CD8+ T_{EMRA} Low Mon$_{INT}$	1.93 (0.97–3.84)	0.06
Low CD8+ T_{EMRA} High Mon$_{INT}$	1.47 (0.72–2.97)	0.29
Low CD8+ T_{EMRA} Low Mon$_{INT}$	1.00	
Age	1.03 (1.01–1.06)	0.001*
Gender (Male)	1.28 (0.81–2.01)	0.29
Diabetes	2.92 (1.86–4.60)	< 0.001*
Albumin (g/dL)	1.03 (0.51–2.08)	0.93
hs-CRP (mg/dL)	1.40 (1.11–1.77)	0.005*
Hemoglobin (g/dL)	1.04 (0.90–1.22)	0.54

Multivariable-adjusted logistic regression models were adjusted for: age, gender, albumin, hemoglobin, DM, hs-CRP and immunophenotype group. The immunophenotype groups were constructed as a categorical variable based on the median-split of the absolute number of CD8+ T_{EMRA} cells and intermediate monocyte number (Mon$_{INT}$), with the Low Mon$_{INT}$ Low CD8+ T_{EMRA} group as the reference group. The results were expressed as odds ratio (OR), 95% confidence interval (CI)
*P value < 0.05

stress and inflammation [27]. Others and our previous study also indicated that higher levels of uremic toxins in ESRD patients were related to atherosclerotic complications and mortality [28, 29]. Because aging-related immune changes positively associated with dialysis vintage, we were curious about the relationships between uremic toxins with the level of CD8+ T_{EMRA} and intermediate monocytes. We measured two major uremic toxins, *p*-cresyl sulfate and indoxyl sulfate, in 100 iESRD participants. As shown in Table 5, we found that levels of uremic toxin *p*-cresyl sulfate significantly correlated with higher levels of CD8+ T_{EMRA} cells in both relative percentage and absolute cell number terms. Nevertheless, levels of indoxyl sulfate were not associated with the

accumulation of CD8+ T_{EMRA} cells, and levels of uremic toxin were not associated with levels of intermediate monocytes (data not shown).

Discussion

The immunity in ESRD, or "iESRD study" was designed with the goal of identifying biomarkers that can accurately assess the health status of ESRD patients undergoing hemodialysis and of investigating the potential mechanism underlying the aggravated aging-related immune changes that may ultimately also apply to the general population. A longitudinal follow-up of the cohort participants is currently being performed to analyze if immune status can predict patients' survival and if these immune changes will evolve over-time.

The baseline analysis found both adaptive and innate immune subset distribution dramatically changed in ESRD patients compared with healthy individuals. Aging-related changes of lymphocytes and monocytes also positively associate with dialysis vintage and other cardiovascular risk factors in ESRD patients. In the current study, we identified the positive association between these changes and systemic inflammation, and identified a combinatorial aging-related immunophenotype is associated with prevalent atherosclerotic cardiovascular disease in ESRD independently from systemic inflammation. The odds ratio of patients with the high CD8+ T_{EMRA} and high intermediate monocyte immunophenotype for CAD and CVD is higher than every 1 mg/dL increase in high-sensitivity CRP and is in a range close to diabetes. Thus, these findings suggest that aggravated immunosenescence significantly impacts on ESRD patients' health.

Our study found both CD4+ and CD8+ T cells differentiations are dramatically enhanced in ESRD patients. Compared to healthy donors, ESRD patients have much fewer naïve T cells but at the same time, higher percentage of memory T cells with advanced differentiation-especially CD8+ T_{EMRA} cells. Overall, enhanced immunosenescence is more evident in CD8+ T cells than CD4+ T cells. Consistent with most published studies, CD4+ T cells tend to be less affected by aging than CD8+ T cells [30]. Compared to CD8+ T cells, naïve CD4+ T cells maintain their absolute cell numbers and memory CD4+ T cells maintain a highly diverse T cell receptor repertoire without significant clonal expansion during aging. However, as recently reviewed by Goronzy et al. [31], it remains largely unknown why CD4+ T cells are less susceptible to aging. While a decrease in naïve T cells potentially affects an individual's response toward new infections and vaccinations [30], memory T cells expressing cytotoxic or terminal differentiation features are increasingly implicated in the pathogenesis of atherosclerotic disease and inflammation [26, 32] although many studies are observational so far.

Table 5 Correlations between uremic toxin levels with levels of CD8+ T$_{EMRA}$ cells

Cell subset	p-cresyl sulfate (µg/ml)		Indoxyl sulfate (µg/ml)	
	Correlation Coeff.	P value	Correlation Coeff.	P value
CD8+ T$_{EMRA}$ (percent CD8+)	0.22	0.027*	−0.01	0.97
CD8+ T$_{EMRA}$ (cell number)	0.22	0.029*	−0.02	0.83

*P value < 0.05

Spearman's correlation test was performed to analyze the relationships between T$_{EMRA}$ cell and uremic toxin levels. Positive relationships were found between p-cresyl sulfate and CD8+ T$_{EMRA}$ cells

For example, unstable atherosclerotic plaques show a 10-fold increase in their T cell content [33]. In patients with chronic kidney disease without dialysis, CD8+ CD57 + T cell (similar to T$_{EMRA}$ cell) fraction positively associates with arterial stiffness [34]. Terminally differentiated T cells are highly proinflammatory and may produce multiple cytokines [35]. In addition, T$_{EM}$ and T$_{EMRA}$ cells express high level of CX3CR1, a chemokine receptor allows T cells to bind to activated endothelial cells through fractalkine [36, 37] and subsequently cause endothelial injury. Recently, an interesting study [38] demonstrated less immunosenescence in ESRD patients received peritoneal dialysis when compared to hemodialysis. Surprisingly, patients received peritoneal dialysis had more acute rejection events after renal transplantation. As a result, accelerated immunosenescence might be harmful for cardiovascular health in dialysis patients but after transplantation it might be associated with better graft survival.

Our study also found that intermediate and non-classical monocytes are both significantly increased in ESRD. These monocytes are key players in atherosclerosis and previous studies have provided ample evidence of their significant predictive value for CAD and CVD in both the general population as well as renal failure [39–41]. Intermediate monocytes exhibit senescence features because they have shorter telomere compared to classical monocytes and have higher expression of β-galactosidase [42]. Similar to terminally differentiated T cells, intermediate monocytes express both high levels of CCR2 and CX3CR1 [43] and thus are preferentially recruited to the vascular endothelium. In our analysis, ESRD patients exhibit a dramatic increase in these cells when compared to the healthy individuals. Patients with longer dialysis vintage also exhibit higher percentage of intermediate monocytes in their blood.

In humans, CMV virus infection is an important driver of T cell senescence [44] and we have recently found that level of CMV-IgG also positively associated with advanced differentiation of T cells in ESRD patients [45]. Since the iESRD participants are more than 99% CMV seropositive, the enhanced aging-related immune changes we observed is not due to CMV infection per se; but host factors might have modulated CMV-specific immunity. By correlation analyses, dialysis vintage was associated with both T$_{EMRA}$ cells and intermediate monocytes independent of age. The result strongly supports the hypothesis that the duration of renal failure (thus dialysis vintage) may determine the degree of immunosenescence. In addition, there was a statistically significant association between uremic toxin p-cresyl sulfate levels with CD8+ T$_{EMRA}$ cells. Although uremic toxin levels did not correlate with monocyte differentiation, one explanation is that one-time, cross-sectional measurement of uremic toxins may not completely capture the complete exposure of uremic milieu. It is important to recognize that the immunosenescent T cell phenotype also does not normalize after successful renal transplantation despite a rapid reduction of uremic toxins [46]. As a result, effects of uremic toxin on immunosenescence might not be reversible by reducing uremic toxin levels.

Our study has several limitations. First, because this is a cross-sectional observational study, the causality between aging-related immune changes and cardiovascular disease cannot be established. Secondly, since the study population is composed of 99% CMV seropositive Taiwanese, it is not known if the findings can be extrapolated to CMV seronegative ESRD patients and to other racial groups. Finally, T cells and monocytes may exhibit aging-related changes in their effector functions that are not reflected by phenotypic changes. In addition, because regulatory T cell differentiation is also affected by renal failure [47], an important direction of further research is to investigate the effects of uremia on regulatory T cells and effector T cells separately.

Conclusions

ESRD patients exhibit accelerated immunosenescence in both T lymphocyte and monocyte compartment and these changes are positively related to inflammation and cardiovascular morbidities. Chronic exposure to the uremic milieu may directly contribute to these immune changes. ESRD may be used as a disease model in the future for investigating how immunosenescence mediates inflammation and vascular health.

Additional file

Additional file 1: Table S1. Relationships between dialysis vintage and immune cell subsets using tertiles of dialysis vintage, least squares regression and robust regression. **Table S2.** Numbers of age-related immune cells correlate with cardiovascular risk factors and systemic inflammation in ESRD patients. **Table S3.** Comparisons of circulatory T cell and monocyte subset cell numbers between ESRD patients with and without diabetes. **Table S4.** End-stage renal disease patients with concurrent coronary artery disease or cardiovascular disease display more immunosenescence. **Table S5.** Logistic regression model for coronary artery disease and cardiovascular disease using subset percentage to characterize the combinatorial immunophenotype. **Figure S1.** Representative staining of lymphocytes and monocytes. **Figure S2.** Correlogram of immune cell subsets among healthy donors and ESRD patients.

Abbreviations
CAD: Coronary artery disease; CMV: Cytomegalovirus; CRP: C-reactive protein; CVD: Cardiovascular disease; ESRD: End-stage renal disease

Acknowledgements
The authors thank Ms. Priscilla Tsai for her expertise and assistance with multicolor flow cytometry.

Funding
This work was supported by Far Eastern Memorial Hospital grant FEMH-2015-C-007, Ministry of Science and Technology grant 104–2314-B-418-017, 105–2314-B-418-002, Far Eastern Memorial Hospital-National Taiwan University collaboration grant 104-FTN17, Far Eastern Memorial Hospital-National Yang Ming University collaboration grant 105-FN13 and 106-DN13.

Authors' contributions
YLC, YFC, NL and KHS initiated the study and major experiments; YLC, FJY and SYP recruited study participants; TYC, FYL, PMC, KHS, KCK and CJL carried out experiments; YLC, FJY, YFC and SB analyzed experiments; NL, MB, GW and JSC edited the manuscript; YLC, SB and YFC wrote the manuscript. All the authors participated in the reading and completion of this manuscript. All authors read and approved the final manuscript.

Competing interests
Non-declared. The authors declare that the research was conducted in the absence of any commercial or financial relationships that serves as a potential competing interest. The results presented in this paper have not been published previously in whole or part, except in abstract format.

Author details
[1]Division of Nephrology, Department of Medicine, Far Eastern Memorial Hospital, Taipei, Taiwan. [2]Graduate Institute of Clinical Medicine, College of Medicine, National Taiwan University , Taipei, Taiwan. [3]Graduate Program in Biomedical Informatics, Yuan Ze University, Taoyuan, Taiwan. [4]Graduate Institute of Immunology, College of Medicine, National Taiwan University , Taipei, Taiwan. [5]Department of Medicine, National Taiwan University Hospital Yun Lin Branch, Douliu, Taiwan. [6]Division of Nephrology, Department of Internal Medicine, Mackay Memorial Hospital, Taipei, Taiwan. [7]Department of Internal Medicine, Nephrology and Transplantation, Erasmus Medical Center, University Medical Center Rotterdam, Rotterdam, Netherlands. [8]International Health Program, National Yang Ming University School of Public Health, Taipei, Taiwan. [9]Biology of Healthy Aging Program, Division of Geriatric Medicine and Gerontology, Johns Hopkins University School of Medicine, Baltimore, MD, USA. [10]Institute of Public Health, National Yang Ming University School of Public Health, Taipei, Taiwan. [11]Preventive Medicine Research Center, National Yang-Ming University, Taipei, Taiwan.

References
1. Kooman JP, Kotanko P, Schols AM, Shiels PG, Stenvinkel P. Chronic kidney disease and premature ageing. Nat Rev Nephrol. 2014;10:732–42.
2. Stenvinkel P, Larsson TE. Chronic kidney disease: a clinical model of premature aging. Am J Kidney Dis. 2013;62:339–51.
3. Puzianowska-Kuznicka M, Owczarz M, Wieczorowska-Tobis K, Nadrowski P, Chudek J, Slusarczyk P, Skalska A, Jonas M, Franek E, Mossakowska M. Interleukin-6 and C-reactive protein, successful aging, and mortality: the PolSenior study. Immun Ageing. 2016;13:21.
4. Stenvinkel P. Inflammation in end-stage renal failure: could it be treated? Nephrol Dial Transplant. 2002;17(Suppl 8):33–8 discussion 40.
5. Larbi A, Franceschi C, Mazzatti D, Solana R, Wikby A, Pawelec G. Aging of the immune system as a prognostic factor for human longevity. Physiology (Bethesda). 2008;23:64–74.
6. McElhaney JE, Effros RB. Immunosenescence: what does it mean to health outcomes in older adults? Curr Opin Immunol. 2009;21:418–24.
7. Sansoni P, Vescovini R, Fagnoni FF, Akbar A, Arens R, Chiu YL, Cicin-Sain L, Dechanet-Merville J, Derhovanessian E, Ferrando-Martinez S, et al. New advances in CMV and immunosenescence. Exp Gerontol. 2014.
8. Henson SM, Riddell NE, Akbar AN. Properties of end-stage human T cells defined by CD45RA re-expression. Curr Opin Immunol. 2012;24:476–81.
9. Koch S, Larbi A, Derhovanessian E, Ozcelik D, Naumova E, Pawelec G. Multiparameter flow cytometric analysis of CD4 and CD8 T cell subsets in young and old people. Immun Ageing. 2008;5:6.
10. Deng Y, Jing Y, Campbell AE, Gravenstein S. Age-related impaired type 1 T cell responses to influenza: reduced activation ex vivo, decreased expansion in CTL culture in vitro, and blunted response to influenza vaccination in vivo in the elderly. J Immunol. 2004;172:3437–46.
11. Swain S, Clise-Dwyer K, Haynes L. Homeostasis and the age-associated defect of CD4 T cells. Semin Immunol. 2005;17:370–7.
12. Betjes MG, Langerak AW, van der Spek A, de Wit EA, Litjens NH. Premature aging of circulating T cells in patients with end-stage renal disease. Kidney Int. 2011;80:208–17.
13. Betjes MG, Huisman M, Weimar W, Litjens NH. Expansion of cytolytic CD4+CD28- T cells in end-stage renal disease. Kidney Int. 2008;74:760–7.
14. Huang L, Litjens NHR, Kannegieter NM, Klepper M, Baan CC, Betjes MGH. pERK-dependent defective TCR-mediated activation of CD4(+) T cells in end-stage renal disease patients. Immun Ageing. 2017;14:14.
15. Schaenman JM, Rossetti M, Sidwell T, Groysberg V, Sunga G, Korin Y, Liang E, Zhou X, Abdallah B, Lum E, et al. Increased T cell Immunosenescence and accelerated maturation phenotypes in older kidney transplant recipients. Hum Immunol. 2018;79(9):659–67. https://doi.org/10.1016/j.humimm.2018.06.006.
16. Hearps AC, Martin GE, Angelovich TA, Cheng WJ, Maisa A, Landay AL, Jaworowski A, Crowe SM. Aging is associated with chronic innate immune activation and dysregulation of monocyte phenotype and function. Aging Cell. 2012;11:867–75.
17. Heine GH, Ulrich C, Seibert E, Seiler S, Marell J, Reichart B, Krause M, Schlitt A, Kohler H, Girndt M. CD14(++)CD16+ monocytes but not total monocyte numbers predict cardiovascular events in dialysis patients. Kidney Int. 2008;73:622–9.
18. Passos S, Carvalho LP, Costa RS, Campos TM, Novais FO, Magalhaes A, Machado PR, Beiting D, Mosser D, Carvalho EM, Scott P. Intermediate monocytes contribute to pathologic immune response in Leishmania braziliensis infections. J Infect Dis. 2015;211:274–82.
19. Rossol M, Kraus S, Pierer M, Baerwald C, Wagner U. The CD14(bright) CD16+ monocyte subset is expanded in rheumatoid arthritis and promotes expansion of the Th17 cell population. Arthritis Rheum. 2011;64:671–7.
20. Gattinoni L, Lugli E, Ji Y, Pos Z, Paulos CM, Quigley MF, Almeida JR, Gostick E, Yu Z, Carpenito C, et al. A human memory T cell subset with stem cell-like properties. Nat Med. 2011;17:1290–7.
21. Pulko V, Davies JS, Martinez C, Lanteri MC, Busch MP, Diamond MS, Knox K, Bush EC, Sims PA, Sinari S, et al. Human memory T cells with a naive phenotype accumulate with aging and respond to persistent viruses. Nat Immunol. 2016;17:966–75.
22. Foley RN, Parfrey PS, Sarnak MJ. Epidemiology of cardiovascular disease in chronic renal disease. J Am Soc Nephrol. 1998;9:S16–23.
23. Collins AJ. Cardiovascular mortality in end-stage renal disease. Am J Med Sci. 2003;325:163–7.
24. Bazeley J, Bieber B, Li Y, Morgenstern H, de Sequera P, Combe C, Yamamoto H, Gallagher M, Port FK, Robinson BM. C-reactive protein and prediction of 1-year mortality in prevalent hemodialysis patients. Clin J Am Soc Nephrol. 2011;6:2452–61.

25. Wikby A, Maxson P, Olsson J, Johansson B, Ferguson FG. Changes in CD8 and CD4 lymphocyte subsets, T cell proliferation responses and non-survival in the very old: the Swedish longitudinal OCTO-immune study. Mech Ageing Dev. 1998;102:187–98.

26. Hansson GK, Hermansson A. The immune system in atherosclerosis. Nat Immunol. 2011;12:204–12.

27. Vaziri ND. Oxidative stress in uremia: nature, mechanisms, and potential consequences. Semin Nephrol. 2004;24:469–73.

28. Wu IW, Hsu KH, Hsu HJ, Lee CC, Sun CY, Tsai CJ, Wu MS. Serum free p-cresyl sulfate levels predict cardiovascular and all-cause mortality in elderly hemodialysis patients--a prospective cohort study. Nephrol Dial Transplant. 2012;27:1169–75.

29. Lin CJ, Chuang CK, Jayakumar T, Liu HL, Pan CF, Wang TJ, Chen HH, Wu CJ. Serum p-cresyl sulfate predicts cardiovascular disease and mortality in elderly hemodialysis patients. Arch Med Sci. 2013;9:662–8.

30. Nikolich-Zugich J. Aging of the T cell compartment in mice and humans: from no naive expectations to foggy memories. J Immunol. 2014;193:2622–9.

31. Goronzy JJ, Weyand CM. Successful and maladaptive T cell aging. Immunity. 2017;46:364–78.

32. Ammirati E, Cianflone D, Vecchio V, Banfi M, Vermi AC, De Metrio M, Grigore L, Pellegatta F, Pirillo A, Garlaschelli K, et al. Effector memory T cells are associated with atherosclerosis in humans and animal models. J Am Heart Assoc. 2012;1:27–41.

33. De Palma R, Del Galdo F, Abbate G, Chiariello M, Calabro R, Forte L, Cimmino G, Papa MF, Russo MG, Ambrosio G, et al. Patients with acute coronary syndrome show oligoclonal T-cell recruitment within unstable plaque: evidence for a local, intracoronary immunologic mechanism. Circulation. 2006;113:640–6.

34. Yu HT, Youn JC, Kim JH, Seong YJ, Park SH, Kim HC, Lee WW, Park S, Shin EC. Arterial stiffness is associated with cytomegalovirus-specific senescent CD8+ T cells. J Am Heart Assoc. 2017;6.

35. Chiu YL, Lin CH, Sung BY, Chuang YF, Schneck JP, Kern F, Pawelec G, Wang GC. Cytotoxic polyfunctionality maturation of cytomegalovirus-pp65-specific CD4 + and CD8 + T-cell responses in older adults positively correlates with response size. Sci Rep. 2016;6:19227.

36. van de Berg PJ, Yong SL, Remmerswaal EB, van Lier RA, ten Berge IJ. Cytomegalovirus-induced effector T cells cause endothelial cell damage. Clin Vaccine Immunol. 2012;19:772–9.

37. Pachnio A, Ciaurriz M, Begum J, Lal N, Zuo J, Beggs A, Moss P. Cytomegalovirus infection leads to development of high frequencies of cytotoxic virus-specific CD4+ T cells targeted to vascular endothelium. PLoS Pathog. 2016;12:e1005832.

38. Ducloux D, Legendre M, Bamoulid J, Rebibou JM, Saas P, Courivaud C, Crepin T. ESRD-associated immune phenotype depends on dialysis modality and iron status: clinical implications. Immun Ageing. 2018;15:16.

39. Rogacev KS, Cremers B, Zawada AM, Seiler S, Binder N, Ege P, Grosse-Dunker G, Heisel I, Hornof F, Jeken J, et al. CD14++CD16+ monocytes independently predict cardiovascular events: a cohort study of 951 patients referred for elective coronary angiography. J Am Coll Cardiol. 2012;60:1512–20.

40. Rogacev KS, Seiler S, Zawada AM, Reichart B, Herath E, Roth D, Ulrich C, Fliser D, Heine GH. CD14++CD16+ monocytes and cardiovascular outcome in patients with chronic kidney disease. Eur Heart J. 2010;32:84–92.

41. Shantsila E, Tapp LD, Wrigley BJ, Pamukcu B, Apostolakis S, Montoro-Garcia S, Lip GY. Monocyte subsets in coronary artery disease and their associations with markers of inflammation and fibrinolysis. Atherosclerosis. 2014;234:4–10.

42. Merino A, Buendia P, Martin-Malo A, Aljama P, Ramirez R, Carracedo J. Senescent CD14+CD16+ monocytes exhibit proinflammatory and proatherosclerotic activity. J Immunol. 2011;186:1809–15.

43. Wildgruber M, Aschenbrenner T, Wendorff H, Czubba M, Glinzer A, Haller B, Schiemann M, Zimmermann A, Berger H, Eckstein HH, et al. The "intermediate" CD14++CD16+ monocyte subset increases in severe peripheral artery disease in humans. Sci Rep. 2016;6:39483.

44. Wertheimer AM, Bennett MS, Park B, Uhrlaub JL, Martinez C, Pulko V, Currier NL, Nikolich-Zugich D, Kaye J, Nikolich-Zugich J. Aging and cytomegalovirus infection differentially and jointly affect distinct circulating T cell subsets in humans. J Immunol. 2014;192:2143–55.

45. Yang FJ, Shu KH, Chen HY, Chen IY, Lay FY, Chuang YF, Wu CS, Tsai WC, Peng YS, Hsu SP, et al. Anti-cytomegalovirus IgG antibody titer is positively associated with advanced T cell differentiation and coronary artery disease in end-stage renal disease. Immun Ageing. 2018;15:15.

46. Meijers RW, Litjens NH, de Wit EA, Langerak AW, Baan CC, Betjes MG. Uremia-associated immunological aging is stably imprinted in the T-cell system and not reversed by kidney transplantation. Transpl Int. 2014;27:1272–84.

47. Schaier M, Leick A, Uhlmann L, Kalble F, Morath C, Eckstein V, Ho A, Mueller-Tidow C, Meuer S, Mahnke K, et al. End-stage renal disease, dialysis, kidney transplantation and their impact on CD4(+) T-cell differentiation. Immunology. 2018.

Permissions

List of Contributors

Shu-Chun Chuang
Institute of Population Health Sciences, National Health Research Institutes, 35 Keyan Road, Zhunan, Miaoli County 35053, Taiwan
Department of Epidemiology and Biostatistics, School of Public Health, Imperial College London, London, UK

Marc Gunter, Yunxia Lu, Amanda J. Cross, Elio Riboli and Paolo Vineis
Department of Epidemiology and Biostatistics, School of Public Health, Imperial College London, London, UK

Bas Bueno-de-Mesquita
Department of Epidemiology and Biostatistics, School of Public Health, Imperial College London, London, UK
The National Institute for Public Health and the Environment (RIVM), Bilthoven, The Netherlands
Department of Gastroenterology and Hepatology, University Medical Centre, Utrecht, The Netherlands
Department of Social and Preventive Medicine, Faculty of Medicine, University of Malaya, Kuala Lumpur, Malaysia

Petra H Peeters
Department of Epidemiology and Biostatistics, School of Public Health, Imperial College London, London, UK
Julius Center for Health Sciences and Primary Care, University Medical Center Utrecht, Utrecht, The Netherlands

Heiner Boeing
Department of Epidemiology, German Institute of Human Nutrition Potsdam-Rehbruecke, Nuthetal, Germany

Stein Emil Vollset
Department of Public Health and Primary Health Care, University of Bergen, Bergen, Norway
Division of Epidemiology, Norwegian Institute of Public Health, Bergen, Norway

Øivind Midttun
Bevital AS, Bergen, Norway

Per Magne Ueland
Department of Clinical Science, University of Bergen, Bergen, Norway
Laboratory of Clinical Biochemistry, Haukeland University Hospital, Bergen, Norway

Martin Lajous, Guy Fagherazzi and Marie-Christine Boutron-Ruault
Inserm, Centre for research in Epidemiology and Population Health (CESP), U1018, Nutrition, Hormones and Women's Health team, F-94805 Villejuif, France
University of Paris Sud, UMRS 1018, F-94805 Villejuif, France
IGR, F-94805, Villejuif, France

Rudolf Kaaks and Tilman Küehn
Division of Cancer Epidemiology, German Cancer Research Center, Heidelberg, Germany

Tobias Pischon
Molecular Epidemiology Group, Max Delbrueck Center for Molecular Medicine (MDC), Berlin-Buch, Germany

Dagmar Drogan
Department of Epidemiology, German Institute of Human Nutrition Potsdam-Rehbrücke, Nuthetal, Germany

Anne Tjønneland
Diet, Genes and Environment, Danish Cancer Society Research Center, Copenhagen, Denmark

Kim Overvad
Department of Public Health, Section for Epidemiology, Aarhus University, Aarhus, Denmark

J Ramón Quirós
Public Health Directorate, Asturias, Oviedo, Spain

Antonio Agudo
Unit of Nutrition, Environment and Cancer, Catalan Institute of Oncology-ICO, IDIBELL, L'Hospitalet de Llobregat, Barcelona, Spain

Esther Molina-Montes
Escuela Andaluza de Salud Pública. Instituto de Investigación Biosanitaria de Granada (Granada.ibs), Granada, Spain
Consortium for Biomedical Research in Epidemiology and Public Health (CIBER Epidemiología y Salud Pública-CIBERESP), Madrid, Spain

José María Huerta
Consortium for Biomedical Research in Epidemiology and Public Health (CIBER Epidemiología y Salud Pública-CIBERESP), Madrid, Spain
Department of Epidemiology, Murcia Regional Health Council, Murcia, Spain

Miren Dorronsoro
Epidemiology and Health Information, Public Health Division of Gipuzkoa, Basque Regional Health Department, San Sebastian, Spain

Aurelio Barricarte
Navarre Public Health Institute, Pamplona, Spain

Kay-Tee Khaw
Clinical Gerontology Unit, Addenbrooke's Hospital, University of Cambridge School of Clinical Medicine, Cambridge, UK

Nicholas J. Wareham
MRC Epidemiology Unit, Institute of Metabolic Science, University of Cambridge School of Clinical Medicine, Cambridge, UK

Ruth C. Travis
Cancer Epidemiology Unit, Nuffield Department of Population Health, University of Oxford, Oxford, UK

Antonia Trichopoulou
Cancer Epidemiology Unit, Nuffield Department of Population Health, University of Oxford, Oxford, UK
Hellenic Health Foundation, Athens, Greece

Dimitrios Trichopoulos
Hellenic Health Foundation, Athens, Greece
Department of Hygiene, Epidemiology and Medical Statistics, University of Athens Medical School, Athens, Greece

Pagona Lagiou
Bureau of Epidemiologic Research, Academy of Athens, Athens, Greece
Department of Hygiene, Epidemiology and Medical Statistics, University of Athens Medical School, Athens, Greece
Department of Epidemiology, Harvard School of Public Health, Boston, USA

Giovanna Masala
Molecular and Nutritional Epidemiology Unit, Cancer Research and Prevention Institute – ISPO, Florence, Italy

Claudia Agnoli
Epidemiology and Prevention Unit, Fondazione IRCCS Istituto Nazionale dei Tumori, Milan, Italy

Rosario Tumino
Cancer Registry and Histopathology Unit, "Civic - M.P. Arezzo" Hospital, ASP Ragusa, Italy

Amalia Mattiello
Dipartamento di Medicina Clinica e Chirurgia, Federico II University, Naples, Italy

Julius Center for Health Sciences and Primary Care, University Medical Center Utrecht, Utrecht, The Netherlands

Elisabete Weiderpass
Department of Community Medicine, Faculty of Health Sciences, University of Tromso, Tromsø, Norway
Department of Research, Cancer Registry of Norway, Oslo, Norway
Department of Medical Epidemiology and Biostatistics, Karolinska Institutet, Stockholm, Sweden
Samfundet Folkhälsan, Helsinki, Finland

Richard Palmqvist
Department of Medical Biosciences, Pathology, Umeå University, Umeå, Sweden

Ingrid Ljuslinder
Department of Radiation Sciences, Oncology, Umeå University, Umeå, Sweden

Krasimira Aleksandrova
Nutrition, Immunity and Metabolism Start-up Lab, Department of Epidemiology, German Institute of Human Nutrition Potsdam-Rehbruecke, Nuthetal, Germany

Lindsay Reynolds, Li Hou, Kurt Lohman, Wei Cui and Yongmei Liu
Department of Epidemiology and Prevention, Public Health Sciences, Wake Forest School of Medicine, Winston-Salem, NC 27157, USA

Jackson Taylor
Department of Epidemiology and Prevention, Public Health Sciences, Wake Forest School of Medicine, Winston-Salem, NC 27157, USA
Department of Internal Medicine, Wake Forest School of Medicine, Winston-Salem, NC 27157, USA
Department of Molecular Biology, Cell Biology, Biochemistry at Brown University, Providence, RI 02912, USA

Stephen Kritchevsky and Charles McCall
Department of Internal Medicine, Wake Forest School of Medicine, Winston-Salem, NC 27157, USA

Sarah McCormack, Shruti Yadav, Upasana Shokal, Eric Kenney, Dustin Cooper and Ioannis Eleftherianos
Insect Infection and Immunity Laboratory, Department of Biological Sciences, Institute for Biomedical Sciences, The George Washington University, 800 Science and Engineering Hall, 22nd Street NW, Washington, D.C. 20052, USA

R. E. Banks and B. M. Wilson
Geriatric Research, Education, and Clinical Center, Louis Stokes Cleveland VA Medical Center, Cleveland, OH, USA

P. Van Epps, H. Aung and D. H. Canaday
Geriatric Research, Education, and Clinical Center, Louis Stokes Cleveland VA Medical Center, Cleveland, OH, USA
Division of Infectious Disease, Case Western Reserve University, Cleveland, OH, USA

T. R. Hornick
Geriatric Research, Education, and Clinical Center, Louis Stokes Cleveland VA Medical Center, Cleveland, OH, USA
Division of Geriatrics, Department of Medicine, Case Western Reserve University, Cleveland, OH, USA

P. A. Higgins and C. Burant
Geriatric Research, Education, and Clinical Center, Louis Stokes Cleveland VA Medical Center, Cleveland, OH, USA
School of Nursing, Case Western Reserve University, Cleveland, OH, USA

D. Oswald
Division of Infectious Disease, Case Western Reserve University, Cleveland, OH, USA

S. Gravenstein
Division of Geriatrics, Department of Medicine, Case Western Reserve University, Cleveland, OH, USA

Giusy Russomanno, Valentina Manzo, Maria Consiglia Calabrese, Amelia Filippelli and Valeria Conti
Department of Medicine, Surgery and Dentistry, University of Salerno, Via S. Allende 43, 84081 Baronissi, Italy

Annibale A. Puca
Department of Medicine, Surgery and Dentistry, University of Salerno, Via S. Allende 43, 84081 Baronissi, Italy
IRCCS MultiMedica, Milan, Italy

Carmine Vecchione
Department of Medicine, Surgery and Dentistry, University of Salerno, Via S. Allende 43, 84081 Baronissi, Italy
Vascular Physiopathology Unit, IRCCS INM Neuromed, Pozzilli, Italy

Graziamaria Corbi
Department of Medicine and Health Sciences, University of Molise, Campobasso, Italy

Nicola Ferrara and Giuseppe Rengo
Department of Translational Medical Sciences, Federico II University of Naples, Naples, Italy

Salvatore Maugeri Foundation, IRCCS, Scientific Institute of Telese Terme, Benevento, Italy

Salvatore Latte
Cardiac Rehabilitation Unit of "San Gennaro dei Poveri" Hospital, Naples, Italy

Albino Carrizzo
Vascular Physiopathology Unit, IRCCS INM Neuromed, Pozzilli, Italy

Ramaroson Andriantsitohaina
INSERM U1063, Stress Oxydant et Pathologies Métaboliques, Institut de Biologie en Santé, Université d'Angers, Angers, France

Walter Filippelli
Department of Institutional Study and Territorial Systems, University of Naples "Parthenope", Naples, Italy

Bart P. X. Grady
Department of Research, Cluster Infectious Diseases, Public Health Service, Amsterdam, The Netherlands
Center for Infection and Immunity Amsterdam (CINIMA), Academic Medical Center, Amsterdam, The Netherlands

Nening M. Nanlohy
Department of Immunology, University Medical Center Utrecht, Utrecht, The Netherlands

Debbie van Baarle
Department of Immunology, University Medical Center Utrecht, Utrecht, The Netherlands
Department of Internal Medicine, University Medical Center Utrecht, Utrecht, The Netherlands
Department of Immune Mechanisms, Center for Infectious Disease Control, National Institute for Public Health and the Environment (RIVM), Bilthoven, The Netherlands

Jan Olsson and Fredrik Elgh
Department of Clinical Microbiology, Virology, Umeå University, Umeå, Sweden

Eloise Kok
Department of Forensic Medicine, University of Tampere, Tampere 33520, Finland

Rolf Adolfsson
Department of Clinical Sciences, Psychiatry, Umeå University, Umeå, Sweden

Hugo Lövheim
Department of Community Medicine and Rehabilitation, Geriatric Medicine, Umeå University, Umeå, Sweden

Kornelis S. M. van der Geest, Qi Wang, Elisabeth Brouwer and Annemieke M. H. Boots
Departments of Rheumatology and Clinical Immunology and Translational Immunology Groningen (TRIGR), University of Groningen, University Medical Center Groningen, Hanzeplein 1, 9700RB Groningen, The Netherlands

Thijs M. H. Eijsvogels and Maria T. E. Hopman
Department of Physiology, Radboud University Medical Centre, Nijmegen, The Netherlands

Hans J. P. Koenen, Irma Joosten and Joannes F. M. Jacobs
Department of Laboratory Medicine, Laboratory Medical Immunology, Radboud University Medical Centre, Nijmegen, The Netherlands

Myeongjoo Son, Hyosang Ahn and Kyunghee Byun
Department of Anatomy and Cell Biology, Graduate School of Medicine, Gachon University, Incheon 21936, Republic of Korea
Functional Cellular Networks Laboratory, Lee Gil Ya Cancer and Diabetes Institute, Gachon University, Incheon 21999, Republic of Korea

Seyeon Oh
Functional Cellular Networks Laboratory, Lee Gil Ya Cancer and Diabetes Institute, Gachon University, Incheon 21999, Republic of Korea

Wook-Jin Chung
Department of Cardiovascular Medicine, Gachon University, Incheon 21999, Republic of Korea
Gachon Cardiovascular Research Institute, Gachon University, Incheon 21999, Republic of Korea

Chang Hu Choi, Kook Yang Park and Kuk Hui Son
Department of Thoracic and Cardiovascular Surgery, Gachon University Gil Medical Center, Gachon University, Incheon 21565, Republic of Korea

Suntaek Hong
Laboratory of Cancer Cell Biology, Department of Biochemistry, School of Medicine, Gachon University, Incheon 21999, Republic of Korea

Marta Jonas and Edward Franek
Department of Human Epigenetics, Mossakowski Medical Research Centre PAS, 5 Pawinskiego Street, 02-106 Warsaw, Poland

Monika Puzianowska-Kuźnicka
Department of Human Epigenetics, Mossakowski Medical Research Centre PAS, 5 Pawinskiego Street, 02-106 Warsaw, Poland
Department of Geriatrics and Gerontology, Medical Centre of Postgraduate Education, 01-826 Warsaw, Poland

Magdalena Owczarz
Department of Human Epigenetics, Mossakowski Medical Research Centre PAS, 5 Pawinskiego Street, 02-106 Warsaw, Poland
PolSenior Project, International Institute of Molecular and Cell Biology, 02-109 Warsaw, Poland

Przemyslaw Slusarczyk and Malgorzata Mossakowska
PolSenior Project, International Institute of Molecular and Cell Biology, 02-109 Warsaw, Poland

Katarzyna Wieczorowska-Tobis
Department of Palliative Medicine, Poznan University of Medical Sciences, 61-245 Poznan, Poland

Pawel Nadrowski
Third Department of Cardiology, Medical University of Silesia in Katowice, 40-635 Katowice, Poland

Jerzy Chudek
Department of Pathophysiology, Faculty of Medicine, Medical University of Silesia in Katowice, 40-752 Katowice, Poland
Deparament of Internal Medicine and Oncological Chemotherapy, Faculty of Medicine, Medical University of Silesia in Katowice, 40-027 Katowice, Poland

Anna Skalska
Department of Internal Medicine and Geriatrics, Jagiellonian University Medical College, 31-351 Cracow, Poland

Agnieszka Przemska-Kosicka, Caroline E. Childs, Sumia Enani, Catherine Maidens, Honglin Dong, Iman Bin Dayel, Margot A. Gosney and Parveen Yaqoob
Department of Food and Nutritional Sciences, University of Reading, PO Box 226Whiteknights, Reading, Berkshire RG6 6AP, UK

Susan Todd
Department of Mathematics and Statistics, University of Reading, Reading, RG6 6AP, UK

Kieran Tuohy
Department of Food Quality and Nutrition, Research and Innovation Centre, Fondazione Edmund Mach, via E. Mach, 1, San Michele all'Adige, Trento 38010, Italy

Ling Huang, Nicolle H. R. Litjens, Nynke M. Kannegieter, Mariska Klepper, Carla C. Baan and Michiel G. H. Betjes
Department of Internal Medicine, Section Nephrology and Transplantation, Erasmus University Medical Center, Rotterdam, the Netherlands

Yun Lin, Jiewan Kim, Huy Nguyen, Thai Truong, Ana Lustig and Nan-ping Weng
Laboratory of Molecular Biology and Immunology, National Institute on Aging, 251 Bayview Blvd., Baltimore, MD 21224, USA

Luigi Ferrucci
Translational Gerontology Branch, National Institute on Aging, National Institutes of Health, Baltimore, MD 21224, USA

E. Jeffrey Metter
Translational Gerontology Branch, National Institute on Aging, National Institutes of Health, Baltimore, MD 21224, USA
Department of Neurology, University of Tennessee Health Science Center, Memphis, TN 38111, USA

Giuseppe Passarino, Francesco De Rango and Alberto Montesanto
Department of Biology, Ecology and Earth Science, University of Calabria, 87036 Rende, Italy

William Galbavy, Yong Lu, Martin Kaczocha, Michelino Puopolo, Lixin Liu and Mario J. Rebecchi
Department of Anesthesiology, School of Medicine, Health Sciences CenterbL4, Stony Brook University, Stony Brook, New York 11794-8480, USA

Annalisa Barera and Calogero Caruso
Pathobiology Department and Biomedical Technologies (DIBIMED), University of Palermo, Palermo, Italy

Marcello Ciaccio
Pathobiology Department and Biomedical Technologies (DIBIMED), University of Palermo, Palermo, Italy
Biomedic Department of Internal and Specialistic Medicine (DIBIMIS), University of Palermo, Palermo, Italy
Department of Experimental Biomedicine and Clinical Neuroscience (BioNeC), University of Palermo, Palermo, Italy
CORELAB, Policlinico Paolo Giaccone, University of Palermo, Palermo, Italy

Silvio Buscemi
Biomedic Department of Internal and Specialistic Medicine (DIBIMIS), University of Palermo, Palermo, Italy

Roberto Monastero
Department of Experimental Biomedicine and Clinical Neuroscience (BioNeC), University of Palermo, Palermo, Italy

Rosalia Caldarella
CORELAB, Policlinico Paolo Giaccone, University of Palermo, Palermo, Italy

Sonya Vasto
Department of Biological Chemical and Pharmaceutical Sciences and Technologies (STEBICEF), University of Palermo, Viale delle Scienze, Building 16, Palermo, Italy
Institute of biomedicine and molecular immunology "Alberto Monroy" CNR, Palermo, Italy

Bjørn Grinde and Bo Engdahl
Department of Aging, Norwegian Institute of Public Health, Box 4404 Nydalen, 0403 Oslo, PO, Norway

Didier Ducloux, Jamal Bamoulid, Cécile Courivaud and Thomas Crepin
INSERM, UMR1098, Federation Hospitalo-Universitaire, INCREASE, Besançon, France
Univ. Bourgogne-Franche-Comté, Faculté de Médecine et de Pharmacie, LabEx LipSTIC, Besançon, France
Univ. Bourgogne-Franche-Comté, Faculté de Médecine et de Pharmacie, LabEx LipSTIC, Dijon, France
CHU Besançon, Department of Nephrology, Dialysis, and Renal Transplantation, Besançon, France

Mathieu Legendre and Jean-Michel Rebibou
INSERM, UMR1098, Federation Hospitalo-Universitaire, INCREASE, Besançon, France
Univ. Bourgogne-Franche-Comté, Faculté de Médecine et de Pharmacie, LabEx LipSTIC, Besançon, France
Univ. Bourgogne-Franche-Comté, Faculté de Médecine et de Pharmacie, LabEx LipSTIC, Dijon, France
CHU Dijon, Department of Nephrology, Dialysis, and Renal Transplantation, Dijon, France

Philippe Saas
INSERM, UMR1098, Federation Hospitalo-Universitaire, INCREASE, Besançon, France
Univ. Bourgogne-Franche-Comté, Faculté de Médecine et de Pharmacie, LabEx LipSTIC, Besançon, France
Univ. Bourgogne-Franche-Comté, Faculté de Médecine et de Pharmacie, LabEx LipSTIC, Dijon, France
EFS Bourgogne Franche-Comté, Plateforme de Biomonitoring, INSERM CIC 1431/UMR1098, Besançon, France

Houfen Su, Sudhanshu Agrawal and Sastry Gollapudi
Program in Primary Immunodeficiency and Aging, Division of Basic and Clinical Immunology, University of California, Irvine, USA

Sudhir Gupta
Program in Primary Immunodeficiency and Aging, Division of Basic and Clinical Immunology, University of California, Irvine, USA

Division of Basic and Clinical Immunology, Medical Sci. I, C-240, University of California at Irvine, Irvine, CA 92697, USA

Monica Neri and Aliaksei Kisialiou
Unit of Clinical and Molecular Epidemiology, IRCCS San Raffaele Pisana, Via di Val Cannuta, 247, 00166 Rome, Italy

Stefano Bonassi
Unit of Clinical and Molecular Epidemiology, IRCCS San Raffaele Pisana, Via di Val Cannuta, 247, 00166 Rome, Italy
Department of Human Sciences and Quality of Life Promotion, San Raffaele University, Rome, Italy

Luigi Sansone and Marco Tafani
Department of Cellular and Molecular Pathology, IRCCS San Raffaele Pisana, Rome, Italy
Department of Experimental Medicine, Sapienza University of Rome, Rome, Italy

Luisa Pietrasanta and Marina Martini
Terme di Genova, Genoa, Italy
Terme di Acqui, AcquiTerme (AL), Italy

Eloisa Cabano
Casa di Cura Villa Montallegro, Genova, Italy

Matteo A. Russo
Consortium MEBIC, San Raffaele University, Rome, Italy

Donatella Ugolini
Department of Internal Medicine, University of Genoa, Genoa, Italy

Kyung Mi Jo, Mee Ae Cheong, Min Hwa Hong and Yoori Kim
Department of Senior Healthcare, BK21 plus program, Graduate School, Eulji University, Daejeon 34824, Korea

In Sik Kim
Department of Senior Healthcare, BK21 plus program, Graduate School, Eulji University, Daejeon 34824, Korea
Department of Biomedical Laboratory Science, School of Medicine, Eulji University, 77, Gyeryoung-ro 771 beon-gil, Jung-Gu, Daejeon 34824, Republic of Korea

Jae Woong Sull
Department of Senior Healthcare, BK21 plus program, Graduate School, Eulji University, Daejeon 34824, Korea
Department of Biomedical Laboratory Science, College of Health Science, Eulji University, Seongnam 13135, Korea

Hyo Kyung Lim
Department of Biomedical Laboratory Science, School of Medicine, Eulji University, 77, Gyeryoung-ro 771 beon-gil, Jung-Gu, Daejeon 34824, Republic of Korea

Eugene Choi
Department of Respiratory Internal Medicine, College of Medicine, Konyang University, Daejeon 35365, Korea

Ji-Sook Lee
Department of Clinical Laboratory Science, Wonkwang Health Science University, Iksan 54538, Republic of Korea

Birgit Weinberger
Universität Innsbruck, Institute for Biomedical Aging Research, Rennweg 10, 6020 Innsbruck, Austria

Divyansh Agarwal
Genomics and Computational Biology, Perelman School of Medicine, University of Pennsylvania, Philadelphia, PA 19104, USA

Kenneth E. Schmader and Susan Doyle
Division of Geriatrics, Duke University Medical Center; Geriatric Research, Education, and Clinical Center, Durham VA Medical Center, Durham, NC 27705, USA

Andrew V. Kossenkov, Raj Kurupati and Hildegund C. J. Ertl
The Wistar Institute, Philadelphia, PA 19104, USA

Ivan Sanz, Silvia Rojo and Raúl Ortiz de Lejarazu
Valladolid National Influenza Centre, Avenida Ramón y Cajal s/n, 47005 Valladolid, Spain
Microbiology and Immunology Unit, Hospital Clínico Universitario de Valladolid, Avenida Ramón y Cajal s/n, 47005 Valladolid, Spain

Jose María Eiros
Valladolid National Influenza Centre, Avenida Ramón y Cajal s/n, 47005 Valladolid, Spain
Microbiology Unit, Hospital Universitario Río Hortega, Calle Dulzaina 2, 47012 Valladolid, Spain

Sonia Tamames
Epidemiology Unit, Consejería de Sanidad, Junta de Castilla y León, Paseo de Zorrilla 1, 47007 Valladolid, Spain

Ying Tang, Peifen Liang, Junzhe Chen, Sha Fu, Bo Liu, Min Feng, Baojuan Lin and Anping Xu
Department of Nephrology, Sun Yat-sen Memorial Hospital, Sun Yat-sen University, Guangzhou, China
Guangdong Provincial Key Laboratory of Malignant Tumor Epigenetics and Gene Regulation, Sun Yat-sen Memorial Hospital, Sun Yat-sen University, Guangzhou, China

Hui Y. Lan
Department of Medicine and Therapeutics, Li KaShing Institute of Health Sciences, the Chinese University of Hong Kong, Hong Kong, SAR, China
Lui Che Woo Institute of Innovative Medicine, the Chinese University of Hong Kong, Hong Kong, SAR, China

Ben Lee
Guangzhou Deling Software Technology Co., Ltd, Guangzhou, China

Richard Aspinall
Rivock Ltd, Bury St Edmunds, UK
3Anglia Ruskin University, Cambridge, UK

Pierre Olivier Lang
Geriatric and Geriatric Rehabilitation Division, Department of Medicine, University Hospital of Lausanne, Lausanne, Switzerland
3Anglia Ruskin University, Cambridge, UK

Marco Casciaro and Sebastiano Gangemi
School and Division of Allergy and Clinical Immunology, Department of Clinical and Experimental Medicine, Azienda Ospedaliera Universitaria Policlinico "G. Martino", University of Messina, Messina, Italy

Eleonora Di Salvo and Elisabetta Pace
IBIM-CNR Institute of Biomedicine and Molecular Immunology, National Research Council, 90100 Palermo, Italy

Elvira Ventura-Spagnolo
Legal Medicine Section, Department for Health Promotion and Mother-Child Care, University of Palermo, Via del Vespro, 129, 90127 Palermo, Italy

Michele Navarra
Department of Chemical, Biological, Pharmaceutical and Environmental Sciences, University of Messina, Messina, Italy

Tzu-Ying Chou, Ping-Min Chen, Fang-Yun Lay, Szu-Yu Pan and Yu-Sen Peng
Division of Nephrology, Department of Medicine, Far Eastern Memorial Hospital, Taipei, Taiwan

Kai-Hsiang Shu
Division of Nephrology, Department of Medicine, Far Eastern Memorial Hospital, Taipei, Taiwan
Graduate Institute of Immunology, College of Medicine, National Taiwan University, Taipei, Taiwan

Yen-Ling Chiu
Division of Nephrology, Department of Medicine, Far Eastern Memorial Hospital, Taipei, Taiwan
Graduate Institute of Clinical Medicine, College of Medicine, National Taiwan University, Taipei, Taiwan
Graduate Program in Biomedical Informatics, Yuan Ze University, Taoyuan, Taiwan

Feng-Jung Yang
Graduate Institute of Clinical Medicine, College of Medicine, National Taiwan University, Taipei, Taiwan
Department of Medicine, National Taiwan University Hospital Yun Lin Branch, Douliu, Taiwan

Kung-Chi Kao and Jean-San Chia
Graduate Institute of Immunology, College of Medicine, National Taiwan University, Taipei, Taiwan

Cheng-Jui Lin
Division of Nephrology, Department of Internal Medicine, Mackay Memorial Hospital, Taipei, Taiwan

Nicolle H R Litjens and Michiel G H Betjes
Department of Internal Medicine, Nephrology and Transplantation, Erasmus Medical Center, University Medical Center Rotterdam, Rotterdam, Netherlands

Selma Bermudez
International Health Program, National Yang Ming University School of Public Health, Taipei, Taiwan

Yi-Fang Chuang
International Health Program, National Yang Ming University School of Public Health, Taipei, Taiwan
Institute of Public Health, National Yang Ming University School of Public Health, Taipei, Taiwan
Preventive Medicine Research Center, National Yang-Ming University, Taipei, Taiwan

George Wang
Biology of Healthy Aging Program, Division of Geriatric Medicine and Gerontology, Johns Hopkins University School of Medicine, Baltimore, MD, USA

Index

A

Acute Rejection, 168, 170-173, 175-176, 270

Adjuvant Therapy, 46

Anti-ageing Molecule, 46

Antibacterial Immune Function, 26

Apoptosis, 12, 15-16, 20, 24, 61, 117, 125, 128, 138, 149, 151, 177-183, 185-187, 207, 229, 255-256, 259, 264

Apoptotis, 178

Asthma Medicine, 161, 163, 165

Autoimmune Disease, 111

B

Balneology, 188

Blood Lymphocyte, 130

Blood Pressure, 1, 3-7, 9, 47-48, 51-52, 73-74, 159, 253

C

C-reactive Protein, 2, 4, 9, 11, 38, 44, 64, 74, 82, 92, 101-102, 156, 159, 240, 242, 245-247, 267, 271

Calorie Restriction, 139, 142, 229

Cardiac Rehabilitation, 46-48, 51-53

Cellular Immune Activity, 1, 33

Central Memory, 62, 77-78, 82-83, 120-124, 126-127, 178, 185, 266-267

Chronic Rhinitis, 188-190, 194-195, 197, 199-200

Coagulation, 37-40, 42-45, 112

Cytokine Receptor, 15, 20-21

Cytokines, 37-38, 40, 42-44, 72, 74, 81, 90-91, 93, 100, 102-103, 130, 135-137, 145, 151, 156, 159, 175, 177, 183, 186, 200, 202-204, 206-208, 223, 243, 250, 252, 261, 270

Cytomegalovirus, 42, 44-45, 65, 67, 69-71, 82-83, 101, 110, 113, 115, 118, 127-129, 135, 138, 169, 176-177, 251, 255, 265, 271-272

D

Dementia, 42, 45, 66, 69-70, 102, 145, 158, 161-167, 246, 261

Dendritic Cell, 128, 223

Dialysis, 117, 119, 121, 127-128, 168-169, 171-173, 175-177, 263, 265-272

E

Endothelial Cell, 47, 49-50, 91, 174, 272

Endothelium, 46, 270, 272

F

Frailty, 13, 37-45, 49, 54, 70, 92-93, 102, 144, 159, 209, 211, 215, 226, 254

G

Gluco-oligosaccharide, 104-105, 112, 114-115

Glycated Hemoglobin, 1, 6

Glycation, 84-85, 88, 91, 159, 189, 200, 261

Gut Microbiota, 93, 101, 104-105, 110

H

Heart Failure, 46-48, 52-53, 101-102, 259, 261

Herpes Virus, 65, 67-68, 219

Human Longevity, 139-141, 143-144, 271

Hyperlipidemia, 1, 3, 9

I

Immune Activation, 1-3, 10-11, 54-55, 58, 60-62, 64, 167, 271

Immune Phenotype, 170-171, 272

Immune System, 3, 10-11, 15, 20, 35, 54, 61, 63, 71-72, 82, 91, 102, 115, 124-125, 128, 130, 138, 148, 150, 152, 156, 168, 186, 200, 212, 218, 224, 226, 247-251, 261, 271-272

Immunometabolism, 2, 10

Immunosenescence, 24, 37, 44, 54, 63, 71-72, 82, 93, 102, 104-105, 108-111, 115, 138, 177, 186, 200, 203, 208-209, 211, 213-215, 217, 226, 238, 246, 254-255, 263, 269-271

Inflammaging, 37, 82, 92-93, 100, 102, 145, 152-153, 166, 261

Inflammatory Index, 37-40, 42-44, 103

Innate Immunity, 24, 26, 35, 177, 189, 193, 200, 207, 223, 267

Insect Pathogen, 26-27, 31, 36

Insulin Receptor, 26-27, 31

Interferon, 1, 9-11, 18, 38, 44, 156, 159, 175-176, 203, 221, 223, 229

Interleukin-6, 37, 44-45, 64, 72, 82, 92-93, 101-102, 144, 159, 176, 186, 240, 245, 271

L

Leukotriene, 161, 164, 167

Lipoprotein Cholesterol, 1-7, 9, 240-242, 245-246

Lumbar Spinal Cord, 145

M

Macrophage Activation, 84

Macrophage Expression, 84, 89

Macrophage Infiltration, 84-87, 90

Mediterranean Diet, 155, 159

Metabolic Syndrome, 1-2, 6-7, 9-11, 158, 167, 244, 246-247

Microglia, 145, 147-148, 150-154

Mitogen-activated Protein Kinase, 116, 128-129, 246
Monocyte, 1, 11, 20, 91, 93, 101, 202, 207, 246, 263-272
Montelukast, 161-167

N
Neopterin, 1-11, 44
Neuropathic, 145-146, 150-154
Neurotoxic Response, 145

O
Octogenarian, 71-72, 79, 81, 138
Oxidative Phosphorylation, 12, 15, 20, 143, 220
Oxidative Stress, 1, 27, 42, 44-47, 49-51, 53, 84-85, 90-91, 147-148, 154-155, 157, 168, 173, 175, 177, 241, 246-247, 256-262, 272

P
Peripheral Blood, 24, 44, 46-47, 58, 64, 71, 74, 78-79, 82-83, 110, 113-114, 118, 127, 130-135, 138, 179, 186, 224, 227-228, 252, 266
Peripheral Immune Cell, 71
Pharyngitis, 188-199
Phosphorylation, 12, 15, 20-21, 63, 116-128, 143, 178-179, 181-182, 185, 220
Photorhabdus, 26-30, 32, 34, 36
Probiotic, 104-105, 108, 110-112, 115
Protein Expression, 13, 49, 188, 193, 197, 199

R
Renal Disease, 91, 116, 120-128, 168, 176-177, 263, 271-272

Respiratory Infection, 213
Respiratory Tract Infection, 114

S
Seasonal Influenza Vaccination, 104, 107, 230-231, 233, 238
Seroepidemiology, 65, 70, 216
Seroprevalence, 65, 67-70
Signal-regulated Kinase, 116, 128
Sinusitis, 188-199
Sirtuin, 46, 48, 52-53, 219, 228-229
Skeletal Muscle, 84-91
Substance Abuse, 54, 158
Systemic Adaptive Immune Activation, 1

T
T Cell, 12-13, 16, 19-25, 56, 58, 60-64, 71-72, 74-75, 77-78, 80, 82-83, 109, 111, 113, 122-130, 135, 145, 147, 149, 151, 153, 180, 183, 202, 211, 213, 216, 229, 263-264, 269-272
T-cell Immune, 54, 128
T-helper Cell, 1, 147
Thrombosis, 37-38, 44
Transcriptome, 13, 145, 150, 154, 217-218, 221, 226
Triglycerides, 1, 4, 6-7, 9, 156, 159

V
Varicella Zoster Virus, 65, 67, 214, 251
Viral Infection, 1, 42, 105, 117, 169

www.ingramcontent.com/pod-product-compliance
Lightning Source LLC
Chambersburg PA
CBHW061330190326
41458CB00011B/3958